PACS AND IMAGING INFORMATICS

PACS AND IMAGING INFORMATICS
BASIC PRINCIPLES AND APPLICATIONS

Second Edition

H. K. Huang, D.Sc., FRCR (Hon.), FAIMBE

Professor of Radiology and Biomedical Engineering
University of Southern California

Chair Professor of Medical Informatics
The Hong Kong Polytechnic University

Honorary Professor, Shanghai Institute of Technical Physics
The Chinese Academy of Sciences

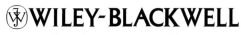WILEY-BLACKWELL

A John Wiley & Sons, Inc., Publication

Library of Congress Cataloging-in-Publication Data:

Huang, H. K., 1939–
    PACS and imaging informatics : basic principles and applications / H.K. Huang. – 2nd ed. rev.
        p. ; cm.
    Includes bibliographical references and index.
    ISBN 978-0-470-37372-9 (cloth)
    1. Picture archiving and communication systems in medicine. 2. Imaging systems in medicine. I. Title.
II. Title: Picture archiving and communication system and imaging informatics.
    [DNLM: 1. Radiology Information Systems. 2. Diagnostic Imaging. 3. Medical Records Systems, Computerized. WN 26.5 H874p 2010]
    R857.P52H82 2010
    616.07'54–dc22
                                                    2009022463

Printed in the United States of America

10 9 8 7 6 5 4 3 2 1

To my wife, Fong, for her support and understanding,
my daughter, Cammy, for her growing wisdom and ambitious spirit, and my
grandchildren Tilden and Calleigh, for their calming innocence.

INTRODUCTION
Chapter 1

PART I MEDICAL IMAGING PRINCIPLES

Imaging Basics Chapter 2	2-D Images Chapter 3	3-D Images Chapter 4	4-D Images & Image Fusion Chapter 5	Compression Chapter 6

PART II PACS FUNDAMENTALS

PACS Fundamentals Chapter 7	Communication & Networks Chapter 8	DICOM, HL7 and IHE Chapter 9

Image/Data Acquisition Gateway Chapter 10	PACS Server & Archive Chapter 11	Display Workstation Chapter 12	HIS/RIS/PACS Integration & ePR Chapter 13

PART III PACS OPERATION

Data Management & Web-Based PACS Chapter 14	Telemedicine & Teleradiology Chapter 15	Fault-Tolerant & Enterprise PACS Chapter 16	Image/Data Security Chapter 17

Implementation & Evaluation Chapter 18	Clinical Experience/ Pitfalls/Bottlenecks Chapter 19

PART IV PACS- AND DICOM-BASED IMAGING INFORMATICS

Medical Imaging Informatics Chapter 20	Computing & Data Grid Chapter 21	Multimedia ePR Chapter 22	DICOM RT ePR Chapter 23	Image-Assisted Surgery ePR Chapter 24

Image-Based CAD Chapter 25	CAD-PACS Integration Chapter 26	Biometric Tracking Chapter 27	Education/ Learning Chapter 28

CONTENTS IN BRIEF

CONTENTS

THE DEFENSE HEALTH CARE SYSTEM PERSONAL'S POINT OF VIEW

Picture Archiving and Communication Systems (PACS) are commonplace in the Defense Health Care System. Within the Army, Navy, Air Force, and the Marines healthcare is accomplished in a PACS-rich imaging environment. Department of the Defense Medical Treatment Facilities (MTFs) transmit digital radiography information between continents, from ships at sea, and from remote battlefields in accordance with security and networking parameters. Nascent and locale specific communications exist between numerous facilities within the healthcare networks of the Department of Defense and the Department of Veterans Affairs. These all are remarkable advances within the relatively short history of digital imaging and PACS. As a pioneering researcher, scientist, and program manager Dr. H.K. (Bernie) Huang has played a critical role in the evolution of digital informatics.

In *PACS Imaging Informatics, Second Edition*, Professor Huang succeeds as few others could by defining the history and evolution of this fascinating technology in clear, concise, and eminently readable terms. He also adeptly summarizes the current state of technology and shares unique insights into the challenges and opportunities of imaging informatics in the 21st Century. The second edition covers all the core concepts of medical imaging principles to include 4D imaging, image fusion, and image compression. Part II elucidates the essentials of PACS architecture, as well as the fundamental healthcare Information Technology standards of DICOM (Digital Imaging and Communications in Medicine) and HL7 (Health Level Seven), and IHE (Integrating the Healthcare Enterprise) workflow profiles, HIS/RIS (Hospital Information System/Radiology Information System) and their relationship with PACS. Part III of this work focuses on the day-to-day operation of the PACS system and highlights the intricacies and challenges of data management in a security-centric era. The focus in Part IV of this excellent text extends well beyond the commodity aspects of Picture Archiving and Communication Systems by bringing the reader into the world of integrated medical informatics, including the application of PACS in Radiation Therapy, Image-guided Surgery (IGS), Computer-Aided Detection (CAD) and the multimedia world of the electronic health care record.

Professor Huang's efforts in this decisive second edition assures that this work will become a standard reference for Radiology in the 21st Century and our "global positioning system" for the development of digital imaging and medical informatics for years to come.

MICHAEL P. BRAZAITIS, M.D.
COL, MC
Chief, Department of Radiology
Walter Reed Army Medical Center, Washington, DC
Radiology and Teleradiology Consultant
North Atlantic Regional Medical Command

xxxix

THE ACADEMIC AND EDITOR-IN-CHIEF OF CARS (COMPUTER ASSISTED RADIOLOGY AND SURGERY) POINT OF VIEW

The information accrued in PACS and imaging informatics in the last 25 years at the CARS and other congresses as well as in numerous peer-reviewed publications has been overwhelming. If there is any comprehensive and adequate coverage of the content of this very large scientific/medical field, it is contained in Bernie Huang's new and revised book.

As in his previous PACS book, Bernie Huang's PACS project work and his related publications are a leading source of reference and learning. The spectrum of topics covered in the book (as outlined in approximately 30 pages of content) is thoroughly selected and discussed in considerable depth. The second edition of this new book provides an excellent state-of-the-art review of PACS and of the rapidly developing field of Imaging Informatics.

PACS is extending increasingly from the now well-established radiology applications into a hospital-wide PACS. New challenges are accompanying its spread into other clinical fields. Particularly important are the modeling and analysis of the workflow of the affected clinical disciplines as well as the interface issues with the image connected electronic patient record. The second edition of Bernie Huang's book, and in particular Part IV, is addressing these new applications very effectively, for example, in computer-aided detection/diagnosis, image-assisted therapy and treatment and specifically minimally invasive spinal surgery, and thereby providing an opportunity to gain insight into new applications of PACS and imaging informatics.

Although the awareness of these application possibilities is increasing rapidly, equally important is the recognition in the professional community that a more rigorous scientific/systems engineering method is needed for system development. Imaging informatics can provide an answer to structured design and implementation of PACS infrastructures and applications.

Image processing and display, knowledge management, computer-aided diagnosis, and image and model guided therapy are a first set of imaging informatics methods and applications. These will certainly be followed by a widespread expansion into therapeutic applications, such as radiation therapy and computer-assisted surgery. Special workflow requirements and the specifics of therapy assist systems need to be considered in a corresponding PACS design. Pre- and intra-operative image acquisition as well as multidimensional presentations rather than image archiving is becoming a central focus in image-assisted surgery systems. These new developments and possibilities are well represented in Bernie Huang's new book.

It is comforting to know that the knowledge generated by Bernie Huang and his many colleagues and co-workers in the field of PACS and imaging informatics is regularly documented in this series of now classic textbooks.

Heinz U. Lemke, PhD
Director, International Foundation of CARS
Professor of Computer Science, Technical University of Berlin, Germany
Visiting Professor for Computer Assisted Surgery, University of Leipzig, Germany
Research Professor of Radiology, University of Southern California, Los Angeles, USA
hulemke@cars-int.org

THE ACADEMIC AND HEALTH CENTER POINT OF VIEW

Dr. H. K. "Bernie" Huang's second edition of his book is highly recommended for practicing physicians and other healthcare providers for department chairs, particularly in radiology and surgical disciplines, and also for other specialty departments like cardiology and orthopedics. Hospital administrators and their staff as well as the chief financial officer of any institution will find this book useful when considering digital imaging and digitization of information for purchases as such.

Bernie Huang with his extensive knowledge of mathematical issues is fully an expert in theoretical aspects of communication and picture archiving communication systems (PACS). His extensive work in practical implementation gives him a unique background to write books that are full of extraordinarily detailed information for those interested in the topic. His students are presently running industry and academic departments.

This book is particularly critical for those interested in practical solutions and improving healthcare. Informatics students should be aware and read this book. This book is a "must" for those students. Similarly people in hospital administration and the finance office interested in cost-effectiveness analysis should read this book. Those institutions planning on establishing outside facilities in imaging like imaging centers connected with their own main practice will benefit from familiarity with this book.

My personal view is that this type of publication would be perfect reading material for policy makers with a vision of implementing electronic medical record across the country. Bernie Huang has already provided a foundation for the PACS programs in many institutions including our own.

Readers would gain fundamental knowledge regarding two-dimensional imaging in the form of traditional X-ray films as well as plate technology and direct radiography. They will also gain necessary knowledge related to three-dimensional and fourth-dimensional imaging, particularly CT and MRI and become familiar with image compression (the latest versions of it) such as wavelet compression.

Professor Hooshang Kangarloo, M.D.
Chairman Emeritus, Department of Radiology, UCLA,
UCLA Medical Faculty Board—Governing Body of UCLA Physicians
Los Angeles, California
hkangarloo@mii.ucla.edu

THE MANUFACTURER'S POINT OF VIEW

In the last dozen years Dr. H. K. "Bernie" Huang has published three comprehensive and insightful texts dealing with PACS and other imaging informatics technologies. Although each text presented state of the art details of existing technologies, as well as new technologies and applications, the three texts were subtly but quite effectively directed to the requirements of different groups of readers.

Bernie's first book, *PACS: Picture Archiving and Communication Systems in Biomedical Imaging*, was primarily directed to the training of medical informatics scientists. The second book, *PACS (Picture Archiving and Communication Systems): Basic Principles and Applications*, was intended for training of those in industry and in the field of healthcare who dealt with the everyday, practical realities of planning, operating and maintaining PAC systems. A third book, *PACS and Imaging Informatics*, summarized and updated the material covered in both of its predecessors and directed it to continued developments in the field of medical informatics. The third book additionally introduced the concept of expanding PACS technology into every aspect of the healthcare enterprise.

Now Bernie Huang gives us a fourth book, the second edition of the previous third book, *PACS and Imaging Informatics*, which updates all of the material covered in previous books but also makes wide excursions into new methods of managing medical information as well as requirements of many new and exciting imaging methods.

PACS and Imaging Informatics, second edition, will therefore be of great interest to clinicians and other members of the healthcare team who apply these technologies in the practice of medicine. All of us—clinicians, healthcare personnel, information scientists and the industry—owe Bernie and his colleagues a great debt of gratitude for creating this text, which will stand as the standard reference source for years to come.

William M. Angus, M.D., Ph.D., FACR, h.c.
Senior Vice President
Philips Medical Systems North America Company
Bothell, Washington

PREFACE

My interest in PACS and imaging informatics was inspired and deeply influenced by Dr. Robert S. Ledley* and initially by his book *Use of Computers in Biology and Medicine* (McGraw-Hill, 1965) the first such book combining principles of biology, medicine, and mathematics. After earning degrees in meteorology and mathematics, I worked for IBM and the space industry as a professional programmer for several years. My goal at that time was to become an astronomer. It was during this fork in the road that I came across Ledley's book and was fascinated by the contents and tangible hypotheses. I made an appointment to see him in Washington, DC, and before the end of the visit he offered me a job (I was not looking for one) and convinced me that I should change my interest from astronomy to biomedical imaging. I soon after went to work for him at the National Biomedical Research Foundation (NBRF), Georgetown University Medical Center, Washington, DC, from 1966 to 1980. During this period of time I also obtained my doctorate in applied mechanics and mathematics, and continued with postdoctoral studies in anatomy, physiology, and radiology.

Dr. Ledley guided me through the design and implementation of several revolutionary medical imaging instrumentation including FIDAC (film input to digital automatics computer), SPIDAC (specimen input to digital automatics computer), and automatic computerized transverse axial (ACTA) whole-body CT scanner. These instruments were the infants of today's film digitizers, digital microscopes, and multislice CT scanners. I also led or worked on research projects in chromosomes karyotyping; classification of pneumoconiosis on chest X-ray films; 3-D image rendering; image subtraction; CT for radiotherapy on bone and body mass densities, diagnosis of pulmonary nodules, and cardiac imaging; and protein sequences medical database. These projects were predecessors of many of today's medical imaging informatics methodologies and database concepts.

I further benefited from working with Dr. Ledley on soliciting for grants, designing a research laboratory, and writing a book. I followed technology transfer from the university research to private industry and entrepreneurship. I had the opportunity to develop innovative interdisciplinary courses combining physical and biological sciences that were taught as electives at Georgetown.

*Dr. Ledley, Professor Emeritus, Georgetown University; President of the National Biomedical Research Foundation, is credited with establishing the field of medical informatics in which computers and information technologies assist physicians in the diagnosis and treatment of patients. He has been awarded more than 60 patents related to this field. Among the many highest honor awards are induction into the National Inventors Hall of Fame, the National Medal of Technology—awarded by the President of the United States of America—and the Morris E. Collen, MD Award from the American College of Medical Informatics.

MY INTEREST IN PACS AND MEDICAL IMAGING INFORMATICS

I joined the Departments of Bioengineering and Radiology at the University of Iowa in 1980 and I developed there my first image processing laboratory. Although my stay at Iowa was short, the concept of bridging the gap between engineering and medicine that was due to Dr. Tony Franklin, then Chair of Radiology, became the mainstay of my academic career. I summarized this learning experience in "Biomedical Image Processing," a single article issue in the *CRC Critical Reviews in Bioengineering* (Vol 5, Issue 3, 1981). From 1982 to 1992, I developed the Medical Imaging Division, headed the Biomedical Physics Graduate Program, and implemented the in-house PACS at UCLA. From 1992 to 2000, I taught medical imaging at UC, Berkeley, developed the Radiological Informatics Lab, implemented the hospital-integrated PACS, and introduced the concept of imaging informatics at UCSF. Since then, I have been overseeing the development of medical imaging informatics at the Hong Kong Polytechnic University (2000–now) and at USC (2000–now). For more than 25 years I have been documenting PACS and imaging informatics research, development, and implementation in a number of books: *Elements of Digital Radiology: A Professional Handbook and Guide* (Prentice-Hall, 1987), *Picture Archiving and Communication Systems in Biomedical Imaging* (VCH Publishers, 1996), *Picture Archiving and Communication Systems: Principles and Applications* (Wiley, 1999), and *PACS and Imaging Informatics: Principles and Applications* (Wiley, 2004).

These earlier books document the developments in new digital technologies that have emerge through the years. The reader not familiar with a certain concept or term in a newer book could find it explained in more detail in an older book.

PACS AND IMAGING INFORMATICS DEVELOPMENT SINCE THE 2004 BOOK

After the 2004 book was published, PACS development trends shifted to imaging informatics, PACS-based CAD, ePR with image distribution, and ePR for therapy and surgery. The milestones were recorded in two special Issues that I edited in 2005 and 2007 for the *Journal of Computerized Medical Imaging and Graphics*, as sequels to the special issues on picture archiving and communication systems, in 1991; on medical image databases, in 1996, and on PACS twenty Years later, in 2003. The previous special issues were mainly on PACS research and development, whereas the two newer issues were on PACS applications. The first was "Imaging Informatics" (2005), and the second was "Computer-Aided Diagnosis (CAD) and Image-Guided Decision Support" (2007).

In the annual RSNA meetings, we have witnessed progressively fewer film-based technical exhibits from the industry, as well as scientific presentations and exhibits by radiologists and scientists throughout these years. At the 2008 RNSA meeting, there were practically none. Many nonclinical presentations and exhibits are now in CAD, imaging informatics related research, ePR, and image-based therapy.

Since the development of PACS has become matured several well-attended annual conferences in PACS like CARS, SPIE, and SCAR have been gradually shifting their interests from PACS to imaging informatics and related topics. The CARS (Computer-Assisted Radiology and Surgery) annual meeting has been changed to a private foundation-sponsored annual congress, with the official journal JCARS accepting manuscripts in imaging informatics and image-assisted surgery and treatment. In the SPIE (International Society for Optical Engineering) the annual medical imaging conference, the PACS conference track has shifted their sessions to more PACS-driven imaging informatics topics. The SCAR (Society for Computer Applications in Radiology) changed their society name to SIIM (Society for Imaging Informatics in Medicine). The conclusions that can be deduced from such evidence are that PACS has completed its original goal and gradually become a commodity, a dc facto integrated imaging tool for image-based diagnoses. PACS-based medical imaging informatics has taken over as the next wave of development to better the patient service and improve healthcare.

PACS AND IMAGING INFORMATICS, THE SECOND EDITION

Medical imaging informatics has evolved from developments in medical imaging, PACS, and medical informatics. Medical imaging is the study of human anatomy, physiology, and pathology based on imaging techniques. The picture archiving and communication system (PACS) consists of medical image and data acquisition, storage, and display subsystems integrated by digital networks and application software. PACS facilitates the systematic utilization of medical imaging for patient care. Medical imaging informatics is a subset of medical informatics that studies image/data information acquisition; processing; manipulation; storage; transmission; security; management; distribution; visualization; image-aided detection, diagnosis, surgery, and therapy; as well as knowledge discovery from large-scale biomedical image/data sets. Over the past six years, we have witnessed a rapid advancement in the research and development of medical imaging technology, PACS, and medical informatics. A revolutionary break through has occurred in image-based healthcare methodologies that benefits the patient in ways never thought possible.

This new edition on PACS and imaging informatics is organized in an introduction and four parts. All together, in the 28 chapters, over 60% to 70% of the materials are based on the new research and development in PACS and imaging informatics from the past six years. All chapters of Parts I and II have been revised, Chapter 5 is a new chapter. Chapters 3, 4, 8, 9, 11, 12, and 13 have been changed substantially. In Part III, web-based PACS, fault-tolerant and enterprise PACS have been rewritten, so has the chapter on image security; the PACS clinical implementation, experience, and pitfalls are based on PACS operation over the past six years. In Part IV, some concepts and research topics that appeared piecemeal in the last edition have been greatly expanded and organized into nine chapters, presenting totally new materials on methodology, results, and clinical experience.

As I wrote in the Preface of the last edition, I would be remiss in not acknowledging the debt of gratitude owed to many wonderful colleagues for this adventure in PACS and Imaging Informatics. I thank former chairmen of radiology at various universities, Drs. Edmund Anthony Franken, Gabriel Wilson, Robert Leslie Bennett, and Hooshang Kangarloo in the United States; and chairmen and deans, Profs. Maurice Yap, George Woo, and Thomas Wong at PolyU, Hong Kong, for their encouragement and generous support. I can never forget my many students and postdoctoral fellows; I have learned much (and continue to learn now) from their challenges and contributions.

Over the past six years, we have received continuous supports from many organizations with a great vision for the future: the National Library of Medicine (NLM), the National Institute of Biomedical Imaging and Bioengineering (NIBIB), other Institutes of the National Institutes of Health (NIH), and the U.S. Army Medical Research and Materiel Command. The private medical imaging industry has encouraged and funded many projects from small to large scale, allowing me and our team to carry out technology transfers from the academy to the real world. The support from these agencies and manufacturers provided us opportunities to go beyond the boundaries of current PACS and Imaging Informatics and open up new frontiers for patient care and healthcare delivery.

In 2006, Mr. Thomas Moore, who took over the Senior Editorship of Medical Sciences at John Wiley and Blackwell, tempted me to write a new edition with color figures and text. It was like bees and honey. I have had the great pleasure of exchanging humorous emails, conversations, and worked with him and his editorial team in developing the concepts and contents of this manuscript.

Selected portions of the book have been used as lecture materials in graduate courses: "Medical Imaging and Advanced Instrumentation" at UCLA, UCSF, and UC Berkeley; "Biomedical Engineering Lectures" in Taiwan, and the People's Republic of China; "PACS and Medical Imaging Informatics" at the Hong Kong Polytechnic University; and required courses in the "Medical Imaging and Informatics" track at the Department of Biomedical Engineering, School of Engineering, USC. It is my greatest hope that this new edition will not only provide guidelines for those contemplating a PACS career but also inspire others to apply PACS-based imaging informatics as a tool toward a brighter future for healthcare delivery.

H.K. (BERNIE) HUANG
Agoura Hills, CA; Berkeley Springs,
WVA; and Hong Kong

PREFACE OF THE LAST EDITION, 2004

In the early 1980s members of the radiology community envisioned a future practice built around the concept of a picture archiving and communication system (PACS). Consisting of image acquisition devices, storage archive units, display workstations, computer processors, and databases, all integrated by a communications network and a data management system, the concept has proved to be much more than the sum of its parts. During the past 20 years, as technology has matured, PACS applications have gone beyond radiology to affect and improve the entire spectrum of healthcare delivery. PACS installations are now seen around the world—installations that support focused clinical applications as well as hospital-wide clinical processes are seen on every continent. The relevance of PACS has grown far beyond its initial conception; for example, these systems demonstrate their value by facilitating large-scale longitudinal and horizontal research and education in addition to clinical services. PACS-based imaging informatics is one such important manifestation.

Many important concepts, technological advances, and events have occurred in this field since the publication of my previous books, *PACS in Biomedical Imaging*, published by VCH in 1996, and *PACS: Basic Principles and Applications* published by John Wiley & Sons in 1999. With this new effort, I hope to summarize these developments and place them in the appropriate context for the continued development of this exciting field. First, however, I would like to discuss two perspectives that led to the preparation of the current manuscript: the trend in PACS, and my personal interest and experience.

THE TREND

The overwhelming evidence of successful PACS installations, large and small, demonstrating improved care and streamlined administrative functions, has propelled the central discussion of PACS from purchase justification to best practices for installing and maintaining a PACS. Simply put, the question is no longer "Should we?" but "*How* should we?" Further spurring the value-added nature of PACS are the mature standards of Digital Imaging and Communication in Medicine (DICOM) and Health Level Seven (HL7) for medical images and health data, respectively, which are accepted by all imaging and healthcare information manufacturers. The issue of component connectivity has gradually disappeared as DICOM conformance components have become a commodity. Armed with DICOM and HL7, the Radiological Society of North America (RSNA) pioneered the concept of Integrating the Healthcare Enterprise (IHE), which develops hospital and radiology workflow profiles to ensure system and component compatibility within the goal of streamlining patient care. For these reasons the readers will find the presentation of the PACS operation in this book shifted from technological development, as in the last two books, to analysis of clinical workflow. Finally, the expansion and development of inexpensive Windows-based PC hardware and software with flat panel display has made it much more feasible to place high-quality diagnostic workstations throughout the healthcare enterprise. These trends set the stage of Part I: Medical Imaging Principles (Chapters 1–5) and Part II: PACS Fundamentals (Chapters 6–12) of the book.

MY PERSONAL INTEREST AND EXPERIENCE

Over the decade since I developed PACS at UCLA (1991) and at UCSF (1995) from laboratory environments to daily clinical use, I have had the opportunity to serve in an advisory role, assisting with the planning, design, and clinical implementation of many large-scale PACS outside of my academic endeavors at, to name several, Cornell Medical Center, New York Hospital; Kaoshung VA Medical Center, Taiwan; and St. John's Hospital, Santa Monica, California. I had the pleasure of engaging in these three projects from conception to daily clinical operation. There are many other implementations for which I have provided advice on planning or reviewed the design and workflow. I have trained many engineers and healthcare providers from different parts of the world, who visit our laboratory for short, intensive PACS training sessions and return to their respective institutes or countries to implement their own PACS. I have learned much through these interactions on a wide variety of issues, including image management, system fault tolerance, security, implementation and evaluation, and PACS training [Part III: PACS Operation (Chapters 13–18)]. My recent three-year involvement in the massive Hong Kong Healthcare PACS and image distribution planning involving 44 public hospitals and 92% of the healthcare marketplace has prompted me to look more closely into questions of the balance between technology and cost in enterprise-level implementation. I am grateful for the fascinating access to the "backroom" PACS R&D of several manufacturers and research laboratories provided by these assignments. These glimpses have helped me to consolidate my thoughts on enterprise PACS (Part V, Chapter 23), Web-based PACS (Chapter 13), and the electronic patient record (ePR) complete with images (Chapters 12, 21).

In the area of imaging informatics, my initial engagement was outcomes research in lung nodule detection with temporal CT images (Section 20.1). In the late 1990s, Dr. Michael Vannier, then Chairman of Radiology at University of Iowa and Editor-in-Chief, *IEEE Transactions of Medical Imaging*, offered me the opportunity as a visiting professor to present some of my thoughts in imaging informatics; while there, I also worked on the IAIMS (Integrated Advanced Information Management Systems) project funded by the National Library of Medicine (NLM). This involvement, together with the opportunity to serve the study section at NLM for four years, has taught me many of the basic concepts of medical informatics, thus leading to the formulation of *PACS-Based Medical Imaging Informatics* (Part IV: PACS-based Imaging Informatics, Chapters 19–22), and the research in large-scale imaging informatics project *Bone Age Assessment with a Digital Atlas* (Section 20.3). The latter project is especially valuable because it involves the complete spectrum of imaging informatics infrastructure from data collection and standardization, image processing and parameter extraction, Web-based image submission and bone age assessment result distribution, to system evaluation. Other opportunities have also allowed me to collect the information necessary to complete Chapters 21 and 22. The Hong Kong Polytechnic University (PolyU) has a formal training program in Radiography leading to certificates as well as BSc, MS, and PhD degrees. With the contribution of the University and my outstanding colleagues there, we have built a teaching-based clinical PACS Laboratory and hands-on training facility. Much of the data in Chapter 22 was collected in this one-of-a-kind resource. My daughter, Cammy, who is at Stanford University developing multimedia distance learning, helped me expand the PACS learning concept with multimedia technology to enrich the contents of Chapter 22. Working with colleagues outside of radiology has allowed me to develop the concepts of the PACS-based radiation therapy server and the neurosurgical server presented in Chapter 21.

In 1991, Dr. Robert Ledley, formerly my mentor at Georgetown University and Editor-in-Chief of the Journal of *Computerized Medical Imaging and Graphics* offered me an opportunity to act as Guest Editor of a Special Issue, *Picture Archiving and Communication Systems*, summarizing the 10-year progress of PACS. In 2002, Bob graciously offered me another opportunity to edit a Special Issue, *PACS: Twenty Years Later*, revisiting the progress in PACS in the ensuing 10 years and looking into the future of PACS research and development trends. A total of 15 papers plus an editorial were collected; the senior authors are Drs. E. L. Siegel, Heinz Lemke, K. Inamura, Greg Mogel, Christ Carr, Maria Y. Y. Law, Cammy Huang, Brent Liu, Minglin Li, Fei Cao, Jianguo Zhang, Osman Ratib, Ewa Pietka, and Stephan Erberich. Some materials used in this book were culled from these papers.

I would be remiss in not acknowledging the debt of gratitude owed many wonderful colleagues for this adventure in PACS, and now imaging informatics. I thank Drs. Edmund Anthony Franken, Gabriel Wilson, Robert Leslie Bennett, and Hooshang Kangarloo for their encouragement and past support. I can never forget my many students and postdoctoral fellows; I have learned much (and continue to learn even now) from their contributions.

Over the past 10 years, we have received support from many organizations with a great vision for the future: NLM, the National Institute of Biomedical Imaging and Bioengineering, other Institutes of the National Institutes of Health, the U.S. Army Medical Research and Materiel Command, the California Breast Research Program, the Federal Technology Transfer Program, and the private medical imaging industry. The support of these agencies and manufacturers has allowed us go beyond the boundaries of current PACS and open new frontiers in research such as imaging informatics.

In 2002, Mr. Shawn Morton, Vice President and Publisher, Medical Sciences, John Wiley, who was the editor of my last book, introduced me to Ms. Luna Han, Senior Editor, Life & Medical Sciences, at Wiley. I have had the pleasure of working with these fine individuals in developing the concepts and contents of this manuscript.

Selected portions of the book have been used as lecture materials in graduate courses, "Medical Imaging and Advanced Instrumentation" at UCLA, UCSF, and UC Berkeley; "Biomedical Engineering Lectures" in Taiwan, Republic of China and the People's Republic of China; and "PACS and Medical Imaging Informatics" at

PolyU, Hong Kong, and will be used in the "Medical Imaging and Informatics" track at the Department of Biomedical Engineering, School of Engineering, USC. It is our greatest hope that this book will not only provide guidelines for those contemplating a PACS installation but also inspire others to apply PACS-based imaging informatics as a tool toward a brighter future for healthcare delivery.

Agoura Hills, CA and Hong Kong

ACKNOWLEDGMENTS

Many people have provided valuable assistance during the preparation of this book, in particular, many of my past graduate students, postdoctoral fellows, and colleagues, from whom I have learned the most. Chapter 1, Introduction, and Part I, Medical Imaging Principles (Chapters 2–6), have been revised substantially from the original book *PACS and Imaging Informatics: Basic Principles and Applications*, published, 2004. Part II, PACS Fundamentals (Chapters 7–13), consists of materials based on revised industrial standards and workflow profiles, updated technologies, and current clinical experience of other researchers and ourselves. Part III, PACS Operation (Chapters 14–19), are mostly our group's personal experience over the past six years in planning, design, implementation, and operating large-scale PAC systems. Part IV, PACS-based and DICOM-based Imaging Informatics (Chapters 20–28), presents systematic overview of current trends in medical imaging informatics research learned from colleagues and other researchers, as well as our own research and development.

Materials retained from the last edition were contributed by K. S. Chuang, Ben Lo, Ricky Taira, Brent Stewart, Paul Cho, Shyh-Liang Andrew Lou, Albert W. K. Wong, Jun Wang, Xiaoming Zhu, Johannes Stahl, Jianguo Zhang, Ewa Pietka, X. Q. Zhou, F.Yu, Fei Cao, Brent Liu, Maria Y.Y. Law, Lawrence Chan, Harold Rutherford, Minglin Li, Michael F. McNitt-Gray, Christopher Carr, Eliot Siegel, Heinz Lemke, Kiyonari Inamura, and Cammy Huang.

For the new materials, I am thankful for contributions by the following individuals: Brent Liu (Chapters 7, 18, 19, 24, Sections 9.4, 9.5, 11.6, 18.6, 18.7.1, 18.7.2, 18.7.3, 18.8, 19.2, 19.3, 19.4, 21.4, 28.3.1), Jianguo Zhang (Sections 12.7), Maria Y.Y. Law (Chapter 23, Section 28.3.2), Cammy Huang (Section 28.5), Michael Z. Zhou (Chapter 17, Sections 8.6, 21.3, 21.4, 21.5, 26.3, 28.2), Lucy Aifeng Zhang (Sections 20.4.3, 26.7, 26.8), Jorge Documet (Sections 8.6, 14.6, Chapter 24, Chapter 27), Anh Le (24.3, 26.3, 26.5), Jasper Lee (Sections 4.9, 5.4.4, 21.6), Kevin Ma (Section 26.8), Bing Guo (Chapter 27, Sections 12.8, 26.5, 26.6), Kevin Wong (Sections 18.7.3, 19.4), John Chiu (Chapter 24), NT Cheung (Sections 16.11, 22.3), Tao Chan (Sections 16.11, 25.4, 25.5), Anthony Chan (Sections 18.7.4). Paymann Moin and Richard Lee contributed discussions in clinical radiology and some art work and images. A special thank you must go to Mariam Fleshman and Ashley Sullivan who contributed some creative art work, read through all chapters to extract the lists of acronyms and the index, and organized the references, to Angleica Virgen for editorial assistance, to Jim Sayre for numerous data collections and statistical analysis, and to Maria Y. Y. Law, who read through and edited the Introduction, and Part I and Part IV chapters.

This book was written with the assistance of the following staff members and consultants of the Imaging Processing and Informatics Laboratory, USC:

Brent J. Liu, Ph.D.
Associate Professor, USC

Jianguo Zhang, Ph.D.
Professor, Shanghai Institute of Technical Physics,
The Chinese Academy of Science,
Visiting Professor, USC

Maria Y. Y. Law, Ph.D. M.Phil., BRS., Teach Dip.,
Associate Professor, Hong Kong Polytechnic University
Visiting Associate Professor, USC

Jorge Document, Ph.D.
Postdoctoral Fellow, USC

Cammy Huang, Ph.D.
Director of Scientific Outreach, WGLN; and Virtual Labs Project Director
Center for Innovations in Learning
Lecturer, Department of Computer Science, Stanford University

H. K. HUANG SHORT BIOGRAPHY

H. K. (Bernie) Huang, FRCR(Hon.); FAIMBE; Professor of Radiology and Biomedical Engineering; Director, Division of Imaging Informatics, Department of Radiology; and Director MS Program, Medical Imaging and Imaging Informatics, Department of Biomedical Engineering, University of Southern California, Los Angeles, Chair Professor of Medical Informatics, The Hong Kong Polytechnic University; and Honorary Professor, Shanghai Institute of Technical Physics, The Chinese Academy of Sciences.

Dr. Huang pioneered in picture archiving and communication system (PACS) and imaging informatics research. He developed the PACS at UCLA in 1991, and the hospital-integrated PACS at UCSF in 1995, and started imaging informatics research in 1999. Dr. Huang has taught at Georgetown University (1971–80); University of Iowa (1981–82); UCLA (1982–92); UC Berkeley and UC San Francisco (1992–99); Hong Kong Polytechnic University (2000–present); and the University of Southern California (2000–present). His current research interests are in tele-imaging and telemedicine, fault-tolerant PACS server, PACS ASP model, Internet 2, PACS-based CAD and surgery, imaging informatics, image recovery during disaster, image integrity, Data Grid, grid computing, HIPAA compliance, patient tracking system, radiation therapy information system, PDA Web-based image management and distribution, ePR, and image-guided minimally invasive spinal surgery. He has co-authored and authored eight books, published over 200 peer-reviewed articles, and received several patents. His book: *PACS and Imaging Informatics* published by John Wiley & Sons in 2004 has been the only textbook in this field. Over the past 25 years Dr. Huang has received over U.S. $21 million dollars in PACS, medical imaging informatics, tele-imaging, and image processing related research grants and contracts, as well as imaging informatics training grants from the U.S. federal and state governments, and private industry. He has mentored 24 PhD students and over 30 postdoctoral fellows from around the world. Dr. Huang has been a consultant for many national and international hospitals, and imaging manufacturers in the design and implementation of PAC systems, enterprise-level ePR with image distribution, and image-based therapy and treatment ePR systems.

Dr. Huang was inducted into the Royal College of Radiologists, London as an Honorary Fellow, for his contribution in PACS research and development, in November 1992; the American Institute of Medical and Biological Engineering as a Founding Fellow, for his contribution in medical imaging, in March 1993; the EuroPACS Society as an Honorary Member for his contribution in PACS, in October 1996; Honorary President, 2003 International CARS Congress, London; and President, 2007 First Iranian Imaging Informatics Conference. Dr. Huang has been Visiting Professor in many leading universities around the world, and a Board Member in leading medical imaging manufacturers.

1-D	one-dimensional
2-D	two-dimensional
3-D	three-dimensional
4-D	four-dimensional
A/D	analog to digital converter
A & E	ambulatory and emergency
ABF	Air Blown Fiber
ACC	Ambulatory Care Center
ACGME	Accreditation Council for Graduate Medical Education
ACR	American College of Radiology
ACR BIRADS	American College of Radiology Beast Imaging Reporting and Data System Atlas
ACR-NEMA	American College of Radiology–National Electric Manufacturer's Association
ADM	an acquisition and display module
ADT	admission, discharge, transfer
AE	application entities
AFBUS	volumetric (3D) automated full breast ultrasound
AFP	alpha-fetal protein—a tumor marker
AIH	acute intracranial hemorrhage
AL	aluminum
AMP	amplifier
AMS	Acquisition Modality Standards Institute
AMS	automatic monitoring system
ANL	Argon National Laboratory
ANOVA	Analysis of Variance
ANSI	American National Standards Institute
AP or PA	Anterior-Posterior, Access Point
API	application Program Interface
APS	antepartum care summary
ARI	access to radiology information
ASCII	American Standard Code for Information Interchange
ASI NATO	Advanced Study Institute
ASIC	Application-Specific Integrated Circuit
ASP	active server pages
ASP	application services provider

AT	Acceptance Testing
ATL	active template library
ATM	asynchronous transfer mode
ATNA	audit trail and node authentication
Az	area under the ROC curve
BAA	bone age assessment
BPP	bit per pixel
BDF	Building Distribution Center
BGO	Bismuth Germanate X-ray detector
BIDG	Breast imaging data grid
BIS	Bispectral Index System
BME	Biomedical Engineering
BMI	Body Mass Index
BNC	a type of connector for 10 Base2 cables
BPPC	basic patient privacy consents
Brachy	brachytherapy
CA	certificate authority
CA	continuous available
CaBIG	cancer Biomedical Informatics grid
CAD	computer-aided detection, diagnosis
CADe	computer-aided detection
CADx	computer-aided diagnosis
CAI	computer-aided instruction
CalREN	California Research and Education Network
CARS	Computer assisted radiology and surgery
CATH	cardiac cath
CC	cancer center
CC	cranio-caudal
CCD	charge-coupled device
CCU	coronary care unit
CDA R2	clinical document architecture release 2
CDDI	copper distributed data interface
CDR	central data repository
CDRH	Center for Devices and Radiological Health
CDS	clinical decision support
CE-MRI	contrast-enhanced MRI
CEN TC251	Comite Europeen de Normalisation–Technical Committee 251–Healthcare Informatics
CF	computerized fluoroscopy
CFR	contrast frequency response
CHG	charge posting
CHLA	Childrens Hospital Los Angeles
CIE	Commission Internationale de L'Eclairag
CNA	Center for Network Authority
CO_2	carbon dioxide
CMS	clinical management system

CNA	campus network authority
COG	children's oncology group
COM	component object model
CORBA	common object request broker architecture
COSTAR	computer-stored ambulatory record
CPI	consistent presentation of images
CPU	central processing unit
CR	computed radiography
CRF	central retransmission facility—headend
CRPS	Clinical Patient Record System
CRT	cathode ray tube
CsF	Cesium Flouride
CSI	California Spine Institute, Thousand Oaks, CA
CSMA/CD	carrier sense multiple access with collision detection
CSS	cascading style sheet
CSU/DSU	channel service unit/data service unit
CT	computed tomography
CT	consistent time
CTN	central test node
CTV	clinical target volume
D/A	digital-to-analog
DAI	data access interface
DASM	data acquisition system manager
DB	a unit to measure the signal loss
DB MRI	dedicated breast MRI
DBMS	Database Management System
DC	direct current
DCM	DICOM
DCT	Discrete Cosine Transform
DCU	DICOM conversion unit
DDR	digital reconstructed radiography
DE	digital envelope
DEC	device enterprise communication
DECRAD	DEC radiology information system
DES	data encryption standard
DEN	distance education network
DF	digital fluorography
DHA	digital hand atlas
DHHS	Department of Health and Human Services
DICOM	Digital Imaging and Communication in Medicine
DICOM-RT	DICOM in radiotherapy
DIFS	distributed image file server
DIMSE	DICOM message service elements
DIN/PACS	digital imaging network/PACS
DLT	digital linear tape
DM	digital mammography

DMR	diabetic mellitus retinopathy
DOD	Department of Defense
DOT	directly observed treatment
DOR	Department of Radiology
DP	display and processing
DQE	Detector Quantum Efficiency
DR	digital radiography
DR11-W	a parallel interface protocol
DRPT	displayable reports
DRR	digitally reconstructed radiograph
DS	digital signature
DS-0	digital service
DSA	digital subtraction angiography
DSA	digital subtraction arteriography
DSC	digital scan converter
DSL	Digital Subscriber List
DSSS	direct sequence spread spectrum
DTD	document type definition
DTI	Diffusion Tensor MRI
DVA	digital video angiography
DVD	digital versatile disks
DVSA	digital video subtraction angiography
DVH	dose volume histogram
DWI	diffusion weighted MR imaging
ECDR	eye care displayable report
ECED	eye care evidence document
ECG	electrocardiogram
ECT	emission computed tomography
ECHO	echocardiography
ED	emergency department
ED	evidence documents
EDER	emergency department encounter record
EDGE	enhanced data rates for GSM evolution
EDH	extradural hemorrhage
EDR	emergency department referral
EHR	electronic health record
EIA	electrical industry association
EMG	electromyography
eMR	electronic medical record
EP	emergency physician
EPI	echo-planar imaging
EPI	electronic portal image
EPID	electronic portal imaging device
EP	electrophysiology
ePR	electronic Patient Record
ESF	edge spread function
EUA	enterprise user authentication

EuroPACS	European Picture Archiving and Communication System Association
EVN	event type segment
EYECARE	eye care
FCR	Fuji CR
FDA	US Food and Drug Administration
FDDI	fiber distributed data interface
FDG	flurodcoxyglucose
FFBA	full frame bit allocation
FFD	Focus to film distance
FFDDM	full-field direct digital mammography
FID	free induction decay
FIFO	first-in-first-out
FLAIR	Fluid attenuated inversion recovery
FM	folder manager
fMRI	functional MRI
FP	false positive
FPD	flat panel detector
FRS	facial recognition system
FRSS	facial and fingerprint recognition system
FSA	functional status assessment
FT	fault tolerance
FFT	fast Fourier transformation
FTE	full time equivalents
FTP	file transfer protocol
FUSION	image fusion
FWHM	full width at half maximum
G & P	Greulich and Pyle bone development atlas
GAP	Grid Access Point
GEMS	General Electric Medical System
GIF	graphic interchange format
GMAS	Grid Medical archive solution
GPRS	general packet radio services
GRAM	grid resource allocation and management
GSM	global system for mobile communication
GT4	Globus toolkit Version 4, open source software for Grid computing
GTV	Gross target volume
GUI	Graphic user interface
GW	gateway
HA	high availability
H & D curve	Hurter & Driffield characteristic curve
H-CAS	HIPAA-compliant auditing system
HCC	Health Consultation Center
HCC II	Health Consultation Center II

HELP	health evaluation though logical processing
HII	Healthcare Information Infrastructure
HIMSS	Healthcare Information and Management Systems Society
HIPAA	Health Insurance Portability and Accountability Act
HI-PACS	hospital integrated-PACS
HIS	hospital information system
HISPP	healthcare information standards planning panel
HK HA	Hong Kong Hospital Authority
HKID	Hong Kong identity card number
HL-7	Health Level 7
HMO	health care maintenance organization
HOI	Health Outcomes Institute
HP	Hewlett Packard
HPCC	high performance computing and communications
HTML	hypertext markup language
HTTP	hypertext transfer protocol
HTTPS	hypertext transfer protocol secured
Hz	Hertz (cycle/sec)
I2	Internet 2
I/O	input/output
IASS	image-assisted surgery system
ICD-9-CM	International Classification of Diseases, ninth edition, Clinical Modification
ICH	intracerebral hemorrhage
ICMP	internet control message protocol
ICT	information and communication technology
ICU	intensive care unit
ID	identification
IDCO	implantable device cardiac observation
IDF	intermediate distribution
IDNET	a GEMS imaging modality network
IEC	international electrotechnical commission
IEEE	Institute of Electrical and Electronics Engineers
IFT	inverse Fourier transform
IG-MISS	Image guided—minimally invasive spinal surgery
IHE	Integrating of Healthcare Enterprise
IHE-RO	Integrating the Healthcare Enterprise, Radiation Oncology
IIS	Internet Information Server
IMAC	a meeting devoted to image management and communication
IMRT	intensity modulated radiation therapy
INC	identifier Names and Codes
InCor	Heart Institute at the University of San Paulo, Brazil
InfoRAD	Radiology information exhibit at RSNA
IOD	information object definition
IP	imaging plate
IP	internet protocol
IPILab	Image Processing and Informatics Laboratory at USC

IRB	Institute Review Board
IRM	imaging routing mechanism
IRWF	import reconciliation workflow
ISCL	integrated secure communication layer
ISDN	integrated service digital network
ISO	International Standards Organization
ISO-OSI	International Standards Organization—Open System Interconnection
ISP	internet service provider
ISSN	integrated image self-scaling network
IT	information technology
ITS	information technology services
IU	integration unit
IUPAC	International Union of Applied Chemistry
IVA	intravenous video arteriography
IVF	intravenous fluid
IVH	intraventricular hemorrhage
IVUS	intravascular ultrasound
JAMIT	Japan Association of Medical Imaging Technology
JAVA	Just another vague acronym, a programming language
JCAHO	Joint Commission on Accreditation of Healthcare Organizations
JCMIG	Journal of Computerized Medical Imaging and Graphics
JIRA	Japan industries association of radiation apparatus
JND	just noticeable difference
JPEG	Joint Photographic Experts Group
KIN	key image note
kVp	kilo-volt potential difference
LAC	Los Angeles County
LAN	local area network
LCD	liquid crystal display
LDMS	legacy data migration system
LDS	Latter-Day Saints Hospital
LDSE	lossless digital signature embedding
LDSERS	lossless digital signature embedding receiving site
LINAC	linear accelerator
L.L.	left lower
LOINC	logical observation identifier names and codes
lp	line pair
LRI	laboratory for radiological informatics
LSB	least significant bit
LSF	line spread function
LSWF	laboratory scheduled workflow
LTCS	LOINC test codes subset
LTVS	location tracking and verification system
LUT	look up table

mA	milli-ampere
MAC	media access control
MAC	message authentication code
MAMMO	mammography image
MAN	metropolitan area network
MB, Mb	megabytes
MDA	monitoring and discovery system
MDF	message development framework
MDIS	medical diagnostic imaging support systems
MEDICUS	medical imaging and computing for unified information sharing
MFC	Microsoft foundation class
MGH	Massachusetts General Hospital
MHS	Message header segment—A segment used in HL7
MIACS	Medical image archiving and communication system
MIDS	Medical image database server
MIII	medical imaging informatics infrastructure
MIME	multipurpose internet mail extension
MIMP	Mediware information message processor—A computer software language for HIS used by the IBM computer
MIP	maximum intensity projection
MITRE	a non-profit defense contractor
MISS	minimally invasive spinal surgery
MIU	modality integration unit
MLO	mediolateral oblique view in a mammograpm
mmHg	millimeters of mercury
MOD	magnetic Optical Disk
MODEM	modulator/demodulator
MMR-RO	multimodality registration for radiation oncology
MOD	magnetic optical disk
MP	megapixels
MP	multi-processors
MPEG	motion picture experts group compression
MPR	multi-planar reconstruction
MR	magnetic resonance
mR	milli-Roentgen
MRA	magnetic resonance angiography
MRI	magnetic resonance imaging
MRMC	multiple-reader multiple-case in ROC analysis
MRS/MRSI	magnetic resonance spectroscopic imaging
MS	multiple sclerosis
MS	medical summaries
MSDS	healthcare message standard developers sub-committee
MSH	message header segment
MSM	mobile site module
MTF	modulation transfer function
MUM	mobile unit modules
MUMPS	Massachusetts General Hospital Utility Multi-Programming System—A computer software language

MZH	Mt. Zion Hospital, San Francisco
NA	numerical aperture
NANT	new Approaches to neuroblastoma therapy
NATO ASI	North Atlantic Treaty Organization—Advanced Science Institutes
NCI	National Cancer Institute
NDC	network distribution center
NDC	national drug codes
NEC	Nappon Electronic Corporation
NEMA	national electrical manufacturers association
NFS	network file system
NGI	next generation Internet
NIE	network interface equipment
NIBIB	National Institute of Biomedical Imaging and Bioengineering
NIH	National Institutes of Health
NINT	nearest integer neighbor
NK1	next of kin segment
NLM	National Library of Medicine
NM	nuclear medicine
NMSE	normalized mean-square error
NPC	nasopharynx carcinoma
NPRM	Notice of Proposed Rule Makings
NSF	National Science Foundation
NTPL-S	normal treatment planning-simple
NTSC	national television system committee
NTW	new territories west cluster, Hong Kong
NVRAM	nonvolatile random access memory
OARs	organs at risk
OC	optical carrier
OD	optical density
ODBC	open database connectivity
OFDM	orthogonal frequency division multiplexing
OGSA	open grid services architecture
OML	orbital-meatal line
OP IC	out patient imaging Center
OR	operating room
OS	operating system
OSI	open system interconnection
PA	posterior-anterior
PACS	picture archiving and communication system
PBR	pathology-bearing region
PC	personal computer
PD	postdoctoral
PDA	personal digital assistant
PDI	portable data for imaging

PDQ	patient demographics query
Perl	practical extraction and report language
PET	positron emission tomography
PGP	presentation of grouped procedures
PHD	personal health data
PHI	protected health information
PHP	hypertext preprocessor
PI	principal investigator
PICT	Macintosh picture format
PIR	portable data for imaging
PID	patient identification segment
PIR	patient information reconciliation
PIX	patient identifier cross-referencing
PL	plastic
PLUS	PACS local user support
PMS	Philips Medical Systems
PMT	photomultiplier tube
PNG	portable network graphics
POH	Pok Oi Hospital, Hong Kong
PolyU	Hong Kong Polytechnic University
PoP	point-of-presence
PP	post processing
PPI	parallel peripheral interface
PPI-ePR	public private interface–electronic patient record
ppm	parts per million
PPM	post processing manager
PPW	post processing workflow
PPHP	pre-procedural history and physical
PRA	patient record architecture
PRF	pulse repetition frequency
PSA	patient synchronized application
PSF	point spread function
PSL	photo-stimulable luminescence
PSNR	peak signal-to-noise ratio
PTD	parallel transfer disk
PTV	planning target volume
PV1	patient visit segment
PVM	parallel virtual machine system
PWF	pathology workflow
PWF	post-processing workflow
PWP	personnel white pages
Q/R	query and retrieve
QA	quality assurance
QC	quality control
QED	query for existing data
R&D	research and development

RAID	redundant array of inexpensive disks
RAM	random access memory
RETMA	Radio-Electronics-Television Manufacturers Association
RF	radio frequency
RFD	retrieve form for data capture
RFP	request for proposals
RGB	red, green and blue colors
RID	request information for display
RIM	reference information model
RIS	radiology information system
RLE	run length encoding
RLS	replica location service in Grid computing
RNp2	Rede Nacional de Ensino e Pesquisa
ROC	receiver operating characteristic
ROI	region of interest
RR	radiologist residents
RS	radiology specialists
RS	receiving site
RS232	recommended electrical device interface standard 232
RSNA	Radiological Society of North America
RT	radiation therapy
RWF	reporting workflow
S-bus	a computer bus used by SPARC
SAH	subarachnoid hemorrhage
SAN	storage area network
SC	screen captured
SCAR	Society of Computer Applications in Radiology
SCH	student health center
SCP	service class provider
SCSII	small computer systems interface II
SCU	service class user
SD	standard deviations
SDH	subdural hemorrhage
SDK	software development toolkit
SEQUEL	structured English query language
SFVAMC	San Francisco VA Medical Center
SIG	special interest group
SIIM	Society for Imaging Informatics in Medicine
simPHYSIO	simulation physiology
SINR	simple image and numeric report
SJHC	Saint John's Healthcare Center
SMIBAF	super medical image broker and archive facility
SMPTE	Society of Motion Picture and Television Engineers
SMZO	Social and Medical Center East, Vienna
SNOMED	systemized nomenclature of medicine
SNR	signal-to-noise ratio

Solaris 2.x	a computer operating system version 2.x used in a SUN computer
SONET	synchronous optical Network
SOP	service-object pairs
SPARC	a computer system manufactured by Sun Microsystems
SPECT	single photon emission computed tomography
SPIE	International Society for Optical Engineering
SPOF	single-point-of failure
SQL	structured query language
SR	structured reporting
SRS/SRT	stereotactic radiosurgery/stereotactic radiotherapy
SS	sending site
SSD	surface shaded display
SSG	service selection gateway
SSL	secure socket layer
ST	a special connector for optical fibers
STIP	Shanghai Institute of Technical Physics
STRESS	stress testing
SUN OP	SUN computer operating system
SWF	scheduled workflow
T-rate	data transmission rate
T1	DS-1 private line
TB, Tb	terabyte
TC	threshold contrast
TCE	teaching file and clinical trial export
TCP/IP	transmission control protocol/internet protocol
TDS	tube distribution system
TFS	teaching file script
TGC	time gain compensation
TIFF	tagged image file format
TLS	transport layer security
TMH	Tuen Mun Hospital, Hong Kong
TMR	triple modular redundancy
TP	true positive
TPS	treatment planning System
TRWF	treatment workflow
UCAID	University Corporation for Advanced Internet Development
UCLA	University of California at Los Angeles
UCSF	University of California at San Francisco
UH	University Hospital
UID	unique identifier
UMDNS	universal medical device nomenclature system
UMLS	unified medical language system
UMTS	universal mobile telecommunications service

UPS	uninterruptible power supply
URL	uniform resource locator
US	ultrasound
USAVRE	United States Army Virtual Radiology Environment
USC	University of Southern California
UTP	unshielded twisted pair
VA	Department of Veterans Affairs
VAHE	United States Department of Veterans Affairs Healthcare Enterprise Information System
VAMC	VA Medical Center
VAS	visual analog scale
VAX	a computer system manufactured by Digital Equipment Corporation (DEC)
VB	visual basic
vBNS	very high-performance backbone network service
VGA	video graphics array
VL	visible light
VM	value multiplicity
VME	a computer bus used by older SUN and other computers
VMS	a computer operating system software used by DEC computers
VPN	virtual private network
VR	value representation
VR	voice recognition
VRAM	video RAM
VRE	virtual radiology environment
VS	virtual simulator
VTK	visualization toolkit
WADO	web access to DICOM persistent objects
WAN	wide area network
WECA	Wireless Ethernet Compatibility Alliance
WEP	wired equivalent privacy
Wi-Fi	wireless fidelity
WLAN	wireless LAN
WORM	write once read many
WS	workstation
WWAN	wireless WAN
WWW	world wide web
XCT	x-ray computed tomography
XD*-LAB	sharing laboratory reports
XDM	cross-enterprise document media interchange
XDR	cross-enterprise document reliable interchange
XDS	cross-enterprise document sharing
XDS-I	cross-enterprise document sharing for imaging

XDS-SD	cross-enterprise sharing of scanned documents
XML	extensible markup language
XPHR	exchange of personal health record content
YCbCr	luminance, and two chrominance coordinates used in color digital imaging
YIQ	luminance, in-phase, and quadrature chrominance color coordinates

Introduction

1.1 INTRODUCTION

PACS (picture archiving and communication system) based on digital, communication, display, and information technologies has revolutionized the practice of
radiology, and in a sense, of medicine during the past fifteen years. This textbook introduces the PACS basic concept, terminology, technological development,
and implementation, as well as PACS-based applications to clinical practice and
PACS-based imaging informatics. There are many advantages of introducing digital, communications, display, and information technologies (IT) to the conventional
paper and film-based operation in radiology and medicine. For example, through digital imaging plate and detector technology, and various energy source digital imaging
modalities, it is possible to improve the modality diagnostic value while at the same
time reducing the radiation exposure to the patient; then through the computer and
display, the digital image can be manipulated for value-added diagnosis. Also digital,
communication, IT technologies can been used to understand the healthcare delivery
workflow, resulting in a speed-up of healthcare delivery and reduction of medical
operation costs.

   With all these benefits, digital communication and IT are gradually changing the
way medical images and related information in the healthcare industry are acquired,
stored, viewed, and communicated. One natural development along this line is the
emergence of digital radiology departments and digital healthcare delivery environment. A digital radiology department has two components: a radiology information
management system (RIS) and a digital imaging system. RIS is a subset of the
hospital information system (HIS) or clinical management system (CMS). When
these systems are combined with the electronic patient (or medical) record (ePR or
eMR) system, which manages selected data of the patient, we are envisioning the
arrival of the total filmless and paperless healthcare delivery system. The digital
imaging system, PACS, involves an image management and communication system
(IMAC) for image acquisition, archiving, communication, retrieval, processing, distribution, and display. A digital healthcare environment consists of the integration of
HIS/CMS, ePR, PACS and other digital clinical systems. The combination of HIS
and PACS is sometime referred to as hospital-integrated PACS (HI-PACS). A PACS

PACS and Imaging Informatics, Second Edition, by H. K. Huang
Copyright © 2010 John Wiley & Sons, Inc.

database contains voluminous health-related data. If organized and used properly, it can improve patient care and outcome. The art and science of utilizing these data is loosely termed as imaging informatics. The cost of healthcare delivery related to PACS, health-related IT, as well as imaging informatics has passed one billion dollars each year (excluding imaging modalities) and is still growing.

Up-to-date information on these topics can be found in multidisciplinary literature, reports from research laboratories of university hospitals and medical imaging manufacturers but not in a coordinated way. Therefore it is difficult for a radiologist, physician, hospital administrator, medical imaging researcher, radiological technologist, trainee in diagnostic radiology, and the student in physics, engineering, and computer science to collect and assimilate this information. The purpose of this book is to consolidate and to organize PACS and its integration with HIS and ePR, as well as imaging informatics-related topics, into one self-contained text. Here the emphasis is on the basic principles and augmented by discussion of current technological developments and examples.

1.2 SOME HISTORICAL REMARKS ON PICTURE ARCHIVING AND COMMUNICATION SYSTEMS (PACS)

1.2.1 Concepts, Conferences, and Early Research Projects

1.2.1.1 Concepts and Conferences   The concept of digital image communication and digital radiology was introduced in the late 1970s and early 1980s. Professor Heinz U. Lemke introduced the concept of digital image communication and display in a paper in 1979 (Lemke, 1979). SPIE (International Society for Optical Engineering) sponsored a Conference on Digital Radiography held at the Stanford University Medical Center and chaired by Dr. William R. Brody (Brody, 1981). Dr. M. Paul Capp and colleagues introduced the idea of photoelectronic radiology department and depicted a system block diagram of the demonstration facility at the University of Arizona Health Sciences Center (Capp, 1981). Professor S. J. Dwyer, III (Fig. 1.1*a*) predicted the cost of managing digital diagnostic images in a radiology department (Dwyer, 1982). However, technology maturation was lacking, and it was not until the First International Conference and Workshop on Picture Archiving and Communication Systems (PACS) at Newport Beach, California, held in January 1982 and sponsored by SPIE (Duerinckx, 1982; Fig. 1.1*b*,*c*), that these concepts began to be recognized. During that meeting, the term PACS was coined. Thereafter, and to this day, the PACS and Medical Imaging Conferences have been combined into a joint SPIE meeting held each February in southern California.

In Asia and Europe a similar timeline has been noted. The First International Symposium on PACS and PHD (Personal Health Data) sponsored by the Japan Association of Medical Imaging Technology (JAMIT) was held in July 1982 (JAMIT, 1983; Fig. 1.1*d*). This conference, combined with the Medical Imaging Technology meeting, also became an annual event. In Europe, the EuroPACS (Picture Archiving and Communication Systems in Europe) has held annual meetings since 1983 (Niinimaki, 2003), and this group remains the driving force for European PACS information exchange (Fig. 1.1*e*,*f*).

Notable among the many PACS-related meetings that occur regularly are two others: the CAR (Computer-Assisted Radiology; Lemke, 2002) and IMAC (Image

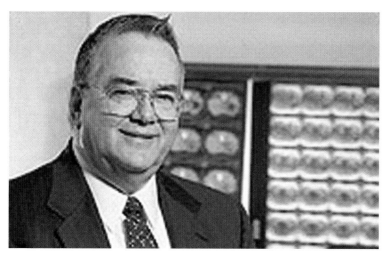

Figure 1.1a The late Samuel J. Dwyer III in front of his early developed workstation.

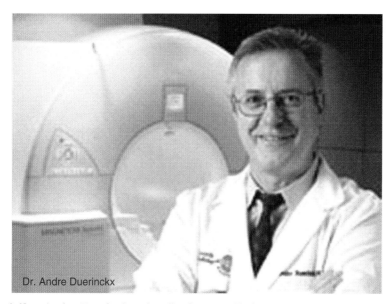

Dr. Andre Duerinckx

Figure 1.1b Andre Duerinckx, the Conference Chairman of the First SPIE Medical Imaging Conference (International Society for Optical Engineering) where the term PACS was coined.

Management and Communication; Mun, 1989). CAR is an annual event organized by Professor Lemke of Technical University of Berlin since 1985 (CAR expanded its name to CARS in 1999, adding Computer-Assisted Surgery to the Congress, and Professor Lemke is now with the University of Southern California). The *Annual Proceeding of CARS* became the *International Journal of CARS* in 2005 (Fig. 1.1*g*). IMAC was started in 1989 as a biannual conference and organized by Professor Seong K. Mun of Georgetown University (Mun, 1989), and its meetings were stopped

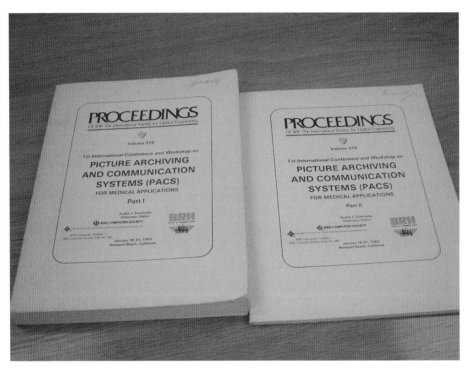

Figure 1.1c First set of PACS Conference Proceedings sponsored by SPIE at Newport Beach, CA, in 1982.

in late 1990s. SPIE, EuroPACS, and CARS annual conferences have been consistent in publishing conference proceedings and journals that provide fast information exchange for researchers working in this field, and many have been benefited from such information sources.

A meeting dedicated to PACS sponsored by NATO ASI (Advanced Study Institute) was a PACS in Medicine Symposium held in Evian, France, from October 12 to 24, 1990. Approximately 100 scientists from over 17 countries participated, and the *ASI Proceedings* summarized international efforts in PACS research and development at that time (Huang, 1991b; Fig. 1.1*h*). This meeting was central to the formation of a critical PACS project: the Medical Diagnostic Imaging Support System (MDIS) project sponsored by the U.S. Army Medical Research and Materiel Command, which has been responsible for large-scale military PACS installations in the United States (Mogel, 2003).

The InfoRAD Section at the RSNA (Radiological Society of North America) Scientific Assembly has been instrumental to the continued development of PACS technology and its growing clinical acceptance. Founded in 1993 by Dr. Laurens V. Ackerman (and subsequently managed by Dr. C. Carl Jaffe, and others), InfoRAD has showcased live demonstrations of DICOM and IHE (Integrating the Healthcare Enterprise) compliance by manufacturers. InfoRAD has repeatedly set the tone for industrial PACS renovation and development. Many refresher courses in PACS during RSNA have been organized by Dr. C. Douglas Maynard, Dr. Edward V. Staab, and subsequently by the RSNA Informatics committee, to provide continuing

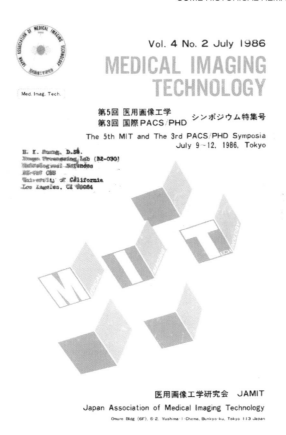

Vol. 4 No. 2 July 1986

MEDICAL IMAGING
TECHNOLOGY

Med. Imag. Tech.

第5回 医用画像工学
第3回 国際PACS/PHD   シンポジウム特集号

The 5th MIT and The 3rd PACS/PHD Symposia
July 9~12, 1986, Tokyo

医用画像工学研究会　JAMIT
Japan Association of Medical Imaging Technology

Figure 1.1d   Cover of *Journal of the Japan Association of Medical Imaging Technology* (*JAMIT*), July 1986 issue.

education in PACS and informatics to the radiology community. When Dr. Roger A. Bauman became editor in chief of the then new *Journal of Digital Imaging* in 1998, the consolidation of PACS research and development peer-reviewed papers in one representative journal became possible. Editor-in-chief Bauman was succeeded by Dr. Steve Horii, followed by Dr. Janice C. Honeyman-Buck. The *Journal of Computerized Medical Imaging and Graphics* (*JCMIG*) published two special Issues on PACS in 1991 (Huang, 1991a); *PACS—Twenty Years Later* summarized in 2003 (Huang, 2003a) the progress of PACS before 2003 in two 10-year intervals (Fig. 1.1*i*).

1.2.1.2   *Early Funded Research Projects by the U.S. Federal Government*   One of the earliest research projects related to PACS in the United States was a teleradiology project sponsored by the U.S. Army in 1983. A follow-up project was the Installation Site for Digital Imaging Network and Picture Archiving and Communication System (DIN/PACS) funded by the U.S. Army and administered by the MITRE Corporation in 1986 (MITRE, 1986). Two university sites were selected for the implementation, University of Washington in Seattle and Georgetown University/George Washington University Consortium in Washington, DC, with the participation of Philips Medical Systems and AT &T. The U.S. National

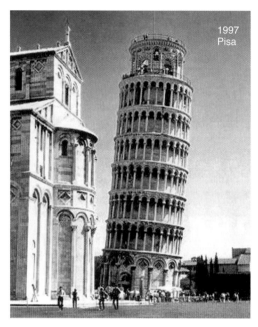

Figure 1.1e EuroPACS Conference held at Pisa, Italy in 1997.

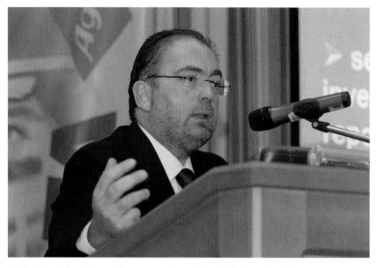

Figure 1.1f Davide Caramella presenting the 25th EuroPACS Anniversary Lecture.

Cancer Institute, National Institutes of Health (NCI, NIH) funded the University of California, Los Angeles (UCLA) several large-scale PACS-related research program projects under the titles of Multiple Viewing Stations for Diagnostic Radiology, Image Compression, and PACS in Radiology started in mid-1980s and early 1990s.

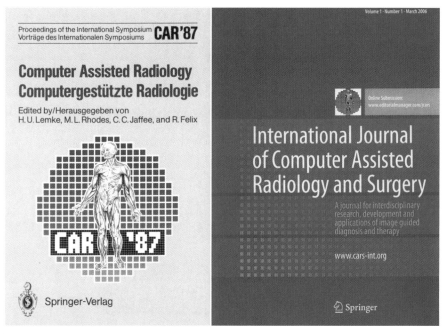

Figure 1.1g   Cover of the *Proceedings of the CAR'87 Annual International Symposium* (left), Cover of the *International Journal of Computer Assisted Radiology and Surgery*, March 2006, the first issue (right).

1.2.2   PACS Evolution

1.2.2.1   In the Beginning   A PACS integrates many components related to medical imaging for clinical practice. Depending on the application, a PACS can be simple, consisting of a few components, or it can be a complex hospital-integrated or an enterprise system. For example, a PACS for an intensive care unit in the early days may comprise no more than a scanner adjacent to the film developer for digitization of radiographs, a base band communication system to transmit, and a video monitor in the ICU (Intensive care unit) to receive and display images. Such a simple system was actually implemented by Dr. Richard J. Steckel (Steckle, 1972) as early as 1972. Nowadays some hospitals install a CT (computed tomography) or MRI (magnetic resonance imaging) scanner connected with a storage device and several viewing stations would also call these components as a PACS. On the other hand, implementing a comprehensive hospital-integrated or enterprise PACS is a major undertaking that requires careful planning and multimillion US dollars of investment.

PACS operating conditions and environments have differed in North America, Europe, and Asia, and consequently has PACS evolution in these regions. Initially PACS research and development in North America was largely supported by government agencies and manufacturers. In the European countries, development was supported through a multinational consortium, a country, or a regional resource. European research teams tended to work with a single major manufacturer, and since most early PACS components were developed in the United States and Japan, they

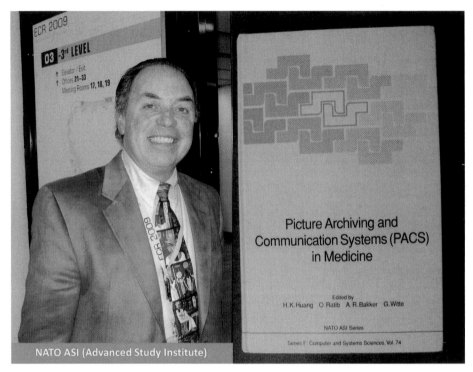

Figure 1.1h Cover of the *Proceedings of the NATO ASI* (Advanced Study Institute): Picture Archiving and Communication Systems (PACS) in Medicine, Series F, Vol 74. Evian France, 1990 (right), Osman Ratib (left) taken during the EuroPACS Annual meeting at Vienna, Austria, March 2009.

were not as readily available to the Europeans. European research teams emphasized PACS modeling and simulation, as well as the investigation of image processing components of PACS. In Asia, Japan led the PACS research and development and treated it as a national project. The national resources were distributed to various manufacturers and university hospitals. A single manufacturer or a joint venture from several companies integrated a PACS system and installed it in a hospital for clinical evaluation. The manufacturer's PACS specifications tended to be rigid and left little room for the hospital research teams to modify the technical specifications.

During the October 1997 IMAC meeting in Seoul, South Korea, three invited lectures described the evolution of PACS in Europe, America, and Japan, respectively. It was apparently from these presentations that these regional PACS research and development enterprises gradually merged and led to many successful international PACS implementation. Five major factors contributed to these successes: (1) information exchanges from the SPIE, CAR, IMAC, and RSNA conferences; (2) introduction of image and data format standards (DICOM) and gradual mature concepts and their acceptance by private industry; (3) globalization of the imaging manufacturers; (4) development and sharing of solutions to difficult technical and clinical problems in PACS; and (5) promotion by RSNA through demonstrations and refresher courses.

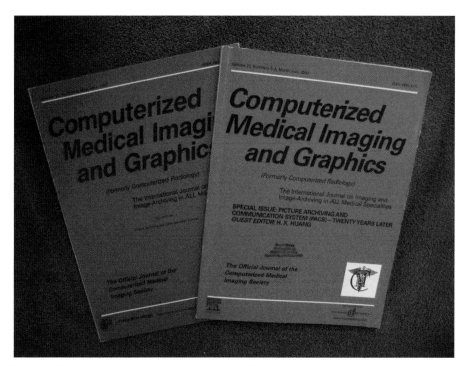

Figure 1.1i Covers of two special Issues: PACS 1991, and PACS—Twenty years later in the 2003 *Journal of Computerized Medical Imaging and Graphics*.

1.2.2.2 Large-Scale PACS The late Roger Bauman, in two papers in the *Journal of Digital Imaging* (Bauman, 1996a, b), defined a large-scale PACS as one that satisfies the following four conditions:

1. Use in daily clinical operation.
2. Augmented by at least three or four imaging modalities connected to the system.
3. Containing workstations inside and outside of the radiology department.
4. Able to handle at least 20,000 radiological procedures a year.

Such a definition loosely separated the large and the small PACS at that time. However, nowadays most PACS installed except teleradiology are meeting these requirements.

Colonel Fred Goeringer instrumented the Army MDIS project, which resulted in several large-scale PACS installations and provided a major stimulus for the PACS industry (Mogel 2003). Dr. Walter W. Hruby opened a completely digital radiology department in the Danube Hospital, Vienna in April, 1992 setting the tone for future total digital radiology departments (Hruby and Maltsidis, 2000; Fig. 1.1*j*). Figure 1.1*k* depicts two medical imaging pioneers, Professor Heniz Lemke (left) and Professor Michael Vannier (right, then editor in chief, *IEEE Transactions on Medical Imaging*) at the Danube Hospital's opening ceremony. These two projects set the stage for the continuing PACS development.

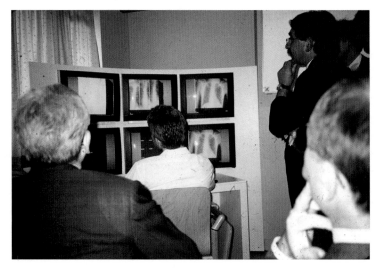

Figure 1.1j W. Hruby (right, in a dark suit), Chairman of Radiology at the Danube Hospital, Vienna, during the PACS Open House Ceremony in 1990.

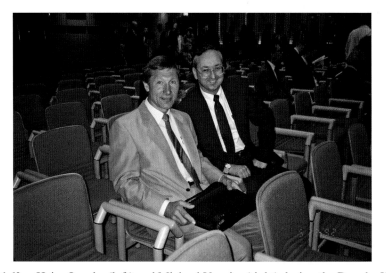

Figure 1.1k Heinz Lemke (left) and Michael Vannier (right) during the Danube Hospital PACS Open House Ceremony, Vienna.

1.2.3 Standards

The ACR-NEMA (American College of Radiology–National Electrical Manufacturers' Association) and later DICOM (Digital Imaging and Communication in Medicine) standards (DICOM, 1996) are the necessary requirements of system integration in PACS. The establishment of these standards and their acceptance by the medical imaging community required the contributions of many people from both industry and academe. On the private industry side, major PACS manufactures

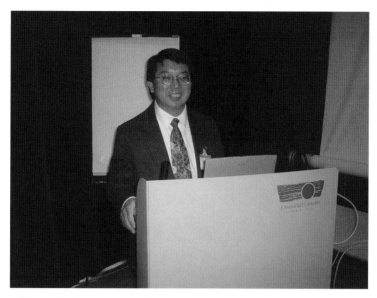

Figure 1.1l Steve Horii presenting one of his DICOM lectures.

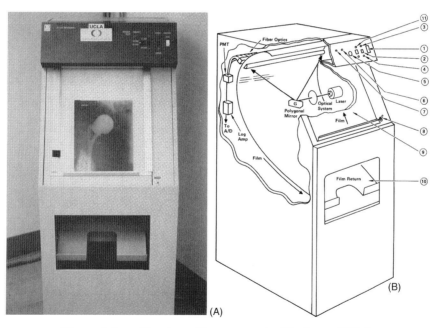

Figure 1.1m First laser film scanner by Konica at UCLA.

often assigned their own personnel to DICOM committees. Participants from academe have been mostly individuals with more altruistic interests. Among these scholars, special mention should be given Professor Steve Horii. His unselfish and tireless efforts in educating others about the concept and importance of DICOM have been vital to the success of PACS (Fig. 1.1*l*).

1.2.4 Early Key Technologies

Many key technologies developed over the past 20 years have contributed to the success of PACS operation. Although many such technologies have since been gradually replaced by more up-to-date technologies, it is instructive for historical purposes to review them. This section only lists these technologies (Huang, 2003a). Because these technologies are well known by now, only a line of introduction for each is given. For more detailed discussions of these technologies, the reader is referred to other Huang references (1987, 1996, 1999, 2004).

The key technologies are as follows:

- The first laser film digitizers developed for clinical use by Konica (Fig. 1.1*m*) and Lumisys, and the direct CR chest unit by Konica (Fig. 1.1*n*).
- Computed radiography (CR) by Fuji and its introduction from Japan to the United States (Fig. 1.1*o*) by Dr. William Angus of Philips Medical Systems of North America (PMS).
- The first digital interface unit using DR11-W technology transmitting CR images to outside of the CR reader designed and implemented by the UCLA PACS team (Fig. 1.1*p*).
- Hierarchical storage integrating a large-capacity optical disk Jukebox by Kodak with the then innovative redundant array of inexpensive disks (RAID), using the AMASS software designed by the UCLA PACS team (Fig. 1.1*q*).

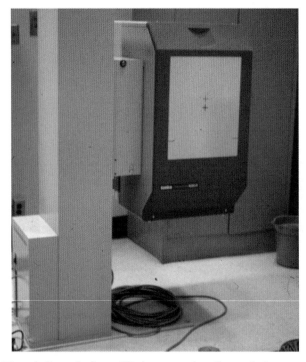

Figure 1.1n First dedicated chest CR (computed radiography) system by Konica at UCLA. The concept matured later and became the DR (digital radiography) system.

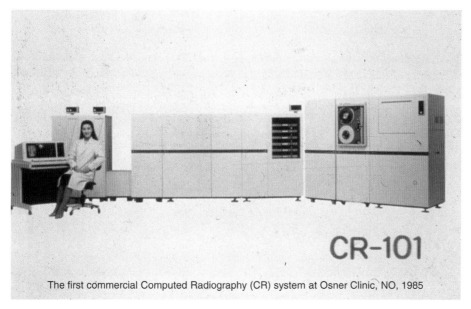

The first commercial Computed Radiography (CR) system at Osner Clinic, NO, 1985

Figure 1.1o   First Fuji CR system, CR-101 at the Osner Clinics, New Orleans.

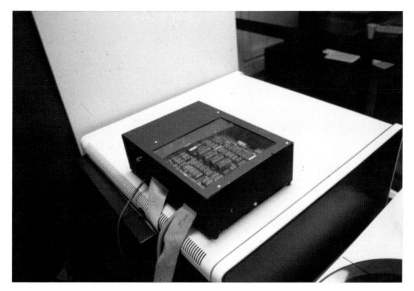

Figure 1.1p   First interface box using the DR-11 W technology transmitting digital CR images out of the PCR-901 and PCR-7000 systems (Philips Medical Systems) to a PACS acquisition computer at UCLA. The concept allowing direct transmission of a full CR image to the outside world as input to PACS was the cornerstone of viewing direct digital projection image on a display monitor.

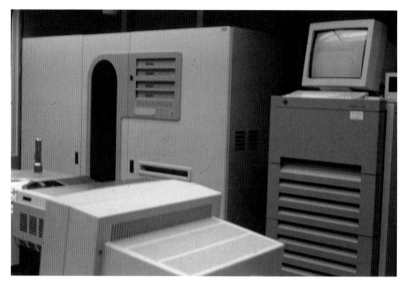

Figure 1.1q Hierarchical storage system of a PACS, consisting of a Kodak Optical Disk Library (left) with one hundred 14-inch disk platters, a RAID (right), and AMASS file management software at UCLA. Similar systems were used in later military MDIS PAC systems.

- Multiple display using six 512 monitors at UCLA (Fig. 1.1r).
- Multiple display using three 1024 monitors (Fig. 1.1s) and the controller (Fig. 1.1t, blue) at UCLA with hardware supported by Dr. Harold Rutherford of the Gould DeAnza.
- Various spatial resolution 512, 1024, 1400 display systems at UCLA (Fig. 1.1u)
- Two 2000-line and 72 Hz CRT monitors display system by MegaScan at UCLA (Fig. 1.1v).
- System integration methods developed by the Siemens Gammasonics and Loral for large-scale PACS in the MDIS project.
- Asynchronous transfer mode (ATM) technology by Pacific Bell, merging the local area network and high-speed wide area network communications for PACS application in teleradiology by the Laboratory for Radiological Informatics, University of California, San Francisco (UCSF; Huang, 1995).

1.2.5 Medical Imaging Modality, PACS, and Imaging Informatics R&D Progress Over Time

Over the past 25 years three developments have mainly propelled the advancement of imaging modalities and the clinical acceptance of PACS. They are sizable funding to academe by the U.S. federal government for early key technology research and development, adoption of medical imaging standards by the imaging community, and manufacturers' developing workflow profiles for large-scale PACS operation. The large amount of imaging/data now available is enabling the next wave of innovation

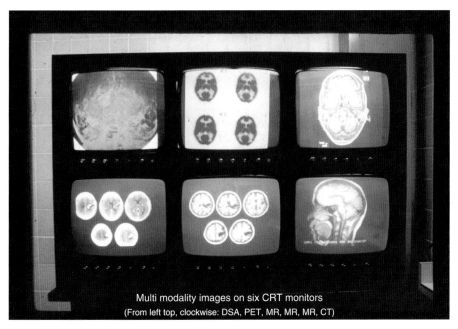

Figure 1.1r Display system showing six 512-line multiple modality images at UCLA.

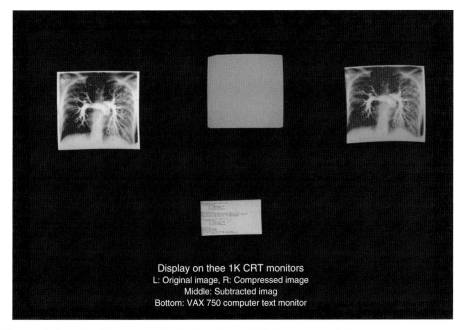

Figure 1.1s Gould system displaying three 1K images used in image compression study at UCLA: The original image (left); compressed (right); subtraction (middle). The system was the first to use for comparing the quality of compressed images with different compression ratios.

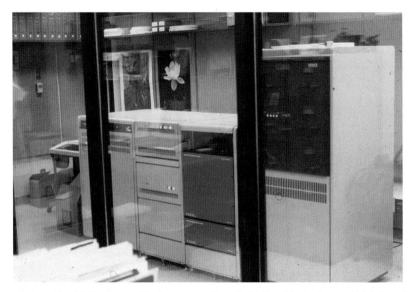

Figure 1.1t Gould DeAnza display controller (middle, blue) for a 1024-line 3-color display system (24 bits/pixel) with the VAX 750 (left) as the control computer.

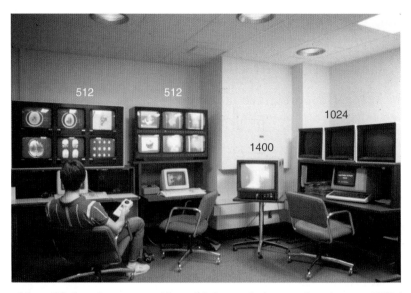

Figure 1.1u Workstation room with multiple resolution workstations at UCLA, with two six-monitor display systems (512 × 512), one three-monitor display system (1K x 1K), and one 1400 line single-monitor system by Mitsubishi. This workstation room was used to perform the first large-scale study in quality of image display with different spatial resolutions.

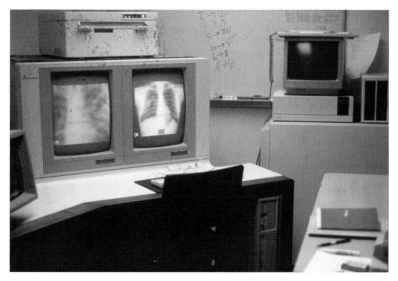

Figure 1.1v   Early display system with two Megascan 2K monitors at UCLA.

and fruition of the concept of medical imaging informatics. Table 1.1 summarizes the progress made in imaging modalities, PACS, and imaging informatics R&D over time.

1.3   WHAT IS PACS?

1.3.1   PACS Design Concept

A picture archiving and communication system (PACS) consists of medical image and data acquisition, storage, and display subsystems integrated by digital networks and application software. It can be as simple as a film digitizer connected to several display workstations with a small image data base and storage device or as complex as an enterprise image management system. PACS developed in the late 1980s were designed mainly on an ad hoc basis to serve small subsets, called modules, of the total operation of a radiology department. Each PACS module functioned as an isolated island unable to communicate with other modules. Although the PACS concepts proved to work adequately for different radiology and clinical services, the piecemeal approach was weak because it did not address connectivity and cooperation between modules. This problem became exacerbated as more PACS modules were added to hospital networks. The maintenance, routing decisions, coordination of machines, fault tolerance, and expandability of the system became increasingly difficult to manage. This inadequacy of the early PACS design was due partially to a lack of understanding by the designers and implementers of PACS's potential for large-scale applications, clearly because at that time the many necessary PACS-related key technologies were not yet available.

PACS design, we now understand, should focus on system connectivity and workflow efficiency. A general multimedia data management system that is expandable, flexible, and versatile in its operation calls for both top-down

TABLE 1.1   Medical imaging, PACS, and imaging informatics R&D progress over time

Decade	R&D Progress
1980s	Medical imaging technology development
	• CR, MRI, CT, US, DR, WS, storage, networking
Late 1980s	Imaging systems integration
	• PACS, ACR/NEMA, DICOM, high-speed networks
Early 1990s	Integration of HIS/RIS/PACS
	• DICOM, HL7, Intranet and Internet
Late 1990s–present	Workflow and application servers
	• IHE, ePR, enterprise PACS, Web-based PACS
2000s–present	Imaging informatics
	• Computer-aided diagnosis (CAD), image contents indexing,
	• Knowledge base, decision support,
	• Image-assisted diagnosis and treatment

management to integrate various hospital information systems and a bottom-up engineering approach to build its foundation (i.e., PACS infrastructure). From the management point of view, a hospital-wide or enterprise PACS is attractive to administrators because it provides economic justification for implementing the system. Proponents of PACS are convinced that its ultimately favorable cost–benefit ratio should not be evaluated as the balance of the resource of the radiology department alone but should extend to the entire hospital or enterprise operation. As this concept has gained momentum, many hospitals, and some enterprise level healthcare entities around the world have been implementing large- scale PACS and have provided solid evidence that PACS does improve the efficiency of healthcare delivery and at the same time saves hospital operational costs. From the engineering point of view, the PACS infrastructure is the basic way to introduce such critical features as standardization, open architecture, expandability for future growth, connectivity, reliability, fault-tolerance, workflow efficiency, and cost effectiveness. This design approach can be modular with an infrastructure as described in the next section.

1.3.2   PACS Infrastructure Design

The PACS infrastructure design provides the necessary framework for the integration of distributed and heterogeneous imaging devices and makes possible intelligent database management of all patient-related information. Moreover it offers an efficient means of viewing, analyzing, and documenting study results, and thus a method for effectively communicating study results to the referring physicians. PACS infrastructure consists of a basic skeleton of hardware components (imaging device interfaces, storage devices, host computers, communication networks, and display systems) integrated by a standardized, flexible software system for communication, database management, storage management, job scheduling, interprocessor communication, error handling, and network monitoring. The infrastructure is versatile and can incorporate more complex research, clinical service, and education needs. The software modules of the infrastructure are embedded with sufficient learning capacity and interactivity at a system level to permit the components to work together as a system rather than as individual networked computers.

Hardware components include patient data servers, imaging modalities, data/modality interfaces, PACS controller with database and archive, and display workstations connected by communication networks for handling the efficient data/image flow in the PACS and satisfying the clinical workflow requirements. Image and data stored in the PACS can be extracted from the archive and transmitted to application servers for various uses. Nowadays PACS should also consider the enterprise level interconnectivity for image/data communication throughout several healthcare providers. Figure 1.2 shows the PACS basic components and data flow. This diagram will be expanded to finer details in later chapters. The PACS application servers and Web servers concepts are shown at the bottom of the diagram; these components enriche the role of PACS in the healthcare delivery system and have contributed to the advancement of PACS utilization over the past several years. These servers are cornerstones of PCAS- and DICOM-based imaging informatics.

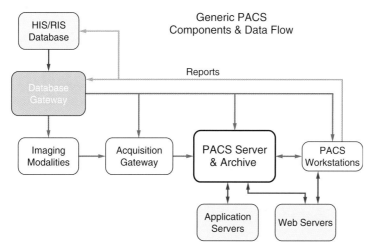

Figure 1.2   PACS basic components (yellow) and data flow (blue: internal; green and orange: external between PACS and other information systems); other information systems (light blue). HIS: Hospital Information System; RIS: Radiology Information System. System integration and clinical implementation are two other components necessary for implementation after the system is physically connected. Application servers and Web servers connected to the PACS server enrich the PACS infrastructure for other clinical, research and education applications.

1.4 PACS IMPLEMENTATION STRATEGIES

1.4.1 Background

The many technical and clinical components of PACS related to medical imaging form an integrated healthcare information technology (IT) system. For the past 20 years many hospitals and manufacturers in the United States and abroad have researched and developed PACS of varying complexity for daily clinical use. These systems can be loosely grouped into six models according to their methods of implementation as described next in the Section 1.4.2.

1.4.2 Six PACS Implementation Models

1.4.2.1 Home-Grown Model Most early PACS models were implemented by university hospitals, academic departments, and research laboratories of major imaging manufacturers. For implementation of a model a multidisciplinary team with technical knowledge was assembled by the radiology department or hospital. The team became a system integrator, selecting PACS components from various manufacturers. The team developed system interfaces and wrote the PACS software according to the clinical requirements of the hospital.

Such a model allowed the research team to continuously upgrade the system with state-of-the-art components. The system so designed was tailored to the clinical environment and could be upgraded without depending on the schedule of the manufacturer. However, a substantial commitment was required of the hospital to assemble the multidisciplinary team. In addition, since the system developed was to be one of a kind, consisting of components from different manufacturers, system service and maintenance proved to be difficult. Today PACS technology has so matured that very few institutions depend on this form of PACS implementation. Nevertheless, the development of specific PACS application servers shown in Figure 1.2 does require knowing the basic concept and construction of the model.

1.4.2.2 Two-Team Effort Model In the two-team model, a team of experts, both from outside and inside the hospital, is assembled to write detailed specifications for the PACS for a certain clinical environment. A manufacturer is contracted to implement the system. Such a model of team effort between the hospital and manufacturers was chosen by US military services when they initiated the Medical Diagnostic Imaging Support System (MDIS) concept in the late 1980s. The MDIS follows military procurement procedures in acquiring PACS for military hospitals and clinics.

The primary advantage of the two-team model is that the PACS specifications are tailored to a certain clinical environment, yet the responsibility for implementing is delegated to the manufacturer. The hospital acts as a purchasing agent and does not have to be concerned with the installation. However, there are disadvantages. Specifications written by a hospital team often tend to be overambitious because they underestimate the technical and operational difficulty in implementing certain clinical functions. The designated manufacturer, on the other hand, could lack clinical experience and thus overestimate the performance of each component. As a result the completed PACS will not meet the overall specifications. Also, because the cost of contracting the manufacturer to develop a specified PACS is high, only one such system can be built. For these reasons this model is being gradually replaced by the partnership model described in Section 1.4.2.4.

1.4.2.3 Turnkey Model   The turnkey model is market driven. The manufacturer develops a turnkey PACS and installs it in a department for clinical use. The advantage of this model is that the cost of delivering a generic system tends to be lower. However, some manufacturers could see potential profit in developing a specialized turnkey PACS to promote the sale of other imaging equipment, like a CR (computed radiography) or DR (digital radiography).

Another disadvantage is that the manufacturer needs a couple of years to complete the equipment production cycle, the fast moving computer and communication technologies may render the PACS becomes obsolete after only several years of use. Further it is doubtful whether a generalized PACS can be used for every specialty in a single department and for every radiology department.

1.4.2.4 Partnership Model   The partnership model is very suitable for large-scale PACS implementation. In this model the hospital and a manufacturer form a partnership to share the responsibility of implementation of a PCAS. Over the past few years, because of the availability of PACS clinical data, healthcare centers have learned to take advantages of the good and discard the bad features of a PACS for their clinical environments. As a result the boundaries between the aforementioned three implementation models have gradually fused resulting in the emergent partnership model. Because the healthcare center forms a partnership with a selected manufacturer or a system integrator, responsibility is shared in its PACS implementation, maintenance, service, training, and upgrading. The arrangement can be a long-term purchase with a maintenance contract, or a lease of the system. A tightly coupled partnership can even include the manufacturer training the hospital personnel in engineering, maintenance, and system upgrade. Financial responsibility is then shared by both parties.

1.4.2.5 The Application Service Provider (ASP) Model   In the ASP model, a system integrator provides all PACS-related services to a client, which can be the entire hospital or a small radiology practice group. No on-site IT specialty is needed by the client. ASP is attractive for smaller subsets of the PACS, for examples, off-site archive, long-term image archive/retrieval or second copy archive, DICOM-Web server development, and Web-based image database. For larger comprehensive PACS implementations, the ASP model requires detailed investigation by the healthcare provider, and a suitable and reliable system integrator must be identified.

1.4.2.6 Open Source Model   As PACS technologies have matured, specialties have gradually migrated to commodities, especially knowledge of the DICOM (Digital Imaging and Communication in Medicine) standard, IHE (Integrating the Healthcare Enterprise) workflow profiles, and Web technology. Many academic centers and some manufacturers R&D personnel have deposited their acquired knowledge in the public domain as open source software. This phenomenon encourages use of the home-grown model described in Section 1.4.2.1 whereby the healthcare providers utilize their in-house clinical and IT personnel to develop PACS application servers and Web servers described in Figure 1.2 These PACS components once were of the manufacturer's domain as the after sale add-on profits earned upon installing a PACS for the healthcare provider. Open source PACS related software has gained momentum in recent years among home-grown teams that develop special applications components of PACS and Web servers. For example, the healthcare provider would purchase off-the-shelf computer and communication hardware and use open source PACS software to develop in-house special PACS applications.

Each of these six models has its advantages and disadvantages. Table 1.2 summarizes the comparisons.

1.5 A GLOBAL VIEW OF PACS DEVELOPMENT

1.5.1 The United States

PACS development in the United States has benefited from four factors:

1. Many university research laboratories and small private companies that have entered the field since 1982 were supported by government agencies, venture capital, and IT industries.
2. The heaviest support of PACS implementation has come from the U.S. Department of Defense hospitals (Mogel, 2003) and the Department of Veterans Affairs (VA) Medical Center Enterprise (see Chapter 22 for more details).
3. A major imaging equipment and PACS manufacturer is US based.
4. Fast moving and successful small IT companies have contributed their innovative technologies to PACS development.

There are roughly 300 large and small PAC systems in use today. Nearly every new hospital being built or designed has a PACS implementation plan attached to its architectural blue prints.

1.5.2 Europe

PACS development in Europe has advanced remarkably:

1. Hospital information system- and PACS- related research and development were introduced to European institutions in the early 1980s.
2. Three major PACS manufactures are based in Europe.
3. Two major PACS-related annual conferences, EuroPACS and CARS, are based in Europe.

Many innovative PACS-related technologies were even invented in Europe. Still there are presently far more working PACS installations in the United States than in Europe. Lemke studied the factors that may account for this phenomenon and came up with results shown in Table 1.3 (Lemke, 2003). However, over the past five years European countries have recognized the importance of PACS contribution to regional healthcare, so inter-hospital communications have led to an enterprise-level PACS concept and development. The United Kingdom, Sweden, Norway, Finland, France, Italy, Austria, Germany, and Spain are all developing PACS for large-scale

TABLE 1.2   Advantages and disadvantages of six PACS implementation models

Method	Advantages	Disadvantages
Home-Grown system	Built to specifications State-of-the-art technology Continuously upgrading Not dependent on a single manufacturer	Difficult to assemble a team One-of-a-kind system Difficult to service and maintain
Two-team effort	Specifications written for a certain clinical environment Implementation delegated to the manufacturer	Specifications overambitious Underestimated technical and operational difficulty Manufacturer lacks clinical experience Expensive
Turnkey	Lower cost Easier maintenance	Too general Not state-of-the-art technology
Partnership	System will keep up with technology advancement Health center does not deal with the system becoming obsolete, but depends on manufacturer's long-term service contract	Expensive to the health center, Manufacturer may not want to sign a partnership contract with less prominent center Center has to consider the longevity and stability of the manufacturer
ASP	Minimizes initial capital cost May accelerate potential return on investment No risk of technology obsolescence Provides flexible growth No space requirement in data center	More expensive over 2–4 year time frame comparing to a capital purchase Customer has no ownership in equipment
Open source	Healthcare provider purchases computer and communication equipment Good for special PACS application server Lower cost	Open source software may not be robust for daily clinical use Maintenance and upgrade of the software may be a problem May not be good for a full large-scale PACS

enterprises, typically at the province or state level; many PACS implementation models have been installed or are in the implementation stage.

1.5.3 Asia

Driving PACS development in Asia are Japan, South Korea, and Taiwan as well as China including Hong Kong. Japan entered PACS research, development, and

TABLE 1.3   Nine positive factors (for the United States) and hindering factors (for Europe) related to PACS implementation

Favorable Factors in USA	Hindering Factors in Europe
Flexible investment culture	Preservation of workplace culture
Business infrastructure of health care	Social service oriented healthcare
Calculated risk mindedness	Security mindedness
Competitive environment control	Government and/or professional associates
Technological leadership drive	No change "if it works manually"
Speed of service oriented	Quality of service oriented
Include PACS experts consultants	"Do it yourself" mentality
"Trial-and-error" approach	"Wait and see" approach
Personal gain driven	If it fails "Find someone to blame"

implementation in 1982. According to a survey by Inamura (2003), as of 2002 there are a total of 1468 PACS in Japan:

- Small: 1174 (fewer than 4 display workstations)
- Medium: 203 (5–14 display workstations)
- Large: 91 (15–1300 display workstations)

Some of the large PACS systems are the result of legacy PAC systems being interconnected with newer PAC systems. Earlier Japan PAC systems were not necessarily DICOM compliant, nor connected to HIS. Recently, however, more PAC systems are adhering to the DICOM standard and coupling HIS, RIS, and PACS.

South Korea's large-scale countrywise PACS development was almost a miracle. Its fast growth path of PACS development over the past seven years occurred despite no domestic X-ray film industry, an economic crisis in 1997, and the National Health Insurance PACS Reimbursement Act. We will return to study this case in more depth in later chapters (Huang, 2003b).

The third major development of PACS in Asia over the past five years involves China, Hong Kong, and Taiwan. China mainland has installed many small- and medium-size PAC systems even though their HIS and RIS are still lacking maturity. A major contribution to PACS in Asia is the ePR (electronic patient record) with image distribution technology developed by the Hong Kong Hospital Authority (HKHA). This system has been gradually implemented hospital-by-hospital in 44 hospitals since the early 2000s (Cheung, 2005). A case study will be described in Chapter 22. Taiwan has had many large- and medium-scale PACSs and ePRs designed and implemented by local PACS manufacturers throughout the island since the late 1990s.

1.6   ORGANIZATION OF THE BOOK

This book consists of an introductory chapter and four parts. Figure 1.3, shows the organization of this book. In Part I are covered the principles of medical imaging

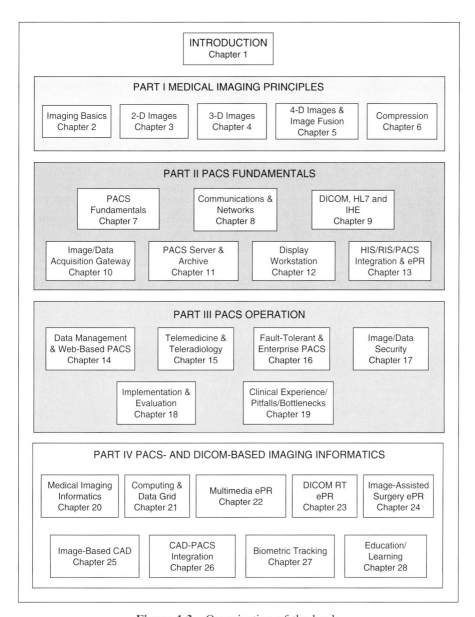

Figure 1.3   Organization of the book.

technology. Chapter 2 describes the fundamentals of digital radiological imaging. It is assumed that the reader already has some basic background in conventional radiographic physics. This chapter introduces the terminology used in digital radiological imaging with examples. Familiarizing oneself with this terminology will facilitate the reading of later chapters.

Chapters 3, 4, and 5 discuss commonly used radiological and medical light imaging acquisition systems. The concepts of patient workflow and data workflow are also introduced. Chapter 3 presents two-dimensional (2-D) projection images. Since radiography still accounts for over 60% of current examinations in a typical radiology department, methods of obtaining digital output from radiographs are crucial for the success of implementing a PACS. For this reason laser film scanner, digital fluorography, laser-stimulated luminescence phosphor imaging plate (computed radiography), and digital radiography (DR) technologies, including full-field direct digital mammography are discussed. In addition 2-D nuclear medicine and ultrasound imaging are presented, followed by 2-D microscopic and endoscopic light imaging; all these are today used extensively in medical diagnosis and image-assisted therapy and treatment.

Chapter 4 presents three-dimensional (3-D) imaging. The third dimension in 3-D imaging can be space (x, y, z) or time (x, y, t). The concept of image reconstruction from projections is first introduced, followed by the basic physics involved in transmission and emission computed tomography (CT), ultrasound (US) imaging, magnetic resonance imaging (MRI), and light imaging.

Chapter 5 discusses four-dimensional (4-D) imaging. If 3-D imaging represents a 3-D space volume of the anatomical structure, the fourth dimension then is the time component (x, y, z, t), and it accounts for the fusion of images from different modalities. Developing effective methods of displaying a 4-D volume set with many images on a 2-D display device is challenging, as is discussed in Chapter 12.

Chapters 3, 4, and 5 nevertheless do not provide comprehensive treatment of 2-D, 3-D, and 4-D imaging. The purpose of these chapters is to review the basic imaging and informatics terminologies commonly encountered in medical imaging; these chapters emphasize the digital and communication aspects, and not of the physics and formation of the images. Understanding the basics of the digital procedure of these imaging modalities facilitates PACS design and implementation, as well as imaging informatics applications. A thorough understanding of digital imaging is essential for interfacing these imaging modalities to a PACS and for utilizing image databases for clinical applications.

Chapter 6 covers image compression. After an image or an image set has been captured in digital form from an acquisition device, it is transmitted to a storage device for long-term archiving. A digital image file requires a large storage capacity for archiving. For example, a two-view computed radiography (CR) or an average computed tomography (CT) study comprises over 20 to 40 Mbytes. Therefore it is necessary to consider how to compress an image file into a compact form before storage or transmission. The concept of reversible (lossless) and irreversible (lossy) compression are discussed in detail followed by the description of cosine and wavelet transformation compression methods. Techniques are also discussed on how to handle 3-D and 4-D data sets that often occur in dynamic imaging.

In Part II PACS fundamentals are introduced. Chapter 7 covers PACS components, architecture, workflow, operation models, and the concept of image-based electronic patient records (ePR). These PACS fundamentals are discussed further in next chapters. Chapter 8 is on image communications and networking. The latest technology in digital communications using asynchronous transfer mode (ATM), gigabit Ethernet, and Internet 2 technologies is described. In Chapter 9 industrial standards and protocols are introduced. For medical data, HL7 (Health Level), is reviewed. For image format and communication protocols ACR-NEMA (American College of Radiology–National Electrical Manufacturers Association) standard is briefly mentioned followed by a detailed discussion of the DICOM

(Digital Imaging and Communication in Medicine) standard that has been adopted by the PACS community. IHE (Integrating of Healthcare Enterprise) workflow protocols, which allow smooth workflow execution between PACS, DICOM components, are described with examples. HL7, DICOM, and IHE have been well documented, the purpose of Chapter 9 is to explain the concepts and guide the reader on how to use the documents and search for details.

Chapter 10 presents the image acquisition gateway. It covers the systematic method of interfacing imaging acquisition devices using the HL 7 and DICOM standards, and discusses automatic error recovery schemes. The concept of the DICOM Broker is introduced, which allows the direct transfer of patient information from the hospital information system (HIS) to the imaging device, eliminating potential typographical errors by the radiographer/technologist at the imaging device console.

Chapter 11 presents the DICOM PACS server and image archive. The PACS image management design concept and software are first discussed, followed by the presentation of storage technologies essential for PACS operation. Four archive concepts: off-site backup, ASP (application service provider) backup, data migration, and disaster recovery are presented.

Chapter 12 is on image display. A historical review of the development of image display is introduced, followed a discussion on types of workstations. The DICOM PC-based display workstation is presented. LCD (liquid crystal display) is gradually replacing the CRT (cathode ray tube) for display of medical images, so a review of this technology is given. The challenges and methods of displaying 3-D and 4-D image set with many images per set, as well as data flow in real-time image-assisted therapy and treatment are discussed.

Chapter 13 describes the integration of PACS with the hospital information system (HIS), the radiology information system (RIS), and other medical databases, including voice recognition. This chapter forms the cornerstones for the extension of PACS modules to hospital-integrated PACS, and to the enterprise-level PACS.

In Part III the chapters focus on PACS operation. Chapter 14 presents PACS data management, distribution, and retrieval. The concept of Web-based PACS and its dataflow are introduced. Web-based PACS can be used to cost-effectively populate the number of image workstations throughout the whole hospital and the enterprise, and be integrated with the ePR system with image distribution.

Chapter 15 describes Telemedicine and teleradiology. State-of-the-art technologies are given, including the Internet 2 and teleradiology service models. Some important issues in teleradiology regarding cost, quality, and medical-legal issues are discussed, as well as current concepts in telemammography and telemicroscopy.

Chapter 16 explains the concept of fault-tolerance and enterprise PACS. Causes of PACS failure are first listed, followed by explanations of no loss of image data and no interruption of the PACS dataflow. Current PACS technology in addressing fault-tolerance is presented. The full discussion of continuous available (CA) PACS design is given along with an example of a CA PACS archive server. The basic infrastructures of enterprise-level PACS and business models are also covered.

Chapter 17 considers the concept of image data security. Data security has become an important issue in tele-health and teleradiology, which use public high-speed wide area networks connecting examination sites with expert centers. This chapter reviews current available data security technology and discusses the concept of image digital signature.

Chapter 18 describes PACS implementation and system evaluation. Both the institutional and manufacturer's point of view in PACS implementation are discussed. Some standard methodologies in the PACS system implementation, acceptance, and evaluation are given.

Chapter 19 describes some PACS clinical experience, pitfalls, and bottlenecks. For clinical experience, special interest is shown for hospital-wise performance. For pitfalls and bottlenecks, some commonly encountered situations are illustrated and remedies recommended.

In Part IV the book ends with much up-dated discussion of PACS- and DICOM-based imaging informatics. This part has been greatly expanded from four chapters in the original book to the current nine chapters. The imaging informatics topics discussed include computing and data grid, ePR, image-assisted therapy and treatment, CADe/CADx (computer-aided detection/diagnosis), biometric tracking, and education. Chapter 20 describes the PACS- and DICOM-based imaging informatics concept and infrastructure. Several examples are used to illustrate components and their connectivity in the infrastructure. Chapter 21 presents Data Grid and its utilization in PACS and imaging informatics.

Chapter 22 presents ePR with image distribution. Two examples are used to illustrate its connectivity to PACS, and methods of image distribution. The discussion picks up the example given in Chapter 16 and follows its PACS workflow to image distribution using the Web-based ePR system.

Chapters 23 and 24 discuss two treatment-based ePR systems, one for radiation therapy (RT) applications and the second for image-assisted surgery. In RT ePR, the DICOM-RT is introduced to form the foundation of a DICOM-based RT ePR. In image-assisted surgery, minimally invasive spinal surgery is used to introduce the concept of digital pre-surgical consultation authoring, real-time intra-operative image/data collection and post-surgical patient outcome analysis. Chapters 25 and 26 are on PACS-based computer-aided detection/diagnosis (CADe/CADx), and CAD-PACS integration, respectively. Chapter 25 focuses on case studies, to demonstrate how a CAD is developed for daily clinical use, starting from problem definition, CAD algorithms, data collection for CAD validation, validation methodology, and ending with clinical evaluation. Chapter 26 presents methods of connecting CAD results to the PACS seamlessly for daily clinical use without interrupting its normal workflow.

Chapter 27 presents the concept of patient and staff member tracking in clinical environment, using the biometric parameters of the subject. In Chapters 22 through 27, the emphasis is on the connectivity of the informatics components with PACS, as shown in Figure 1.3. In these chapters the theory, concept, and goals are first defined, followed by methodology used for solving the problems, and concluded with actual examples.

Chapter 28 first discusses PACS training, and then expands the training methodology to include medical imaging informatics. Five topics are presented: new directions in PACS and imaging informatics education and training; examples of PACS and Imaging Informatics Training Program; concept of the PACS Simulator; teaching Medical Imaging Informatics for interdisciplinary candidates; and changing PACS learning with new interactive and media-rich learning environments.

References

Bauman RA, Gell G, Dwyer SJ III. Large picture arching and communication systems of the world—Parts 1 and 2. *J Digital Imag* 9(3,4): 99–103, 172–7; 1996.

Brody WR., ed. Conference on Digital Radiography. *Proc SPIE* 314: 14–16; 1981.

Capp MP, Nudelman S, et al. Photoelectronic radiology department. *Proc SPIE* 314: 2–8, 1981.

Cheung NT, Lam A, et al., Integrating Images into the electronic patient record of the Hospital Authority of Hong Kong. *Comp Med Imag Graph* 29(2–3): 137–42; 2005.

Digital Imaging and Communications in Medicine (DICOM). National Electrical Manufacturers' Association. Rosslyn, VA: NEMA, 1996; PS 3.1.

Duerinckx A, ed. Picture archiving and communication systems (PACS) for medical applications. *First Int Conf Workshop. Proc SPIE* 318(1–2); 1982.

Dwyer SJ III, et al. Cost of managing digital diagnostic images. *Radiology* 144: 313; 1982.

Hruby W, Maltsidis A. A view to the past of the future—a decade of digital revolution at the Danube hospital. In: Hruby W, ed. *Digital Revolution in Radiology*. Vienna: Springer; 2000.

Huang HK. *Elements of Digital Radiology: A Professional Handbook and Guide*. Englewood Cliffs, NJ: Prentice-Hall; 1987.

Huang HK. 1991a. Editorial: Picture and communication systems. *Comp Med Imag Graph* 15(3): 133; 1991a.

Huang HK, Ratib O, et al. *Picture Archiving and Communication System (PACS)*. Berlin: Springer 1991b.

Huang HK. *Picture Archiving and Communication Systems: Principles and Applications*. New York: Wiley; 1999, p. 521.

Huang HK. 2003a. Editorial: Some historical remarks on picture and communication systems. *Comp Med Imag Graph* 27(2–3): 93–9; 2003a.

Huang HK. Enterprise PACS and image distribution. *Comp Med Imag Graph* 27(2–3): 241–53; 2003b.

Huang HK. *PACS and Imaging Informatics: Principles and Applications*. Hoboken, NJ: Wiley; 2004.

Inamura K. PACS development in Asia. *Comp Med Imag Graph* 27(2–3): 121–8; 2003.

JAMIT. First International Symposium on PACS and PHD. *Proc. Med Imag Tech* 1; 1983.

Law M, Huang HK. Concept of a PACS and imaging informatics-based server for radiation therapy. *Comp Med Imag Graph* 27: 1–9; 2003.

Lemke HU, A network of medical work stations for integrated word and picture communication in clinical medicine. Technical report. Technical University Berlin; 1979.

Lemke HU, Vannier MW, et al. Computer assisted radiology and surgery (CARS). *Proc 16th Int Congr Exhibit* Paris. CARS 2002.

Lemke HU. PACS development in Europe. *Comp Med Imag Graph* 27(2–3): 111–20; 2003.

MITRE/ARMY. RFP B52-15645 for University Medical Center Installation Sites for Digtial Imaging Network and Picture Archiving and Communication System (DIN/PACS), October 18, 1986.

Mogel GT. The role of the Department of Defense in PACS and telemedicine research and development. *Comp Med Imag Graph* 27(2–3): 129–35; 2003.

Mun SK, ed. Image management and communication. *The First International Conference* Washington, DC: 1989. IEEE Computer Society Press; 1989.

Niinimaki J, Ilkko E, Reponen J. *Proc 20th EuroPACS* Oulu, Finland, EuroPACS; 2002

Steckel RJ. Daily X-ray rounds in a large teaching hospital using high-resolution closed-circuit television. *Radiology* 105: 319–21; 1972.

PART I

MEDICAL IMAGING PRINCIPLES

CHAPTER 2

Digital Medical Image Fundamentals

2.1 TERMINOLOGY

Medical imaging involves radiological, nuclear, photon and positron emission, nuclear magnetic resonance, ultrasound and light photon images. However, concepts and image quality measurement techniques of these various types of image are derived from conventional radiographic imaging and fundamental digital image processing principles. For an extensive review of the these concepts and quality measuring techniques, see: Bankman (2008), Barrett and Swindell (1981), Benedetto, Huang, and Ragan (1990), Bertram (1970), Beutel et al. (2000), Bracewell (1965), Brigham (1979), Cochran et al. (1967), Curry, Dowdey, and Murry (1987), Dainty and Shaw (1984), Dhawan (2003, 2008), Gonzalez and Cointz (1982), Hendee and Wells (1997), Huang (1987, 1996, 1999, 2004), Leondes (1997), Prince and Links (2006), Robb (1995), Rosenfeld and Kak (1976), and Rossman (1969).

2.1.1 Digital Image

A digital image is a two-dimensional array of nonnegative integer function, $f(x, y)$, where $1 \leq x \leq M$ and $1 \leq y \leq N$, and M and N are positive integers representing the number of columns and rows, respectively. For any given x and y, the small square in the image represented by the coordinates (x, y) is called a picture element, or a pixel, and $f(x, y)$ is its corresponding pixel value. If $M = N$, then f becomes a square image; most sectional images in a three-dimensional (3-D) image volume used in medicine are square images. If the digital image $f(x, y, z)$ is 3-D, then the picture element is called a voxel. As $f(x, y, z)$ is collected through time t, the collection becomes a four-dimensional image set where the fourth dimension is t. Throughout this book, we use the symbols f and p interchangeably, f is used when mathematics is presented, and p when picture or image is being emphasized.

2.1.2 Digitization and Digital Capture

Digitization is a process that quantizes or samples analog signals into a range of digital values. Digitizing a picture means converting the continuous gray tones in the picture into a digital image. About 60% to 70% of radiological examinations, including skull, chest, breast, abdomen, bone, and mammogram are captured on X-ray films or radiographs, computed radiography (CR), and digital radiography (DR) techniques. The process of projecting a three-dimensional body into a two-dimensional image is called projection radiography. An X-ray film can be converted to digital numbers with a film digitizer. The laser scanning digitizer is the gold standard among digitizers because it can best preserve the resolutions of the original analog image. A laser film scanner can digitize a standard X-ray film (14 × 17 in.) to 2000 × 2500 pixels with 12 bits per pixel. A CR or DR image is already in digital form when it is formed. The CR uses a laser-stimulated luminescence phosphor imaging plate as an X-ray detector. The imaging plate is exposed and a latent image is formed in it. A laser beam is used to scan the exposed imaging plate. The latent image is excited and emits light photons that are detected and converted to electronic signals. The electronic signals are converted to digital signals to form a digital X-ray image. Recently developed direct X-ray detectors can capture the X-ray image without going through an additional medium like the imaging plate. This method of image capture is sometimes called direct digital radiography (DR). Chapter 3 will discuss projection radiography in more detail.

Images obtained from the other 30% to 40% of medical imaging examinations—including computed tomography (CT), nuclear medicine (NM), positron emission tomography (PET), single photon emission computed tomography (SPECT), ultra-sonography (US), magnetic resonance imaging (MRI), digital fluorography (DF), and digital subtraction angiography (DSA)—are already in digital format when they are generated. Digital color microscopy and color endoscopy use a CCD camera and an A/D (analog-to-digital) converter to convert the light signals to digital electronic signals. The characteristics of these images will be explored in Chapters 3, 4, and 5.

2.1.3 Digital Medical Image

The aforementioned images are collectively called digitized or digital medical images: digitized if the image is obtained through a digitizer, or digital if it is generated digitally. The pixel (voxel) value (or gray level value, or gray level) can range from 0 to 255 (8-bit), 0 to 511 (9-bit), 0 to 1023 (10-bit), 0 to 2045 (11-bit), and 0 to 4095 (12-bit), depending on the digitization procedure or the medical image generation procedure used. These gray levels represent physical or chemical properties of the state of anatomical structures or physiological processes when the image was captured. For example, in an image obtained by digitizing an X-ray film, the gray level value of a pixel represents the optical density of the small square area of the film. In the case of X-ray computed tomography (XCT), the pixel value represents the relative linear attenuation coefficient of the tissue; in magnetic resonance imaging (MRI), it corresponds to the magnetic resonance signal response of the tissue; and in ultrasound imaging, it is the echo signal of the ultrasound beam when it penetrates the tissues.

2.1.4 Image Size

The dimensions of a two-dimensional (2-D) projection image are the ordered pair (M, N), and the size of the image is the product $M \times N \times k$ bits where 2^k equals the gray level range. In sectional images of a 3-D volume, most of the time $M = N$. The exact dimensions of a digital image sometimes are difficult to specify because of the design constraints imposed on the detector system for various examination procedures. Therefore, for convenience, we call a 512×512 image a 512 image, a 1024×1024 image a 1 K image, a 2048×2048 image a 2K image, even though the image itself may not be exactly 512, 1024, or 2048 square. Also, in computers, 12 bits is an odd number for the computer memory and storage device to handle. For this reason 16 bits or 2 bytes are normally allocated to store a 12 bit data of the pixel. Table 2.1 lists the sizes of some conventional 2-D, 3-D, and 4-D medical images.

2.1.5 Histogram

The histogram of an image is a plot of the pixel value (abscissa) against the frequency of occurrence of the pixel value in the entire image (ordinate). For an image with 256 possible gray levels, the abscissa of the histogram ranges from 0 to 255 levels. The total pixel count under the histogram is equal to $M \times N$ (see Section 2.1.1). The histogram represents the frequency of pixel value distribution in the image, an important characteristic of the image (see Fig. 6.4B, D, E, for examples).

2.1.6 Image Display

A digital image can be printed on film or paper as a hard copy, or it can be displayed on a cathode ray tube (CRT) video monitor or a liquid crystal display(LCD) as a soft copy. The soft-copy display is volatile, since the image disappears once the display device is turn off. To display a soft-copy digital medical image, the pixel values are first converted to analog signals, called digital-to-analog (D/A) conversion, similar to conventional video signals used in the television industry. Current software display device can display up to a 2K image on one screen. No commercially available display system can handle a 4K image as of now. In order to display a 4K image, such as a 4K digital mammogram, subsample or split-screen methods are used. Figure 2.1 shows a perspective of image size compared with number of pixels in a 128, 256, 512, 1024, 2048, and 4096 image. It also depicts the concept of 3-D and 4-D images, and image fusion.

2.2 DENSITY RESOLUTION, SPATIAL RESOLUTION, AND SIGNAL-TO-NOISE RATIO

The quality of a digital image is measured by three parameters: spatial resolution, density resolution, and signal-to-noise ratio. The spatial and density resolutions are related to the number of pixels and the range of pixel values used to represent the object of interest in the image. In a square image $N \times N \times k$, N is related to the spatial resolution, and k to the density resolution. A high signal-to-noise ratio means that the image has a strong signal and little noise and is very pleasing to the eye, hence a better quality image.

Figure 2.2 demonstrates the concept of spatial and density resolutions of a digital image using a CT body image ($512 \times 512 \times 12$ bits) as an example. Figure 2.2A shows the original and three images with a fixed spatial resolution (512×512) but

TABLE 2.1   Sizes of some common 2-D, 3-D, 4-D and fusion medical images

2-D Modality	One Image (bits)	No. Images/ Examination	One Examination (MB)
Nuclear Medicine (NM)	$128 \times 128 \times 12$	30–60	1–2
Digital Subtraction Angiography (DSA)	$512 \times 512 \times 8$	30–40	8–10
Digitized Film	$2048 \times 2048 \times 12$– $1780 \times 2160 \times 12$	1	8
Computed/Digital Radiography	$2048 \times 2048 \times 12$– $3520 \times 4280 \times 10$	1	8–28
Digital Mammography	$2560 \times 3328 \times 12$– $4000 \times 5000 \times 12$	4	68–160
Digital Color Microscopy	$512 \times 512 \times 24$	1 up	0.8 up
Digital Color Endoscopy	$512 \times 512 \times 24$	1 up & movie loop	0.8 up & movie loop
3-D Modality			
Positron Emission CT (PET)—Whole body	$168 \times 168 \times 16$–	500	28
Body Regions	$256 \times 256 \times 16$	20 up	2.5 up
Magnetic Resonance Imaging (MRI) Head: 3 Sequences—Proton, T1 and T2	$256 \times 256 \times 12$– $320 \times 320 \times 12$	Multiple sequences 100–1000	60 up
Single Photon Computed Tomography (SPECT)	$512 \times 512 \times 12$	Head: 10 up	5 up
Computed Tomography (CT) Multislide CT (256 Slides)/Rotation	$512 \times 512 \times 12$	Head: 10 up Body: 40 – 1000 256/rotation	5 up 20 up 134
Ultrasound (US)	$512 \times 512 \times 8$	30 f/s video	8
Ultrasound True Color	$480 \times 640 \times 24$	30 f/s video	28
Ultrasound Pseudo-Color	$716 \times 537 \times 8$	30 f/s video	12
4-D Modality			3-D × time
Fusion			2 × images/ modality

Black: Standard
Blue: Examples of the size of an image or examination performed at USC.

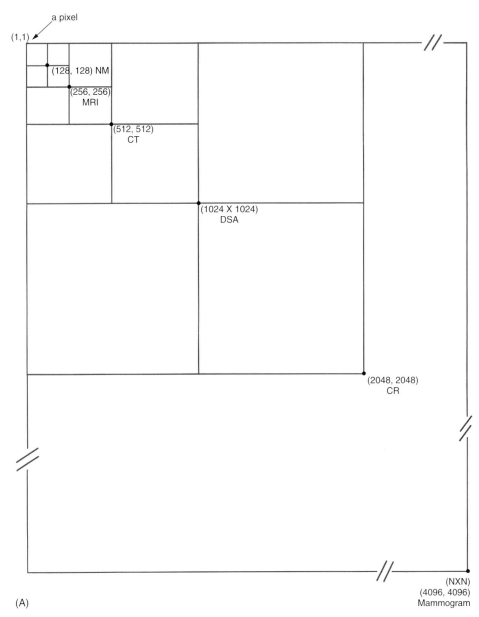

(A)

Figure 2.1 (*A*) Terminology used in medical images: image types, sizes, and number of pixels/image. ($N \times N$): total number of pixels of a 2-D image; (x, y): coordinates of the pixel in the 2-D image; $f(x, y)$: gray level value in (x, y), which can be from 8 to 12 bits in gray level or 24 bits in color image. The total number of bits per image is commonly denoted by ($N \times N \times 12$) or ($N \times N \times 24$). For 12 bits/pixel, the pixel value is stored in 2 bytes. (*B*) 3-D image set. (*i*) a 3-D spatial image set with z as the third dimension; (*ii*) a 3-D temporal image set with t (time) as the third dimension. (*C*) 4-D image set. A 4-D image set consisting of a sequential 3-D spatial sets with t as the fourth dimension. (*D*) Fusion images. (*i*) PET fuses with CT: physiology (color) on anatomy (grey level); (*ii*) MR (color) fuses with CT (grey level): enhancement of soft tissue definition on anatomy.

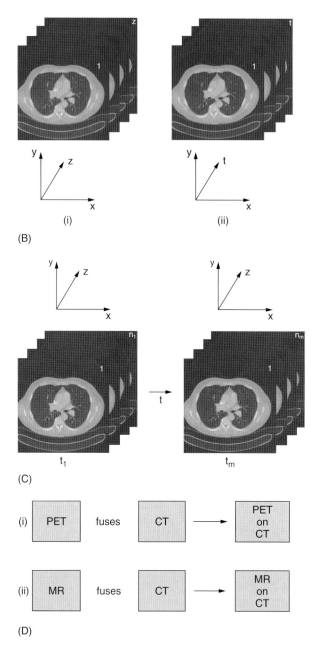

(B)

(C)

(D)

Figure 2.1 *(Continued)*

three variable density resolutions (8, 6, and 4 bits/pixel, respectively). Figure 2.2*B* shows the original and three images with a fixed density resolution (12 bits/pixel) but three variable spatial resolutions (256×256, 128×128, and 32×32 pixels, respectively). Figure 2.2*C* illustrates the deteriorating quality of the CT body image after noise was introduced. Clearly, in all three cases the quality of the CT image is decreasing starting from the original. Spatial resolution, density resolution, and signal-to-noise ratio of the image should be adjusted properly when the image is acquired. A higher resolution image normally requires more storage space to archive and longer time for image processing and transmission. A more detailed discussion of these topics is given in the following sections.

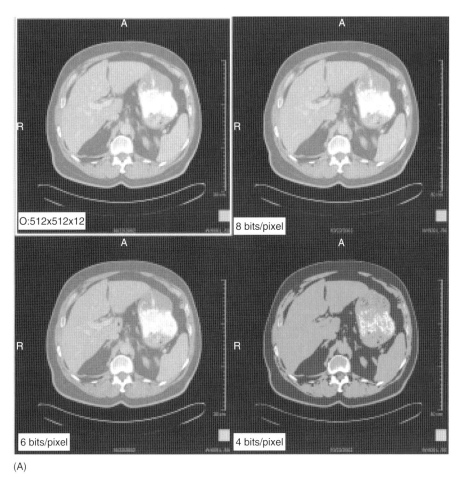

(A)

Figure 2.2   Illustration of spatial and density resolutions, and signal-to-noise ratio using an abdominal CT image ($512 \times 512 \times 12$ bits) as an example. (*A*) Four images with a fixed spatial resolution (512×512) but variable density resolutions: 12, 8, 6, and 4 bits/pixel, respectively). (*B*) The original and three images with a fixed density resolution (12 bits/pixel) but variable spatial resolutions: 512×512, 256×256, 128×128, and 32×32 pixels, respectively. (*C*) The abdominal CT image ($512 \times 512 \times 12$) shown in (*A*). Random noises were inserted in 1,000 pixels, 10,000 pixels, and 100,000 pixels, respectively. The coordinates of each randomly selected noise pixel within the body region were obtained from a random generator. The new pixel value, selected from a range between 0.7 to 1.3 that of the original value is determined by a second random generator. Clearly, the quality of the CT image is decreasing progressively starting from the original.

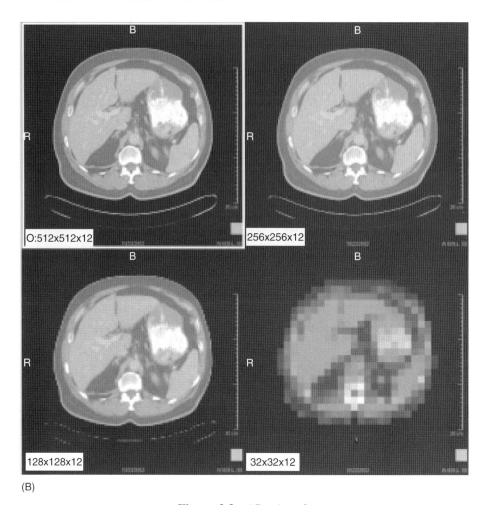

(B)

Figure 2.2   *(Continued)*

2.3   TEST OBJECTS AND PATTERNS FOR MEASUREMENT OF IMAGE QUALITY

Test objects or patterns (sometimes called phantoms) used to measure the density and spatial resolutions of radiological imaging equipment can be either physical phantoms or digitally generated patterns.

A physical phantom is used to measure the performance of a digital radiological device. It is usually constructed with different materials shaped in various geometrical configurations embedded in a uniform background material (e.g., water or plastic). The commonly used geometrical configurations are circular cylinder, sphere, line pairs (alternating pattern of narrow rectangular bars with background of the same width), step wedge, and star shape. The materials used to construct these configurations are lead, various plastics, water, air, and iodine solutions of various

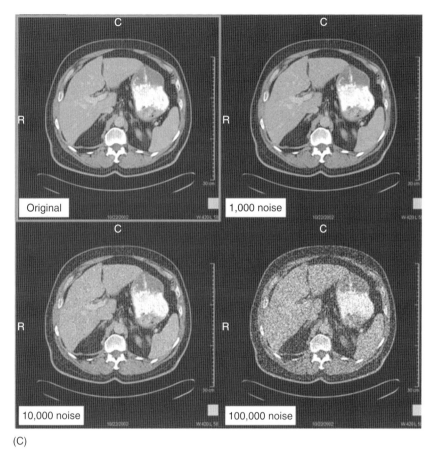

(C)

Figure 2.2   *(Continued)*

concentrations. If the radiodensity of the background material differs greatly from the test object, it is called a high- contrast phantom; otherwise, it is a low-contrast. The circular cylinder, sphere, and step-wedge configurations are commonly used to measure spatial and density resolutions. Thus the statement that the X-ray device can detect a 1-mm cylindrical object with 0.5% density difference from the background means that this particular radiological imaging device can produce an image of the cylindrical object made from material that has an X-ray attenuation difference from the background of 0.5%; thus the difference between the average pixel value of the object and that of the background is measurable or detectable.

A digitally generated pattern, on the other hand, is used to measure the performance of the display component of a light photon or radiological device. In this case the various geometrical configurations are generated digitally. The gray level values of these configurations are inputted to the display component according to certain specifications. A digital phantom is an ideal digital image. Any distortion of these images observed from the display is a measure of the imperfections of the display component. The most commonly used digital phantom is the SMPTE (Society of Motion Picture and Television Engineers) phantom/pattern. Figure 2.3 shows some commonly used physical phantoms, their corresponding X-ray images, and the SMPTE digitally patterns.

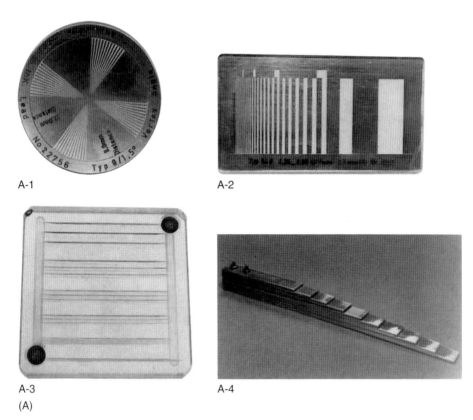

A-1   A-2

A-3   A-4

(A)

Figure 2.3 Some commonly used physical test objects and digitally generated test patterns. (*A*) Physical: *A*-1, star-shaped line pair pattern embedded in water contained in a circular cylinder; *A*-2, high contrast line pair (aluminum against water); *A*-3, low contrast line pair (contrast media against water); *A*-4, aluminum step wedge. (*B*) Corresponding X-ray images of *A*; morie patterns can be seen in *B*-1. (*C*) Digitally generated 512 images: *C*-1, high-contrast line pair: gray level = 0, 140; width (in pixel) of each line pair = 2, 4, 6, 8, 10, 12, 14, 16, 32, 64, and 128 pixels; *C*-2, low contrast line pair: gray level = 0, 40; width in pixel of each line pair = 2, 4, 8, 16, 20 and 28 pixels. The line pair (LP) indicated in the figure shows the width of 16 pixels. (*D*) Softcopy display of the 1024 × 1024 SMPTE phantom (Society of Motion Picture and Television Engineers) using the JPEG format (see Chapter 6) depicts both contrast blocks [0 (black)–100 (white)%], and high-contrast and low-contrast line pairs (four corners, and middle). *D*-1, display adjusted to show as many contrast blocks as possible resulted in the low-contrast line pairs barely discerned; *D*-2, adjusted to show the low-contrast line pairs resulted in indistinguishable contrast blocks (0–40%, and 60–100%). The manipulation of softcopy display is discussed in Chapter 12.

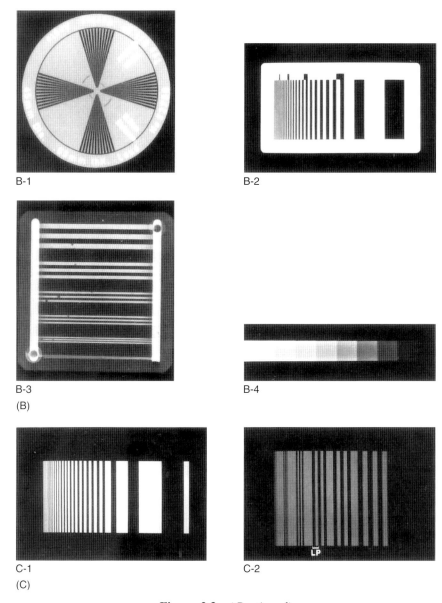

Figure 2.3 *(Continued)*

2.4   IMAGE IN THE SPATIAL DOMAIN AND THE FREQUENCY DOMAIN

2.4.1   Frequency Components of an Image

If pixel values $f(x, y)$ of a digital medical image represent anatomical structures or physiological functions in space, one can say that the image is defined in the spatial domain. The image, $f(x, y)$, can also be represented as its spatial frequency components (u, v) through a mathematical transform (see Section 2.4.2). In this

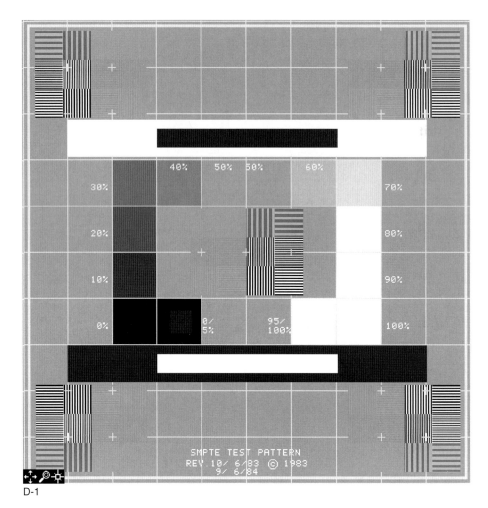

D-1

Figure 2.3   *(Continued)*

case we use the symbol $F(u, v)$ to represent the transform of $f(x, y)$ and say that $F(u, v)$ is the frequency representation of $f(x, y)$ and that it is defined in the frequency domain. $F(u, v)$ is again a digital image, but it bears no visual resemblance to $f(x, y)$ (see Fig. 2.4). With proper training, however, one can use information shown in the frequency domain, and not easily that in the spatial domain, to detect some inherent characteristics of each type of medical, image. For examples, if the image has many edges, then there would be many high-frequency components. On the other hand, if the image has only uniform materials, like water or plastic, then it has low-frequency components.

The concept of using frequency components to represent anatomical structures might seem strange at first, and one might wonder why we even have to bother with this representation. To understand this better, consider that a medical image is composed of many two-dimensional sinusoidal waves, each with individual amplitude and frequency. For example, a digitally generated "uniform image" has no

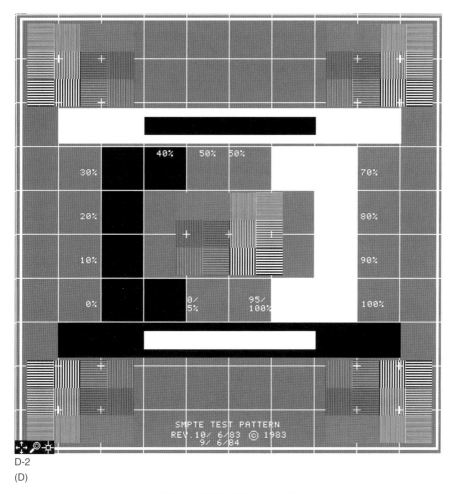

D-2
(D)

Figure 2.3 *(Continued)*

frequency components, only a constant (DC) term. An X-ray image of the hand is composed of many high-frequency components (edges of bones) and few low-frequency components, while an abdominal X-ray image of the gall bladder filled with contrast material is composed of many low-frequency components (the contrast medium inside the gall bladder) but very few high-frequency components. Therefore the frequency representation of a radiological image gives a different perspective on the characteristics of the image under consideration.

Based on this frequency information in the image, we can selectively change the frequency components to enhance the image. To obtain a smoother appearing image, we can increase the amplitude of low-frequency components, whereas to enhance the edges of bones in the hand X-ray image, we can magnify the amplitude of the high-frequency components.

Manipulating an image in the frequency domain also yields many other advantages. For example, we can use the frequency representation of an image to measure its quality. This requires the concepts of point spread function (PSF), line spread

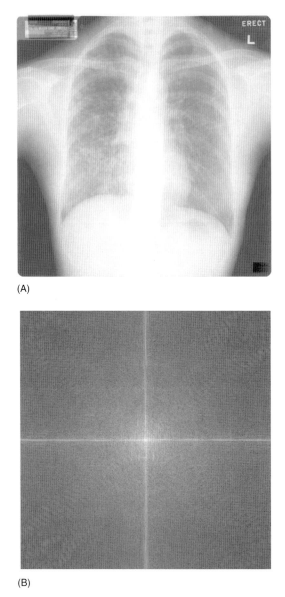

(A)

(B)

Figure 2.4 (*A*) Computed radiography (CR; see Chapter 3) chest X-ray image represented in spatial domain (x, y). (*B*). Same CR chest X-ray image represented in the
Fourier frequency domain (u, v). The low-frequency components are in the center and
the high-frequency components are on the periphery.

function (LSF), and modulation transfer function (MTF), discussed in Section 2.5.
In addition medical images obtained from image reconstruction from projections are
based on the frequency component representation. Utilization of frequency representation gives an easier explanation of how an MRI image is reconstructed from

magnetic signals, and how an image can be compressed. (This is discussed in Chapters 4, 5, and 6.)

2.4.2   The Fourier Transform Pair

As discussed above, a medical image defined in the spatial domain (x, y) can be transformed to the frequency domain (u, v). The Fourier transform is one method for doing this. The Fourier transform of a two-dimensional image $f(x, y)$, denoted by $F\{f(x, y)\}$, is given by

$$\Im\{f(x, y)\} = F(u, v) = \int\limits_{-\infty}^{\infty} \int f(x, y) \exp[-\mathbf{i}2\pi(ux + vy)]\,dxdy$$

$$= Re(u, v) + \mathbf{i}\,Im(u, v)$$

(2.1)

where $\mathbf{i} = \sqrt{-1}$, and $Re(u, v)$ and $Im(u, v)$ are the real and imaginary components of $F(u, v)$, respectively.

The magnitude function

$$|F(u, v)| = [Re^2(u, v) + Im^2(u, v)]^{1/2}$$

(2.2)

is called the Fourier spectrum, and $|F(u, v)|^2$ the energy spectrum of $f(x, y)$, respectively. The function

$$\Phi(u, v) = \tan^{-1}\frac{Im(u, v)}{Re(u, v)}$$

(2.3)

is called the phase angle. The Fourier spectrum, the energy spectrum, and the phase angle are three parameters derived from the Fourier transform that can be used to represent the properties of an image in the frequency domain. Figure 2.4B, with the low-frequency components in the center, shows the Fourier spectrum of the chest image in Figure 2.4A.

Given $F(u, v)$, $f(x, y)$ can be obtained by using the inverse Fourier transform

$$\Im^{-1}[F(u, v)] = f(x, y)$$

$$= \int\limits_{-\infty}^{\infty} \int F(u, v) \exp[\mathbf{i}2\pi(ux + vy)]\,dudv$$

(2.4)

The two functions $f(x, y)$ and $F(u, v)$ are called the Fourier transform pair. The Fourier and the inverse transform enable the transformation of a two-dimensional image from the spatial domain to the frequency domain, and vice versa. In digital imaging, since the image function is represented by a discrete integer function, we use the discrete Fourier Transform for computation instead of using Eq. (2.1), which is continuous. Fourier transform can also be used in three-dimensions by adding the

z-component in the equation, it can transform a 3-D image from spatial to frequency domain, and vice versa.

2.4.3 The Discrete Fourier Transform

Fourier transform is a mathematical concept. In order to apply it to a digital image, the equations must be converted to a discrete form. The discrete Fourier transform is an approximation of the Fourier transform. For a square digital medical image, the integrals in the Fourier transform pair can be approximated by summations as follows:

$$F(u, v) = \frac{1}{N} \sum_{x=0}^{N-1} \sum_{y=0}^{N-1} f(x, y) \exp\left[\frac{-\mathbf{i}2\pi(ux + vy)}{N}\right] \tag{2.5}$$

for $u, v = 0, 1, 2, \ldots, N - 1$, and

$$f(x, y) = \frac{1}{N} \sum_{u=0}^{N-1} \sum_{v=0}^{N-1} F(u, v) \exp\left[\frac{\mathbf{i}2\pi(ux + vy)}{N}\right] \tag{2.6}$$

for $x, y = 0, 1, 2, \ldots, N - 1$.

The $f(x, y)$ and $F(u, v)$ shown in Eqs. (2.5) and (2.6) are called the discrete Fourier transform pair. It is apparent from these two equations that once the digital radiologic image $f(x, y)$ is known, its discrete Fourier transform can be computed with simple multiplication and addition, and vice verse.

2.5 MEASUREMENT OF IMAGE QUALITY

Image quality is a measure of the performance of an imaging system that produces the image for a specific medical examination. Although the process of making a diagnosis from a medical image is often subjective, higher quality image does yield better diagnostic information. We will describe some physical parameters for measuring image quality based on the concepts of density and spatial resolutions and signal-to-noise level introduced above.

In general, the quality of an image can be measured from its sharpness, resolving power, and noise level. Image sharpness and resolving power are related and inherited from the design of the instrumentation, whereas image noise arises from photon fluctuations from the energy source and detector system used, and electronic noise accumulated through the imaging chain. Even if there were no noise in the imaging system (a hypothetical case), the inherent optical properties of the imaging system might well prevent the image of a high-contrast line pair phantom from giving sharp edges between black and white areas. By the same token, even if a perfect imaging system could be designed, the nature of random photon fluctuation in the energy source and detector would introduce noise into the image.

Sections 2.5.1 and 2.5.2 discuss the measurement of sharpness and noise based on the established theory of measuring image quality in diagnostic radiological devices. Certain modifications are included to permit adjustment for digital imaging terminology.

2.5.1 MEASUREMENT OF SHARPNESS

2.5.1.1 Point Spread Function (PSF) Consider the following experiment: A very small perfect circular hole is drilled in the center of a lead plate (phantom) that is placed between an X-ray tube (energy source) and an image receptor. An image of this phantom is obtained, which can be recorded on a film, or by digital means (CR or DR) be displayed on a video monitor (see Fig. 2.5*A*). The gray level distribution of this image (corresponding to the optical density) is comparatively high in the center of the image where the hole is located, and it decreases radially outward, becoming zero at a certain radial distance away from the center. Ideally, if the circular hole is small enough and the imaging system is perfect, we would expect to see a perfectly circular hole in the center of the image with uniform gray level within the hole and zero elsewhere. The size of the circle in the image would be equal to the size of the circular hole in the plate if no magnification were introduced during the experiment. However, in practice, such an ideal image never exists. Instead, a distribution of the gray level, as described above, will be observed.

This experiment demonstrates that the image of a circular hole in the phantom never has a well-defined sharp edge but has instead a certain *unsharpness*. If the circular hole is small enough, the shape of this gray level distribution is called the

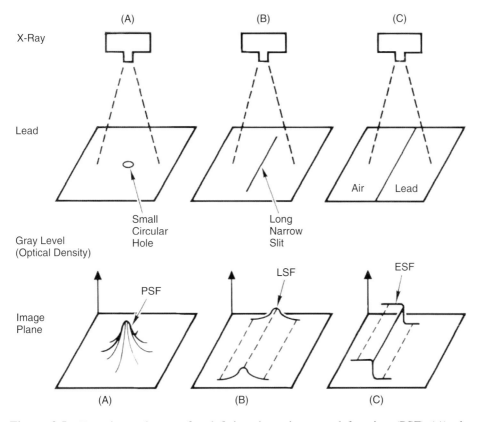

Figure 2.5 Experimental setup for defining the point spread function (PSF) (*A*), the line spread function (LSF) (*B*), and the edge spread function (ESF) (*C*).

point spread function (PSF) of the imaging system (consisting of the X-ray source, the image receptor, and the display). The point spread function of the imaging system can be used as a measure of the *unsharpness* of an image produced by this imaging system. In practice, however, the point spread function of an imaging system is difficult to measure. For the experiment described in Figure 2.5*A*, the size of the circular hole must be chosen very carefully. If the circular hole is too large, the image formed in the detector and seen in the display would be dominated by the circular image, and one would not be able to measure the gray level distribution anymore. On the other hand, if the circular hole is too small, the image formed becomes the image of the X-ray focal spot, which does not represent the complete imaging system. In either case the image cannot be used to measure the PSF of the imaging system.

Theoretically, the point spread function is a useful concept in estimating the sharpness of an image. Experimentally, the point spread function is difficult to measure because of constraints just noted. To circumvent this difficulty in determining the point spread function of an imaging system, the concept of the line spread function is introduced.

2.5.1.2 Line Spread Function (LSF)
Replace the circular hole with a long narrow slit in the lead plate (slit phantom) and repeat the experiment. The image formed on the image receptor and seen on the display becomes a line of certain width with non-uniform gray level distribution. The gray level value is high in the center of the line, decreasing toward the sides of the width until it assumes the gray level of the background. The shape of this gray level distribution is called the line spread function (LSF) of the imaging system. Theoretically, a line spread function can be considered as a line of continuous holes placed very closely together. Experimentally, the line spread function is much easier to measure than the PSF. Figure 2.5*B* illustrates the concept of the line spread function of the system.

2.5.1.3 Edge Spread Function (ESF)
If the slit phantom is replaced by a single step wedge (edge phantom) such that half of the imaging area is lead and the other is air, then the gray level distribution of the image is the edge spread function (ESF) of the system. For an ideal imaging system, any trace perpendicular to the edge of this image would yield a step function

$$
\begin{aligned}
\text{ESF}(x) &= 0 \qquad x_0 > x \geq -B \\
&= A \qquad B \geq x \geq x_0
\end{aligned}
\tag{2.7}
$$

where x is the direction perpendicular to the edge, x_0 is the location of the edge, $-B$, and B are the left and right boundaries of the image, and A is a constant. Mathematically the line spread function is the first derivative of the edge spread function given by the equation

$$
\text{LSF}(x) = \frac{d[\text{ESF}(x)]}{dx}
\tag{2.8}
$$

It should be observed that the edge spread function is easy to obtain experimentally, since only an edge phantom is required to set up the experiment. Once the image has been obtained with the image receptor, a gray level trace perpendicular to the edge yields the edge spread function of the system. To compute the line spread function of the system, it is only necessary to take the first derivative of the edge spread function. Figure 2.5C depicts the experimental setup to obtain the edge spread function.

2.5.1.4 Modulation Transfer Function (MTF)

Now substitute the edge phantom with a high-contrast line pair phantom with different spatial frequencies, and repeat the preceding experiment. In the image receptor, an image of the line pair phantom will form. From this image, the output amplitude (or gray level) of each spatial frequency can be measured. The modulation transfer function (MTF) of the imaging system, along a line perpendicular to the line pairs, is defined as the ratio between the output amplitude and the input amplitude expressed as a function of spatial frequency

$$\text{MTF}(u) = \left(\frac{\text{Output amplitude}}{\text{Input amplitude}} \right)_u \tag{2.9}$$

where u is the spatial frequency measured in the direction perpendicular to the line pairs. Mathematically the MTF is the magnitude (see Eq. 2.2) of the Fourier transform of the line spread function of the system given by the following equation:

$$\text{MTF}(u) = \left| \Im[\text{LSF}(x)] \right| = \left| \int_{-\infty}^{\infty} [\text{LSF}(x) \exp(-\text{i}2\pi xu)] \, dx \right| \tag{2.10}$$

It is seen from Eq. (2.9) that the MTF measures the modulation of the amplitude (gray level) of the line pair pattern in the image. The amount of modulation determines the quality of the imaging system. The MTF of an imaging system, once determined, can be used to predict the quality of the image produced by the imaging system. For a given frequency U, if $\text{MTF}(u) = 0$ for all $u \geq U$, then the imaging system under consideration cannot resolve spatial frequency (cycle/mm) or line pair equal to or higher than U. The MTF so defined is a one-dimensional function; it measures the spatial resolution of the imaging system only in the direction perpendicular to the ESF (x in Eq. 2.8). Extreme care must be exercised to specify the direction of measurement when the MTF is used to describe the spatial resolution of the system.

Notice that the MTF of a system is multiplicative; that is, if an image is obtained by an imaging system consisting of n components (e.g., energy source, detector, A/D, D/A, and display), each having its own MTF_i, then the effective MTF of the imaging system is expressed by the equation

$$\text{MTF}(u) = \prod_{i=1}^{n} \text{MTF}_i(u) \tag{2.11}$$

where Π is the multiplication symbol. It is obvious that a low $\text{MTF}_i(u)$ value in any given component i will contribute to an overall low $\text{MTF}(u)$ of the complete system.

2.5.1.5   Mathematical Relationship among ESF, LSF, and MTF   The MTF described in Section 2.5.1.4 is sometimes called the high-contrast response of the imaging system because the line pair phantom used is a high-contrast phantom (see Fig. 2.3*A*-2, and *D*-1 at four corners and the midright line pairs). By "high-contrast," we mean that the object (lead) and the background (air) yield high radiographic or image contrast. On the other hand, MTF obtained with a low-contrast phantom (Fig. 2.3*A*-3, and *D*-1, midleft line pairs) constitutes the low-contrast response of the system. The MTF value obtained with a high-contrast phantom is always larger than that obtained with a lower contrast phantom for a given spatial frequency; therefore, when the MTF of a system is presented, the contrast of the line pair used to measure the MTF should also be given.

With this background we are ready to describe the relationships among the edge spread function, the line spread function, and the modulation transfer function. Let us set up an experiment to obtain the MTF of a digital imaging system composed of a light table, a CCD camera, a digital chain that converts the video signals into digital signals (A/D) to form the digital image, and a D/A converts the digital image to video signal to display on a output monitor. The experimental steps are as follows:

1. Cover half the light table with a sharp-edged, black-painted metal sheet (edge phantom).
2. Obtain a digital image of this edge phantom with the CCD camera of the imaging system, as shown in Figure 2.6*A*. Then the ESF(x) has a gray level distribution (as shown in Fig. 2.6*B* arrows), which is obtained by taking the average value of several lines (a–a) perpendicular to the edges. Observe the noise characteristic of the ESF(x) in the figure.
3. The line spread function (LSF) of the system can be obtained by taking the first derivative of the edge spread function (ESF) numerically (Eq. 2.8), indicated by the three arrows shown in Figure 2.6*B*. The resulting LSF is depicted in Figure 2.6*C*.
4. To obtain the MTF of the system in the direction perpendicular to the edge, a 1-D Fourier transform (Eq. 2.10) is applied to the line spread function shown in Figure 2.6*C*. The magnitude of this 1-D Fourier transform is then the MTF of the imaging system in the direction perpendicular to the edge. The result is shown in Figure 2.6*D*.

This completes the experiment of obtaining the MTF from the ESF and the LSF. In practice, we can take 10% of the MTF values as the minimum resolving power of the imaging system. In this case, the MTF of this imaging system is about 1.0 cycle/mm, or can resolve one line pair per millimeter.

2.5.1.6   Relationship between Input Image, MTF, and Output Image
Let $A = 1$, $B = \pi$, and $x_0 = 0$, and extend the edge spread function described in Eq. (2.7) to a periodic function with period 2π shown in Figure 2.7*A*. This periodic function can be expressed as a Fourier series representation, or more explicitly, a sum of infinitely many sinusoidal functions, as

$$\mathrm{ESF}(x) = \frac{1}{2} + \frac{2}{\pi}\left[\sin + \frac{(\sin 3x)}{3} + \frac{(\sin 5x)}{5} + \frac{(\sin 7x)}{7} + \cdots\right] \qquad (2.12)$$

The first term, 1/2, in this Fourier series is the DC-term. Subsequent terms are sinusoidal, and each is characterized by an amplitude and a frequency.

If the partial sum of Eq. (2.12) is plotted, then it is apparent that the partial sum will approximate the periodic step function more closely as the number of terms used to form the partial sum increases (Fig. 2.7*B*). We can also plot the amplitude spectrum or the spatial frequency spectrum shown in Figure 2.7*C*, which is a plot of the amplitude against the spatial frequency (Eq. 2.12). From this plot we can observe that the periodic step function ESF(x) can be decomposed into infinite components, each having an amplitude and frequency. To reproduce this periodic function ESF(x) exactly, it is necessary to include all the components. If some of the components are missing or have diminished amplitude values, the result is a diffused or unsharp edge. A major concern in the design of an imaging system is how to avoid missing frequency components or diminished amplitudes in the frequency components in the output image.

The MTF of a system can be used to predict missing or modulated amplitudes. Consider the lateral view image of a plastic circular cylinder taken with a perfect X-ray imaging system. Figure 2.8*A* shows an optical density trace perpendicular to

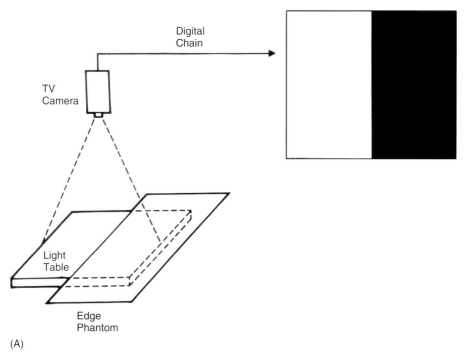

(A)

Figure 2.6   Relationships among ESF, LSF, and MTF (modulation transfer function). (*A*) Experimental setup. The imaging chain consists of a light table, a video or CCD camera, a digital chain that converts the video signals into digital signals (A/D) and forms the digital image, and a D/A that converts the digital image to video so that the it can been displayed on a display monitor. The object under consideration is an edge phantom. (*B*) The ESF (arrows) by averaging several lines parallel to a–a. (*C*) The LSF. (*D*) The MTF (c/mm = cycle/mm).

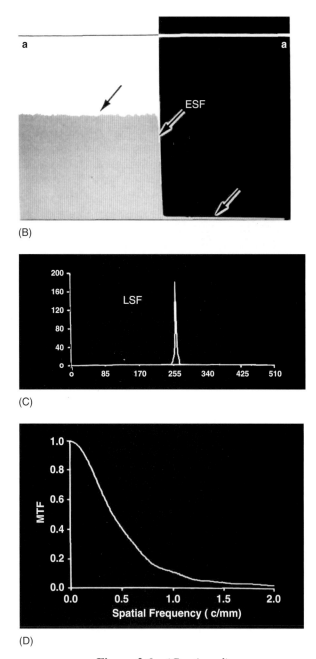

(B)

(C)

(D)

Figure 2.6 *(Continued)*

the axis of the circular cylinder in the perfect image. How would this trace look if the image is digitized by the CCD camera system described in Section 2.5.1.5?

To answer this question, we first take the Fourier transform of the trace from the perfect image, which gives its spatial frequency spectrum (Fig. 2.8B). If this frequency spectrum is multiplied by the MTF of the imaging system shown in

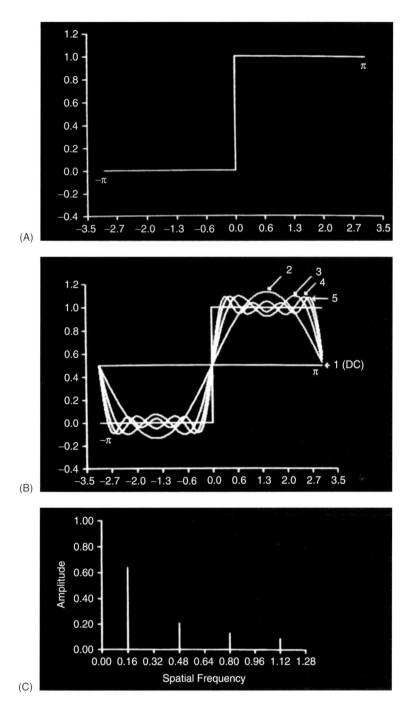

(A)

(B)

(C)

Figure 2.7   Sinusoidal functions representation of an edge step function. (*A*) The ideal edge step function (*x*-axis: distance, *y*-axis: values of the edge). (*B*) Partial sums of sinusoidal functions; numerals correspond to the number of terms summed, described in Eq. (2.12). (*C*) Amplitude spectrum of the step function.

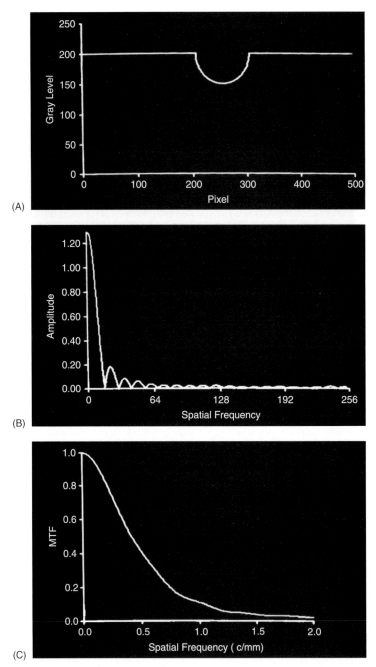

Figure 2.8   Relationships among the input function, MTF of the imaging system, and the output function. (*A*) A line profile from a lateral view of a circular cylinder from a perfect imaging system, MTF = 1. (*B*) The spatial frequency spectrum of A. (*C*) MTF of the imaging system described in Figure 2.6*D*. (*D*) The output frequency response (*B* × *C*). (*E*) The predicted line trace from the imperfect imaging system obtained by an inverse Fourier transform of *D*. (*F*) Superposition of *A* and *E* showing the rounding of the edges (arrows) due to the imperfect imaging system.

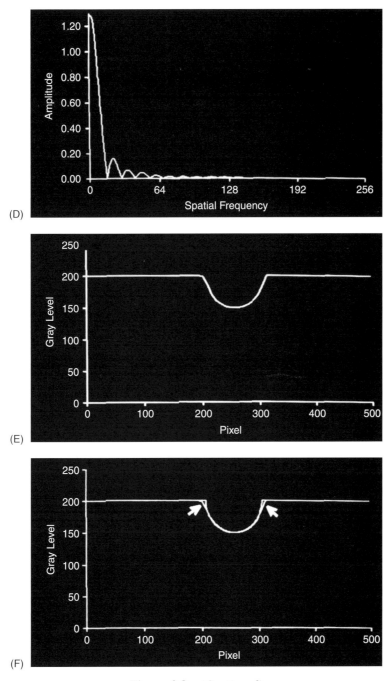

(D)

(E)

(F)

Figure 2.8   *(Continued)*

Figure 2.6D, which is reproduced as Figure 2.8C, frequency by frequency, the result is the output frequency response of the trace (Fig. 2.8D, after normalization) obtained with this digital imaging system. It is seen from Figure 2.8B and D that there is no phase shift; that is, all the zero crossings are identical between the input and the output spectra. The output frequency spectrum has been modulated to compensate for the imperfection of the CCD camera digital imaging system. Figure 2.8E shows the expected trace. Figure 2.8F is the superposition of the perfect and the expected trace. It is seen that both corners in the expected trace (arrows) lose their sharpness.

This completes the description of how the concepts of point spread function, line spread function, edge spread function, and modulation transfer function of an imaging system can be used to measure the unsharpness of an output image. The concept of using the MTF to predict the unsharpness due to an imperfect system has also been introduced.

2.5.2 Measurement of Noise

MTF is often used as a measure of the quality of the imaging system. By definition, it is a measure of certain optical characteristics of an imaging system, namely the ability to resolve fine details. It provides no information regarding the effect of noise on the contrast of the medical image. Since both unsharpness and noise can affect the image quality, an imaging system with large MTF values at high frequencies does not necessarily produce a high-quality image if the noise level is high. Figure 2.2C, at the upper left, shows an excellent quality abdominal CT image, and the remaining three images depict the same CT image with various degrees of random noise added. On comparing these figures, it is clearly seen that noise degrades the quality of the original image. The study of the noise that arises from quantum statistics, electronic noise, optical diffusion, and film grain represents another measure on the image quality. To study the noise, we need the concept of power spectrum, or Wiener spectrum, which describes the noise characteristics produced by an imaging system. Let us make the assumption that all the noises N are random in nature and do not correlate with the signals S that form the image; then the signal-to-noise power ratio

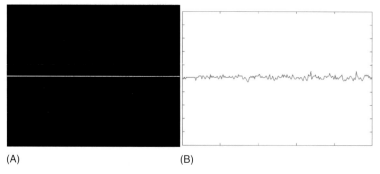

(A)   (B)

Figure 2.9 (A) Example demonstrating the signal and the noise in a line trace (white) on a uniform digital light photo image (black). (B) The small variations (blue) adjacent to the profile is the noise. If there were no noise, the line trace would be a straight line.

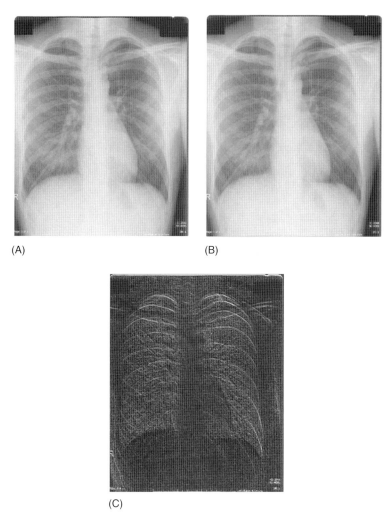

(A)   (B)

(C)

Figure 2.10 Subtraction between a chest X-ray image digitized once and the average digitized 16 times. (*A*) Chest X-ray film as digitized once with a laser film digitizer; (*B*) digital image of the same chest X-ray film digitized 16 times and then averaged; (*C*) image *B* subtracted from image *A*. A very narrow window (see Chapter 12) was used to display the subtracted image to highlight the noise.

spectrum, or the signal-to-noise power ratio P(*x*, *y*), of each pixel is defined by

$$P(x, y) = \frac{S^2(x, y)}{N^2(x, y)} \tag{2.13}$$

Figure 2.9 illustrates a signal and the associated random noise in a line trace on a uniform background image. A high signal-to-noise ratio (SNR) means that the image is less noisy. A common method to increase the SNR (i.e., reduce the noise in the image) is to obtain many images of the same object under the same conditions and average them. This, in a sense, minimizes the contribution of the random noise to the image. If M images are averaged, then the average signal-to-noise power ratio $\overline{P}(x, y)$ becomes

$$\overline{P}(x, y) = \frac{M^2 S^2(x, y)}{M \ N^2(x, y)} = M P(x, y) \qquad (2.14)$$

The SNR is the square root of the power ratio

$$\mathrm{SNR}(x, y) = \sqrt{\overline{P}(x, y)} = \sqrt{M}\sqrt{P(x, y)} \qquad (2.15)$$

Therefore the signal-to-noise ratio increases by the square root of the number of images averaged.

Equation (2.15) indicates that it is possible to increase the SNR of the image by this averaging technique. The average image will have less random noise, which gives a smoother visual appearance. For each pixel, the noise $N(x, y)$ defined in Eq. (2.13) can be approximated by using the standard deviation of the image under consideration $p(x, y)$ and the computed average image $\overline{P}(x, y)$.

Figure 2.10 illustrates how the SNR of the imaging system is computed. Take a chest X-ray image $p(x, y)$ (Fig. 2.10A), digitize it with an imaging system M times and average the results, pixel by pixel, to form the average image $\overline{P}(x, y)$ or the signal (Fig 2.10B). The noise of each pixel $N(x, y)$ can be approximated by the standard deviation of $\overline{P}(x, y)$ and $p_i(x, y)$, where p_i is a digitized image, and $M \geq i \geq 1$; then the SNR for each pixel can be computed by using Eqs. (2.13) and (2.15). Figure 2.10A, B, and C shows a digitized image $p_i(x, y)$, the average image $\overline{P}(x, y)$ with $M = 16$, and the difference image between $p_i(x, y)$ and $\overline{P}(x, y)$. After the display parameters are adjusted to highlight the difference image, it shows faint radiographic shadows of the chest illustrating anatomical structures like the ribs, clavicles, mediastinum, heart, and diaphragm. The noise, which is most prominent in the anatomical edges, is not random but systematic due to the existence of anatomical structures that contribute to the imaging system noise.

References

Bankman IN. *Handbook of Medical Imaging Processing and Analysis*, 2nd ed. San Diego: Academic Press; 2008.

Barrett HH, Swindell W. *Radiological Imaging: The Theory of Image Formation, Detection, and Processing*. San Diego: Academic Press; 1981.

Benedetto AR, Huang HK, Ragan DP. *Computers in Medical Physics*. New York: American Institute of Physics; 1990.

Bertram S. On the derivation of the fast Fourier transform. *IEEE Trans Audio Electroacoust* 18: 55–58; 1970.

Beutel J, Kundel H, Van Metter RL. *Handbook of Medical Imaging. Vol. 1. Physics and Psychophysics*. Bellingham, WA: SPIE Press; 2000.

Bracewell R. *The Fourier Transform and its Applications*. New York: McGraw-Hill; 1965.

Bracewell RN. Strip integration in radio astronomy, *Austr J Phys* 9: 198– 217; 1956.

Brigham EO. *The Fast Fourier Transform*. Englewood Cliffs, NJ: Prentice-Hall, 1974, pp. 148–183.

Cochran WT, et al. What is the fast Fourier transform? *IEEE Trans Audio Electroacoust* 15: 45–55; 1967.

Curry TS III, Dowdey JE, Murry RC Jr. *Introduction to the Physics of Diagnostic Radiology*, 4th ed. Philadelphia: Lea and Febiger; 1990.

Dainty JC, Shaw R. *Image Science*. San Diego: Academic Press; 1974, ch. 5.

Dhawan AT. *Medical Image Analysis*. Hoboken, NJ: Wiley/IEEE; 2003.

Dhawan AP, Huang HK, Kim D-S, 2008. *Principles and Advanced Methods in Medical Imaging and Image Analysis*, Edited. World Scientific Publishing: New Jersey, London, Singapore. 850 pages.

Gonzalez RG, Wood RE. *Digital Image Processing*, 2nd ed. Reading, MA: Addison-Wesley; 2002.

Hendee WR, Wells PNT. *The Perception of Visual Information*, 2nd ed. New York: Springer; 1997.

Huang HK. *Elements of Digital Radiology: A Professional Handbook and Guide*. N.J.: Prentice-Hall, Inc., April 1987.

Huang HK. *PACS: Picture Archiving and Communication Systems in Biomedical Imaging*. New York: VCH/Wiley; 1996.

Huang HK 1999. *Picture Archiving and Communication Systems: Principles and Applications*. Wiley & Sons, NY, p. 521.

Huang HK, March, 2004. *PACS and Imaging Informatics: Principles and Applications*. John Wiley & Sons, Hoboken New Jersey, 704 pages.

Kim Y, Horii SC. *Handbook of Medical Imaging. Vol. 3 Display and PACS*. Bellingham, WA: SPIE Press; 2000.

Leondes CT. *Medical Systems Techniques and Applications*. London: Gordon and Breach Science Publishers; 1997.

Prince JL, Links JM. *Medical Imaging Signals and Systems*. Englewood Cliffs, NJ: Prentice Hall; 2006.

Robb RA. *Three-Dimensional Biomedical Imaging*. New York: VCH/Wiley; 1997.

Rosenfeld A, Kak AC. *Digital Picture Processing*, 2nd ed. San Diego: Academic Press, 1997.

Rossman K. Image quality. *Radiolog Clin N Am* 7(3); Saunders Company, Philadelphia, Penn 1969.

Sonka M, Fitzpatrick JM. *Handbook of Medical Imaging. Vol. 2. Medical Imaging Processing and Analysis*. Bellingham, WA: SPIE Press; 2000.

CHAPTER 3

Two-Dimensional Medical Imaging

In this chapter two-dimensional (2-D) medical imaging are presented, including the following topics: conventional projection radiography, and computed and digital radiography; 2-D nuclear medicine and ultrasound imaging, and 2-D light imaging. The discussion emphasizes the digital aspect of these modalities and not the imaging physics. Interested readers should refer to proper references on the imaging physics of each modality.

3.1 PRINCIPLES OF CONVENTIONAL PROJECTION RADIOGRAPHY

Conventional projection radiography accounts for 60% to 70% of the total number of diagnostic imaging procedures. Therefore, to transform radiology from a film-based to a digital-based operation, we must understand (1) radiology workflow, (2) conventional projection radiographic procedures, (3) analog-to-digital conversion, and (4) digital radiography. This chapter discusses these four topics.

3.1.1 Radiology Workflow

Picture archiving and communication system (PACS) is a system integration of both patient workflow and diagnostic components and procedures. A thorough understanding of radiology workflow should allow efficient system integration, and hence a better PACS design for the radiology department and the hospital operation. Radiology workflow can vary from department to department and hospital to hospital. For these reasons workflow analysis is the first step for PACS design and implementation. Figure 3.1 shows a generic radiology workflow before PACS. Among the 14 steps, steps 4, 8, 9, 10, 12, and 14 are no longer needed in the PACS operation, and this renders a more efficient radiology workflow.

1. New patient arrives at hospital for radiological examination (exam).
2. Patient registers in Radiology area. If the patient is new, patient is registered in the Hospital Information System (HIS).
3. Exam ordered at Radiology Information System (RIS) upon arrival at Radiology registration desk. Exam accession number is automatically assigned, and a requisition is printed.

PACS and Imaging Informatics, Second Edition, by H. K. Huang
Copyright © 2010 John Wiley & Sons, Inc.

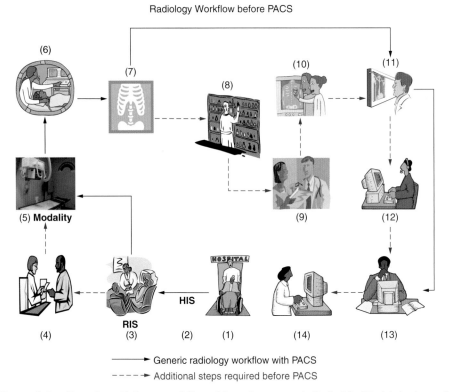

Radiology Workflow before PACS

———→ Generic radiology workflow with PACS

- - - -→ Additional steps required before PACS

Figure 3.1 Generic radiology workflow. Note that steps 4, 8, 9, 10, 12, 14 (→) can be replaced by PACS, thus providing more efficient workflow.

4. Technologist receives information from clerk and calls the patient in the waiting area for exam.
5. Patient escorted into the modality room.
6. Examination is performed by a technologist.
7. Examination is completed.
8. Clerk pulls out old films.
9. Clerk prepares all necessary papers and films for radiologist.
10. Films are hanged for radiologist's review.
11. Radiologist reviews films (images), check examination record and dictates reports.
12. Transcriptionist types the draft report from the dictation.
13. Radiologist reviews the report and signs it off.
14. Final reports are input into RIS for clinician viewing.

3.1.2 Standard Procedures Used in Conventional Projection Radiography

Conventional X-ray imaging procedures are used in all subspecialties of a radiology department, including out-patient, emergency, pediatric, neuroimaging, chest,

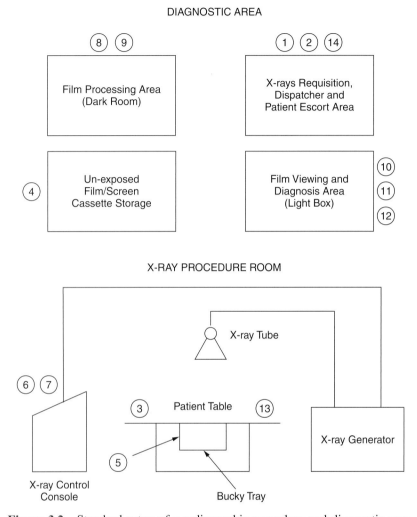

Figure 3.2   Standard setup of a radiographic procedure and diagnostic area.

genitourinary, gastrointestinal, cardiovascular, musculoskeletal, and breast imaging. In each subspecialty procedure, two major work areas are involved: the X-ray procedure room and the diagnostic area. These two areas may share subspecialties. Although the detailed exam procedures may differ among subspecialties, the basic steps can be summarized. Figure 3.2 shows a standard setup of a conventional radiographic procedure room and a diagnostic area (for diagnosis and reporting). The numbers in the figure correspond to the workflow steps of a table-top examination described in the following:

1. Transfer patient related information from HIS and RIS to the X-ray procedure room before the examination.
2. Check patient X-ray requisition for anatomical area under consideration for imaging.

3. Set patient in the proper position, stand up or on table top, for X-ray examination, and adjust X-ray collimator for the size of exposed area, or field size.

4. Select a proper film-screen cassette.

5. Place the cassette in the holder located behind the patient, or on the table under the patient.

6. Determine X-ray exposure factors for obtaining the optimal quality image with minimum X-ray dose to the patient.

7. Turn on X rays to obtain a latent image of the patient on the screen/film cassette.

8. Process exposed film through a film processor.

9. Retrieve developed film from the film processor.

10. Inspect quality of radiograph (developed film) through a light box for proper exposure or other possible errors (e.g., patient positioning, or movement).

11. Repeat steps 3 to 10 if image quality on radiograph is unacceptable for diagnosis. Always keep in mind that the patient should not be subjected to unnecessary additional X-ray exposure.

12. Submit radiograph to a radiologist for approval.

13. Remove patient from the table after radiologist has determined that quality of the radiograph is acceptable for diagnosis.

14. Escort patient out of the exam area.

Observe that if digital radiography with PACS is used (see Section 3.6), three components in the diagnostic area—film processing (8, 9), storage (4), and film viewing (10, 11, 12 replaced by workstations)—can be eliminated resulted in a saving of space as well as a more effective and efficient operation.

3.1.3 Analog Image Receptor

Radiology workflow gives a general idea on how the radiology department handles the patient coming in for examination, and how the imaging examination results are reviewed and archived. This section discusses equipment used for radiographic examination, and some physics principles of imaging.

After the patient is exposed to X rays during an examination, the attenuated X-ray photons exiting the patient carry the information of an image or the latent image. The latent image cannot be visualized by the human eyes and has to be converted to a light image used an analog image receptor. Two commonly used analog image receptors are the image intensifier tube and the screen/film combination cassette.

3.1.3.1 Image Intensifier Tube The image intensifier tube is used often as the image receptor in projection radiography especially for low X-ray dose dynamic imaging. The image intensifier tube is particularly useful for fluorographic and digital subtraction angiography procedures, which allow real-time imaging of moving structures in the body and their dynamic processes. If X-ray films were used for these types of examinations, the dose exposure to the patient would be very high and not be acceptable. The use of an image intensifier renders quality dynamic images from

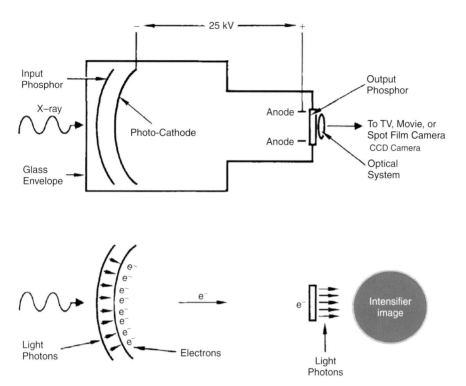

Figure 3.3 Schematic of the image intensifier tube and the formation of an image on the output screen.

the study, although lower than that of film/screen, but minimizes the X-ray exposure to the patient. An image intensifier tube is shown schematically in Figure 3.3.

The formation of the image is as follows: X-rays penetrate the patient; exited X-rays carry patient image information enter the image intensifier tube through the glass envelope and are absorbed in the input phosphor intensifying screen. The input screen converts X-ray photons to light photons that are not sufficient to render a sufficient quality light image for visualization. Thus these light photons must be amplified or intensified. To do this, the light photons emitted from the screen next strike the light-sensitive photocathode, causing the emission of photoelectrons. These electrons are then accelerated across the tube attracted by the anode with a difference of 25,000 Volts. This stream of electrons is focused and converges on an output phosphor screen. This way the attenuated X-ray photons are converted to proportional accelerated electrons. When the electrons strike the anode phosphor, they are absorbed by the output phosphor screen and converted once again to light photons, but in a much larger quantity (brightness gain) than the light output from the input phosphor, hence the term image intensifier. Image intensifiers are generally listed by the diameter of the input phosphor, ranging from 4.5 to 14 inches.

The light from the output phosphor is then coupled to an optical system for recording using a movie camera (angiography), a video camera or CCD camera (fluorography), or a spot film camera.

There are three approaches to convert an analogy-based radiographic image to digital form. The first method is to digitize the X-ray film to a digital image. The second method utilizes existing equipment in the radiographic procedure room and only changing the image receptor component. Two technologies—computed radiography (CR), using the photostimulable phosphor imaging plate technology, and digital fluorography—are in this category. This approach does not require any modification in the procedure room and is therefore easily adopted for daily clinical practice. The third method is to redesign the conventional radiographic procedure equipment, including the geometry of the X-ray beams and the image receptor. This method is therefore more expensive to adopt, but it offers the advantages of more efficient workflow and special features like low X-ray scatter that would not otherwise be achievable in the conventional procedure. Examples are digital radiography and digital mammography. These technologies are to be discussed in the following sections.

3.1.3.2 Screen/Film Combination Cassette

A screen/film combination cassette consists of a double-emulsion radiation-sensitive film sandwiched between two intensifying phosphor screens housed inside a light tight cassette (Fig. 3.4). The X-ray film of silver halide crystals suspended with a gelatin medium, which is coated on both sides by an emulsion, consists of a transparent (polyethylene terephthalate) plastic substrate called the base. A slightly blue tint is commonly incorporated in the base to give the radiograph a pleasing appearance. A photographic emulsion can be exposed to X rays directly, but it is more sensitive to light photons of much less energy ($\sim$2.5–5 eV). For this reason an intensifying screen is used first to absorb the attenuated X rays.

The screen, which is made of a thin phosphor layer (e.g., crystalline calcium tungstate), is sensitive to the diagnostic X-ray energy in the range of 20–90 keV. The X-ray photons exiting the patient impinge onto an intensifying screen causing

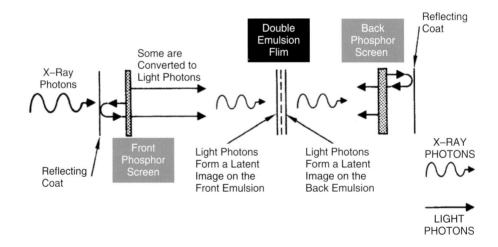

PRINCIPLE OF OPERATION

Figure 3.4 Schematic of a screen/film cassette (not in scale) and the formation of a latent image on the film. Distances between the front screen, film, and the back screen shown in the drawing are for illustration purposes; they are actually in contact with each other.

it to emit visible light photons, which are collected by the film to form a latent image. X-ray photons that are not absorbed by the front screen in the cassette can be absorbed by the back screen. The light emitted from this second screen then exposes the emulsion on the back side of the film. The double emulsion film thus can effectively reduce the patient exposure by half. With the screen/film as the image detector, the patient receives much lower exposure than when film alone is used. Image blur due to patient motion can also be minimized with a shorter exposure time if screen/film combination is used. The film is then developed, forming a visible X-ray film, or a radiograph. Figure 3.4 presents physics of the film/screen detector and its interaction with X-ray photons.

3.1.3.3   X-ray Film

Optical Density of the X-ray Film   The number of developed silver halide crystals per unit volume in the developed film determines the amount of light from the viewing light box that can be transmitted through a unit volume. This transmitted light is referred to as the optical density of the film in that unit volume. Technically the optical density (OD) is defined as the logarithm base 10 of 1 over the transmittance of a unit intensity of light.

$$OD = \log_{10} \left(\frac{1}{transmittance} \right) \qquad (3.1)$$

$$= \log_{10} \left(\frac{I_o}{I_t} \right)$$

where

I_o = light intensity at the viewing box before transmission through the film
I_t = light intensity after transmission through the film

The film optical density is used to represent the degree of film darkening due to X-ray exposure.

Characteristic Curve of the X-ray Film   The relationship between the amount of X-ray exposure received and the film optical density is called the *characteristic curve* or the *H and D curve* (after F. Hurter and V. C. Driffield, who first published such a curve in England in 1890). The logarithm of relative exposure is plotted instead of the exposure itself, partly because it compresses a large linear to a manageable logarithm scale that makes analysis of the curve easier. Figure 3.5 shows an idealized curve with three segments, the toe (A), the linear segment (B), and the shoulder (C).

The toe is the based density or the base-plus-fog level (usually $OD = 0.12 - 0.20$). For very low exposures the film optical density remains at the fog level and is independent of exposure level. Next is a linear segment over which the optical density and the logarithm of relative exposure are linearly related (usually between $OD = 0.3$ and 2.2). The shoulder corresponds to high exposures or overexposures where most of the silver halides are converted to metallic silver (usually $OD = 3.2$). The film becomes saturated, and the optical density is no longer a function of exposure level.

The characteristic curve is usually described by one of the following terms: the film gamma, average gradient, film latitude, or film speed. The film gamma (γ) is

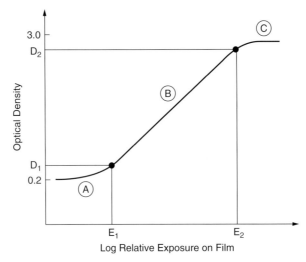

Figure 3.5 Relationship between logarithm of relative X-ray exposure and the film optical density plotted as a curve, the characteristic curve or the H and D curve.

the maximum slope of the characteristic curve, and is described by the formula

$$\text{Gamma } (\gamma) = \frac{D_2 - D_1}{\log_{10} E_2 - \log_{10} E_1} \tag{3.2}$$

where

> $D_2 =$ the highest *OD* value within the steepest portion of the curve (see Fig. 3.5)
> $D_1 =$ the lowest *OD* value within the steepest portion of curve
> $E_2 =$ exposure corresponding to D_2
> $E_1 =$ exposure corresponding to D_1

The average gradient of the characteristic curve is the slope of the characteristic curve calculated between optical density 0.25 and 2.00 above base plus fog level for the radiographic film under consideration. The optical density range between 0.25 to 2.00 is considered acceptable for diagnostic radiology application. For example, assume a base and fog level of 0.15. Then the range of acceptable optical density is 0.40 to 2.15. The average gradient can be represented by the following formula:

$$\text{Average gradient } = \frac{D_2 - D_1}{\log_{10} E_2 - \log_{10} E_1} \tag{3.3}$$

where

> $D_2 = 2.00 +$ base and fog level
> $D_1 = 0.25 +$ base and fog level
> $E_2 =$ exposure corresponding to D_2
> $E_1 =$ exposure corresponding to D_1

The film latitude describes the range of exposures used in the average gradient calculation. Thus, as described in Eq. (3.3), the film latitude is equal to $\log_{10} E_2 - \log_{10} E_1$. The film speed (unit: 1/roentgen) can be defined as follows:

$$\text{Speed} = \frac{1}{E} \tag{3.4}$$

where E is the exposure (in roentgens) required to produce a film optical density of 1.0 above base and fog. Generally speaking:

1. The latitude of a film varies inversely with film contrast, film speed, film gamma, and average gradient.
2. Film gamma and average gradient of a film vary directly with film contrast.
3. Film fog level varies inversely with film contrast.
4. Faster films require less exposure to achieve a specific density than slower films.

3.2 DIGITAL FUOROGRAPHY AND LASER FILM SCANNER

3.2.1 Basic Principles of Analog-to-Digital Conversion

Currently 60% to 70% of the conventional procedures performed in a radiology department are 2-D projection radiography that traditionally uses either film or an intensifier tube as the output medium. This section discusses two methods to convert these analog images to digital images: a video or CCD camera coupled with an A/D converter, and the laser film scanner.

Take the film image as an example. When film is digitized, the shades of gray are quantized into a two-dimensional array of nonnegative integers called pixels. Two factors determine if the digitized image truly represents the original analog image: the quality of the scanner and the aliasing artifact. A low-quality digitizer or scanner with a large pixel size and insufficient bits/pixel will yield a bad digitized image. Even when a better quality scanner is used, it may sometimes still produce aliasing artifact in the digitized image due to some special inherent patterns, such as grid lines and edges, in the original film. The aliasing artifact can best be explained with the concept of data sampling. The well-known sampling theorem states:

If the Fourier transform of the image $f(x, y)$ vanishes for all u, v where $|u| \geq 2f_N$, $|v| \geq 2f_N$, then $f(x, y)$ can be exactly reconstructed from samples of its nonzero values taken $(1/2)\,f_N$ apart or closer. The frequency $2f_N$ is called the Nyquist frequency.

The theorem implies that if the pixel samples are taken more than $1/2\,f_N$ apart, it will not be possible to reconstruct the original image completely from these samples because some information in the original image is lost. The difference between the original image and the image reconstructed from these samples is caused by the aliasing error. The aliasing artifact creates new frequency components in the reconstructed image called Moiré patterns. For example, in a radiograph when the physical star phantom contains radial patterns with frequency higher than the X-ray machine can resolve the star phantom X-ray image creates Moiré patterns near the center of the star shown in Figure 2.3*B*-1. The Nyquist frequency principle can be applied to digitize a radiograph when the scanner cannot resolve some patterns in the radiograph.

3.2.2 Video/CCD Scanning System and Digital Fluorography

The video scanning system is a low-cost X-ray digitizer that produces either a 512 or 1 K to 2 K digitized image with 8 to 10 bits per pixel. The system consists of three major components: a scanning device with a video or a CCD (charge-coupled device) camera that scans the X-ray film, an analog/digital converter that converts the video signals from the camera to gray level values, and an image memory to store the digital signals from the A/D converter.

The image stored in the image memory is the digital representation of the X-ray film or image in the image intensifier tube obtained by using the video scanning system. If the image memory is connected to a digital-to-analog (D/A) conversion circuitry and to a TV monitor, this image can be displayed back on the monitor (which is a video image). The memory can be connected to a peripheral storage device for long-term image archive. Figure 3.6 shows a block diagram of a video scanning system. The digital chain shown is a standard component in all types of scanner.

A video scanning system can be connected to an image intensifier tube to form a digital fluoroscopic system. Digital fluorography is a method that can produce dynamic digital X-ray images without changing the radiographic procedure room drastically. This technique requires an add-on unit in the conventional fluorographic system. Figure 3.7 shows a schematic of a digital fluorographic system with the following major components:

1. *X-ray source*: X-ray tube and a grid to minimize X-rays scatter
2. *Image receptor*: An image intensifier tube
3. *Video camera plus optical system*: The output light from the image intensifier goes through an optical system, which allows the video camera to be adjusted

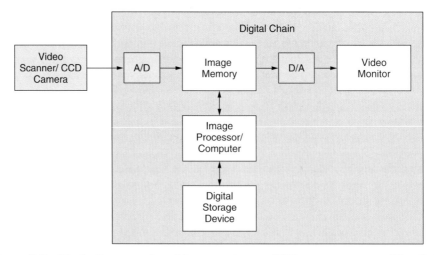

Figure 3.6 Block diagram of a video scanning or CCD camera system. The digital chain is a standard component in all types of scanner.

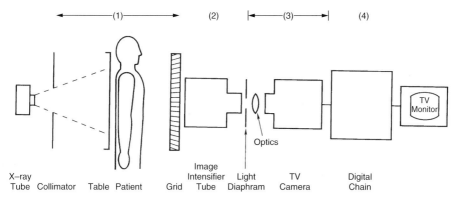

Figure 3.7 Schematic of a digital fluorographic system coupling the image intensifier and the digital chain.

for focusing. The amount of light going into the camera is controlled by means of a light diaphragm. The camera used is usually a plumbicon or a CCD (charge couple device) with 512 or 1024 scan lines.

4. Digital chain: The digital chain consists of an A/D converter, image memories, image processor, digital storage, and video display. The A/D converter, the image memory, and the digital storage can handle $512 \times 512 \times 8$-bit image at 30 frames per second, or $1024 \times 1024 \times 8$-bit image at 7.5 frames per second. Sometime the RAID (redundant array of inexpensive disks) is used to handle high-speed data transfer.

Fluorography is used to visualize the motion of body compartments (e.g., blood flow, heart beat), the movement of a catheter, as well as to pinpoint an organ in a body region for subsequent detailed diagnosis. Each exposure required in a fluorographic procedure is very minimal compared with a conventional X-ray procedure.

Digital fluorography used to be considered to as an add-on system because a digital chain can be added to an existing fluorographic unit. This method utilizes the established X-ray tube assembly, image intensifier, video scanning, and digital technologies. Most current digital radiographic system combines the video scanning and A/D conversion as a single unit forming a direct digital video output. The output from a digital fluorographic system is a sequence of digital images displayed on a video monitor. Digital fluorography has an advantage over conventional fluorography in that it gives a larger dynamic range image and can remove uninterested structures in the images by performing digital subtraction.

When image processing is introduced to the digital fluorographic system, dependent on the application, other names are used, for example, digital subtraction angiography (DSA), digital subtraction arteriography (DSA), digital video angiography (DVA), intravenous video arteriography (IVA), computerized fluoroscopy (CF), and digital video subtraction angiography (DVSA).

3.2.3 Laser Film Scanner

Laser scanner is the gold standard in film digitization. It normally converts a 14 in. $\times$ 17 in. X-ray film to a $2K \times 2.5K \times 12$-bit image. The principle of laser scanning is

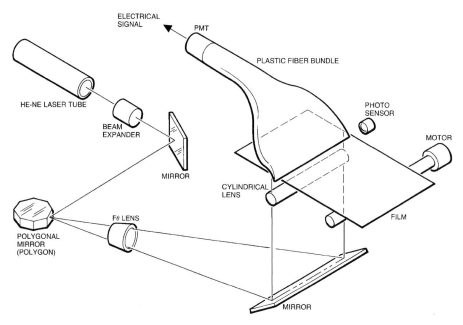

Figure 3.8 Scanning mechanism of a laser film scanner.

shown in Figure 3.8. A rotating polygon mirror system is used to guide a collimated low-power (5 mW) laser beam (usually helium-neon) to scan across a line of the radiograph in a light-tight environment. The radiograph is advanced and the scan is repeated for the second lines, and so forth. The optical density of the film is measured from the transmission of the laser through each small area (e.g., 175 × 175 microns) of the radiograph using a photomultiplier (PMT) tube and a logarithmic amplifier. This electronic signal is sent to a digital chain where it is digitized to 12 bits from the A/D converter. The data are then sent to a computer where a storage device is provided for the image. Figure 3.9 shows the schematic block diagram of a laser scanner system. Table 3.1 gives the specifications of a generic scanner.

Before a scanner is ready for clinical use, it is important to evaluate its specifications and to verify the quality of the digitized image. Several parameters are of importance:

- Relationship between the pixel value and the optical density of the film
- Contrast frequency response
- Linearity
- Flat field response

Standard tests can be set up for such parameter measurements (Huang, 1999).

3.3 IMAGING PLATE TECHNOLOGY

Sections 3.3, 3.4, and 3.5 describe three methods of eliminating the X-ray film in conventional radiography exam. In this section we first discuss imaging plate

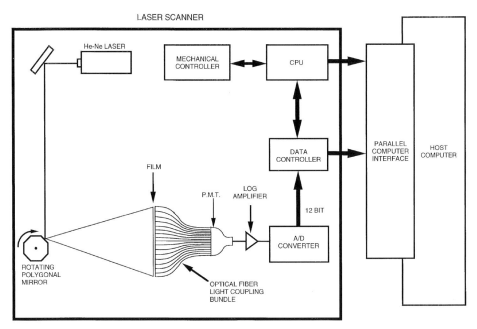

Figure 3.9 Block diagram of a laser film scanner interfacing to a host computer.

TABLE 3.1 Specifications of a laser film scanner

Film size supported (in. × in.)	14 × 17, 14 × 14, 12 × 14, 10 × 12, 8 × 10
Pixel size, μm	50–200
Sampling distance, μm	50, 75, 100, 125, 150, 175, 200
Optical density range	0–2, 0–4
Bits/pixel	12 bits
Hardware interface	SCSII,[a] Other faster interfaces
Laser power	5 mW
Scanning speed	200–400 lines/s
Data Format	DICOM[b]

[a]SCSII: Small computer systems interface.
[b]See Chapter 9

technology. Imaging plate system, commonly called computed radiography (CR), consists of two components: the imaging plate and the scanning mechanism. The imaging plate (*laser-stimulated luminescence phosphor plate*) used for X-rays detection, is similar in principle to the phosphor intensifier screen used in the screen/film receptor described in Section 3.1.3.2. The scanning of a laser-stimulated luminescence phosphor imaging plate also uses similar scanning mechanism (the reader) as that of a laser film scanner. The only difference is that instead of scanning an X-ray film, the laser scans the imaging plate. This section describes the principle of the imaging plate, specifications of the system, and system operation.

3.3.1 Principle of the Laser-Stimulated Luminescence Phosphor Plate

The physical size of the imaging plate is similar to that of a conventional radiographic screen; it consists of a support coated with a photo-stimulable phosphorous layer made of $BaFX:Eu^{2+}$ (X=Cl, Br, I), Europium-activated barium-fluorohalide compounds. After the X-ray exposure, the photo-stimulable phosphor crystal is able to store a part of the absorbed X-ray energy in a quasi-stable state. Stimulation of the plate by a 633 nanometer wavelength helium-neon (red) laser beam leads to emission of luminescence radiation of a different wavelength (400 nanometer), the amount of which is a function of the absorbed X-ray energy (Figure 3.10B).

The luminescence radiation stimulated by the laser scanning is collected through a focusing lens and a light guide into a photomultiplier tube, which converts it into electronic signals. Figure 3.10A and B shows the physical principle of the laser-stimulated luminescence phosphor imaging plate. The size of the imaging plate can be from 8 × 10, 10 × 12, 14 × 14, to 14 × 17 square inches. The image produced is 2000 × 2500 × 10 bits. For mammographic study the image size can be as high as 4000 × 5000 × 12 bits.

3.3.2 Computed Radiography System Block Diagram and Principle of Operation

The imaging plate is housed inside a cassette just like a screen/film receptor. Exposure of the imaging plate (IP) to X-ray radiation results in the formation of a latent image on the plate (similar to the latent image formed in a screen/film receptor). The exposed plate is processed through a CR reader to extract the latent image—analogous to the exposed film developed by a film developer. The processed imaging plate can be erased by bright light and be reused thousands of times. The imaging plate can be removable or nonremovable. An image processor is used to optimize the display (look-up tables, see Chapter 12) based on types of exam and body regions.

The output of this system can be one of two forms: a printed film or a digital image; the digital image can be stored in a digital storage device and be displayed on a video or LCD monitor. Figure 3.11 illustrates the dataflow of an upright CR system with three un-removable rotating imaging plates. Figure 3.12 shows the FCR XG5000 system with removable imaging plate and its components, including a reader with a stacker accommodating four image cassettes and a quality assurance display workstation.

3.3.3 Operating Characteristics of the CR System

A major advantage of the CR system compared to the conventional screen/film system is that the imaging plate has a linear response with a large dynamic range between the X-ray exposure and the relative intensity of the stimulated phosphors. Hence, under a similar X-ray exposure condition, the image reader is capable of producing images with density resolution comparable or superior to those from the conventional screen/film system. Since the image reader automatically adjusts the amount of exposure received by the plate, over- or underexposure within a certain threshold does not affect the appearance of the image. This useful feature can best be explained by the two examples given in Figure 3.13.

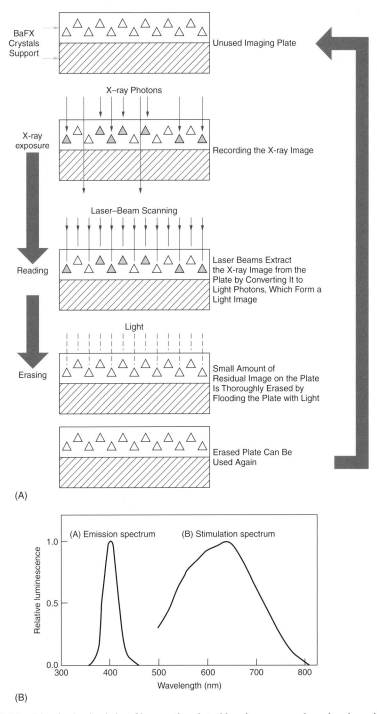

Figure 3.10 Physical principle of laser-stimulated luminescence phosphor imaging plate. (*A*) From the X-ray photons exposing the imaging plate to the formation of the light image. After the light image is converted to a digital image, a high-intensity flood light is used to erase the residue image in the plate allowing it to be reusable. (*B*) The wavelength of the scanning laser beam (*b*) is different from that of the emitted light (*a*) from the imaging plate after stimulation. (Courtesy of J. Miyahara, Fuji Photo Film Co., Ltd.)

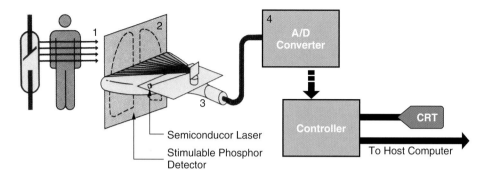

Figure 3.11   Dataflow of an upright CR system with nonremovable imaging plates (IP). (1) Formation of the latent image on the IP; (2) IP being scanned by the laser beam; (3) light photons converted to electronic signals; (4) electronic signals converted to the digital signals that form a CR image. (Courtesy of Konica Corporation, Japan)

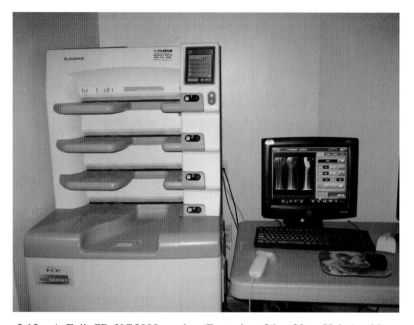

Figure 3.12   A Fuji CR XG5000 reader (Footprint: $26 \times 29 \times 58$ in.) with a stacker accommodating four image cassettes (left) and image processing workstation and quality assurance monitor (right).

In quadrant *A* of Figure 3.13, example I represents the plate exposed to a higher relative exposure level but with a narrower exposure range ($10^3 - 10^4$). The linear response of the plate after laser scanning yields a high level but narrow light intensity (photo-stimulable luminescence, PSL) range from 10^3 to 10^4. These light photons are converted into electronic output signals that represent the latent image stored on the image plate. The image processor senses a narrow range of electronic signals and selects a special look-up table (the linear line in Fig. 3.13*B*), which converts

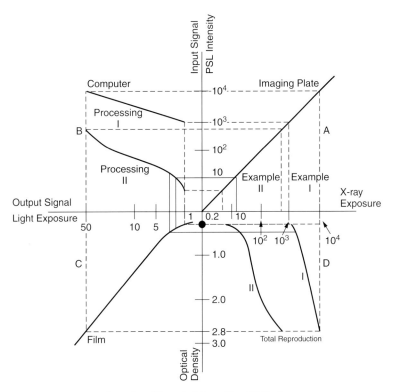

Operating Characteristics of the CR System

Figure 3.13 Two examples of the operating characteristics of the CR system and how it compensates for over- and underexposures with examples shown in Figure 3.14.

the narrow dynamic range of 10^3 to 10^4 to a large light relative exposure of 1 to 50 (Fig. 3.13*B*). If hardcopy is needed, a large latitude film can be used that covers the dynamic range of the light exposure from 1 to 50, as shown in quadrant *C*, these output signals will register the entire optical density (*OD*) range from *OD* 0.2 to *OD* 2.8 on the film. The total system response including the imaging plate, the look-up table, and the film subject to this exposure range is depicted as curve I in quadrant *D*. The system-response curve, relating the relative exposure on the plate and the *OD* of the output film, shows a high gamma value and is quite linear. This example demonstrates how the system accommodates a high exposure level with a narrow exposure range. When film is not needed, curve I in quadrant *D* can be converted to digital numbers with a range of 10 to 12 bits.

   Consider example II, in which the plate receives a lower exposure level but with wider exposure range. The CR system automatically selects a different look-up table in the image processor to accommodate this range of exposure so that the output signals again span the entire light exposure range form 1 to 50. The system-response curve is shown as curve II in quadrant *D*. The key in selecting the correct look-up table is that the range of the exposure has to span the total light exposure from 1 to 50. Note that in both examples the entire useful optical density range for diagnostic radiology is utilized.

If a conventional screen/film combination system is used, exposure on example I in Figure 3.13 would only utilize the higher optical density region of the film, whereas in example II it would utilize the lower region. Neither case would utilize the full dynamic range of the optical density in the film. From these two examples it is seen that the CR system allows the utilization of the full optical density dynamic range, regardless whether the plate is overexposed or underexposed. Figure 3.14 shows an example comparing the results of using screen/film versus CR under identical X-ray

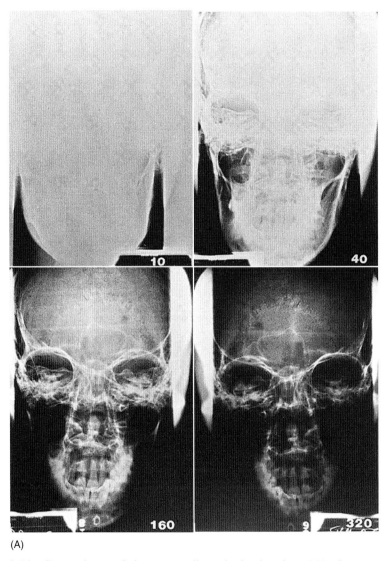

(A)

Figure 3.14 Comparison of image quality obtained using (A) the conventional screen/film method and (B) CR techniques. Exposures were 70 kVp; 10, 40, 160, 320 mAs on a skull phantom, respectively. Note that the CR technique is nearly dose (mAs) independent. (Courtesy of Dr. S Balter)

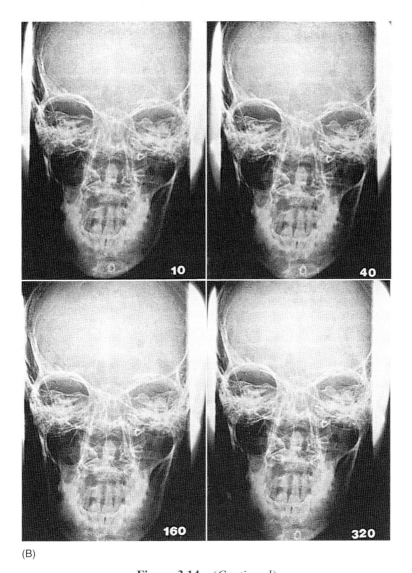

(B)

Figure 3.14 (*Continued*)

exposures. The same effect is achieved if the image signals are for digital output, and not for hard copy film. That is, the digital image produced from the image reader and the image processor will also utilize the full dynamic range from quadrant D to produce 10 to 12 bit digital numbers.

3.3.4 Background Removal

3.3.4.1 What Is Background Removal? Under normal operating conditions, images obtained by projection radiography contain unexposed areas due to X-ray collimation: for example, areas outside the circle of the imaging field in digital fluorography (DF), and areas outside the collimator of CR for skeletal and pediatric

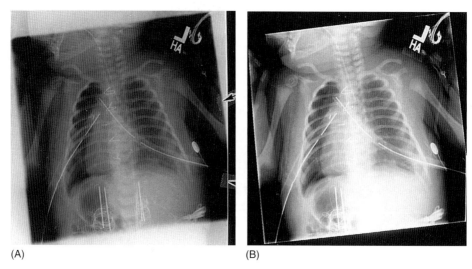

(A)   (B)

Figure 3.15 (*A*) A pediatric CR image, with white background (arrows) as seen on a video monitor. (*B*) A better visual quality image after the white background is automatically removed.

radiology. In digital images, unexposed areas appearing white on a display monitor is defined as background in this context. Figure 3.15*A* is a pediatric CR image with white background as seen on a monitor. Background removal in this context means that the brightness of the background is converted from white to black. Figure 3.15*B* shows that the white background in Figure 3.15*A* has been removed automatically.

3.3.4.2 Advantages of Background Removal in Digital Radiography

There are four advantages to using background removal in digital projection radiography. First, background removal immediately provides lossless data compression because the background is no longer in the image, an important cost-effective parameter in digital radiography when dealing with large-size images. Second, a background-removed image has better image visual quality for the following reason: diagnosis from radiography is the result of information processing based on visualization by the eyes. Since the contrast sensitivity of the eyes is proportional to the Weber ratio $\Delta B/B$, whereas B is brightness of the background, and ΔB is brightness difference between the region of interest in the image and the background, removing or decreasing the unwanted background in a projection radiography images makes the image more easily readable and greatly improves its diagnostic effect. Once the background is removed, a more representative look-up table (see Chapter 12) pertinent to only the range of gray scales in the image and not the background can be assigned to the image. Thus it can improve the visual quality of the images. Third, often in portable CR, it is difficult to examine the patient in an anatomical position aligned with the standard image orientation for reading because of the patient condition. As a result the orientation of the image during reading may need to be adjusted. In film interpretation, it is easy to rotate or flip the film. But in soft copy display, to automatically recognize and make orientation correction of the digital image is not a simple task: sophisticated software programs are needed. These software algorithms often fail if the background of the image is not removed. A background removed image will improve the successful rate of automatic image orientation. And fourth, because background removal is a crucial preprocessing step in computer-aided detection and diagnosis (CAD, CADx). A background-removed image can improve the diagnostic accuracy of CAD algorithms as the cost functions in the algorithms can be assigned to the image only rather than to the image and its background combined.

In the cases of digital fluorography and the film digitizer, the background removal procedure is straight forward. In the former, since the size of the image field is a predetermined parameter, the background can be removed by converting every pixel outside the diameter of the image field to black. In the latter, since the digital image is obtained in a two-step procedure (first a film is obtained, then the film is digitized), the boundaries between the background and the exposed area can be determined interactively by the user, and the corner points may be inputted during the digitizing step.

In the case of CR, background removal is a more complex procedure, since it has to be done automatically during image acquisition or preprocessing time. Automatic removal of CR background is difficult because the algorithm has to recognize different body part contours as well as various collimator sizes and shapes. Since the background distribution in CR images is complex and the removal is an irreversible procedure, it is difficult to achieve a successful high ratio of full background removal and yet ensure that no valid information in the image had been discarded. Background removal is sometimes called a "shutter" in commercial arena. Current methods based on a statistical description of the intensity distribution of the CR background can achieve up to 90% successful rate (Zhang, 1997). Background removal is also being used in digital radiography (to be discussed in the next section) as well as in image display.

3.4 DIGITAL RADIOGRAPHY

3.4.1 Some Disadvantages of the Computed Radiography System

Through the years CR has gradually replaced many conventional screen/film projection radiography procedures, and it has been successfully integrated in PACS operation. The advantages are that it produces a digital image, eliminates the use of films, requires a minimal change in the radiographic procedure room, and the image quality is acceptable for most examinations. However, the technology has certain inherent limitations. First, it requires two separate steps to form a digital image, a laser to release the light energy in the latent image from the IP, and a photomultiplier to convert the light to electronic signals. Second, although the IP is a good image detector, its signal-to-noise ratio and spatial resolution are still not ideal for some specialized radiographic procedures. Third, the IP requires a high intensive light to erase the residue of the latent image before it can be reused. This requirement adds on an extra step in the imaging acquisition operation. Also many IPs are needed during the CR installation just like many screens (cassettes) are required in the screen/film detector system. IP has a limited number of exposure expectancy, is breakable especially in the portable unit, and is expensive to replace. Manufacturers are working diligently for its improvement.

3.4.2 Digital Radiography Image Capture

Over the past five years research laboratories and manufacturers have expended tremendous energy and resources in investigating new digital radiography systems other than CR. The main emphases are to improve the image quality and operation efficiency, and to reduce the cost of projection radiography examination. Digital radiography (DR) is an ideal such candidate. In order to compete with conventional screen/film and CR, a good DR system should:

- have a high detector quantum efficiency (DQE) detector with 2 to 3 or higher line pairs/mm spatial resolution, and a higher signal to noise ratio,
- produce digital images of high quality,
- deliver low dosage to patients,
- produce the digital image within seconds after X-ray exposure,
- comply with industrial standards,
- have an open architecture for connectivity,
- be easy to operate,
- be compact in size, and
- offer competitive cost savings.

Depending on the method used for the X-ray photon conversion, DR can be loosely categorized into direct and indirect image capture methods. In indirect image capture, attenuated X-ray photons are first converted to light photons by the phosphor or the scintillator, from which the light photons are converted to electronic signals to form the DR image. The direct image capture method generates a digital image directly from X-ray photons to electronic signal without going through the light photon conversion process. Figure 3.16 shows the difference between the direct and the indirect digital capture method. The advantage of the direct image capture

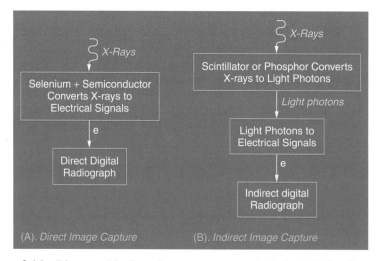

Figure 3.16 Direct and indirect image capture methods in digital radiography.

method is that it eliminates the intermediate step of light photon conversion. The disadvantages are that the engineering involved in direct digital capture is more elaborate, and that it is inherently difficult to use the detector for dynamic image acquisition due to the necessity of recharging the detector after each readout. The indirect capture method uses either the amorphous silicon phosphor or scintillator panels. The direct capture method uses the amorphous selenium panel. It appears that the direct capture method has the advantage over the indirect capture method, since it eliminates the intermediate step of light photon conversion. Recent development in the indirect capture method has been in eliminating active devices in the light photon conversion step, which makes the whole system appeared as if the detector system is direct capturing. The full-field direct digital mammography (FFDDM) to be discussed in the next section belongs to this hybrid digital radiography system.

Two prevailing scanning modes in digital radiography are slot and areal scanning. The digital mammography system discussed in the next section uses the slot-scanning method. Current technology for areal detection mode uses the flat-panel sensors. The flat panel can be one large or several smaller panels put together. The areal scan method has the advantage of being fast in image capture, but it also has two disadvantages, one being the high X-ray scattering. The second is the manufacturing of the large flat panels is technically difficult.

Digital radiography (DR) design is flexible and can be used as an add-on unit in a typical radiography room or a dedicated system. In the dedicated system some design can be used as a table-top unit attached to a C-arm radiographic device for variable angle exam or as an upright unit shown in Figure 3.17.

Figure 3.18*A* illustrates the formation of a DR image (compare with Fig. 3.11 on that of a CR image). Figure 3.18*B* shows an add-on unit in an existing table-top radiographic system. A typical DR unit produces a $2000 \times 2500 \times 12$-bit image instantaneously after the exposure. Figure 3.19 shows the system performance in terms of ESF (edge spread function), LSF (Line spread function), and MTF (modulation transfer function) of a DR unit (see Section 2.5.1) [X. Cao 2000]. In this system the 10% MTF at the center is about 2 lp/mm.

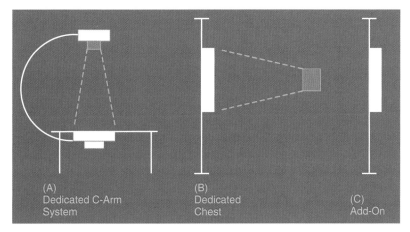

Figure 3.17   Three configurations of digital radiography design. The first two designs include the X-ray unit.

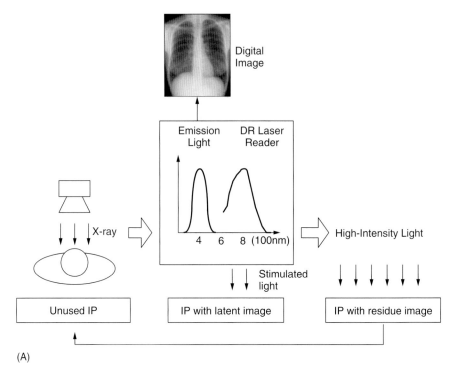

(A)

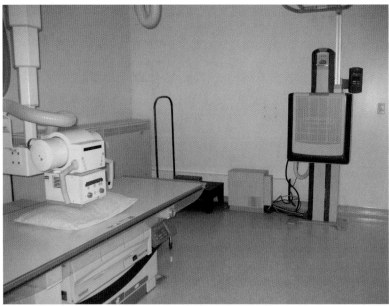

(B)

Figure 3.18   (*A*) Steps in the formation of a digital radiography (DR) image, comparing it with that of a CR image shown in Figure 3.11. (*B*) An add-on DR system utilizing the existing X-ray unit.

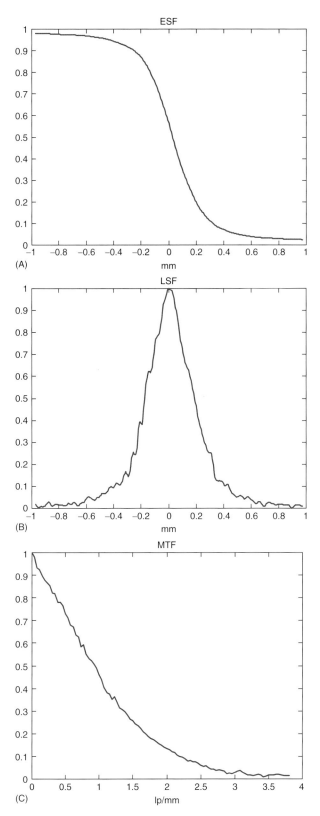

Figure 3.19   The ESF, LSF, and MTF of a digital radiography unit.

3.5 FULL-FIELD DIRECT DIGITAL MAMMOGRAPHY

3.5.1 Screen/Film Cassette and Digital Mammography

Conventional screen/film mammography produces a very high quality mammogram on an 8×10 sq in. film. However, some abnormalities, like calcification, in the mammogram require 50 µm spatial resolution to be recognized. For this reason it is difficult to use CR or a laser film scanner to convert a mammogram to a digital image, hindering the integration of the modality images to PACS. Yet mammography examinations account for about 8% of all diagnostic procedures in a typical radiology department. Over the past 10 years, in the United States as well as world wide, to better women's health has become a major social issue. As a result joint research efforts between academic institutions and private industry, supported by the US National Cancer Institute and Army Medical Research and Development Command, have propelled the development of some very good quality digital mammography systems. Many of these systems are in daily clinical use. In the next section we describe the principle of digital mammography, a very critical component of total digital imaging operation in a hospital.

3.5.2 Slot-Scanning Full-field Direct Digital Mammography

There are two methods of obtaining a full-field direct digital mammogram, one is the imaging plate technology described in Section 3.3, but with higher resolution imaging plate made from different materials with higher quantum efficient detection. The other is the slot-scanning method, which can be a direct or indirect digital radiography system. This section summarizes the hybrid direct slot-scanning method.

The slot-scanning technology modifies the image receptor of a conventional mammography system by using a slot-scanning mechanism and detector system. The slot-scanning mechanism scans a breast by an X-ray fan beam, and the image is recorded by a charged couple device (CCD) camera encompassed in the Bucky antis-catter grid of the mammography unit. Figure 3.20 shows a picture of a full-field direct digital mammography (FFDDM) system; the word "direct" requires some explanations in the following as the system is actually leaning toward a hybrid direct digital radiography system. The X-ray photons emitted from the X-ray tube are shaped by a collimator to become a fan beam. The width of the fan beam covers one dimension of the imaging area (e.g. x-axis) and the fan beam sweeps in the other direction (y-axis). The movement of the detector system is synchronous with the scan of the fan beam. The detector system of the FFDDM shown is composed of a thin phosphor screen directly coupled with four CCD detector arrays via a tapered fiber-optic bundle. Each CCD array is composed of 1100×300 CCD cells. The gap between any two adjacent CCD arrays requires a procedure called "butting" to minimize the loss of pixels. The phosphor screen converts the penetrated X-ray photons (i.e., the latent image) to light photons. The light photons pass through the fiber-optic bundle, reach the CCD cells, and then are transformed to electronic signals. The more light photons received by each CCD cell, the larger is the signal that is transformed. The electronic signals are quantized by an analog-to-digital converter to create a digital image. Finally, the image pixels travel through a data channel to the system memory of the FFDDM acquisition computer. Although there are several energy conversion steps, the whole system does not require active devices to perform the energy conversions.

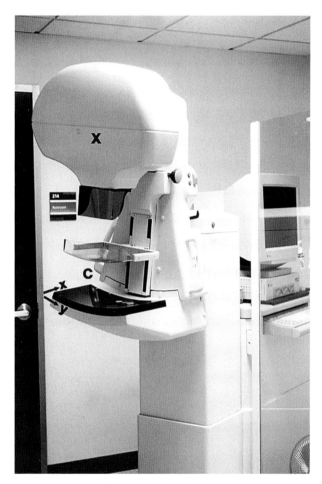

Figure 3.20   A slot-scanning digital mammography system. The slot with the 300-pixel width covers the x-axis (4400 pixels). The X-ray beam sweeps (arrow) in the y direction, producing over 5500 pixels. X: X-ray and collimator housing; C: breast compressor.

Figure 3.21 left shows a 4K × 5K × 12-bit digital mammogram obtained with the system shown in Figure 3.20, and Figure 3.21 (right) depicts a localized smaller size digital mammogram for biopsy purpose. A standard screening mammography examination requires four images, two for each breast (the cranio-caudal [CC] and mediolateral oblique [MLO] views) producing a total of 160 Mbytes of image data.

3.6 DIGITAL RADIOGRAPHY AND PACS

3.6.1 Integration of Digital Radiography with PACS

A major advantage of DR is that it can minimize the number of steps in patient workflow, which translates to a better healthcare delivery system. To fully utilize this capability, DR should be integrated with the PACS or teleradiology operation.

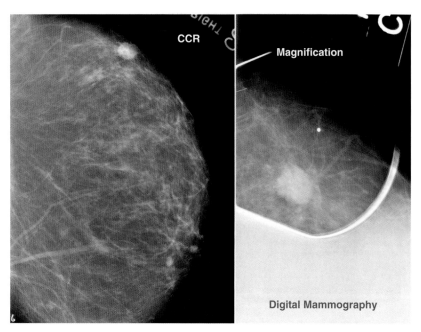

Figure 3.21 A 4K × 5K × 12-bit CCR view digital mammogram shown on a 2K × 2.5K monitor (left). A localized digital mammogram for needle biopsy verification (right).

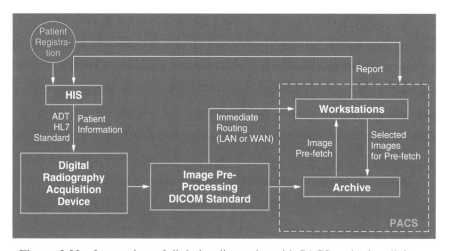

Figure 3.22 Integration of digital radiography with PACS and teleradiology.

The main criterion of an effective integration is to have the DR images available for display as soon as they are captured. Figure 3.22 shows a method of integration.

Following Figure 3.22, while the DR image is being generated, the hospital information system (HIS) transmits ADT (admission, discharge, and transfer) information in the HL7 standard (see Chapter 9) to the PACS archive. From there, it triggers the prefetch function to retrieve relevant images/data from the patient historical examinations and appends them to the patient folder in the archive. The folder is forwarded to the workstations after the examination. If the network used is local area network (LAN), the integration is with PACS. If wide area network (WAN) is used, the integration is with teleradiology.

After the DR image is available from the imaging system, the DICOM (digital imaging and communication in medicine; see Chapter 9) standard should be used for system integration. Certain image preprocessing is performed to enhance its visual quality. For example, in digital mammography, preprocessing functions include the segmentation of the breast from the background, and the determination of the ranges of pixel value of various breast tissues for automatic window and level adjustment. In digital radiography, removal the background in the image due to X-ray collimation (see Section 3.3.4), along with automatic lookup table generation for various parts of the anatomical structure, are crucial.

After preprocessing, the image is routed immediately to proper workstations pertinent to the clinical applications; from there the image is appended to the patient folder which has already been forwarded by the archive. The current DR image and historical images can be displayed simultaneously at the workstations for comparison. The current image with the patient folder is also sent back to PACS for long-term archive.

Another critical component in the DR system integration is the display workstation. The workstation should be able to display DR images with the highest quality possible. The image display time should be within several seconds and with pre- and instantaneous- window and level adjustments. The flat-panel LCD (liquid crystal display) should be used because of its excellent display quality, high brightness, lightweight and small size, and easy-to-tilt angle to accommodate the viewing environment (see Chapter 12).

3.6.2 Applications of Digital Radiography in Clinical Environment

Outpatient clinic, emergency room, and ambulatory care clinical environment are perfect for DR applications. Figure 3.23 shows a scenario of patient workflow in a filmless outpatient clinic.

1. Patient registers, changes garments, queues up for the examination, walks to the DR unit, get x-rayed, changes back to street clothes, walks to the assigned physician room where the DR images are already available for viewing.
2. In the background, while the patient registers, HIS sends the patient's information to the PACS outpatient server.
3. The server retrieves relevant historical images, waits until the DR images are ready, appends new images to the patient image folder.
4. The server forwards the patient's image folder to the assigned physician's room (Rm 1, Rm 2), where images are displayed automatically when the patient arrives.
5. Images can also be sent to the off-site expert center through teleradiology for diagnosis.

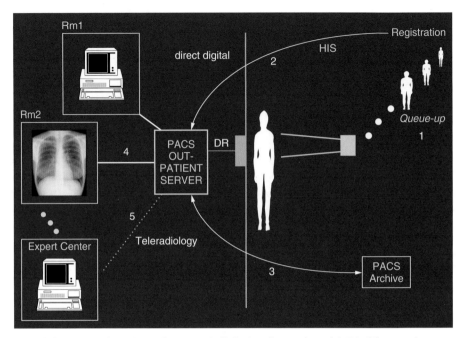

Figure 3.23 Workflow in an integrated digital radiography with PACS outpatient operation environment.

This patient workflow is efficient and cost-effective because the operation is entirely automatic, filmless, and paperless. It eliminates all human intervention, except during the X-ray procedure. We will revisit this scenario in later chapters.

3.7 NUCLEAR MEDICINE IMAGING

3.7.1 Principles of Nuclear Medicine Scanning

The nuclear imaging (NM) technique can be used to generate both 2-D and 3-D images. In 2-D imaging, it produces a projection image. In 3-D imaging, the combined nuclear imaging and tomography techniques can generate an emission CT (ECT). This section will discuss 2-D NM imaging, an ECT will be presented in Chapter 4. The formation of a NM image is by administering a radiopharmaceutical agent that can be used to differentiate between a normal and an abnormal physiological process. A radiopharmaceutical agent consists of a tracer substance and a radionuclide for highlighting the tracer's position. The tracer typically consists of a molecule that resembles a constituent of the tissue of interest, a colloidal substance that is taken up by reticuloendothelial cells, for example, or a capillary blocking agent. A gamma camera (see the next section) is then used to obtain an image of the distribution of the radioactivity in an organ.

The gamma emitter is chosen on the basis of its specific activity, half-life, energy spectrum, and ability to bond with the desired tracer molecule. Its radionuclide half-life is important because, in general, one would like to perform scans in the shortest possible time while still accumulating sufficient statistically meaningful nuclear decay counts. Further a reasonably short half-life minimizes the radiation dose to the patient. The energy spectrum of the isotope is important because if the energy emitted is too low, the radiation will be severely attenuated when passing through the body, so the photon count statistics will be poor or scan times unacceptably long. If the energy is too high, there may not be enough photoelectric interaction, so absorption in the detector crystal will be low. Typical isotopes used in nuclear medicine have γ-ray emission energies of 100 to 400 keV.

3.7.2 The Gamma Camera and Associated Imaging System

As with most imaging systems, a nuclear medicine imager (e.g., a gamma camera) contains subsystems for data acquisition, data processing, data display, and data archiving. A computer is used to control the flow of data and coordinate these subsystems into a functional unit. The operator interactively communicates with the computer control via graphical user interface (GUI) or predefined push buttons on the system's control paddle. Figure 3.24 shows a schematic of a generic nuclear medicine gamma camera. Typical matrix sizes of nuclear medicine image are 64 × 64, 128 × 128 or 256 × 256 by 8 to 12 bits, with a maximum of 30 frames per second in cardiac imaging. In gated cardiac mode, useful parameter values such as ejection fraction and stroke volume can be calculated. In addition the frames of a cardiac cycle can be displayed consecutively and rapidly in cine fashion to evaluate heart wall motion. Some older nuclear imager do not have the DICOM standard (see Chapter 9). Figure 3.24*B* shows a generic NM bone scan image.

3.8 2-D ULTRASOUND IMAGING

Ultrasound imaging is used in many medical specialties including obstetrics, gynecology, pediatrics, ophthalmology, mammography, abdominal imaging, and cardiology, as well as in imaging smaller organs such as the thyroid, prostate, and testicles, and

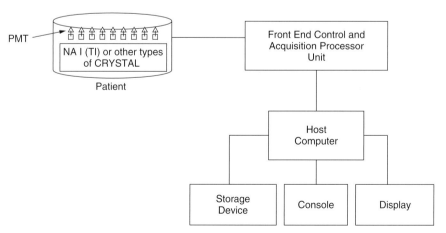

Figure 3.24   Schematic of a general gamma camera used in nuclear medicine imaging. (See Figure 4.13 for some PET (position emission tomograph) images).

recently in intravascular ultrasound endoscopy (see Section 3.9). Its wide acceptance is partially due to its noninvasiveness, its use of non-ionizing radiation, and its lower equipment and procedural costs compared with XCT and MRI. An ultrasound examination is often used as the first step in attempting to diagnose a possible ailment due to its noninvasive nature. Recently developed handheld portable US scanners are popular for applications in emergency situations.

3.8.1 Principles of B-Mode Ultrasound Scanning

B-mode ultrasound imaging is used to generate a sectional view of an area of interest of the patient by detecting the amplitudes of acoustical reflections (echoes) occur at the interfaces of tissues of different acoustical properties.

Pulses of high-frequency ultrasonic wave from a transducer are introduced into the structures of interest in the body by pressing it against the skin. A coupling gel is used to provide efficient transfer of acoustical energy into the body. The acoustical wave propagates through the body tissues, and its radiation pattern will demonstrate high directivity in the near field or Fresnel zone close to the body surface (see Fig. 3.25), and begin to diverge in the far field or Fraunhoffer zone. The range of the near and far fields is determined mainly by the wavelength λ of the sonic waves used and the diameter of the transducer. In general, it is preferable to image objects that are within the Fresnel zone, where the lateral resolving power is better.

The fate of the acoustical wave is dependent on the acoustical properties of the medium in which the wave is propagating. The speed of the wave in media depends on the elasticity and density of the material and affects the degree of refraction (deviation from a straight path) that occurs at a boundary between tissues. The characteristic impedance of the material, which determines the degree of reflection

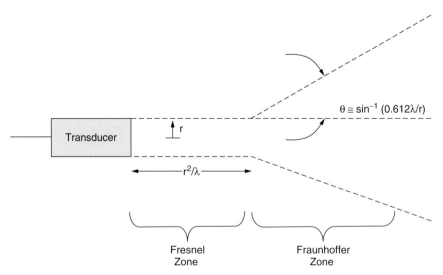

Figure 3.25 Principle of 2-D ultrasound imaging. The ultrasound waves produced by a transducer made of piezoelectric material penetrate the tissues of interest, the reflection waves (echoes) from boundaries between different tissue types received by the transducer form a B-mode ultrasound image. λ: wavelength of the sound wave used.

that occurs when a wave is incident at a boundary, is dependent on the material's density and the speed of sound in the material. The larger the difference between the acoustic impedances of two materials forming a boundary, the greater will be the strength of the reflected wave.

3.8.2 System Block Diagram and Operational Procedure

Figure 3.26 shows a general block diagram of a typical B-mode ultrasound scanner. It is made up of a transducer, a high-voltage pulse generator, a transmitter circuit, a receiver circuit with time gain compensation (TGC), a mechanical scanning arm with position encoders, a digital scan converter (DSC), and a video display monitor.

Acoustical waves are generated by applying a high-voltage pulse to a piezoelectric crystal. A longitudinal pressure sonic wave results, and the rate at which its pulses are supplied by the transmitter circuit to the transducer, as determined by a transmission clock, is called the pulse repetition frequency (PRF). Typical PRF values range from 0.5 to 2.5 kHz. The frequency of the acoustic wave, which is determined by the thickness of the piezoelectric crystal, may range from 1 to 15 MHz. The transducer can serve as an acoustic transmitter as well as a receiver, since mechanical pressure waves interacting with the crystal will result in the creation of an electrical signal.

Received echo amplitude pulses, which eventually form an ultrasound image, are transferred into electrical signals by the transducer. A radio frequency receiver circuit then amplifies and demodulates the signal. The receiver circuit, a crucial element in an ultrasound scanner, must have a huge dynamic range (30–40 dB) to be able to

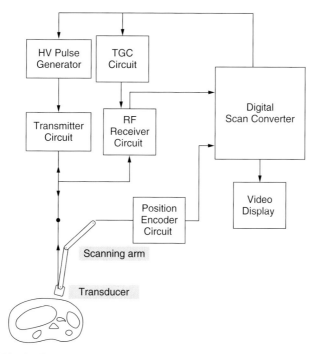

Figure 3.26   Block diagram of a B-mode ultrasound scanner system. TGC: Time gain compensation; RF: radio frequency; HV: high voltage.

detect the wide range of reflected signals, which are typically 1 to 2 volts at interfaces near the surface and microvolts at deeper structures. In addition the receiver must introduce little noise and have a wide amplification bandwidth.

The time gain compensator circuit allows the ultrasound user to interactively amplify the echoed signal according to its depth of origin. This feature compensate for the higher attenuation of the signal seen in the echoes originating from deeper interfaces and results in a more uniform image (i.e., interfaces are not darker closer to the body surface on the image display solely on the basis of being closer to the transducer). The operator is able to obtain the best possible image by controlling the amount of gain at a particular depth.

The output of the receiver is fed into the digital scan converter (DSC) and used to determine the depth (z direction) at which the echo occurred. The depth at which the echo originated is calculated by determining the time that the echo takes to return to the transducer. The depth of the reflector can be obtained because time and depth are related, and the depth is half the time interval from the transmission of the signal pulse to signal return times the velocity of sound in the traversal medium.

The encoding of the x and y positions of the face of the transducer and angular orientation of the transducer with respect to the normal of the scanning surface is determined by the scanning arm position encoder circuit. In 2-D US, the scanning arm is restricted to the movement in one linear direction at a time. The arm contains four potentiometers whose resistance will correspond to the x and y positions and cosine and sine directions (with angle with respect to the normal of the body surface) of the transducer.

For example, if the transducer is moved in the y direction while keeping x and the angle of rotation fixed, then only the Y potentiometer will change its resistance. Position encoders on the arm will generate signals proportional to the position of the transducer and the direction of the ultrasound beam. The x, y, and z data are fed into the digital scan converter to generate the x, y position, and the z depth that will permit the echo strength signals to be stored in the appropriate memory locations.

The digital scan converter performs A/D conversions of data, data preprocessing, pixel generation, image storage, data post processing, and image display. The analog echo signals from the receiver circuit are digitized by an analog-to-digital converter in the DSC, typically to 8 to 12 bits (256–4096 gray levels). Fast A/D converters are normally used because most ultrasound echo signals have a wide bandwidth, and the sampling frequency should be at least twice the highest frequency of interest in the image. Typical A/D sampling rates range from 10 to 20 MHz. The DSC image memory is normally $512 \times 512 \times 8$ bits, for a color Doppler US image, it can be $512 \times 512 \times 24$ bits (see Section 3.8.4).

The data may be preprocessed to enhance the visual display of the data and to match the dynamic range of the subsequent hardware components. Echo signals are typically rescaled, and often nonlinear (e.g., logarithmic) circuits are used to emphasize and de-emphasize certain echo amplitudes.

3.8.3 Sampling Modes and Image Display

Three different sampling modes are available on most ultrasound units: the *survey mode*, in which the data stored in memory is continually updated and displayed, *the static mode*, in which only maximum US echo signals (values) during a scanning session are stored and displayed, and an *averaging mode*, in which the average of all scans for a particular scan location are stored and displayed.

Once stored in memory, the digital data are subjected to postprocessing operations of several types. These can be categorized according to changes in the gray level display of the stored image, temporal smoothing of the data, or spatial operations. Gray scale mean and windowing and nonlinear gray scale transformations are common.

Image display is performed by a video processor and controller unit that can quickly access the image memory and modulate an electron beam to show the image on a video monitor. The digital scan converter allows for echo data to be read continuously from the fast access image memory.

3.8.4 Color Doppler Ultrasound Imaging

Ultrasound scanning using Doppler principle can detect the movement of blood inside vessels. In particular, it can detect whether the blood is moving away or toward the scanning plane. When several blood vessels are in the scanning plane, it is advantageous to use different colors to represent the blood flow direction and speed with respect to the stationary anatomical structures. Thus colors coupling with the gray scale ultrasound image results in a duplex Doppler ultrasound image. This coupling permits simultaneously imaging of anatomical structures as well as characterization of circulatory physiology from known reference planes within the body. The resulting image is called color Doppler or color-flow imaging. A color Doppler image needs $512 \times 512 \times 24$ bits. Figure 3.27 shows a color Doppler US blood flow image demonstrating pulmonary vein inflow convergent.

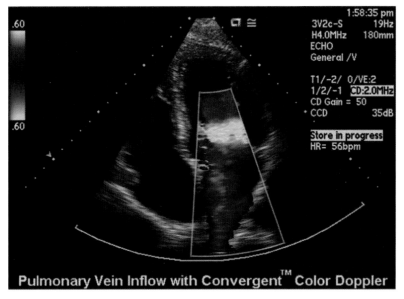

Figure 3.27   Color Doppler ultrasound of blood flow showing convergent pulmonary vein inflow. (Courtesy of Siemens Medical Imaging Systems) http://www.siemens-medical.com/webapp/wcs/stores/servlet/PSProductImageDisplay?productId=17966&storeId=10001&langId=-1&catalogId=-1&catTree=100001,12805,12761*559299136.

3.8.5 Cine Loop Ultrasound Imaging

One advantage of ultrasound imaging over other imaging modalities is its noninvasive nature, which permits the accumulation of ultrasound images continuously through time without adverse effects to the patient. Such images can be played back in a cine loop, which can reveal the dynamic motion of a body organ, for example, the heart beat (see also Section 4.3.3 on multislice CT). Several seconds of cine loop ultrasound images can produce a very large image file. For example, a 10 s series of color Doppler cine loop ultrasound images will yield $(10 \times 30) \times 0.75 \times 10^6$ bytes ($= 225$ Mbyte) of image information. In general, unless the study is related to dynamic movement like the cardiac motion, very seldom is the complete cine loop archived. The radiologist or clinician in charge previews all images and discards most but the most relevant few for the patient record.

3.9 2-D LIGHT IMAGING

Light imaging is to use various light sources to generate images for diagnosis or image-guided treatment. Two common use light images for medical applications are microscopy and endoscopy, both generate real color images. These two modalities are quite different in the nature of the method used in image generation; the former is in microscopic and the latter in anatomical scale. However, after the light image is obtained, they use a similar digital chain for image preprocessing, analysis, display, and archive. Microscopic image capture is more involved in instrumentation because it could include various types of microscope, namely among these fluorescence and confocal, and the skill of using them, whereas endoscopy only involves a cannula, a light source with a light guide assembly, and a CCD camera. We first describe the digital chain and the basics of color imaging.

3.9.1 The Digital Chain

After the light source creates an image and is captured by a CCD camera, the image is transmitted to a digital chain. The digital chain consists of an A/D converter, image memory, computer, storage, and display shown in Figure 3.28, which is identical to that of a digital fluorography shown in Figure 3.6. The hardware components' special specifications may not be identical due to the different nature of image capture, but their functions are the same. For example, the method of capturing a color image is different from that of a gray scale image. The next section describes the basic of color image and color memories in both microscopy and endoscopy.

3.9.2 Color Image and Color Memory

Light images are mostly colored. In the digitization process the image is digitized three times with a red, blue, and green filter, in three separate but consecutive steps. The three color-filtered images are then stored in three corresponding image memories—red, blue, and green, each of which with eight bits. Thus a true color image has 24 bits/pixel. The computer treats the content of the three image memories as individual microscopic images and processes them separately. The real color image can be displayed back on a color monitor from these three memories with a

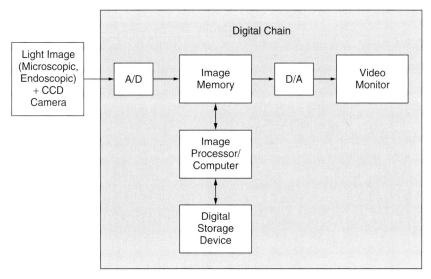

Figure 3.28 Block diagram showing the instrumentation of a digital light imaging system. The digital chain is inside the enclosed rectangle at the right, which is almost identical to that shown in Figure 3.6, except for the input component specifications.

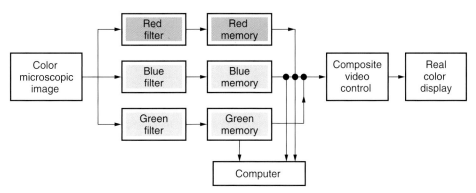

Figure 3.29 Color image processing block diagram. Red, blue, and green filters are used to filter the image before digitization. The three digitized, filtered images are stored in the red, blue, and green memories, respectively. The real color image can be displayed back on the color monitor from these three memories through the composite video control.

color composite video control. Figure 3.29 shows the block diagram of a true color imaging processing block diagram. Figure 3.30 shows a case of two diabetic mellitus retinopathy (DMR) images from an ophthalmoscope attached to a CCD camera during an eye examination.

3.9.3 2-D Microscopic Image

3.9.3.1 Instrumentation   Digital microscopy is used to extract sectional quantitative information from biomedical microscopic slides. A digital microscopic imaging system consists of the following components:

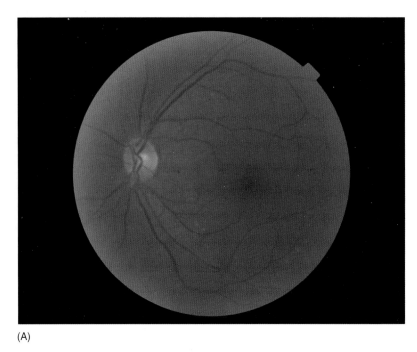

(A)

(B)

Figure 3.30 Two color images showing diabetic mellitus retinopathy (DMR) from an ophthalmoscope attached to a CCD camera during an eye examination. (*A*) No DMR; (*B*) severe DMR with prior panretinal photocoagulaton. (Courtesy of Prof. M Yap, Hong Kong Polytechnic U)

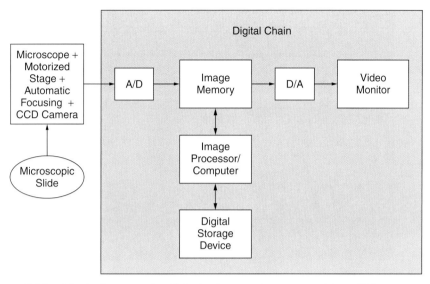

Figure 3.31 Block diagram of a digital microscopic system with a CCD camera connected to the digital chain. Compare to Figure 3.28.

- A compound, or other types, microscope with proper illumination for specimen input
- A motorized stage assembly and an automatic focusing device
- A CCD camera for scanning microscopic slide
- A digital chain

The motorized stage assembly and the automatic focusing device are for effective quantitative analysis. Figure 3.31 shows the block diagram of the instrumentation, and Figure 3.32*A* and *B* illustrate a digital microscopic system which can be used for tele-microscopy applications (see Chapter 15).

3.9.3.2 Resolution   The resolution of a microscope is defined as the minimum distance between two objects in the specimen which can be resolved by the microscope. Three factors determine the resolution of a microscope:

1. The angle subtended by the object of interest in the specimen and the objective lens: the larger the angle, the higher the resolution.
2. The medium between the objective lens and the cover slip of the glass slide: the higher the refractive index of the medium, the higher the resolution.
3. The wavelength of light employed: the shorter the wavelength, the higher the resolution. A narrow wavelength light source also yields better resolution.

These three factors can be combined into a single equation (Ernst Abbe 1840–1905):

$$D = \frac{\lambda}{2(NA)} = \frac{\lambda}{2n \sin \theta} \tag{3.5}$$

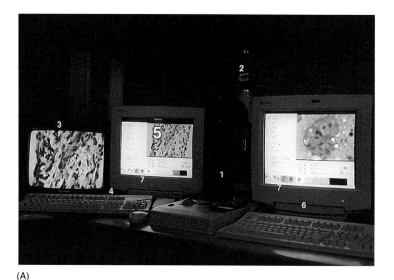

(A)

(B)

Figure 3.32 A digital tele-microscopic system. (*A*, left): Image acquisition workstation: automatic microscope (1), CCD camera (2), video monitor (3), computer with an A/D converter attached to the CCD, image memory, and a database to manage the patient image file (4), the video monitor (3) showing a captured image from the microscope being digitized and shown on the workstation monitor (5). (*A*, right) Remote diagnostic workstation (6). Thumb nail images at the bottom of both workstations are the images sent to the diagnostic workstation (7) from the acquisition workstation (7). (*B*) Closeup of the acquisition workstation. Pertinent data related to the exam are shown in various windows. Icons on the bottom right (8) are six simple click-and-play functions: transmit, display, exit, patient information, video capture, digitize, and store. Six images had been captured and stored shown in the lower icons. The last captured image (9) is displayed on the workstation monitor. (Prototype telemicroscopic imaging system at the Laboratory for Radiological Informatic Lab, UCSF. Courtesy of Drs. S. Atwater, T. Hamill, and H. Sanchez [images], and Nikon Res. Corp. and Mitra Imag. Inc. [equipment])

where D is the distance between two objects in the specimen that can be resolved (a small D means that the imaging system has the resolution power to separate two very close objects), λ is the wavelength of the light employed, n is the refractive index of the medium, θ is the half-angle subtended by the object at the objective lens, and NA is the numerical aperture commonly used for defining the resolution (the larger the NA, the higher the resolution).

Therefore, to obtain a higher resolution for a microscopic image, use an oil immersion lens (large n) with a large angular aperture and select a shorter wavelength light source for illumination.

3.9.3.3 Contrast
Contrast is the ability to differentiate various components in the specimen with different intensity levels. Black-and-white contrast is equivalent to the range of the gray scale (the larger the range, the better the contrast). Color contrast is an important parameter in microscopic image processing; in order to bring out the color contrast from the image, various color filters may be used with adjusted illumination.

It is clear that the spatial and density resolutions of a digital image are determined by the resolution and contrast of a microscope.

3.9.3.4 Motorized Stage Assembly
The motorized stage assembly allows rapid screening and locating the exact position of objects of interest for subsequent detailed analysis. The motorized stage assembly consists of a high precision x-y stage with a specially designed holder for the slide to minimize the vibration due to the movement of the stage. Two stepping motors are used for driving the stage in the x and the y directions. A typical motor step is about 2.5 µm with an accuracy and repeatability to within ± 1.25 µm. The motors can move the stage in either direction with a nominal speed of 650 step per second, or 0.1625 cm/s, or better. The two stepping motors can either be controlled manually or automatically by the computer.

3.9.3.5 Automatic Focusing
Automatic focusing ensures that the microscope is focusing after the stepping motors move the stage from one field to another. It is essential to have the microscope in focus before the CCD camera starts to scan.

Among several methods for automatic focusing are the use of a third stepping motor in the z direction, an air pump, and a confocal microscope. The first method is to use a z-direction motor that moves the stage up and down with respect to the objective lens. The z movements are nested in larger $+z$ and $-z$ values initially and gradually to smaller $+z$ and $-z$ values. After each movement a scan of the specimen is made through the microscope and certain optical parameters are derived from the scan. A focused image is defined if these optical parameters are within certain threshold values. The disadvantage of this method is that the focusing process is slow since the nesting movements requires computer processing time.

Using an air pump for automatic focusing is based on the assumption that in order to have automatic focusing, the specimen lying on the upper surface of the glass slide must be on a perfect horizontal plane with respect to the objective lens all the time. The glass slide is not of uniform thickness, however, and when it rests on the horizontal stage, the lower surface of the slide will form a horizontal plane with respect to the object, but the upper surface will not, contributing to the imperfect focus of the slide. If an air pump is used to create a vacuum from above such that the upper surface of the slide is suctioned from the above forming a perfect horizontal plane with respective to the objective, then the slide will be focused all the time. Using an air pump for automatic focusing does not require additional time during operation, but it does require precision machinery.

In a fluorescence confocal microscope, it uses a narrow wavelength light like a laser beam to focus, excite, and scan fluorescence objects of interest point by point to obtain depth discrimination from other objects. It uses a confocal pinhole to reject none-focused fluorescence that originates outside the plane of focus by using a "confocal" pinhole. Confocal microscope can be used to obtain 3-D images, as will be discussed in the next chapter.

3.9.4 2-D Endoscopic Imaging

An endoscopic examination is a visual inspection of the inside of the body conducted by inserting an endoscopic tube with a light source and light guides into the lumen. The examiner can look into the light guides through an eyepiece from outside of the apparatus or use a CCD camera to capture real-time endoscopic images displayed

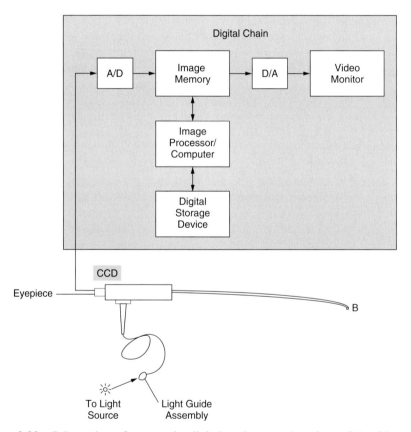

Figure 3.33 Schematics of a generic digital endoscope (not in scale) with a CCD camera; the digital chain and color digitization are standard as shown in Figures 3.28 and 3.31.

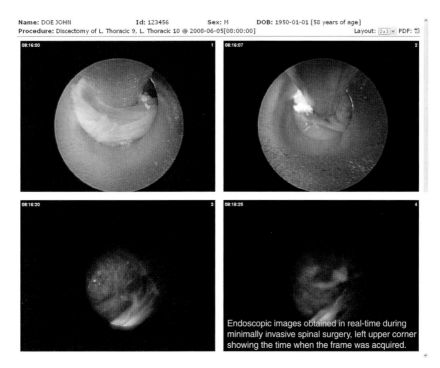

Name: DOE JOHN   Id: 123456   Sex: M   DOB: 1950-01-01 [58 years of age]
Procedure: Discectomy of L. Thoracic 9, L. Thoracic 10 @ 2008-06-05[08:00:00]   Layout: 2x3 ▾ PDF: ⎙

Endoscopic images obtained in real-time during minimally invasive spinal surgery, left upper corner showing the time when the frame was acquired.

Figure 3.34   Endoscopic images of thoracic vertebrae 9 and 10 acquired in real time during image-guided minimally invasive spinal surgery. (Courtesy of Dr. J Chiu, California Spine Institute)

on a LCD monitor to make proper diagnosis. If the insertion is, for example, in the throat, tracheobronchial, upper gastrointestinal, colon, and rectum, the procedure is called laryngoscope, bronchoscope, gastro scope, colonoscopy, and sigmoid scope, respectively. If a digital chain is attached to the light guide so that the image can be seen on a display system, and be archived in a storage device, the system is call digital endoscope. The digital chain consists of a CCD camera, A/D converter, image memory, computer, display, and endoscopic analysis software. The hardware components were described in Section 3.2.2 and shown in Figure 3.28, although their specifications may be different due to the method of image capture. Figure 3.33 illustrates the schematic of a generic digital endoscopic system. Figure 3.34 shows a sequence of four real-time color endoscopic images of thoracic vertebrae 9 and 10 under minimally invasive spinal surgery.

References

Cao X, Huang HK. Current status and future advances of digital radiography and PACS. *IEEE Eng Med Bio* 19(5): 80–8; 2000.

Huang HK, Lou SL. Telemammography: a technical overview. *RSNA Categorical Course Breast Imag* 273–281; 1999.

Zhang J, Huang HK. Automatic background recognition and removal (ABRR) of computed radiography images. *IEEE Trans Med Imag* 16(6): 762–71; 1997.

CHAPTER 4

Three-Dimensional Medical Imaging

Most three-dimensional (3-D) Medical images are generated by using image reconstruction, or tomography, techniques with data from projections that are collected from detectors coupled with various energy sources (Fig. 4.1). These energies can be from X-ray, single-photon emission, positron emission, ultrasound, nuclear magnetic resonance (MR), and light photon. The image so formed is called X-ray-computed tomography (CT, or XCT), single-photon emission tomography (SPECT), positron emission tomography (PET), 3-D ultrasound (3-D US), magnetic resonance imaging (MRI), or 3-D light imaging, respectively. If the projections are 1-D (See Fig. 4.2, left, (Θ)), then the image formed is a 2-D sectional image, $f(x, y)$. A collection of combined multiple sectional images becomes a 3-D image volume. If the projections are 2-D, for example (see Fig. 4.5, (Θ, z)), where z is the body axis, then the reconstruction result will be a fully 3-D image volume.

Recent advances in these techniques produce very large 3-D image volume data. It is not unusual to have hundreds and even thousands of CT or MR images in one examination. Archiving, transmission, display, and management of these large data volume sets become a technical challenge. Refer to Chapter 2, Table 2.1, for the sizes and number of images per examination of these sectional and 3-D imaging modalities.

Since most sectional images, like MRI and CT, are generated based on image reconstruction from projections, we first summarize in Section 4.1 the 2-D Fourier projection theorem, algebraic reconstruction, and filtered back-projection methods with simple numerical examples; followed by Section 4.2, the concept of image reconstruction from 3-D data set, before the discussion of various imaging modalities.

Sections 4.3, 4.4, 4.5, 4.6, 4.7, and 4.8 present various 3-D imaging modalities including CT, SPECT, PET, US, MRI, and light imaging. The last Section 4.9 is on 3-D small animals imaging.

4.1 2-D IMAGE RECONSTRUCTION FROM 1-D PROJECTIONS

4.1.1 The 2-D Fourier Projection Theorem

Let us start with 2-D image reconstruction. Let $f(x, y)$ be a two-dimensional (2-D) cross-sectional image of a three-dimensional object. The image reconstruction theorem states that $f(x, y)$ can be reconstructed from the cross-sectional

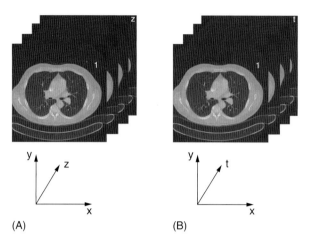

Figure 4.1   Two 3-D image coordinate systems. (*A*) A 3-D spatial image set with z as the third dimension. Images from 1 to z show the anatomical changes of the cross-sectional chest (*B*) A 3-D temporal image set with t (time) as the third dimension. Images from 1 to t show the same anatomy as image 1, the difference would be, for example, the flow of the contrast media injected to the patient from time 1 to t.

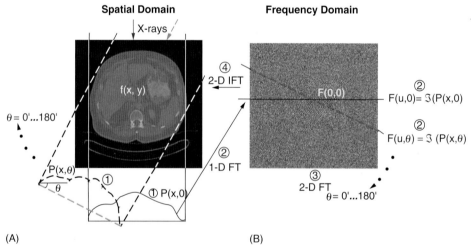

Figure 4.2   Principle of the Fourier projection theorem for image reconstruction from projections. $f(x, y)$ is the image to be reconstructed, $F(0, 0)$ is at the center of the 2-D FT; low-frequency components are located at the center region, and high-frequency components are at periphery. $P(x, \theta)$: X-rays projection at angle θ (green), x is the distance from left to right of the projection. $F(u, \theta)$: 1-D Fourier transform of $P(x, \theta)$; red and green are corresponding projections in the spatial domain, and its 1-D Fourier transforms (1-DF) in the frequency domain, respectively. IFT: inverse Fourier transform.

one-dimensional projections. In general, 180 different projections in one degree increments are necessary to produce an image with satisfactory quality, and the reconstruction with more projections always results to a better quality image.

Mathematically the image reconstruction theorem can be described with the help of the Fourier transform (FT) discussed in Section 2.4. Let $f(x, y)$ represent the two-dimensional image to be reconstructed, and let $p(x)$ be the one-dimensional projection of $f(x, y)$ onto the horizontal x-axis, which can be measured experimentally (see Fig. 4.2, left, for the zero-degree projection). In the case of X-ray CT, we can consider $p(x)$ as the total linear attenuation of tissues transverses by a collimated X-ray beam at location x. Then

$$p(x, 0) = \int_{-\infty}^{+\infty} f(x, y) dy \tag{4.1}$$

The 1-D Fourier transform, $P(u)$, of $p(x)$ has the form

$$P(u) = \int_{-\infty}^{+\infty} \left(\int_{-\infty}^{+\infty} f(x, y) dy \right) \exp(-i2\pi ux) dx \tag{4.2}$$

where u is the frequency parameter. Equations (4.1) and (4.2) imply that the 1-D Fourier transform of a one-dimensional projection of a two-dimensional image is identical to the corresponding central section of the two-dimensional Fourier transform of the object. For example, the two-dimensional image can be a transverse (cross) sectional X-ray image of the body, and the one-dimensional projections can be the X-ray attenuation profiles (projection) of the same section obtained from a linear X-ray scan at certain angles. If 180 projections at one degree increments (Fig. 4.2, left) are accumulated and their 1-D FTs performed (Fig. 4.2, right), each of these 180 1-D Fourier transform represents a corresponding central line of the two-dimensional Fourier transform of the X-ray cross-sectional image. The collection of all these 180 1-D Fourier transform is the 2-D Fourier transform of $f(x, y)$.

The steps of a 2-D image reconstruction from its 1-D projections shown in Figure 4.2 are as follows:

1. Obtain 180 1-D projections of $f(x, y)$, $p(x, \theta)$ where $\theta = 1, \ldots, 180$.
2. Perform the FT on each 1-D projection.
3. Arrange all these 1-D FTs according to their corresponding angles in the frequency domain. The result is the 2-D FT of $f(x, y)$
4. Perform the 2-D IFT, Inverse of the 2-D FT, of step 3, to obtain $f(x, y)$

The Fourier projection theorem forms the basis of tomographic image reconstruction. Other methods to reconstruct a 2-D image from its projections are discussed later in this section. We emphasize that the reconstructed image from projections is not always exact; it is only an approximation of the original image. A different reconstruction method will give a slightly different version of the original image. Since all these methods require extensive computation, specially designed image reconstruction hardware is normally used to implement the algorithm. The term "computerized (computed) tomography" (CT) is often used to represent that the image is obtained from its projections using a reconstruction method. If the 1-D projections are obtained from X-ray transmission (attenuation) profiles, the procedure is called X-ray CT; from single photon γ-ray emission, positron emission, or ultrasound signals, they are called SPECT, PET, 3-D US, respectively. In the following subsections, we present the algebraic and filtered back-projection methods illustrated with simple numerical examples.

4.1.2 Algebraic Reconstruction Method

The algebraic reconstruction method is often used for the reconstruction of images from an incomplete number of projections (i.e., <180°). We use a numerical example to illustrate the method.

Let $f(x, y)$ be a 2 × 2 image with the following pixel values:

$$f(x, y) = \begin{array}{|c|c|} \hline 1 & 2 \\ \hline 3 & 4 \\ \hline \end{array}$$

The four projections of this image are as follows:

$\quad$ 0° projection $\quad$ 4, 6
$\quad$ 45° projection $\quad$ 5 (1 and 4 are ignored for simplicity)
$\quad$ 90° projection $\quad$ 3, 7
$\quad$ 135° projection $\quad$ 5 (3 and 2 are ignored for simplicity)

Combining this information, one obtains:

0° projections:

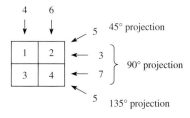

The problem definition is to reconstruct the 2 × 2 image $f(x, y)$, which is unknown, from these four given projections obtained from direct measurements. The algebraic reconstruction of the 2 × 2 image from these four known projections proceeds stepwise as follows:

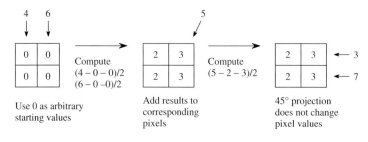

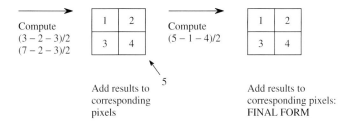

From the last step it is seen that the result is an exact reconstruction (a pure chance) of the original 2×2 image $f(x, y)$. It requires only four projections because $f(x, y)$ is a 2×2 image. For a 512×512 image, it will require over 180 projections, each with sufficient data points in the projection, to render a good quality image.

4.1.3 The Filtered (Convolution) Back-projection Method

The filtered back-projection method requires two components, the back-projection algorithm, and the selection of a filter to modify the projection data. The selection of a proper filter for a given anatomical region is the key in obtaining a good reconstruction from filtered (convolution) back-projection method. This is the method of choice for almost all X-ray CT scanners.

4.1.3.1 A Numerical Example   Consider the same example introduced in the last section. We now wish to reconstruct the 2×2 matrix $f(x, y)$ from its four known projections using the filtered back-projection method. The procedure is to first select a filter function, convolve it with each projection, and then back-project the convoluted data to form an image.

For this example, the filter function $(-1/2, 1, -1/2)$ is selected. This means that when each projection is convolving with this filter function, the data point of the projection under consideration will be multiplied by 1, and both points one pixel away from the data point under consideration will be multiplied by $-1/2$. Thus, when the projection [4, 6] is convolved with $(-1/2, 1, -1/2)$, the result is $(-2, 1, 4, -3)$, since

$$+ \frac{\begin{array}{rrrr} -2 & 4 & -2 & \\ & -3 & 6 & -3 \end{array}}{\begin{array}{rrrr} -2 & 1 & 4 & -3 \end{array}}$$

Back-projecting this result to the picture, we have

-2	1	4	-3
-2	1	4	-3

The data points $-2, -3$ outside the domain of the 2×2 reconstructed image, called reconstructed noise, are truncated. The result of the following step-by-step illustration of this method, is an exact reconstruction (again, by pure chance) of the original $f(x, y)$:

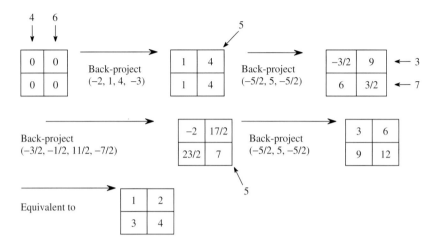

4.1.3.2 *Mathematical Formulation*   The mathematical formulation of the filtered back-projection method is given in Eqn. (4.3):

$$f(x, \ y) \ = \ \int_0^\pi h(t) * m(t, \ \theta)d\theta \tag{4.3}$$

where $m(t, \ \theta)$ is the t sampling point at θ angle projection, $h(t)$ is the filtered function, and $*$ is the convolution operator.

4.2   3-D IMAGE RECONSTRUCTION FROM 3-D DATA SET

4.2.1   3-D Data Acquisition

Over the past several years, with hardware advances in energy beam shaping, development of smaller but efficient linear array and 2-D areal detector technologies, and scanning gantry with moving-bed design, we have been able to collect 2-D data set for image reconstruction and to extend that to the realm of 3-D data collection. The third dimension is mostly in the body axis z direction. The 3-D data acquisition concept allows:

1. a larger cone beam X-ray for CT design—the multislice CT scanner;
2. a larger field-of-view multiring detectors for emission tomography—the whole body SPECT and PET scanners;
3. a faster scanning protocol—minimizing body motion artifact for better quality large body region and whole body imaging;
4. more efficient and effective data collection—shortening the time required for larger body region and whole body imaging;
5. lower dose exposure to the patient—due to Item 4 above; and

6. synchronizing the timing between scanning with patient bed movement, with the possibility of 4-D (x, y, z, t) data collection—4-D imaging and image fusion.

The geometry of various types of 3-D scanning will be discussed in the next sections as their multimodalities are presented.

4.2.2 3-D Image Reconstruction

Advances in 3-D data acquisition require better image reconstruction methods. Conventional 2-D fan-beam reconstruction methods are no longer sufficient to properly reconstruct 3-D data sets acquired by 3-D cone-beam or multi-ring technologies. The main characteristic of 3-D data is that each voxel is contributed not only by a single sectional data set but also by farther away sectional data adjacent to the section. Therefore the image reconstruction algorithm needs to be augmented with certain mathematical models derived from scanner geometry, global and local human anatomical structures, and physiological phenomena in order to optimally reconstruct 3-D voxels. In some cases the 3-D data set may also need to be reconstituted, for example, by data interpolation, recombination, and rearrangement, before the reconstruction. The goals of a good 3-D reconstruction algorithm are very fast speed and better image quality.

The trends in 3-D image reconstruction methods center in two main classes, analytic and iterative. Analytic approach is favored for X-ray cone-beam reconstruction, whereas iterative approach is more suitable for SPECT and PET data. There are two general analytic approaches. The first method is to use 3-D mathematical models and general strategies for exact and numerical inversion of the 3-D object from its 3-D dataset obtained from cone-beam detectors. Equation (4.3) can be extended to 3-D to reconstruct a three-dimensional image $f(x, y, z)$ from a 3-D data set. The second method is to factorize the 3-D problem into a set of independent 2-D sectional tasks for more efficient data and reconstruction management.

The iterative approach takes advantages of a priori knowledge of the objects being reconstructed, including the patient's anatomy, physiology, and pathology. Speed of reconstruction is the key in iterative approach. For further discussion of 3-D reconstruction algorithms development, refer to *Fully 3-D Reconstruction of Medical Imaging*, a special issue of *IEEE Transactions of Medical Imaging*. In this chapter many 3-D medical images are shown, including CT, MRI, and PET to illustrate the quality and fine details of the 3-D anatomy, physiology, and pathology.

4.3 TRANSMISSION X-RAY COMPUTED TOMOGRAPHY (CT)

4.3.1 Convention X-ray CT

A CT scanner consists of a scanning gantry housing an X-ray tube and a detector unit, and a movable bed that can align a specific cross section of the patient with the scanning gantry. The gantry provides a fixed relative position between the X-ray tube and the detector unit with the section of the patient to be scanned. A scanning mode is the procedure of collecting X-ray attenuation profiles (projections) from a transverse (cross) section of the body. From these projections the CT scanner's computer program or back-projector hardware reconstructs the corresponding cross-sectional image of the body. A schematic of the two most popular CT scanners (third and fourth generations) is provided in Figure 4.3*A* and *B*; both scanners use an X-ray fan beam. These types of XCT take about 1 to 5 seconds for a sectional scan, and more time for image reconstruction.

4.3.2 Spiral (Helical) CT

Three other configurations can improve scanning speed: the cine CT, the helical (spiral) CT, and the multislice CT (Section 4.3.3). Cine CT, whose scanning is by an electron beam X-ray tube, was replaced by multislice CT four years ago and is no longer used in the clinical environment. The design of the helical CT is based on the third- and fourth-generation scanner, and the multislice CT uses a cone beam instead of a fan beam. Multislice CT is the prefered configuration, gradually replaces the older helical CT.

The CT configurations shown in Figure 4.3*A* and *B* have one common characteristic: the patient's bed remains stationary during the scanning. After a complete scan, the patient's bed advances a certain distance, and the second scan resumes. The start-and-stop motions of the bed slow down the scanning operation. If the patient's bed could assume a forward motion at a constant speed while the scanning gantry rotates continuously, the total scanning time of a multiple section examination could be reduced. Such a configuration was not possible in the cine CT of the CT configurations shown in Fig. 4.3, because the scanning gantry is connected to an external high energy transformer with power supply through cables. The spiral or helical CT design got rid of the cables requirement through X-ray slip-ring technology.

Figure 4.4 illustrates the principle of a spiral CT. There are two possible scanning modes: single helical and cluster helical. In the early single helical mode, the bed advances linearly while the gantry rotates in sync for a period of time, say 30 seconds. In the cluster helical mode, the simultaneous rotation and translation lasts only 15 seconds, whereupon both motions stop for 7 seconds before resuming again. The single helical mode is used for patients who can hold their breath for a longer period of time, while the cluster helical mode is for patients who need to take a breath after 15 seconds. Current helical scanning technology allows flexible start and stop time modes, providing opportunity for multislice scanning of up to hundreds of slices per scan.

The design of the helical CT, introduced in the late 1980s, is based on three technological advances: the slip-ring gantry, improved detector efficiency, and greater X-ray tube cooling capability. The slip-ring gantry, containing a set of rings and electrical components that rotate, slide and make contact to generate both high energy (to supply the X-ray tube and generator) and standard energy (to supply powers to other electrical and computer components). For this reason no electrical cables are necessary to connect the gantry and external components. During the helical scanning, the term "pitch" is used to define the relationship between the X-ray beam collimation and the velocity of the bed movement:

$$\text{Pitch} = \frac{\text{Table movement in mm per gantry rotation}}{\text{Slice thickness}}$$

Thus when pitch equals 1, the gantry rotates a complete $360°$ as the bed advances 1.5 mm in one second, and this gives a slice thickness of 1.5 mm. During this time

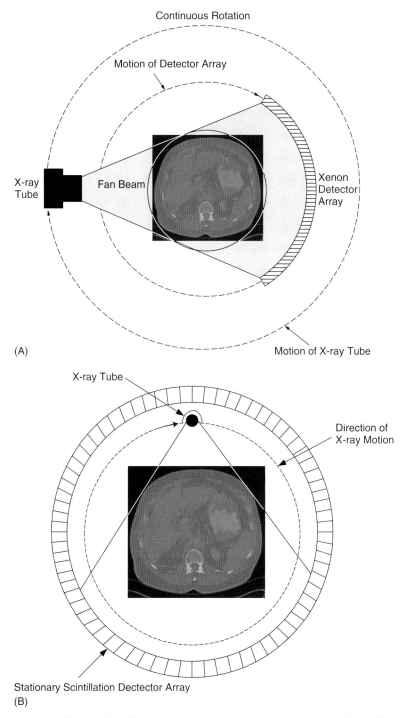

Figure 4.3 (*A*) Schematic of the rotation scanning mode using a fan-beam X ray. The detector array rotates with the X-ray tube as a unit. (*B*) Schematic of the rotation scanning mode with a stationary scintillation detector array, only X-ray source rotates.

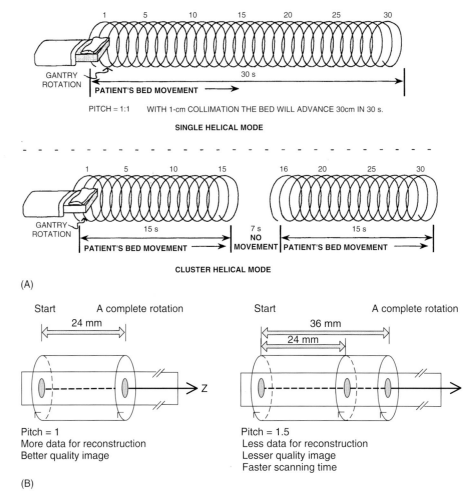

Figure 4.4   (*A*) Spiral (Helical) CT scanning modes: single helical mode and cluster helical mode. The helical scanning concept remains valid in the recent multislice CT scanner (Fig. 4.5), which uses an array detector to reduce the scanning time. (*B*) Concept of "pitch" in a multislice CT scanner. Example of $N = 16$ multislice CT scanner with $T = 1.5$ mm thickness slice (16 images/gantry rotation with 1.5-mm slice thickness). Two scanning protocols: For pitch = 1.0, in one gantry rotation the bed moves 24 mm/s, generating 16 slices that are 1.5-mm thick. Data results are sufficient for reconstruction, yielding better image quality. For pitch = 1.5, the bed moves 36 mm per rotation, and the scanner provides a faster scanning speed but lower quality images. (Courtesy of F. Cheung)

raw data are collected covering the 360 degrees for the 1.5-mm contiguous slices. Assuming one rotation takes one second, then for the single helical scan mode, 30 seconds of raw data are continuously collected while the bed moves 45 mm. After the data collection phase, the raw data are interpolated and/or extrapolated to sectional projections. These organized projections are used to reconstruct individual sectional images. In this case they are 1.5-mm thick, but the reconstruction slice thickness can be from 1.5 mm to 1 cm, depending on the interpolation and extrapolation methods used. Once the given thickness sectional images have been reconstructed, other thicknesses sectional images can be reconstructed, again from the raw data. However, once the raw data have been deleted, only sectional images are in the archive. In PACS applications, users have to understand the difference between archiving raw data and sectional images. In clinical usage, mostly the sectional images are archived.

Two major advantages of the spiral CT scan are high-speed scanning and the selection of slice orientation and thickness for reconstruction. The latter allows for a contiguous 3-D raw data set to be chosen in reconstructing slices: (1) with peak contrast in a contrast injection study, (2) retrospective creation of overlapping or thin slices, (3) orthogonal or oblique section reconstruction, and (4) 3-D rendering. The disadvantages are the helical design can cause reconstruction artifacts due to data interpolation and extrapolation can result in potential object boundary unsharpness.

4.3.3 Multislice CT

4.3.3.1 Principles In spiral CT, the patient's bed moves during the scan, but the X-ray beam is in the form of a fan beam perpendicular to the patient's axis, and the detector system is built to collect data for the reconstruction of one slice. If the X-ray beam is shaped to a 3-D cone beam with the z-axis parallel to the patient's axis, and if a multiple detector array (in the z direction) system is used to collect the data, then we have a multislice CT scanner (see Fig. 4.5). Multislice CT, in essence, is also spiral scan, except that the X-ray beam is shaped to a cone-beam geometry. Multislice CT can obtain many images in one examination with a very rapid acquisition time, for example, 160 images in 20 seconds, or 8 images per second, or 4 MB/s of raw data. Figure 4.5 shows the schematic. Note in this figure that a full rotation of the cone beam is necessary to collect sufficient projection data to reconstruct the number of slides equal to the z-axis collimation of the detector system (see below for a definition). Multislice CT uses several new hardware and software technologies:

- New detector. The ceramic detector has replaced the traditional crystal detector. The ceramic detector has the advantages of more light photons in the output, less afterglow time, and higher resistance to radiation and mechanical damage; it can also be shaped much thinner (1/2) for equivalent amount of X-ray absorption, compared with crystal scintillators.

- Real-time dose modulation. The dose delivered to the patient is minimized by the cone beam geometry in modulating the mAs (milliampere-seconds) of the X-rays beam during the scan.

- High-speed data output channel. For example, with a 256-slice CT scanner much more data have to be collected during a single examination. Fast I/O data channels from the detector system to image reconstruction are necessary.

- Cone-beam geometry image reconstruction algorithm. This enables efficient collection and recombination of cone-beam X-ray projections (raw data) for sectional reconstruction (see Section 4.2).

If the patient's bed is moving linearly, but the gantry does not rotate, the result is a digital fluorographic image with better image quality than that discussed in Section 3.2.2.

4.3.3.2 *Terminology Used in Multislice XCT* Recall the term "pitch" defined in spiral CT. With cone-beam and multidetector scanning, because of the multi-detector arrays in the z direction (see Fig. 4.5) the table movement can be many

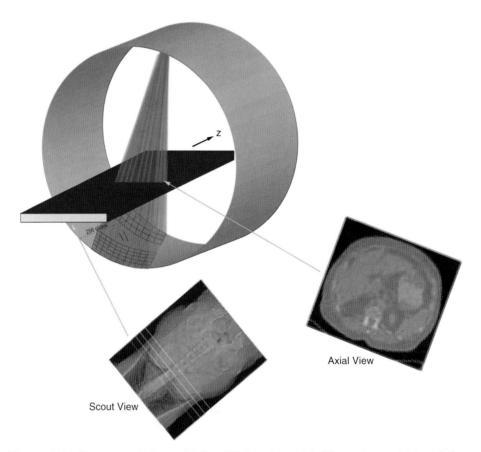

Axial View

Scout View

Figure 4.5 Geometry of the multislice CT (not in scale). The patient axis (parallel to the bed) is in the z direction. The X-ray source (X), shaped as a collimated cone beam, rotates continuously around the z-axis $360°$ in sync with the patient's bed movement in the z direction. The detector system is a combination of detector arrays on a concave surface (not in scale) facing the X-ray beam. The number of slices per $360°$ rotation are determined by two factors: the number of detector arrays (channels) in the z direction and the method used to recombine the cone beam projection data into transverse sectional projections (see Fig. 4.2). The standard reconstructed images are in transverse (axial) view perpendicular to the z-axis; the projection raw data can also be recombined to reconstruct sagittal, coronal, or oblique view images. If the cone beam does not rotate while the patient's bed is moving, the reconstructed image is equivalent to a digital projection image (scout view).

times the thickness of an individual slice. To see this, take the 16×1.5-mm detector system (16 arrays with 1.5 mm thickness per array), with the slice thickness of an individual image being 1.5 mm. Then apply the definition of pitch to a spiral scan:

$$\text{Pitch} = \frac{\text{Table movement in mm per gantry rotation}}{\text{Slice thickness}} = 16$$

$$= \frac{(16 \times 1.5 \text{ mm/rotation})}{1.5 \text{ mm}} = \frac{(24 \text{ mm/rotation})}{1.5 \text{ mm}}. \qquad (4.4)$$

Clearly, the table moves 24 mm/rotation, so with a reconstructed slice thickness of 1.5 mm, the pitch would be 16 (see Section 4.3.2). This case also represents contiguous scans.

Compare this example with that shown in Section 4.3.2 Figure 4.4*A* for a single slice scan. The definition of pitch shows some discrepancy, but this discrepancy is due to the number of data channels available in the multidetector arrays. Since different manufacturers produce different numbers of data channels in multidetector arrays, use of the word pitch can be confusing. For this reason the International Electrotechnical Commission (IEC) accepts the following definition of pitch (now often referred to as the IEC pitch):

z-**Axis collimation (T).** The width of the tomographic section (slice thickness) along the *z*-axis imaged by one data channel (array). In multidetector row (multislice) CT scanners, several detector elements may be grouped together to form one data channel (array).

Number of data channels (N). The number of tomographic sections imaged in a single axial scan (one rotation).

Table speed or increment (I). The table increment per axial scan or the table increment per rotation of the x-ray tube in a helical (spiral) scan:

$$\textbf{Pitch(P)} = \text{table speed I(mm/rotation)}/(\textbf{N} \times \textbf{T})$$

Recall the example discussed earlier in this section. Let the $\textbf{N} = 16$ data channel scanner have slice thickness $\textbf{T} = 1.5$ mm,

Scanning Protocol 1   Pitch $\textbf{P} = 1.0$ means that the table speed $\textbf{I} = 24$ mm/rotation because $\textbf{P} = 1 = 24/(16 \times 1.5)$. This protocol generates 16 contiguous images with 1.5-mm thickness without gaps in between. The raw data collected cover every square millimeter of the subject being scanned in 360 degrees. The images so obtained will have sufficient data for reconstruction and hence better quality than any $\textbf{P} > 1$ protocol.

Scanning Protocol 2   Pitch $\textbf{P} = 1.5$ means that the table speed $\textbf{I} = 36$ mm/rotation because $\textbf{P} = 1.5 = 36/(16 \times 1.5)$. In this protocol, in one full rotation the table moves 36 mm. The result suggests a faster scanning time, but the images so reconstructed will have less image quality than that obtained with $\textbf{P} = 1$. It is because the X-ray beam in one rotation covers more than 24 mm (i.e., 36 mm) and thus cannot cover each square millimeter of an object with 360 angles. Figure 4.4*B* illustrates the concept of "pitch" used in a multislice CT scanner.

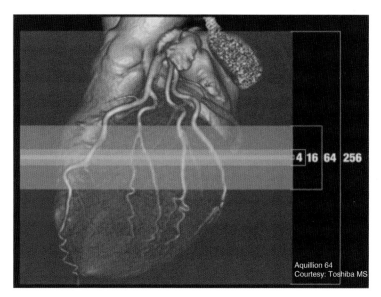

Figure 4.6 Extent of z-dimension scanning of the human anatomy of a multislice CT scanner using the size of the heart as a scaling factor. Slices range from 4, to 16, 64, to 256. For 1-mm thick slices, a $360°$ rotation in a 256-slice scanner can capture a complete heart, minimizing any moving artifact in the image caused by the heart beat. (Courtesy of Toshiba Medical Systems)

Figure 4.6 shows the extent of z-dimension scanning of the human anatomy by variable multislice scanners currently in the commercial market, with array detectors ranging from 4, 16, 64, to 256. In the 256 array detector system, for example, one full rotation of the X ray can capture the entire heart (256 mm), so this multislice architecture can minimize the possible heart beat artifacts, whereas, in the 16 mm architecture, 16 rotations are required.

4.3.3.3 Whole Body CT Scan The scanning speed of the multislice CT scanner allows for fast whole body CT trauma studies in emergency situations as well as health checkup. The patient's whole body is scanned from head to toes, and the contiguous CT images are used for screening review. In PACS and imaging informatics, then, such whole body scanning would result in a very large data set for each examination and so will require special consideration for archiving and data transmission. We will return to this topic in Parts II and III.

4.3.4 Components and Data Flow of a CT Scanner

Figure 4.7 shows the main components and the data flow in a CT scanner. Included are a gantry housing the X-ray tube, the detector system, and signal processing/conditioning circuits; a front-end preprocessor unit for the cone- or fan-beam projection data corrections and recombination to transverse sectional projection data; a high-speed computational processor; a hardware back-projector unit; and a video controller for displaying images. The CT number, or Hounsfield number, or pixel/voxel value, represents the relative X-ray attenuation coefficient of

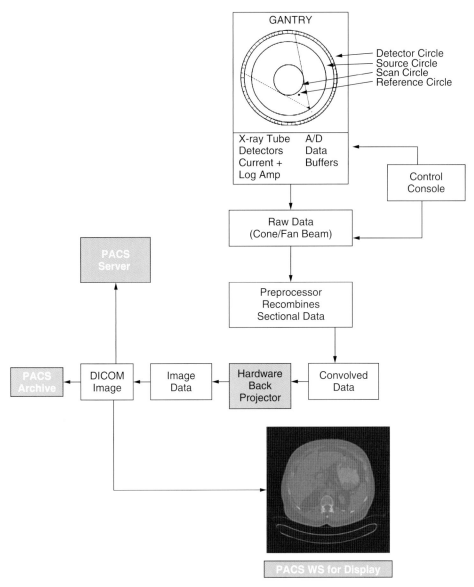

Figure 4.7   Data flow components of an X-ray CT scanner. The scanning and data collection times, in general, are shorter than the image reconstruction time. A hardware back-projector (bottom shaded box) is used to speed up the reconstruction time.

the tissue in the pixel/voxel, defined as follows:

$$\text{CT number} = \frac{K\,(\mu - \mu_{\mathrm{w}})}{\mu_{\mathrm{w}}}$$

where μ is the attenuation coefficient of the material under consideration, μ_{w} is the attenuation coefficient of water, and K is a constant set by the manufacturer.

4.3.5 CT Image Data

4.3.5.1 Isotropic Image and Slice Thickness Current multislice CT scanners can configure up to 256 or even 512 detectors in an array. In a spiral scan, multiple slices of 3-D data can be acquired simultaneously for different detector sizes, and 0.75-, 1-, 2-, 3-, 4-, 5-, 6-, 7-, 8-, and 10-mm slice thickness can be reconstructed. If the x and y resolutions of the pixel are the same as the slice thickness, then the voxel is isotropic. So the transverse, sagittal, and coronal images are of the same resolution, or isotropic, in the multiplannar reconstruction.

4.3.5.2 Image Data File Size Consider a standard chest CT image exam, which covers between 300 and 400 mm generating from 150 to 200 2-mm slices and up to 600 to 800 0.5-mm slices, depending on the slice thickness, or data sizes from 75 MB up to 400 MB. A whole body CT scan for screening can produce up to 2500 images or 1250 MB (1.25 GB) of data, with each image being $512 \times 512 \times 2$ bytes.

4.3.5.3 Data Flow/Postprocessing Both fan- and cone-beam raw data are obtained by an acquisition host computer. The slice thickness reconstructions are performed on the raw data. Once the set of images is acquired in DICOM format (see Chapter 9), any future postprocessing is performed on the DICOM data. This includes multiplanar reconstruction (Fig. 4.8) of transverse, sagittal, coronal, and oblique slice, CTA (angiography, Fig. 4.9A, B, C), as well as 3-D rendering (Fig. 4.10A, B) postprocessing. Sometimes the cone-beam raw data are saved for future reconstruction of the different slice thicknesses.

The reconstruction process is time-consuming. Some scanners feature a secondary computer that shares the database and functions as an acquisition host computer. This secondary computer can perform the same postprocessing functions while the scanner continues acquiring new patient data from scanning. This secondary computer also can perform image transmission through network to PACS or another DICOM destination (e.g., highly specialized 3-D processing workstation), alleviating the acquisition host computer from these functions and thus improving system scanning throughput.

4.4 SINGLE PHOTON EMISSION COMPUTED TOMOGRAPHY

4.4.1 Emission Computed Tomography (ECT)

Emission computed tomography (ECT) has many characteristics in common with transmission X-ray CT, but the main difference is the radiation source used for imaging. In ECT, the radionuclide administered to a patient, in the form of radiopharmaceuticals either by injection or by inhalation, is used as the emission energy source inside of the body instead of an external X-ray beam. Basically ECT consists in nuclear medicine scanning, as discussed in Section 3.7.1.

Selecting a dose-efficient detector system for an ECT system is important for two reasons. First, the quantity to be measured in ECT involves the distribution of the radionuclide in the body, and this changes with time as a result of the flow and biochemical kinetics in the body. So all necessary measurements must be made in a short period of time. Second, the amount of isotope administered has to be minimal

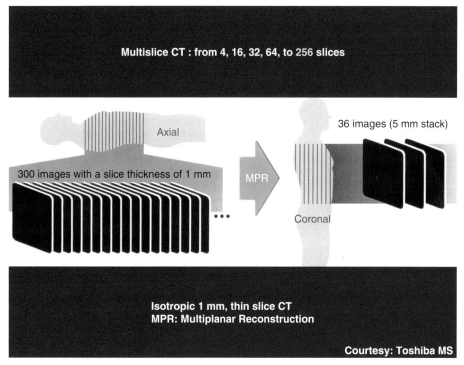

Figure 4.8   Concept of isotropic voxel and multiplanar reconstruction (MPR). In multislice CT scanning with 1-mm isotropic axial images (i.e., 1 mm × 1 mm pixel size with 1 mm thickness, or $1 \times 1 \times 1$ mm^3 (transverse × sagittal × coronal) volex size. MPR reconstruction is from the isotropic data set to reconstruct other sectional image of various thicknesses, for example, from 300 $1 \times 1 \times 1$ mm^3 transverse images to 60 $1 \times 5 \times 1$ mm^3 coronal sectional images with 5 mm thick where axial and sagittal direction pixels remain as 1 mm. Since the body dimension perpendicular to the coronal direction is smaller than the other two dimensions, there are only 36 coronal sections with 5-mm thickness that are usable data. MPR can also be performed for oblique sections to conform with the internal organ under consideration. In this case the 3-D data set needs to be interpolated and extrapolated to fit the contour outlines of oblique sections before the reconstruction. MPR reconstruction should not be confused with the picture reconstruction methods using projections discussed in Section 4.1. (Courtesy of Toshiba Medical Systems)

to limit the dose delivered to the patient. Therefore detector efficiency is a crucial consideration in selecting the detector system.

The basic principle of image reconstruction is the same in ECT as in transmission CT except that the signal in ECT is composed of γ-rays that become attenuated during their flight from the emitting nuclei to the detectors. To minimize the contribution from scattered radiation, the ECT uses the characteristics of monoenergetic energy in setting up a counting window to discriminate the lower energy scattered radiation from the high-energy primary radiation. There are two major categories in ECT: single photon emission CT (SPECT) and positron emission CT (PET).

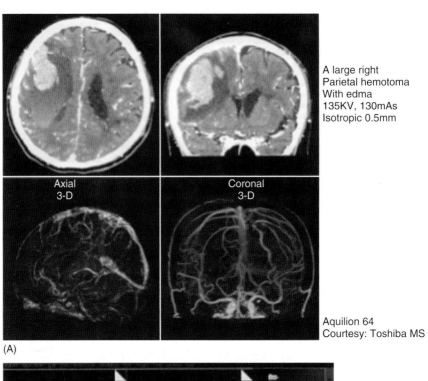

A large right
Parietal hemotoma
With edma
135KV, 130mAs
Isotropic 0.5mm

Axial
3-D

Coronal
3-D

Aquilion 64
Courtesy: Toshiba MS

(A)

Courtesy of Siemens MS

(B)

Figure 4.9   (*Continued*)

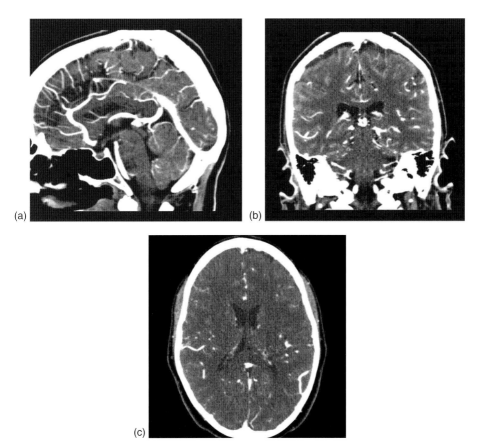

Figure 4.9 (*A*) 3-D multislice CT showing a large right parietal hemotoma with edma: (upper left) Transverse; (right) coronal. The bottom images are CT angiorams showing the 2-D sagittal view (left) and the coronal view (right) extracted from the 3-D CT 0.5-mm isotropic data set. (Courtesy of Toshiba Medical Systems) (*B*) 3-D neuro digital subtraction angiogram: (top two and left bottom) sagittal, coronal, and transverse contrast CT images; (bottom right) 3-D angiogram obtained by tissue and bone subtraction from the 3-D CT images. (Courtesy of Siemens Medical Systems) (*C*) Multiplanar reconstruction CT images. The 16-slice helical CT of the head and neck was obtained during a bolus of intravenous contrast administration. Volumetric data was then transferred to a Vitrea 3-D workstation© for postprocessing, including 3-D volumetric rendering and multiplanar reconstructions (MPR) in the transverse, (*a*) sagittal, (*b*) coronal, and (*c*) transverse planes. This study was conducted in an adult female with transient ischemic attacks. The patient was found to have significant unilateral internal carotid artery stenosis due to atherosclerotic plaque. (Courtesy of Dr. P. Moin)

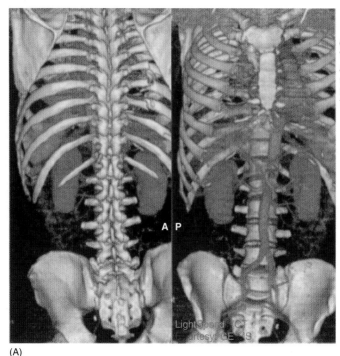

Cage Trauma
Volume Render
A & P Views
reveal fractures
Posterior
7th-10th Ribs

(A)

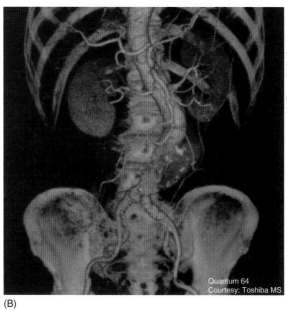

Infra-renal
Abdominal aortic
Aneurysm with
Mural thrombus
135KV, 175mAs,
0.5 s/rot
325 mm scan range
12 s.

(B)

Figure 4.10 (*A*) 3-D CT data set can also be used to produce 3-D volume rendering images. Left and right show the anterior-posterior (A–P) and posterior–anterior (P–A) views of the thoracic cage, revealing fractures of ribs 7 to 10 in the P–A view. (Courtesy of GE Medical Systems) (*B*) 3-D CT abdominal data set obtained by using a 64 multislice scanner showing 3-D volume rendering of bone, blood vessels, and kidneys, and in particular, an infra-renal abdominal aortic aneurysm with mural thrombus. The scan protocol used was a 135 KVp, 175 mAS, 325-mm scan range taking 12 seconds. (Courtesy of Toshiba Medical Systems)

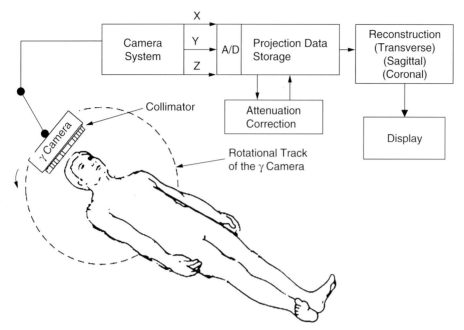

Figure 4.11   Schematic of a single photon emission CT (SPECT). Refer to Figure 3.24 for nuclear medicine scanning.

4.4.2 Single Photon Emission CT (SPECT)

There are several designs for SPECT, but only the rotating gamma camera system is discussed here (see Fig. 4.11) because it is commercially available. In a rotating camera system the gamma camera is rotated around the object, and the multiple 2-D images series are reconstructed and stored for postprocessing. The camera is composed of a large scintillation crystal of diameter 30 to 50 cm and a number of photomultiplier tubes (PMTs) attached to the opposite surface of the crystal. When a γ-ray photon interacts with the crystal, the light generated from the photoelectric effect is uniformly distributed among the neighboring PMTs. By measuring the relative signal of each PMT, the camera can locate the interactive position for each event. The drawback of this system is the difficulty of maintaining a uniform speed of rotation with the rather heavy camera. Figure 4.11 shows the schematic of a SPECT.

Since a typical tomographic study takes 15 to 20 minutes to accomplish, it is important to maintain patient immobilization. To provide the best sensitivity and resolution, it is desirable to have the camera as close to the patient as possible. Since the dimension of body width is greater than body thickness, an elliptical orbit of rotation of the camera tends to produce a higher resolution image. Different collimators are used for different applications. In general, the reconstruction algorithm must be modified and the attenuation values corrected for each type of collimator. For example, a single-plane converging collimator will need a fan-beam reconstruction algorithm, and a parallel collimator will need a parallel-beam algorithm.

Three methods of correcting attenuation values based on the assumption of a constant attenuation value are summarized as follows:

1. *Geometric mean modification.* Each data point in a projection is corrected by the geometric mean of the projection data, which is obtained by taking the square root of the product of two opposite projection data points.
2. *Iterative modification.* The same as with the iteration reconstruction method for CT described earlier, a reconstruction without corrections is first performed, and each pixel in the reconstructed image is compensated by a correction factor that is the inverse of the average measured attenuation from that point to the boundary pixels. The projections of this modified image are obtained, and the differences between each of the corrected projections and the original measured projections are computed. These difference projections are reconstructed to obtain an error image. The error image is then added back to the modified image to form the corrected image.
3. *Convolution method.* Each data point in the projection is modified by a factor that depends on the distance from a centerline to the edge of the object. The modified projection data points are filtered with a proper filter function and then back-projected with an exponential weighting factor to obtain the image (see Section 4.1.3).

Today, SPECT is mostly used for studies of the brain, including brain blood volume (^{99m} Tc- labeled blood cells), regional cerebral blood flow (^{123}I-labeled iodoantipyrine or inhaled ^{133}Xe), and physiological condition measurements.

4.5 POSITRON EMISSION TOMOGRAPHY (PET)

Positron emission tomography (PET) uses a positron instead of a single photon as the radionuclide source. The positron emitted from the radionuclide is rapidly slowed down and annihilated, yielding of two 511 keV γ-ray photons oriented 180 degrees to each other. The PET system utilizes this unique property of positrons by employing a detector system that requires simultaneous detection of both photons from annihilation, and thus it avoids the need for collimators. So a pair of detectors is placed at the opposite sides of the patient, and only events that are detected in coincidence are recorded. Simultaneous detection of two annihilation photons by the detector system thus signals the decay of a positron anywhere along a line connecting the two points of detection (Fig. 4.12). With this multiple coincidence logic, PET systems have higher sensitivity than SPECT.

The correction of attenuation is easier in PET than in SPECT due to the probability that the annihilated photons will reach both detectors simultaneously as a function of the thickness of the body between the two opposite detectors. The correction factor can be obtained by means of a preliminary scan of the body with an external γ-ray source, or by means of a correction table based on a simple geometric shape resembling the attenuation medium to be used. Patient movements, oversimplified geometric shape, and non-uniform medium can cause errors in the correction of attenuation.

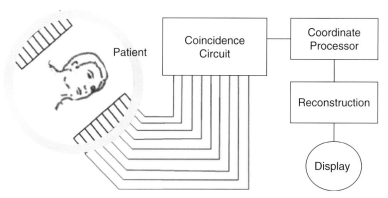

Figure 4.12   Block diagram of a positron emission tomography (PET) system showing two array banks of the detectors.

Thallium-drifted sodium iodide NaI(T1), bismuth germanate (BGO), and cesium fluoride (CsF) are some materials being used for the detector. Because of the high energy of the annihilation photon, detector efficiency is a crucial factor in selecting a scintillator for a PET system. Bismuth germanate is the most prominent PET detector material because of its high detection efficiency, which is due to its high physical density (7.13 g/cm^3) and large atomic number (83), and because of its nonhygroscopicity, which makes for easy packing, and minimal afterglow.

A typical whole body PET scanner consists of 512 BGO detectors placed in 16 circular array banks with 32 detectors in each bank. During the scanning the system is capable of wobbling to achieve higher resolution via finer sampling. The image spatial resolution for the stationary and wobbled modes are 5 to 6 mm and 4.5 to 5 mm, respectively.

In the whole-body imaging technique, PET produces tomographic images of the entire body with equal spatial resolution in the three orthogonal image planes. Since the body longitudinal axis is, in general, longer than the other two axes, the patient bed is required to advance during the scanning process to permit the entire body length to be scanned. A sophisticated data acquisition system in synchrony with the bed motion is necessary to monitor the data collection process. This data collection scheme is very similar to that of the multislice CT. Figure 4.13*A* shows the transverse, coronal, and sagittal planes of a PET scan of the brain. Figure 4.13*B* illustrates images of the transverse, coronal, and sagittal orthogonal planes, as well as the anterior-posterior projection image of the whole body PET scan with a fluoride ion isotope (^{18}F$^-$).

4.6 3-D ULTRASOUND IMAGING (3-D US)

Comparing to other imaging modalities, 2-D US imaging has several limitations, among them are (1) 2-D US images do not provide a fixed origin that can pinpoint the position of the anatomy and the pathology and (2) 2-D US images cannot measure the exact volume of a tumor. 3-D US can be used to remove these weaknesses. 3-D US uses a high data rate (15–60 images per second) to collect tomographic plane

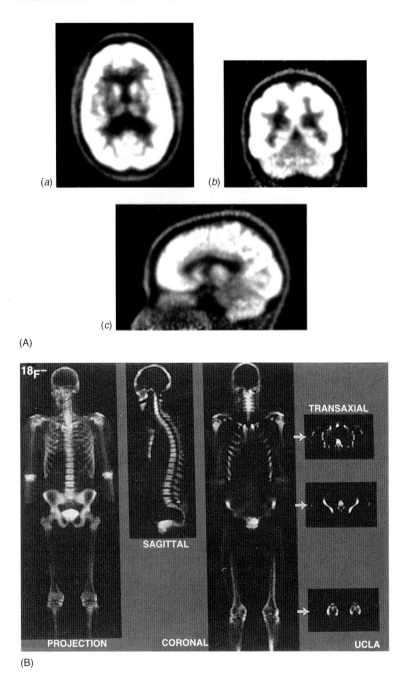

Figure 4.13 (*A*) Positron emission tomography (PET) study of the brain. 18F-fluorodeoxyglucose (18F-FDG) was administered to the patient, and approximately 60 minutes later the patient was positioned on a PET scanner and images (*a*: transverse, *b*: coronal, and *c*: sagittal) were obtained from the skull apex to the skull base. Causes of cognitive impairment, such as Alzheimer's disease, are among the indications for brain 18F-FDG PET. (Courtesy of Dr. P. Moin) (*B*) Images of transverse, coronal, and sagittal orthogonal planes (right to left), as well as the posterior-anterior projection image (leftmost) of the whole body PET image with fluoride ion ($^{18}F^{-}$). (Courtesy of Dr. R.A. Hawkins)

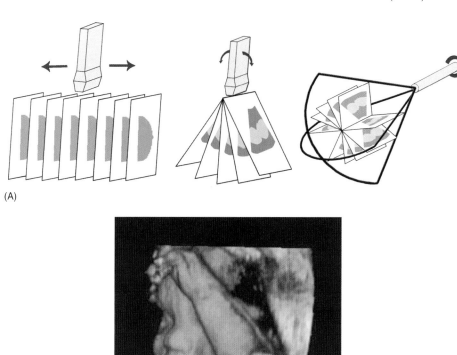

(A)

(B)

Figure 4.14 (*A*) Three scanning modes of 3-D US scanning: (left) linear translation; (middle) tilt scanning; (right) rotational scanning. (*B*) 3-D ultrasound image of a 25 week fetal face. (Courtesy of Philips Medical Systems: http://www.medical.philips.com/ main/products/ultrasound/assets/images/image_library/3d_2295_H5_C5-2_OB_3D.jpg).

(or oblique plane) images under the operator's control of the position and orientation of the images. If an array of ultrasound transducers with a fixed center of translation and/or rotation is used to scan the object of interest, the resulting echo signals are similar to those of a sectional CT image. The scanning modes in 3-D US imaging include linear translation 3-D scanning, tilt 3-D scanning, and 3-D motorizing scanning (Fig. 4.14*A*). These 2-D oblique plane images can be recombined according to the scanning mode and direction, forming a 3-D US image set. Such 3-D US images can be used for breast imaging, obstetrics imaging for fetus, and carotid artery scanning, among other types of scans. Figure 4.14*B* depicts a 3-D rendering of a 26-week fetal face from a set of 3-D US images.

Another type of 3-D US imaging technique is the endovascular 3-D US, in which a miniature US transducer is inserted into the vascular lumen to perform 3-D US imaging. An example is the intravascular ultrasound (IVUS) technology, a technique used to identify blockages in arteries, most commonly near the heart. The technique involves inserting a catheter into the circulatory system through the thigh, and up to the heart, using ultrasound signals to obtain a 3-D map of the arteries.

4.7 MAGNETIC RESONANCE IMAGING (MRI)

4.7.1 MR Imaging Basics

The magnetic resonance imaging (MRI) modality forms images of objects by measuring the magnetic moments of protons using radio frequency (RF) and a strong magnetic field. Information concerning the spatial distribution of nuclear magnetization in the objects is determined from RF signal emission by these stimulated nuclei. The received signal intensity is dependent on five parameters: hydrogen density, spin-lattice relaxation time (T_1), spin-spin relaxation time (T_2), flow velocity (e.g., arterial blood), and chemical shift.

MR imaging collects spatial (anatomical) information from the returned RF signals through a filtered back-projection reconstruction or a Fourier analysis and displays it as a two-dimensional (2-D) section or a three-dimensional (3-D) volume of the objects. There are some distinct advantages to using MRI over other modalities (e.g., CT) in certain types of examination:

1. The interaction between the static magnetic field, RF radiation, and atomic nuclei is free of ionizing radiation; therefore the imaging procedure is relative noninvasive compared with the use of other ionizing radiation sources.
2. The scanning mechanism is either electrical or electronical, requiring no moving parts to perform a scan.
3. It is possible to obtain two-dimensional slices of the coronal, sagittal, and transverse planes, and any oblique section, as well as a 3-D data volume.
4. MRI can use various pulse sequences for imaging to enhance different tissues under consideration.

The two disadvantages at present in MRI, as compared to CT images, are that MRI, in general, has lower spatial resolution, whereas CT has better image quality in some body regions. In current clinical practice, MRI and CT have complementary use, each depending on the case exam under investigation.

4.7.2 Magnetic Resonance Image Production

Figure 4.15 shows the components for the production, detection, and display of MR signals in a simplified block diagram of a generic MR imaging system:

1. A magnet to produce the static magnetic B_0 field,
2. RF equipment to produce the magnitude of the *RF* magnetic field (transmitter, amplifier, and coil for transmitting mode) and then detect the free induction

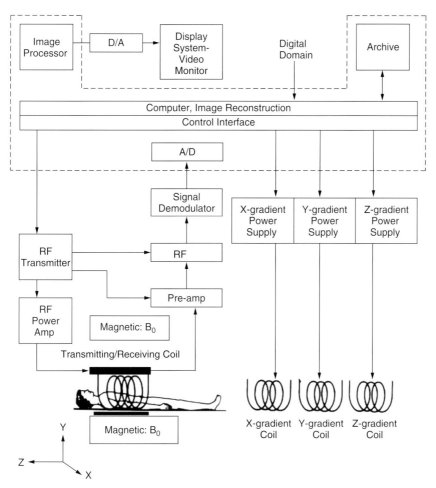

Figure 4.15 Block diagram of a generic magnetic resonance imaging (MRI) system. Dotted line separates the digital domain from the MR signal generation.

decay (FID) of the nucleus, which is the response of the net magnetization to an RF pulse (coil for receiving mode, preamplifier, receiver and signal demodulator).

3. x, y, and z gradient power supplies and coils providing the magnetic field gradients needed for encoding spatial position.

4. The electronics and computer facility to orchestrate the whole imaging process (control interface with computer), convert the MR signals to digital data (A/D converter), reconstruct the image (computer algorithms), and display it (computer, disk storage, image processor and display system).

4.7.3 Steps in Producing an MR Image

An MR image is obtained by using a selected pulse sequence that perturbs the external magnetic field B_0 (e.g., 1.5 and 3.0 Telsa). This set of MR images is named based on the selected pulse sequence. Some useful pulse sequences in radiology applications are therefore spin echo, inversion recovery, gradient echo, and echo planar, as each pulse sequence highlights certain chemical compositions in the tissues under consideration.

We will use a spin-echo pulsing sequence to illustrate how an MR image is produced. First, the object is placed inside of an RF coil situated in the homogeneous portion of the main magnetic field, B_0. Next, a pulsing sequence with two RF pulses is applied to the imaging volume (hence spin echo). At the same time a magnetic gradient is applied to the field B_0 in order to identify the relative position of the spin-echo-free induction decay (FID) signals. Note that FID is composed of frequency components (see Section 2.4.1). The FID signal is demodulated from the RF signal, sampled with an analog-to-digital converter, and stored in a digital data array for processing. This set of data is analogous to one set of projection data in CT. After the repetition time has elapsed, the pulsing sequence is applied and a new FID is obtained and sampled repeatedly with alternate gradient magnitudes until the desired number of projections are acquired.

During and after data collection, the selected tomographic reconstruction algorithm described in Section 4.1, either the filtered back-projection or inverse two-dimensional fast Fourier transform (Inverse FT, Section 4.1.1), is performed on all the acquired projections (digital FID data). The result is a spin-echo image of the localized magnetization in the spatial domain. The pixel values are related to the hydrogen density, relaxation times, flow, and chemical shift. This procedure can be represented as follows:

$$\text{Frequency spectrum} \xrightarrow{\text{FT}} \text{FID} \xrightarrow{\text{Inverse FT}} \text{Spatial distribution(MR image)}$$

This digital image can then be archived and displayed. Figure 4.16 illustrates the data flow in forming an MR image. Figure 4.17 shows a commercial $3T$ MRI scanner through the window of a magnetic field shielded MRI exam room.

4.7.4 MR Imaging (MRI)

MR scanner can reconstruct transverse (like CT), sagittal, coronal, or any oblique plane images (Fig. 4.18) as well as three-dimensional images of other body regions, including the fetus (Figure 4.19) and the breasts (Figure 4.20.) Besides reconstructing images in various planes, MR scanner can selectively emphasize different MR properties of the objects under consideration from the FID. Thus we can reconstruct T_1 and T_2, proton density MR images, and other combinations. The challenge of MRI is to decipher the abundance of information in FID (ρ_H, T_1, T_2,) flow velocity and chemical shift, and to adequately display all this information as images.

4.7.5 Other Types of Images from MR Signals

This section describes several early clinical and work-in-progress MR image types that can be generated from MR signals. The emphasis is not on a discussion of the physics and chemistry aspect of the image acquisition but on the informatics relevant after the images have been acquired.

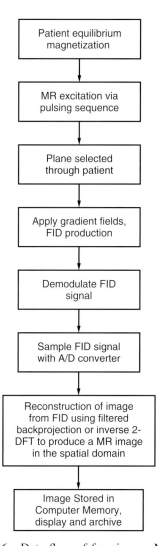

Figure 4.16   Data flow of forming an MR image.

4.7.5.1 MR Angiography (MRA)

4.7.5.1 MR Angiography (MRA) Current MRI scanners have the capability to acquire 3-D volumetric MR angiogram data. The Fourier nature of 3-D MR data acquisition involves collecting the entire 3-D data set prior to reconstruction of any of the individual sections. Phase encoding is employed to spatially encode the y-axis as well as the z-axis position information. The section thickness can be reduced to less than 1 mm, providing a sufficient signal-to-noise ratio. Repetition and echo times are shortened, making it possible to collect large 3-D volumes of high-resolution data or multiple successive lower resolution volumes in 20 to 40 seconds.

A standard MRA study can vary from a typical head/neck study of 100 images to a lower extremity runoff study of 2000 images that produces a data size of between 25 and 500 MB. Performancewise, it depends on the scanner hardware and can yield studies that vary in time from 15 to 40 seconds. Figure 4.21 shows an MRA

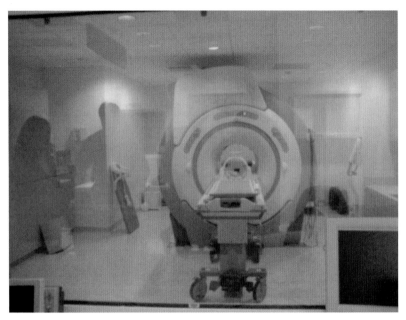

Figure 4.17   Clinical $3T$ MR imaging system in a magnetic shielded room at the Health Science Campus, USC.

study containing abdominal slices, using a maximum projection display method to highlight the contrasting blood vessels in the entire study.

4.7.5.2 Other Pulse-Sequences Image   Over the past decade more than 30 pulse sequences were developed to enhance a certain tissue or image contrasts. The major reason for enhancing pulse sequences is for faster imaging. The idea is to read the signal after RF excitation fast enough before it decays. The latest developments in this direction are in echo-planar imaging (EPI) and spiral imaging readout techniques, which are used for very fast imaging of the heart in motion (cardiac MRI), imaging of multi-voxel chemical profiles, magnetic resonance spectroscopic imaging (MRS and MRSI), and imaging the physiological response to neural activation in the brain (functional MRI, or fMRI). Fast data acquisition and image reconstruction allows 30 to 60 slices to be obtained in 2 to 4 seconds. The increase in field strength from today's 1.5 and 3.0 Tesla to even higher Telsa will increase the signal sensitivity (signal to noise, SNR), which results in smaller image matrices and thus higher resolution. Based on the pulse sequences, certain imaging protocols and image data characteristics have been established for specific application. Below we follow two examples to illustrate the state-of-the-art pulse sequences that are in the verge of being used for daily clinical applications.

Functional MRI (fMRI)   Among these new types of images derived from MR, functional MRI is the closest to daily clinical applications. The image formation consists in 3-D MRI volume acquisition plus selective activation of different functions like motor, sensory, visual or auditory and their location inside the brain to produce a 4-D fMRI data set. Typically an fMRI experiment consists of four series,

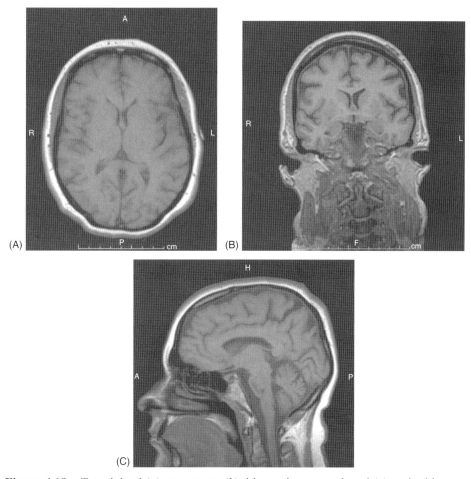

Figure 4.18 T_1 weighted (*a*) transverse, (*b*) thin section coronal, and (*c*) sagittal images from an MRI performed to evaluate a possible structural cause for this patient's recent onset of seizures. Thin-section coronals were obtained to allow better visualization of the hippocampi, a region of interest in the imaging evaluation of seizures. A: Anterior; P: posterior; R: right; L: left; F: front.

each taking about 5 minutes with 100 acquisitions. A whole adult brain is covered by 40 slices with a slice thickness of 3 mm, with each slice having 64×64 or 128×128 voxels. While 2-D and 3-D acquisition techniques exist, in both cases the resulting raw data is a stack of 2-D slices. The average fMRI experiment adds up to 400 volumes, each volume $64 \times 64 \times 40 \times 2$ bytes or about 330 KB, amounting to a total of roughly 130 MB. When using 128×128 matrices the total data volume is increased to around 520 MB per subject.

Because the DICOM standard (Chapter 9) is inefficient for many small images like fMRI, the data are mainly reconstructed as a raw data stack and processed offline on a workstation. Therefore no standard data communication or processing scheme exists so far. A DICOM standard extension, supplement 49, was introduced in mid-2002, but no vendor has yet implemented it for daily clinical operation.

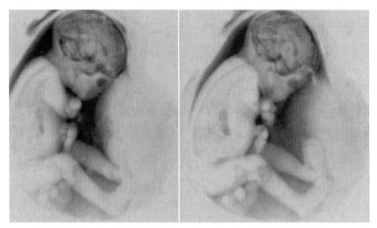

Fetal MR Scans using ultra fast sequences, complementary to US
Courtesy of National Center for Child Health Development, Tokyo, Japan
Diag Imag, 8/2004 P.55

Figure 4.19   Two 3-D fetal $3T$ MR images using ultra fast sequences. (Courtesy of National Center for Child Helath Development, Tokyo, Japan. *Diag Imag* 8/2004, p. 55)

The fMRI data can be efficiently displayed as a color-coded map on the corresponding anatomical image (Fig. 4.22*A*). As this is not possible with the existing PACS and display workstation environment, new ways of fMRI display have to be developed that can facilitate fMRI to be displayed in specialized 3-D workstations.

Clinicians prefer the 2-D mosaic plot (Fig. 4.22*A*) of a structural MRI overlaid with the functional map. Neuroscientists prefer an atlas-based 3-D display in a standard coordinate system or a rendered 3-D projection onto the brain surface (Fig. 4.22*B*).

Diffusion Tensor MRI (DTI)   Another work-in-progress MRI application is in the neurosciences, in particular, diffusion-weighted MR imaging (DWI). DWI uses MR signals based on the structural properties of neural tissue as local water molecular displacements. One type of DWI is a gradient-direction encoded diffusion tensor imaging (DTI) that can reveal neuroanatomical connections in a noninvasive manner. The implication of the availability of this diagnostic tool is that we may be able to characterize neural tissue properties such as cortical thinning, demyelination, and nerve degeneration and regeneration following injury. Figure 4.22*C* shows a tractographic reconstruction of neural connections via MRDTT.

4.8 3-D LIGHT IMAGING

A convention 2-D microscope can be extended to 3-D light imaging using the concept of confocal microscope discussed in Section 3.9.3. A schematic diagram of a fluorescence confocal microscope is shown in Figure 4.23. First, the focusing mechanism, a laser beam as the light source (Fig. 4.23, left) is used to scan (x-y scanning mirrors), focus (objective lens), and excite fluorescence objects of interest in order to obtain depth discrimination from other objects in the sample. Only the in-focus

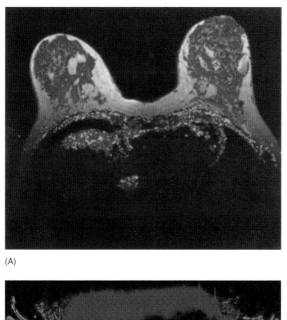

(A)

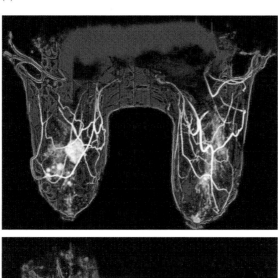

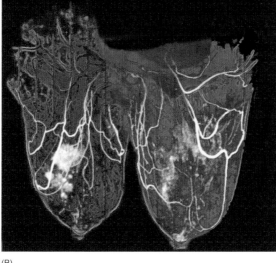

(B)

Figure 4.20 (*A*) Sectional view of a 3*T* CE-MRI (contrast-enhanced) exam of two breasts. (Courtesy of *Diag Imag* 9/2004, p. 53). (*B*) Two views of 3-D Dedicated breast MR angiogram (1.5T). (Courtesy of Dr. X. Hong, Aurora)

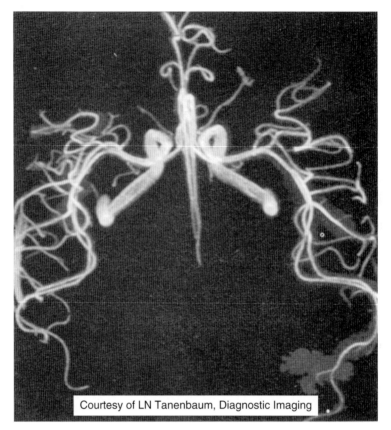

Courtesy of LN Tanenbaum, Diagnostic Imaging

Figure 4.21 MRA using a 3T MRI scanner, approaching image resolution possible with DSA (see Section 3.2.2). (Courtesy of LN Tanenbaum. *Diag Imag* 11/2004, p. 74)

emission from the sample will pass the pinhole mechanism and be recorded by the detector. In operation, the object can be scanned horizontally point by point by x-y scanning mirrors. The pinhole aperture can systematically allow the in-focus emission from the object in contiguous sections in the z direction to pass and be received by the detector. The result is a contiguous 3-D fluorescence image set of the object in the microscopic slide, or a 3-D light imaging volume set.

Although the size of a 2-D color microscopic image is less than 1 MB, we can extrapolate it to 3-D volumes from many objects of interest in a field, and to many fields in the entire microscopic slide; the storage requirement of 3-D light microscopic imaging is enormous. Image storage will be a major challenge to consider.

4.9 3-D MICRO IMAGING AND SMALL ANIMAL IMAGING CENTER

Small animal experiments are performed routinely before a new concept is advanced from bench research to clinical validation. Without micro imaging, animals have to be sacrificed at each stage of the experiment in order to periodically observe the change of conditions. Micro scanners can have a tremendous impact on the design of animal models, for example, for in vivo evaluation of the growth of tumors and the effectiveness of drug treatment to the tumors. With the micro scanners the animal does not have to be sacrificed for validation after each stage of treatment as in the traditional method; the animal can be kept alive under observation during the complete treatment cycle.

CT, MRI, and PET are used mainly for examination of the human; their design is not for small animal studies. One recent advance in CT, MRI, and PET is in the

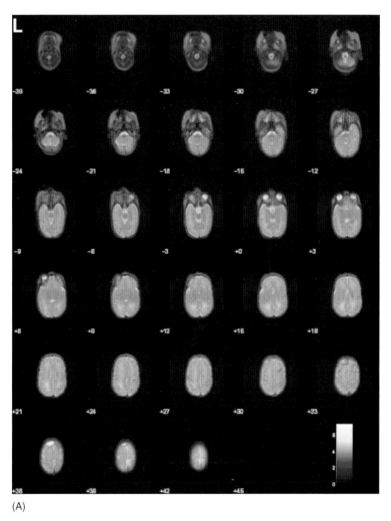

(A)

Figure 4.22 (*A*) Brain activation map overlaid onto the structural T_2 weighted MRI image of a child; color codes represent the degree of activation. (Courtesy of Dr. S. Erberich) (*B*) Brain activation map warped onto 3-D atlas brain; the 3-D reconstruction was based on a series of fMRI images. Color codes represent the degree of activation. (Courtesy of Dr. S. Erberich). (*C*) MRI DTI Tractographic reconstruction of neural connections via DTI, (Courtesy Source: Diffusion MRI - Wikipedia, the free encyclopedia http://en.wikipedia.org/wiki/Diffusion_MRI)

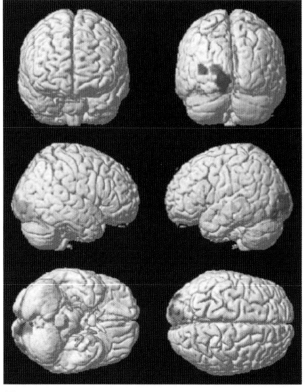

(B)

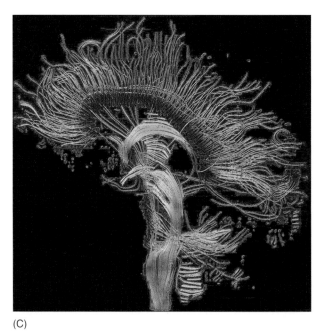

(C)

Figure 4.22   (*Continued*)

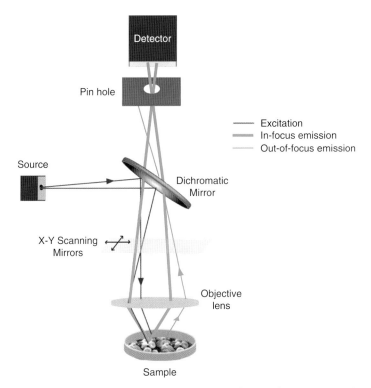

Figure 4.23 Principles of the 3-D fluorescence confocal microscope used to generate serial sections of an object of interest from the specimen. x-y scanning mirrors guide a laser beam (red lines) that excites objects attached with fluorescent dye molecules (yellow) in the sample (size not in scale). The dichromatic mirror only allows excited light (green) to pass. The optical pinhole mechanism accepts in-focus excited emission light (thick green lines) to be recorded by the detector, and rejects out-of-focus emission (thin green line). (Courtesy of M. Fleshman)

development of micro-imaging scanners specially designed for small animal studies involving rats and mice. Major design differences of such micro scanners from clinical sectional imaging systems are their small bore housing of small animals (20–50 g), lower radiation energy input, and smaller size but more sensitive detector system. For a single complete animal experiment, for example, the micro CT scanner can produce 1000 images of 50 μm spatial resolution, or 500 MB of image data. Figure 4.24A shows a 3-D display of a rat scanned by a micro CT scanner with 50-μm resolution, with the skeletal structure emphasized in the display. Figure 4.24B is the 3-D projection molecular images of a mouse with prostate tumor cells in bone marrow, with time as the third dimension. The top row time series shows no intervention, whereas the bottom rows show chemotherapy intervention. The two time series are from weeks 1, 2, 3, and 5.

With the advancements in small animal scanners, the traditional small animal laboratory will have to be renovated to accommodate these scanners, and this has led to the development of the small animal imaging center. Figure 4.24C shows the schematic of such a conceptual small animals imaging center with CT, MRI, PET,

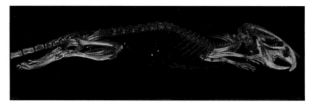

Courtesy of ORNL

(A)

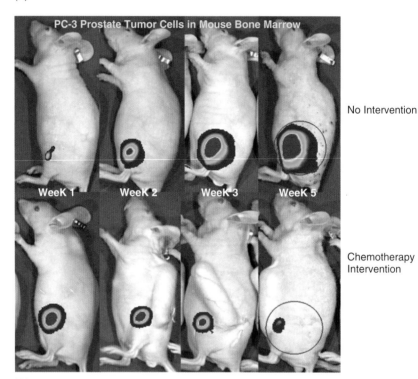

(B)

Figure 4.24 (A) 3-D rendering of the skeleton of a rat with a set of 1000 slices scanned by a micro XCT scanner with 50 micro pixel. 500 MB of image data were generated. The skeletal structure demonstrates the 3-D rendering of the display. (Courtesy of ORNL) (*B*) Two time series—weeks 1, 2, 3, and 5—of molecular images of a mouse with prostate tumor cells in its bone marrow. The three dimensions are projections of the *x*-*y* plane over time: (top row) No intervention; the tumor was growing fast after injection to week 5. (bottom row) With chemotherapy the tumor as seen at week 5 starting to respond, and it shrinks continuously after one week. (Courtesy of Dr. J. Pinski and G. Dagliyan, Molecular Imaging Center, USC) (*C*) Conceptual small animals imaging center at USC where most of the small animals imaging modalities have been acquired and installed. The conceptual model integrates all the modalities utilizing the DICOM standard: PACS, ePR (electronic patient record), and data grid technologies; and the clinical trial imaging model. Instead of ePR, the term has been changed to EAR for electronic animal model (refer to Parts II and III of the book for other PACS/ePR terminology used). (Courtesy of J. Lee)

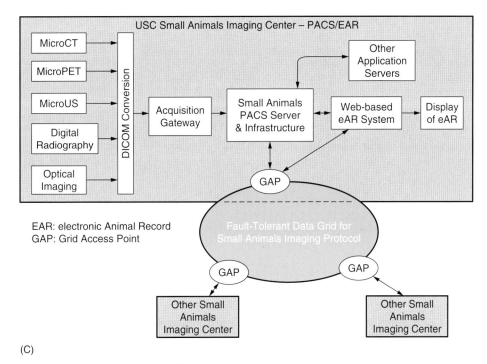

EAR: electronic Animal Record
GAP: Grid Access Point

(C)

Figure 4.24   (*Continued*)

US, molecular imaging, and other imaging modalities. Currently few of the existing small animal imaging centers have implemented the concept of system integration that we have learned from PACS, ePR, and the DICOM standard. This schematic suggests such a system integration concept as the infrastructure of the animals imaging center. In Part IV, where we discuss imaging informatics, we will return to this topic.

References

Beekman FJ, Kachelriesz M. Fully 3-D reconstruction of medical imaging. *IEEE Trans Medi Imag*, 27(7); 2008, 877–879.

Dhawan A P, Huang HK, Kim DS. Future trends in medical and molecular imaging. In: Dhawan AP, Huang HK, Kim DS, eds. *Principles and Advanced Methods in Medical Imaging and Image Analysis* Singapore: World Scientific; 2008, 829–43.

Feldkamp LA, Davis LC, Kress JW. Practical cone-beam algorithm. *J Opt Soc Am* 1: 612–9; 1984.

Fenster A, Downey DB. Three-diemnsional ultrasound imaging. In: Beutel J, Kundel HL, Van Metter RL, eds. *Handbook of Medical Imaging. Vol 1. Physics and Psychophysics*. Bellingham, WA: SPIE Press, shington; 2008, 463–509.

Kim DS. Recent advances in functional magnetic resonance imaging. In: Dhawan AP, Huang HK, Kim DS, eds. *Principles and Advanced Methods in Medical Imaging and Image Analysis*. Singapore; World Scientific; 2008; 267–87.

Kim DS, Ronen I. Recent advances in diffusion magnetic resonance imaging. In Dhawan AP, Huang HK, Kim DS, eds. *Principles and Advanced Methods in Medical Imaging and Image Analysis*. Singapore: World Scientific; 2008, 289–309.

Patwardhan SV, Akers WJ, Bloch S. Florescence molecular imaging: microscopic to macroscopic. In: Dhawan AP, Huang HK, Kim DS, eds. *Principles and Advanced Methods in Medical Imaging and Image Analysis*. Singapore: World Scientific; 2008, 311–36.

Stahl JN, Zhang J, Chou TM, Zellner C, Pomerantsev EV, Huang HK. A new approach to teleconferencing with intravascular ultrasound and cardiac angiography in a low-bandwidth environment. *RadioGraphics* 20: 1495–1503; 2000.

Taguchi K, Aradate H. Algorithm for image reconstruction in multi slice helical CT. *Med Phys* 25(4): 550–61; 1998.

Tanenbaum LN, MRA at 3T approaching image resolution possible with DSA eight-channel surface coils multislab 3 time-of-flight *Diag Imag* 11: 74; 2004.

Von Ramm OT, Smith SW. Three-dimensional imaging system. United States Patent 4694434, 1987.

Wikipedia, the free encyclopedia, Diffusion MRI http://en.wikipedia.org/wiki/Diffusion_MRI.

CHAPTER 5

Four-Dimensionality, Multimodality, and Fusion of Medical Imaging

5.1 BASICS OF 4-D, MULTIMODALITY, AND FUSION OF MEDICAL IMAGING

In Chapter 2 we introduced the concept of multidimensional medical images from 2-D, 3-D, to 4-D. Figure 5.1A revisits two types of 3-D image with z and t as the third dimension, respectively. The details of 3-D imaging were discussed in Chapter 4. This chapter presents 4-D imaging, which can take on several forms. One possible extension from 3-D imaging to 4-D imaging would be adding the fourth dimension of time t to the 3-D (x, y, z) spatial imaging shown in Figure 5.1B. Another form of 4-D imaging is the fusion of two modality anatomical structures, or one anatomical and one physiological modality 3-D image sets depicted in Figure 5.1C. Section 5.1 presents the basics of 4-D imaging, including its formation, multimodality image registration, fusion, and display. Section 5.2 discusses specific 4-D imaging for diagnostic and therapy purposes in daily clinical operation. Section 5.3 introduces multimodality imaging and methods of image registration. Section 5.4 considers the relationship between multimodality image registration with image fusion and display, and some applications. The many examples given in Sections 5.2, 5.3, and 5.4 demonstrate applications of the concepts described in Section 5.1.

5.1.1 From 3-D to 4-D Imaging

Consider a CT contrast study of the heart of a patient, Figure 5.1B, left, shows a 3-D CT image set, 1 to n_1, of the chest taken at time t_1; after a time interval t_m, as the contrast medium travels through the blood stream, a new set of 3-D CT is obtained as depicted in Figure 5.1B right. The combination of both sets and other possible 3-D CT set, obtained at over time t, between t_1 to t_m, forms a 4-D imaging set. The contents of this 4-D image set reveal the contrast media distribution through the 3-D anatomy from $t_1, \ldots, t, \ldots, t_m$. This type of 4-D image set is the most popular in daily clinical practice.

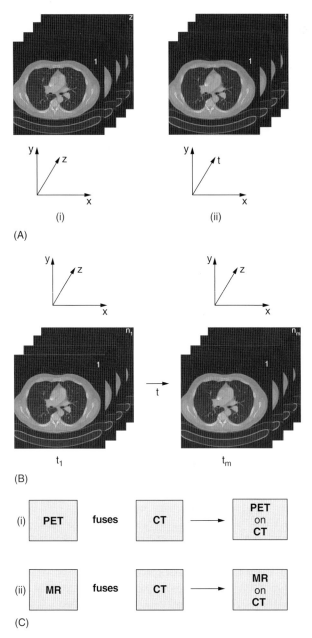

Figure 5.1 (*A*) Two 3-D image coordinate systems: (i) A 3-D spatial image set with z as the third dimension. Images from 1 to z show the anatomical changes of the cross-sectional chest (ii) A 3-D temporal image set with t (time) as the third dimension. Images from 1 to t show the same anatomy as image 1, the difference would be, for example, the flow of the contrast media injected to the patient from time 1 to t. (*B*) A 4-D image set consisting of a sequential 3-D spatial sets, with t as the fourth dimension. (*C*) (i) PET fuses with CT: physiology on anatomy; (ii) MR fuses with CT: enhancement of soft tissue definition on anatomy. (Adapted from Fig. 2.1*B–D*)

For example, to obtain the 4-D CT imaging shown in Figure 5.1*B*, the multislice CT scanner described in Section 4.3.3 is used. In this case the 3-D image consists of multislice CT images in one rotation; a fourth dimension *t* consists of the patient's bed being moved back to the original scanning position and the same scan repeated while the contrast media flows through the anatomical structure of interest, such as the heart.

5.1.2 Multimodality 3-D and 4-D Imaging

Multimodality imaging loosely means that different imaging modalities are used to exam the same anatomical region of interest. Because different modality imaging techniques can reveal tissue characteristics not obtainable by certain imaging techniques, information from multimodality images can enhance the diagnostic or therapeutic process. For example, CT can be used to obtain high-resolution anatomical images, whereas PET can be used to obtain in vivo physiological images that lack anatomical details. So, in combination, PET and CT images can yield a very powerful two-modality tool for high-quality spatial resolution functional imaging. Certain imaging modalities like CT, US, MRI, and PET can be used for obtaining either 3-D or 4-D images. The second imaging modality used to augment the first imaging modality for diagnosis could be conceptually an added dimension (but not necessary in the time domain) to the original 3-D or 4-D images. To avoid confusion of terminology, we will use the terms "multimodality 3-D" and "multimodality 4-D" in this chapter.

Another type of multimodality imaging is to use the same modality to scan the patient; then the energy used during the scanning is split into two energy levels, such as high and low energies. The images generated by the second energy are then treated as if they are from a second modality. So, after one scan, two sets of images are generated, the high and low energy image sets. Figure 5.2 shows the dual energy CT scanning technology in which high-energy and low-energy images are generated in one scan. Both the high- and low-energy images can be combined to identify the lesion inside the circle to be lipid degeneration. Dual energy CT imaging can also be used for identifying bone and soft tissues more readily from both images.

Multimodality imaging always produces multiple images of the same anatomical region. In two-modality imaging, it produces two images as shown in Figure 5.2. In PACS image archive, however, there is the potential of large data accumulation to result from multimodality imaging.

5.1.3 Image Registration

Given two sets of 3-D or 4-D images, in order to maximize their potential use for enhancing the diagnostic and therapeutic process, they need to be registered, fused, and properly displayed. This section discusses principles of image registration.

Image registration means that two sets of images are aligned and matched, and so coincide either in anatomical outline and structure or in the targeted lesion location and specifics. The former type of registration is called global, and the latter local. The alignment and matching can be 2-D, 3-D, or 4-D. In the case of 2-D, two images are registered section by section; 3-D registration is to align two 3-D volumes. The registration in 4-D not only requires 3-D volume registration but also for the images to be in sync with the time dimension.

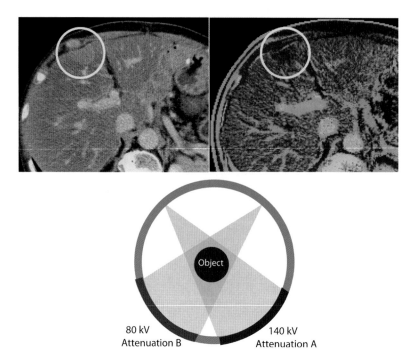

Figure 5.2   Dual X-ray energy CT scan in a gantry producing high- and low-energy images that can distinguish among tissue types. Single energy scan (left) without enough information to differentiate a lipid degeneration (right, inside the white circle), which is shown nicely (left) in the dark red color coded inside the white circle. (Courtesy of Siemens Medical Systems)

Image registration first defines the reference (or primary) image set, and then transforms the secondary (floating) image set to align, match, and coincide with the reference image set. In general, the higher spatial resolution image is used as the primary image (e.g., CT), and the lower resolution is used as the secondary image (e.g., PET). In the transformation, if only translation and rotation are required, it is called a rigid transformation. On the other hand, if a subvolume structure in one image set needs to be warped (or deformed) in order to match the other set, then it is called a nonrigid transformation. Rigid body transformation is much easier to perform compared to nonrigid transformation.

There are, in general, four steps in image registration:

1. The reference image set is defined to include the data format, resolutions, dimensions, slice thickness, scaling factors, and other image parameters; these image properties are normally in the DICOM image header (see Chapter 9). The secondary image set is then reformatted to match the reference image set.

2. Image registration is performed next between the reference image set and the reformatted secondary image set using global or local alignment, with rigid or nonrigid transformation.

3. Criteria are determined to evaluate the "goodness" of the image registration result.

4. Iterative methods can be used to optimize the registration result.

Image registration results as the two image sets are aligned, matched, and correspond one to one. Major hurdles to overcome have been patient movement, in particular:

1. transferring the patient from one modality gantry to the second modality gantry can alter the patient positioning, and
2. patient movement during the time lag between the collections of the two image sets can change the relative positions of internal organs with respect to the body outline.

In earlier clinical image registration applications, for example, image registration between CT and PET was performed as follows: The patient was first scanned by CT, and then by PET; the two data sets were then retrieved from both archiving systems, and image registration was done on a separate computer with the registration software. This method has sometimes been called the software approach. The two aforementioned hurdles of shifting bodily parts have hindered the potential applications of image registration. Over the past several years, multislice PET-CT combined hardware forming a single imaging device became commercially available, and it immediately removed these two obstacles of PET-CT image registration. This method is sometimes called the hardware approach; an example will be presented in Section 5.4.2.

5.1.4   Image Fusion

After two 3-D image sets have been properly registered, the next step is to overlay the two sets and display the result, a process called image fusion. The basic principle is to overlay the secondary 3-D set using a lookup table (LUT) on the secondary 3-D set to highlight specific features on the primary 3-D set obtained from its own LUT. Effective look-up table (LUT) pairs have the primary set in gray scale and the secondary in color. Both LUTs need to use a customized graphical user interface (GUI; see Chapter 12) to manually adjust the overlaid display by optimizing its effectiveness for the specific application. This customized LUT set can then be used as the default for future display of the same application.

In clinical applications, for example, PET-CT fusion is used to map the physiological parameters from PET onto the detailed anatomy CT. In the radiation therapy treatment plan for the prostate gland, to prevent overdosing critical organs, the MRI of the prostate, which has higher soft tissue definition that allows for a precise maximum dose to be delivered to the target organ, is fused onto the CT, which shows the overall anatomical details. This is a case of image fusion of local anatomy with a high-density resolution (MRI) onto a global anatomy with high spatial resolution (CT). Another radiation therapy application is the overlay of dose distribution onto the anatomy shown on a CT in accord with a treatment plan. These examples will be revisited in more detail in the following sections.

5.1.5   Display of 4-D Medical Images and Fusion Images

Currently the best way to display 4-D images is to use the video format. If the fourth dimension is time, then the video will show 3-D images with time frames moving forward and backward. Many commercial products for displaying video are readily available for this purpose. If the PACS workstation (WS) does not have this display feature (see Chapter 12), the 4-D image set may need to be packaged for postprocessing display first; then the user logs out from the PACS WS and uses some standard Web-based video display software.

For image registration and fusion display, the integrated result is to display on the PACS WS, or other specialized postprocessing WS (see Chapter 12). Take the example of PET-CT. The LUT of PET is in color, and the LUT of CT is in gray-scale, each of which has its own GUI. The two GUIs are two sliders allowing for an interactive adjustment of the color for PET and gray scale for CT. When the two customized GUI sliders have been accepted for a given clinical application, they may be combined as one single slider to facilitate interactive fine-tuning adjustments of the display during viewing.

For more effective imaging registration and fusion results, since the displays have multimodality images, it is advantageous to use a color LCD (liquid crystal display) device, with the gray scale component assigned to the LUT of CT, and the color component to the LUT of PET.

5.2 4-D MEDICAL IMAGING

With the time coordinate added to the three-dimensional space, sectional 3-D images can generate 4-D medical images. The time duration may be very short, less than seconds in capturing physiological changes like blood flow or organ movements like the heart beat. But the time duration may also be very long, for example, weeks, to obtain the molecular image shown in Figure 4.24*B*. Therefore we have to be careful in specifying the duration of the time parameter when time is the fourth dimension so that 4-D images are acquired and identified properly.

5.2.1 4-D Ultrasound Imaging

In Section 4.6 we discussed various ways that 3-D ultrasound (US) imaging can be used to steer the US transducer and the detector system automatically in generating 3-D US images. Although the image quality of 3-D US is inferior to that generated by CT and MRI, the advantage of 3-D US, in addition to its noninvasiveness, is that it can produce very fast images compared to CT and MRI. For this reason 4-D US imaging with time as the fourth dimension is practical for certain time essence screening and diagnostic applications. There is an increasing interest in visualizing 4-D US data for use in medical diagnosis.

Already 4-D maternity US scans can provide expectant and eager parents with the very first images of their baby, from a yawn to the heart beats, arms and legs stretch, and other movements at week 12 and on. 4-D US can therefore be used to follow the growth of the fetus in the mother's womb. 4-D US images are most effectively used in dynamic mode such as the video format. For this reason its integration with PACS operation requires special consideration. Figure 5.3 gives a comparison between 2-D, 3-D, and 4-D US fetus images.

5.2.2 4-D X-ray CT Imaging

We used cardiac imaging in Section 5.1.1 as an example to describe 4-D X-ray CT I. Recall Figure 4.6 where we showed 3-D heart volume with 256 images in one

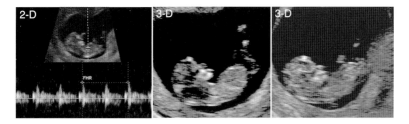

(A)

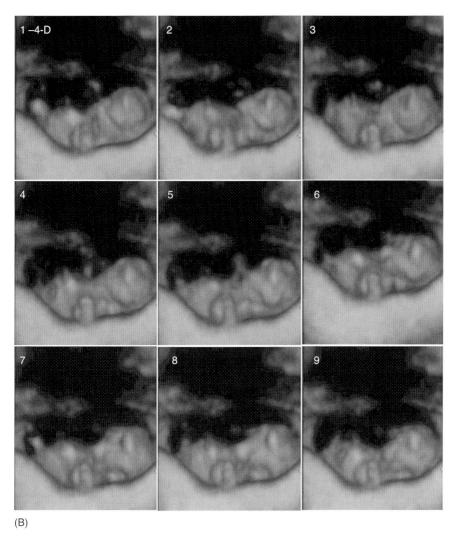

(B)

Figure 5.3 Fetus images taken with 2-D, 3-D, and 4-D US imaging. 2-D, 3-D and 4-D US images can be used to monitor the growth of the fetus before the baby is born. (*A*) 2-D US image with heart beat audio at the bottom. The two 3-D US images reveal the breathing movement of the chest wall and the stretching of the legs. (*B*) Sequence of nine 4-D US image frames (not in equal time intervals) showing the movements of the legs, turning of the body and the face (frames 5, 6, 7), and movement of the arms and legs. (Courtesy of Dr. C. Huang; art work by A. Sullivan)

compete rotation of the X-ray gantry using the 256 multislice CT scanner. Suppose that X-ray contrast enhanced media is injected into the patient, and with the patient and the bed remaining stationary, we perform an EKG gated study of the heart allowing only the X-ray gantry to rotate in sync with the diastole and systole cycles of the heart. We would then obtain a 4-D CT image set with the fourth dimension as the time synchronized with the systolic and diastolic cycles of the heart. In this scanning mode the dynamic of the 3-D heart beat at systole and diastole can be visualized in 3-D anatomy with the contrast enhanced. To realize such potential clinical applications of the 4-D X-ray CT in cardiac imaging, several parameters need to be considered:

1. The multislice CT should have a cone-beam X ray to cover the full heart, and a 256 array detector system, each array with 1000 detectors to receive sufficient data to perform image reconstruction.
2. A gating mechanism to trigger the on and off of the X ray in the rotation gantry.
3. A data transfer rate between the data acquisition system and the display system increased to roughly 1.0 GB/s.
4. A revolutionized display method for 4-D cardiac images.

4-D X-ray CT can produce images in the gigabyte range per examination. Methods of archive, communication, and display are challenging topics in PACS design and implementation. For more on multimodality 4-D cardiac imaging with PET and CT, see Section 5.4.

5.2.3   4-D PET Imaging

3-D PET scanner can generate 3-D physiological images but at a slower rate compared with the 3-D X-ray CT. For this reason the 3-D PET data accumulation is averaged over the period of duration and not in real time. For example, in a whole body PET it takes about 23 minutes in a 64 multislice PET-CT scanner (see Fig. 5.8*B*). Thus 3-D PET averages the images over the time period that the data are collected. At about one second the resulting 3-D PET images compared with those of CT are quite different in terms of the t variable. In a gated 4-D PET cardiac study, as is the case of the gated 64 multislice CT scanner study described in Section 5.2.2, the generated 4-D PET data set has each time unit as the average of many minutes of PET raw data before the images' reconstruction.

5.3   MULTIMODALITY IMAGING

5.3.1   2-D and 3-D Anatomy — An Integrated Multimodality Paradigm for Cancer in Dense Breasts

5.3.1.1   *2-D US, Digital Mammography, 3-D US, and 3-D MRI for Breast Exam*   More than 250,000 women are newly diagnosed with breast cancer in the United States each year. In general, conventional mammography, sometimes accompanied by 2-D ultrasound imaging, is the imaging modality of choice to detect early

stages of breast cancer as well as to evaluate the breast cancer to determine the course of surgery. Specifically, if the cancer in the breast is too large or too extensive within the breast tissue, it may necessitate mastectomy surgery to remove the entire breast. In some cases the breast may be saved from mastectomy if the cancer is properly identified and characterized early. The current standard of clinical practice is to perform breast imaging examinations and then verify the malignancy with tissue samples obtained from a biopsy. Because conventional and digital mammography is the imaging modality of choice, there is one significant weakness in that the accuracy of mammography to detect cancer decreases as breast density increases, which is common in premenopausal women. To support digital mammography (DM; see Section 3.5) in dense breast cases, contrast-enhanced MRI (CE-MRI; see Fig. 4.20*A*, *B*) and 2-D ultrasound (see Section 3.8) have been used for further detecting, identifying, characterizing, and measuring cancer in dense breasts. CE-MRI is a very costly procedure (US$1000), and it has a high rate of false positives. 2-D US is operator-dependent, and the image quality is inconsistent. Volumetric (3-D) automated full-breast US (AFBUS) is an emerging technology and has shown to have better image quality and consistent results than the 2-D US, since it is automatic, systematic, and operator independent. The combination of the four different imaging modalities, 2-D US, DM, AFBUS, and CE-MRI could be crucial in helping to improve the detection, identification, and characterization of abnormalities in dense breasts. This section briefly describes the imaging component of an integrated multimodality paradigm by bringing all four imaging modality data together to guide diagnostic and treatment paths for detection and characterization of abnormalities in dense breast. The imaging informatics component with decision-support and quantified knowledge will be presented in Part IV.

5.3.1.2 *Use of Volumetric 3-D Automated Full-breast US (AFBUS) and Dedicated Breast MRI for Defining Extent of Breast Cancer*

3D AFBUS   As a potential adjunct to mammography in evaluating breast abnormalities, 3-D AFBUS has similar clinical benefits to 2-D US. However, use of a targeted conventional handheld US produces inconsistent image quality and findings due to operator dependency even with the potential benefits that US has in imaging of dense breast cases. Because it is automatic and operator-independent, 3-D AFBUS provides repeatable US image data that are similar to traditional volume-based imaging, such as MRI, in yielding accurate volumetric (3-D) and multislice and multiplanar US image data. The added benefit of low cost and its non-invasive nature as compared to CE-MRI (contrast-enhanced) makes it a potentially significant imaging alternative for identifying and characterizing abnormalities in dense breast tissue. 3-D AFBUS has been used for clinical research as a screening tool and demonstrated concordance with known benign breast conditions and the capability to provide documentation of new benign findings. Because 3-D AFBUS is an emerging technology, its sensitivity and specificity have not yet been properly defined and validated. Figure 5.4 shows a 3-D AFBUS image.

DB MRI   Dedicated breast 3-D MRI differs from the whole body CE-MRI in that the design of the DB MRI is for examining the breasts only. The MRI technology used is normally 1.5 T with a smaller bore gantry compared with the whole body MRI. The system has a specially designed patient bed and breast coils. Because this

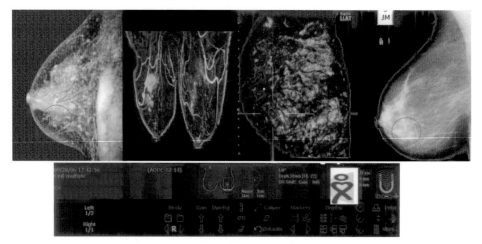

Figure 5.4 GUI (graphical user interface) of a decision-support system with automatic identification and quantification of the dense breast abnormality in multimodality coherence views of, from left to right, CE-MRI, DB 3-D angiograms, 3D AFBUS, and digital mammogram, by location as part of the multimodality paradigm based on BI-RADS shown in bottom row. (Data Sources: U-Systems and Aurora)

design is customized for breast screening especially for dense breasts, its workflow is streamlined for fast and accurate scanning with the breast biopsy capability. The system has the potential to become the screening tool for high risk patients. Currently there are about 60 DB MRI being used in breast imaging centers, hospitals and medical centers. Figure 4.20*B* shows two 3-D views of the DB 3-D MR angiograms, and Section 21.6 will describe the DB MRI system in more detail.

3-D Breast Imaging Decision-Support Tools   Both AFBUS and DB MRI require decision-support viewing tools allowing multimodality breast images to be displayed and compared on the same viewing workstation (see Chapter 12). A decision support viewing system can be tailored to a multimodality paradigm that can bring added value to the diagnostic and treatment path for the breast cancer patient. Figure 5.4 shows a GUI (graphical user interface) of a decision-support system with automatic identification and quantification of a dense breast abnormality in the multimodality views of CE-MRI, BD 3-D MR angiograms, 3D AFBUS, and digital mammography (DM), which are correlated by location as part of the multimodality paradigm based on BI-RADS (*Breast Imaging Reporting and Data System standard*, 4th edition). BI-RADS terminology can be used to categorize lesions on mammograms and sonograms, MRI and MRA as is shown in the bottom row. To accommodate multimodality images like DM, 3-D US, and 3-D MRI into PACS environment for the breast imaging exam, two parameters need to be considered: (1) an effective database for image archive and (2) an image display format on a PACS workstation with user friendly GUI. These topics will be covered in Part II.

5.3.2 Multimodality 2-D and 3-D Imaging in Radiation Therapy (RT)

5.3.2.1 Radiation Therapy Workflow   External beam radiation therapy (RT) calls for treatment planning as well as treatment delivery. Over 90% of the workload in radiation therapy is dedicated to planning radiation therapy and this involves an intensive image and computer graphic process. In the RT planning process patient information is needed in order to plan a treatment; also image registration is needed to identify regions to be treated, and markers are used to align images. Multimodality images from projection X rays, computed tomography (CT), magnetic resonance imaging (MRI), positron emission tomography (PET), and linear accelerator are used for tumor localization and organ identification. Images must include the shape, size, and location of the targets and the radiosensitive vital organs. Sometime 3-D and 2-D images must be fused to identity better the outlines of the tumor and adjacent organ's anatomy. The images are then overlaid with computer graphics derived from the treatment plan and the dose distribution, to verify that the site of delivery of a uniform high dose would target the tumor and avoid adjacent critical structures. Next carefully monitoring of the treatment, optimization, and dose calculation is essential for successful patient treatment outcomes. In all these processes, PACS and imaging informatics technologies are used extensively. Radiation therapy is prepared for the individual patient, so it is important that informatics be utilized to optimize RT workflow and patient treatment outcomes. The RT workflow in Figure 5.5 depicts a generic treatment plan and delivery of prostate cancer treatment. The multimodalities of the imaging component of RT treatment planning and delivery includes, in particular, (1) image acquisition, (2) field planning at the treatment planning system, and (3) generation of DRR (digitally reconstructed radiography), and (6) verification: comparing portal image and reference DRR image, described in the yellow boxes of the workflow. The informatics component will be discussed in more detail in Chapter 23.

5.3.2.2 2-D and 3-D RT Image Registration

Imaging Component in Treatment Planning: Steps 1 to 5   A treatment plan's objective is to deliver as high and uniform as possible a radiation dose to the prostate tumor bearing site but as little as possible dose to the surrounding healthy tissues, especially the surrounding critical and radiosensitive structures. In this example these are the urinary bladder and the rectum of the patient with prostate cancer.

To start with the workflow, the oncologist orders a set of CT images of the patient's pelvis either in the CT simulator (a CT scanner) at the radiation oncology department or a CT scanner at the radiology department. The patient's information is delivered to the CT simulator room where the radiation therapist sets the patient up in his treatment position for scanning.

Step 1. Pelvic CT images (Fig. 5.5 step 1) are generated as DICOM images (see Chapter 9) and stored either in a PACS or the workstation there.

Step 2. The acquired CT images are transferred to a computerized treatment planning system (TPS) for radiation field planning. Previous available diagnostic images—CT, MRI, or PET images—are also retrieved as a reference to aid in the delineation of tumor volume. Image registration and fusion may be needed in this step (see Section 5.3.3 for an example). At the TPS workstation the tumor volume and the organs at risk (OARs) (urinary bladder and rectum) are delineated interactively by a medical physicist (Fig. 5.6*A*). Treatment fields of appropriate size and gantry/collimator angles are positioned (Fig. 5.6*B*). The TPS computes the radiation dose distribution within the bodily region to be treated

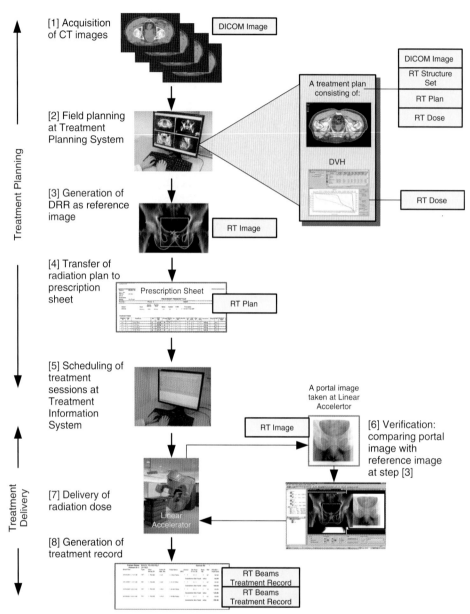

Figure 5.5   Generic external beam radiation therapy workflow, including treatment planning and delivery using prostate gland cancer as an example. RT Information is scattered at where it is generated. The yellow boxes indicate the RT-related images and data that could be generated in the workflow. Treatment planning steps 1, 2, and 3; and treatment delivery step 6 shown in yellow boxes are described in the text. Step 2 in RT treatment plan with radiation dose distribution involves the superposition of the radiotherapy treatment parameters: RT plan, RT structure set and RT dose upon the corresponding set CT images. DRR: digital reconstructed radiograph; DVH: dose volume histogram. (Courtesy of Dr. M Law)

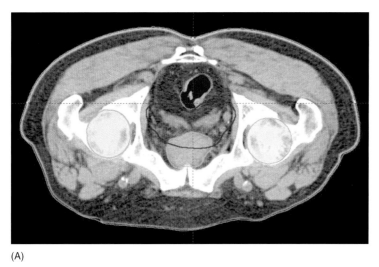

(A)

Figure 5.6 (*A*) RT structure set (see Chapter 9): tumor volume (red), organs at risk (femoral head in green and pink, rectum in purple, bladder in blue), and body contour. The structures in this diagram have the CT image as their frame of reference and are superimposed on the CT image. (*B*) RT plan: includes treatment beam details, fractionation scheme, and prescription (above). On the left is a graphic display of information from the RT plan and RT structure set, both superimposed on the CT image. There are nine radiation beams (attribute of the RT plan), each represented by a red label and three yellow lines in the diagram. (*C*) RT dose: on the left are the radiation dose data from a TPS. Isodose curves (yellow, pink, green, magenta, and blue) are displayed with reference to the CT image and the tumor volume (red shading) from an RT structure set. (*D*) Dose volume histogram (DVH): belongs to the RT dose object in (*C*) for treatment plan evaluation. This is key to evaluating whether proper radiation dose is applied to the target tumor while limiting dose to the surrounding critical healthy tissue and organs. The red line shows that most of the tumor volume receives >7500cGy of radiation dose. Other colors show the dose received by other OARs. (*E*) Web client application page showing a comparison between the reference image (left) and the electronic portal image (right) used to verify the treatment field. The reference image DRR was generated from the CT scans, and the electronic portal image from the linear accelerator. Note that there is an icon marked "X" to indicate approval by the radiation oncologist. (*F*) Three different types of RT 2-D images for verification of the treatment accuracy: (left) Projectional simulator image with delineator showing the field to be irradiated; (middle) reference DRR reconstructed from CT images; (right) portal images from the linear accelerator. Portal images are compared with the reference images from the simulator or the DRRs to verify the accuracy of the treatment portal. (Courtesy of Dr. M Law)

(Fig. 5.6*C*). A dose–volume histogram (DVH) may be generated to show the dose received by the tumor and OARs (Fig. 5.6*D*).

Step 3. DDR (digitally reconstructed radiograph) images similar to X-ray projection images are reconstructed from the CT slices to show the treatment field positions (Fig. 5.5, step 3, and Fig. 5.6*E*).

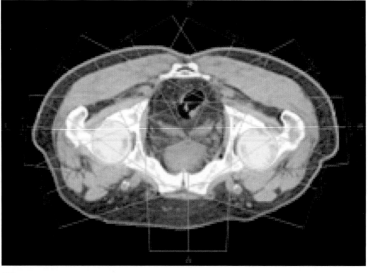

(B)

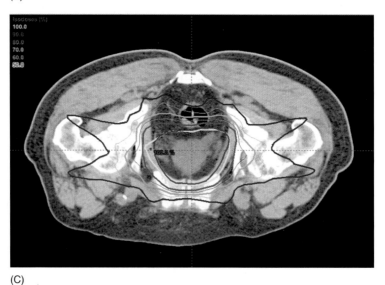

(C)

Figure 5.6 (*Continued*)

Step 4. The finished plan is presented to the radiation oncologist for evaluation and approval. If the plan is found to be satisfactory, the oncologist prescribes the treatment in the RT prescription sheet.

Step 5. A treatment record with all treatment details is prepared with the prescription. Treatment sessions is scheduled at the treatment information system.

Imaging Component in Treatment Delivery: Step 6 At step 6 the approved treatment plan is transferred to the radiation treatment unit or linear accelerator

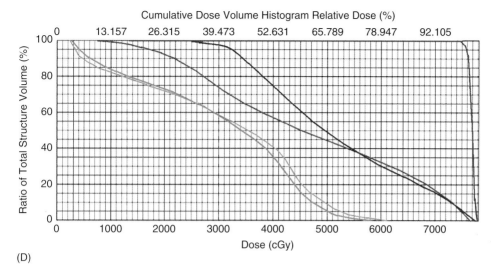

(D)

(E)

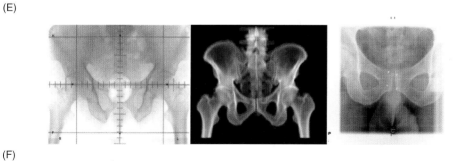

(F)

Figure 5.6   (*Continued*)

(LINAC). Before the radiation treatment can begin, the treatment plan with respect to the DRR (which serves as a reference image) needs to be verified at the LINAC for accuracy in terms of field sizes, setup, and shielding positions, and so forth. For such verification, a portal image by an electronic portal imaging device (EPID, a device installed in the LINAC for taking digital portal images) is taken at the LINAC. It is then compared with the reference DRR images described in step 3 (Fig. 5.6E). When the portal images are found to match the reference images in aligning with the treatment field, the oncologist approves the verification. Radiation treatment can then proceed in accord with step 7. Otherwise, a repeat portal image may be requested. Usually the patient is treated five times a week for seven to eight weeks. Each treatment beam is recorded at each treatment session and as well as the cumulative dose to-date described in step 8. Over the course of treatment the patient will have weekly verification images acquired to ensure the accuracy of the treatment.

3-D and 2-D Image Registration Several 3-D and 2-D imaging processing methods are used to expedite the RT workflow from treatment planning steps 1, 2, and 3 to treatment delivery step 6. For the patient with prostate cancer shown in Figure 5.5, we recapitulate the RT workflow with attention paid to the image registration:

1. Exam of the pelvic using the CT simulator.
2. A physicist uses a computer treatment planning system (TPS) to generate the outlines of the tumor and adjacent organ from the CT images interactively (Fig. 5.6A); then planning of the radiation treatment begins (Fig. 5.6B). TPS computes radiation dose distribution of the target cancer and organs (Fig. 5.6C) and the dose–volume histogram (DVH) (Fig. 5.6D). These information are converted to computer graphics and overlaid on the proper CT images (Fig. 5.6C), and as DVH plots of the individual organs in the vicinity of the tumor (Fig. 5.6D).
3. The TPS reconstructs DDR (digitally reconstructed radiographs) (Fig. 5.6E, *left*) using conical geometry because of the cone-beam X-ray output of the CT scanner, which yields 2-D DDRs.
4. Three different types of RT 2-D images used for verification of the treatment accuracy are shown in Figure 5.6F: projection simulator image with the delineator showing the field to be irradiated (left), the reference DRR reconstructed from the CT images (middle), and portal images from the linear accelerator (right). Portal images are used to compare them with reference images from the simulator or the DRRs and thus to verify the accuracy of the treatment portal, shown in Figure 5.6E.
5. These DDRs are used to compare with electronic portal images of the patient taken from an electronic portal imaging device in the LINAC for patient positioning in the LINAC.

Critical to these processes are (1) various image reconstruction methods from 3-D data to 2-D images, (2) image registration algorithms between the 2-D DDRs and portal images, and (3) proper coordinates transformation between computer graphic outlines and the overlay on 3-D CT images. Because different imaging modalities in

RT generate different images, each with its own image format, data collection using a standardization format is a critical consideration in the PACS related informatics environment.

5.3.3 Fusion of 3-D MRI and 3-D CT Images for RT Application

In step 2 we mentioned that the acquired CT images are transferred to a computer treatment planning system (TPS) for radiation field planning, and that previous diagnostic images, CT, MRI, or PET images, are also retrieved as a reference in the delineation of tumor volume. In the prostate cancer example, there was no previous CT, MRI, or PET to be retrieved to aid in the delineation of the tumor's volume. In this section we give an example of a brain tumor in which the patient had both CT and MRI examinations. In this case CT provides a better image of the overall anatomy of the brain and the head, and is considered the primary image set; although MRI can delineate better the separation between the tumor and brain tissues, it is assigned to the secondary image set. The challenge of this example is to fuse the secondary 3-D MRI volume with the primary 3-D CT volume for a more accurate tumor delineation. The first step is to perform the image registration between the 3-D MRI and the 3-D CT sets.

Recall that in Sections 5.1.3 and 5.1.4 image registration required transforming the secondary 3-D MR image set (Fig. 5.7*A*, right) to align, match, and correspond with the reference 3-D CT image set (Figure 5.7*A*, left). After two 3-D image sets have been properly registered, the next step is to fuse the two 3-D sets by overlaying them, one over the other, and displaying the result. One sectional image each from the 3-D MRI and the 3-D CT is used as an example. One of the most effective lookup table (LUT) pairs is to have the primary in gray scale and the secondary in color. Thus the MRI 3-D set using a reddish LUT highlighting the brain tumor outline is overlaid onto the 3-D CT set with a gray scale LUT, with result shown in Figure 5.7*B*. After satisfaction from the viewing, the target tumor can be outlined interactively, with more accuracy, as shown by the black contour. Note the difficulty to outline the tumor using either the CT image or the MRI alone from Fig. 5.7*A*. In Chapter 23 we will revisit this topic and describe how image fusion results can be integrated with other imaging informatics methods to facilitate RT planning and treatment.

5.4 FUSION OF HIGH-DIMENSIONAL MEDICAL IMAGING

5.4.1 Software versus Hardware Multimodality Image Fusion

In this section we present two advances in X-Ray CT and PET imaging techniques that combine physiology and anatomy for healthcare delivery and for basic animal research. The first is a combination of the CT and PET scanners for image fusion, and the second combines the micro PET and CT scanners. In Sections 5.1.3 and 5.1.4 we saw that one major obstacle in image registration is patient movement as one scanner is replaced by another during two separate examinations. For this reason heavy software and scanning protocols need to be used to obtain the best registration result by a method called the software approach. A hardware method that also can be used to minimize this obstacle is to develop a combined modalities scanner. Below we use a combined CT and PET scanner to explain the principle behind this method and illustrate some results.

5.4.2 Combined PET-CT Scanner for Hardware Image Fusion

X-Ray CT is excellent for anatomical delineation with fast scanning time, while PET is slow in obtaining physiological images with poorer spatial resolution but good for the differentiation between benign from malignant tumors, and for observing physiological phenomena. PET requires attenuation correction in image reconstruction, and the fast CT scan time can provide the necessary anatomical tissue attenuation in seconds during the scan to be used as a base for PET data correction. Thus the

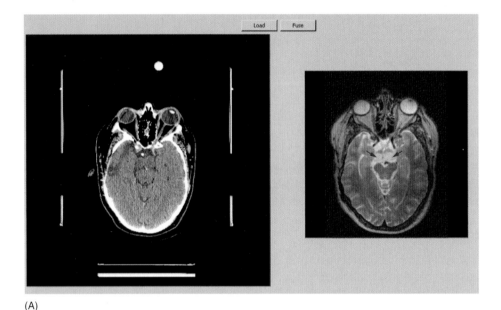

(A)

Figure 5.7 (*A*) MR-CT image fusion used for more accurate tumor delineation. One image each from the 3-D MRI and the 3-D CT is presented for illustration. (*Right*) A transverse section of the 3-D MRI volume in a gray scale LUT showing the brain tumor (arrows). (Left) The corresponding anatomical transverse section of the 3-D CT volume with a gray scale LUT. Two registration points are used for image registration, one point at the tip of the nose and the second at the posterior skull. Since the CT (512 × 512) and the MR (256 × 256) images are of different pixel sizes, the registration requires resizing and scaling to perform a proper mapping. Once the registration is completed, the next step is to display the fused MR and CT images. (*B*) The MR/CT fusion screenshot from a PACS workstation showing the fused MR and CT images. A slider bar at the bottom allows interactively viewing of each image overlaid. The fused image shows the CT image (grayish color) as well as the MR image (reddish color) with the preference color washing to enhance the target tumor tissue. The viewed target tumor can be outlined interactively more accurately as shown by the black contour. Note the difficulty to outline the tumor in the CT image or in the MRI, individually and independently, from Figure 5.7A. (Courtesy of Drs. J. Documet and B. Liu)

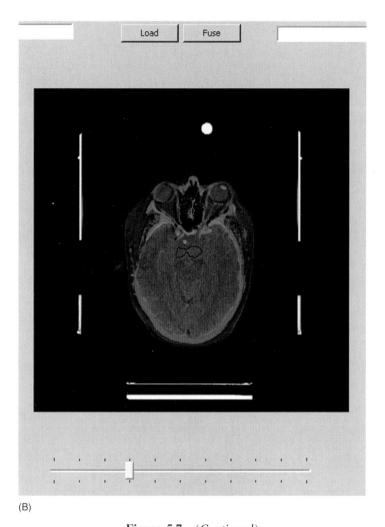

(B)

Figure 5.7   (*Continued*)

combination of a CT and a PET scanner together form a single PET-CT (or PET/CT) scanner, so the patient does not need to be moved to the second scanning gantry during a PET-CT study. While neither tool alone is able to provide such a result, their combination can provide a very powerful diagnostic tool and improve clinical accuracy. The two scanners have to be combined as one system; otherwise, the mis-registration between CT and PET images could at times give misleading information. A PET-CT fusion scanner is a hybrid scanner that generates CT images first, followed by PET images during an examination. The PET images so obtained actually have better resolution than those obtained without using the CT data attenuation correction. The output of a PET-CT fusion scanner is three sets of images: CT images, PET images, and fused PET-CT physiology/anatomy images. These images are aligned by the same spatial coordinate system. The hardware fusion method minimizes any patient positional change and movement during the image registration before fusion occurs. Figure 5.8*A* shows a PET-CT scanner with 64 CT multislices per rotation

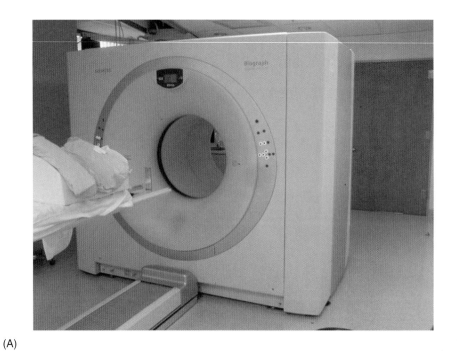

(A)

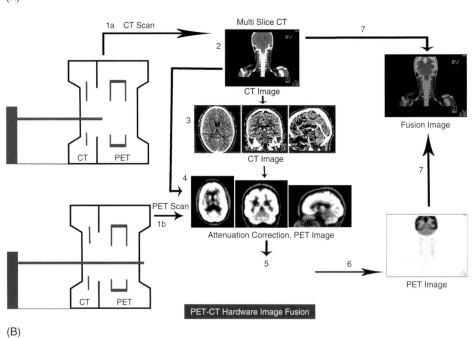

(B)

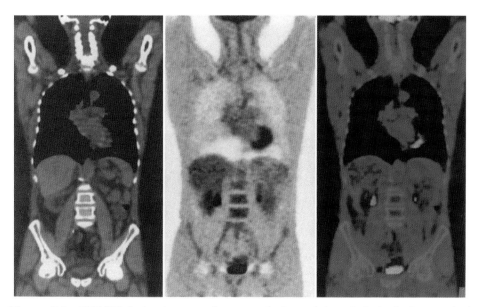

Figure 5.9   PET/CT fusion images of a coronal view of the whole body from a dual gantry CT/PET scanner indicating normal distribution of FDG (18-F fluorodeoxyglucose). (*Left*) CT image; (*middle*) PET image; (*right*) fusion image with pseudo-color look-up table (LUT) PET image (physiology) overlaying CT image (anatomy); FDG accumulation shown in cerebral-cerebellar cortex, myocardium, liver, kidneys, renal pelvis, bone marrow, and urinary bladder. (Courtesy of Dr. R. Shrestha and of L. Kostakoglu, etal. *Radiographics* 2004;24:1411–31)

Figure 5.8   (*A*) PET-CT system with 64 slices at the Nuclear Medicine Division, Department of Radiology, USC. (*B*) Hardware image fusion with a PET/CT combined scanner. The hardware fusion method minimizes patient position change and movement during image registration before fusion. The mockup shows a PET/CT scan of a patient one hour after injection of 18-F fluorodeoxyglucose. The patient was positioned in a positron emission tomography/computed axial tomography (PET/CT) scanner. Workflow steps: (1a) 64 Multislice CT followed by (1b) a PET scan; (2) 3-D CT images of a full reconstructed coronal section along with (3) brain transverse, coronal, and sagittal sections; (4) 3-D CT data used to perform attention correction of PET data; (5) 3-D PET image reconstruction; (6) 3-D PET images obtained showing a coronal, (7) registered and fused CT and PET images with the corresponding coronal section. The "fused" PET/CT images allow for increased sensitivity in the detection of neoplastic disease by combining identified abnormal physiologic activity (PET) with precise anatomic localization (CT). (Courtesy of Dr. P. Moin; artwork by A Sullivan)

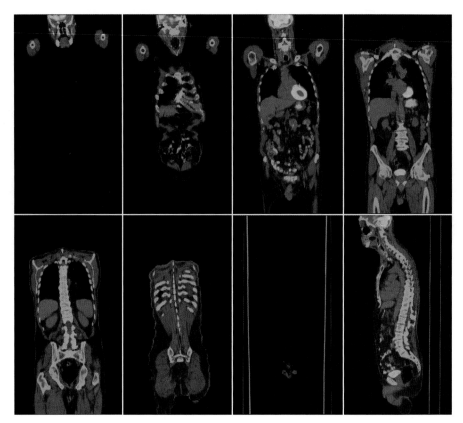

Figure 5.10   PET/CT hardware combined fusion coronal sectional images with 18F-FDG. Of the 25 equal spaced 1.0-cm sequential images, 00, 04, 08, 12, 16, 20, and 24 are shown. A sagittal section is also displayed. (Courtesy of M. Fleshman, artwork)

in clinical operation at USC. Figure 5.8*B* depicts the schematics of the combined scanner and the workflow steps. Workflow starts with the CT scan and CT image reconstruction, followed by the PET scan. Step 4 illustrates that after the PET scan is completed, the PET image reconstruction takes advantage of the already existing CT image data for PET data attenuation correction, which improves the quality of the PET images. The last step is the fusion of PET and CT images. Here we use a coronal view as an example. Figure 5.9 depicts an example of a coronal CT image (anatomy), a PET image (physiology), and a PET and CT fused image (physiology overlaid anatomy).

5.4.3 Some Examples of PET-CT Hardware Image Fusion

Our PET-CT study included investigating fusion of high-dimensional multimodality medical images using a combined PET-CT imaging system. 18-F fluorodeoxyglucose (FDG) was administered to the patient, and one hour after injection the patient was positioned in a PET-CT scanner. The patient was first scanned with CT from head to the pelvis region in about 60 seconds, and then the same regions by PET in about 23 minutes as described in Figure 5.8*B*. In about 24 minutes, three sets of 3-D

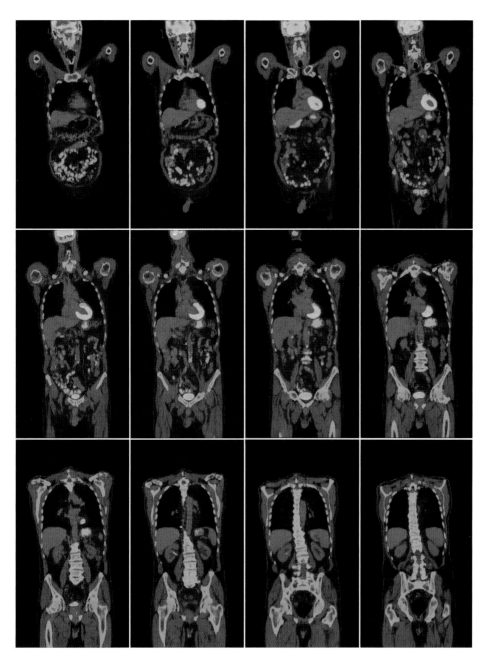

Figure 5.11   Same study as in Figure 5.10. PET/CT hardware combined fusion coronal sectional images with 18F-FDG. Of the 25 equally spaced sequential images, 12 consecutive 1.0-cm sections are displayed. Observe the 18F-FDG distribution in the heart one hour after injection plus 24-minute scanning time. (Courtesy of M. Fleshman, artwork)

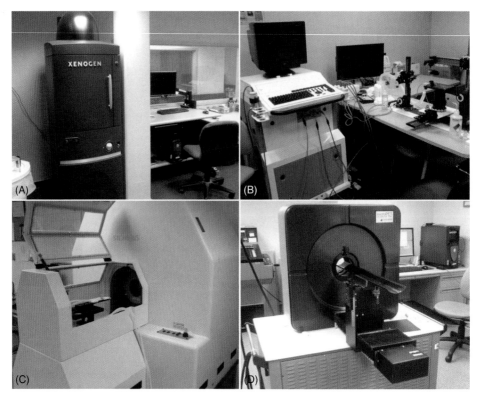

Figure 5.12   (*A*) Optical Imaging device; (*B*) micro US canner; (*C*) micro CT, and D. micro PET at the Molecular Imaging Center (MIC), USC. (Courtesy of the MIC)

images—CT, PET, and fusion CT and PET—were obtained. Notice that the times quoted for the scanning procedures are approximate; they depend on the scanning protocols used and quality of the images required. Twenty-six 1.0-cm equally spaced coronal sections (00, 01, ..., 25) and one mid-sagittal section are displayed for illustration purposes.

Figure 5.10 shows seven equally spaced, about 4.0 cm apart, sequential coronal images: 00, 04, 08, 12, 16, 20, 24, from the most anterior to the posterior of the body; and one mid-sagittal image. The bluish gray color shows the average 18F-FDG whole body distribution, from the front to back of the body, one hour after injection over 24 minutes of scanning time. The brain, the heart, and the urinary bladder have the greatest amount of concentration, followed by the kidneys.

Figure 5.11 depicts 12 consecutive 1.0-cm sections covering the heart from anterior to posterior of the body. The emphasis is to observe the 18F-FDG distribution in the normal heart and the excretion system, including the urinary bladder and the kidneys. Starting from the leftmost image to the eighth image, anterior to posterior, one hour after the injection and 24 minutes of scanning time, it is evident that although a large amount of 18F-FDG has collected in the urinary bladder, there is still much within the heart. So 18F-FDG appears to be a good radiopharmaceutical agent for examining the cardiac system.

CT PET PET/CT Fusion

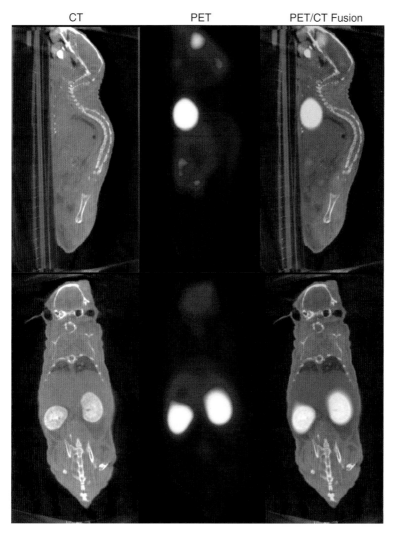

Figure 5.13 Fusion of micro PET and CT 3-D images of a mouse showing (from left to right) CT, PET, and fusion image of a mouse; (from top to bottom) mid-lateral and Mid-top views. (Courtesy of A. Tank, Molecular Imaging Center, USC)

5.4.4 Multimodality 3-D Micro Scanners — Software Image Fusion

In the animal imaging research center discussed in Section 4.9 and shown in Figures 4.23, 4.24*A*, *B*, *C*, imaging modalities mainly included optical imaging, digital radiography, micro US, micro PET, micro CT, and micro MRI. Some of these imaging modalities are shown in Figure 5.12. Image fusion was also performed on the images from some of these modalities, among them the micro PET-CT image fusion. Because there does not yet exist any hardware image fusion mechanism in the micro imaging domain, the image fusion had to be done with software processing. Figure 5.13 shows some of the results obtained from an animal study with the two separate CT and PET scanners presented in Figure 5.12.

References

Baines CJ. A tangled web: Factors likely to affect the efficacy of screening mammography. *J Nat Cancer Inst* 91: 833–8; 1999.

Behrens S, Laue H, Althaus M, et al. Computer assistance for MR based diagnosis of breast cancer: present and future challenges, *J.Comp Med. Imag. Graphics* 31: 236–247; 2007.

Boyd D, et al. Mammographic densities and breast cancer risk. *Cancer Epid Biomark Prev* 7: 1133–44; 1998.

Burhenne HJ, et al. Interval breast cancers in the screening mammography program of British Columbia: analysis and classification. *AJR* 162: 1067–71; 1994.

Chou YH, Tiu CM, Chen JY, Chang RF. Automatic full-field breast ultrasonography: the past and the future. *J Med Ultrasound* 15(1): 31–44; 2007.

Dhawan AP, Huang HK, Kim DS. Future trends in medical and molecular imaging. In: Dhawan AP, Huang HK, Kim DS, eds. *Principles and Advanced Methods in Medical Imaging and Image Analysis*. Singapore: World Scientific; 829–43.

Hendee WR. Medical Imaging for the 21st Century. In: Xie NZ, ed. *Medical Imaging and Precision Radiotherapy*. Guangzhou, China: Foundation of International Scientific Exchange; 2000, 24–30.

Jemal A, et al. Cancer statistics 2002. *CA Cancer J Clin* 52: 23–57; 2002.

Kim DS, Ronen I. Recent advances in diffusion magnetic resonance imaging. In: Dhwan AP, Huang HK, Kim DS, eds. *Principles and Advanced Methods in Medical Imaging and Image Analysis*. Singapore: World Scientific; 2008, 289–309.

Kuzmak PM, Dayhoff RE. The use of digital imaging and communications in medicine (DICOM) in the integration of imaging into the electronic patient record at the Department of Veterans Affairs. *J Digital Imag* 13 (2 Suppl 1): 133–7; 2000.

Law, MYY. A model of DICOM-based electronic patient record in radiation therapy. *J Comput Med Imag Graph* 29: 125–136; 2005.

Law, MYY, Huang HK. Concept of a PACS and Imaging Informatics-based Server for Radiation Therapy. *J Comput Med Imag Graph* 27: 1–9; 2003.

Law, MYY. DICOM-RT and its utilization in radiation therapy. *J Radiograph*; 29: 655–667; 2009.

Law, MYY, Brent JL. DICOM-RT-Based ePR (Electronic Patient Record) Information System for Radiation Therapy. *J Radiograph*; 29: 961–972; 2009.

Law, MYY. Image guidance in radiation therapy. In: Dhawan AP, Huang HK, Kim DS, eds. *Principles and Advanced Methods in Medical Imaging and Image Analysis*. Singapore: World Scientific; 2008, 635–62.

Orel SG, et al. MR imaging of the breast for the detection, diagnosis, and staging of breast cancer. *Radiology* 220: 13–30; 2001.

Raxche V, Mansour M, Reddy V, et al. Fusion of three-dimensional X-ray angiography and three-dimensional echocardiography. *Int J CARS* 2: 293–303; 2008.

Robb RA. Three dimensional biomedical imaging. In: *The Calculus of Imaging*. Cambridge, UK: VCH; 1995, 188–206.

Solbiati L. Image fusion system fast, reliable guide for treatment. *RSNA News* (March): 12–13; 2008.

Song Y, Li G. Current and future trends in radiation therapy. In: Dhawan AP, Huang HK, Kim DS, eds. *Principles and Advanced Methods in Medical Imaging and Image Analysis*. Singapore: World Scientific; 2008, 745–81.

Sternick ES. Intensity Modulated Radiation Therapy. In Xie NZ, ed. *Medical Imaging and Precision Radiotherapy*. Guangzhou, China: Foundation of International Scientific Exchange; 2000, 38–52.

Winchester DP, et al. Standards for diagnosis and management of invasive breast carcinoma. *CA Cancer J Clin* 48: 83–107; 1998.

Zanzonico P. Multimodality image registration and fusion. In: Dhawan AP, Huang HK, Kim DS, eds. *Principles and Advanced Methods in Medical Imaging and Image Analysis*. Singapore: World Scientific; 2008, 413–35.

Zuckier LS. Principles of nuclear medicine imaging modalities. In: Dhawan AP, Huang HK, Kim DS, eds. *Principles and Advanced Methods in Medical Imaging and Image Analysis*. Singapore: World Scientific; 2008, 63–98.

CHAPTER 6

Image Compression

A compressed medical image can **reduce** the image size (see Chapter 2, table 2.1) as well as shorten the transmission time and decrease an image's storage requirement. But a compressed image may compromise the image's original quality and affect its diagnostic value. This chapter describes some compression techniques that are applicable to medical images, and their advantages and disadvantages. In addition recent trends on using image compression in clinical environment are presented.

6.1 TERMINOLOGY

The half-dozen definitions that follow are essential to an understanding of image compression/reconstruction.

- *Original image in 2-D, 3-D, and 4-D.* A two-dimensional (2-D) original digital medical image $f(x, y)$ is a nonnegative integer function where x and y can be from 0 to 255, 0 to 511, 0 to 1023, 0 to 2047, or 0 to 4095 (see Section 2.1). In three-dimensional (3-D) image, $f(x, y, z)$ is a 3-D spatial data block, or $f(x, y, t)$ with spatial 2-D and the time as the third dimension. In the case of four-dimensional image (4-D), $f(x, y, z, t)$ is a sequence of multiple 3-D spatial data blocks collected at different times (see Sections 3.1, 4.1, and 5.1). Image compression of the original 2-D image (a rectangular array), 3-D image (a three-dimensional data block), or 4-D image data set (a time sequence of 3-D data blocks), respectively, is to compress it into a one-dimensional data file.

- *Transformed image.* The transformed image $F(u,v)$ of the original 2-D image $f(x, y)$ after a mathematical transformation is another two-dimensional array data set. If the transformation is the forward discrete cosine transform, then (u, v) are nonnegative integers representing the frequencies (see Sections 2.4, 4.2.1, and 5.1). In the 3-D case, the transformed data block is a 3-D data block, and in a sequence of 4-D image data sets, the transformed sequence is also a sequence of 4-D data sets.

- *Compressed image file.* The compressed image file of any 2-D, 3-D, or 4-D image is a one-dimensional (1-D) encoded information data file derived from the original or the transformed image by an image compression technique.

PACS and Imaging Informatics, Second Edition, by H. K. Huang
Copyright © 2010 John Wiley & Sons, Inc.

- *Reconstructed image from a compressed image file.* The reconstructed image (or image set) from a compressed image file is a two-dimensional rectangular array $f_c(x, y)$, a 3-D data block $f_c(x, y, z)$, or a 4-D $f_c(x, y, z, t)$ image set. The technique used for the reconstruction (or decoding) depends on the method of compression (encoding). In the case of error-free (or reversible, or lossless) compression, the reconstructed image is identical to the original image, whereas in irreversible or lossy image compression, the reconstructed image loses some information of the original image. The term "reconstructed image," which is obtained from a compressed image file, should not be confused with the term "image reconstruction," which is obtained from projections used in computed tomography as described in Chapter 4. Thus the reconstructed image in this chapter means that the image is reconstructed from a compressed file.

- *Encoding and decoding.* We often use the term "encoded" for the image that has been compressed. The term "decoded" is used for the compressed image that has been reconstructed.

- *Difference image.* The difference image is defined as the subtracted 2-D image, the subtracted 3-D data block, or the subtracted 4-D image sequence between the original and the reconstructed image, $f(x, y) - f_c(x, y)$, $f(x, y, z) - f_c(x, y, z)$, or $f(x, y, z, t) - f_c(x, y, z, t)$. In the case of error-free compression, the difference image is the zero image (image set). In the case of irreversible (lossy) compression, the difference image is the pixel-by-pixel, voxel-by-volex, or time and volex-by-volex differences between the original image and the reconstructed image. The amount of the difference depends on the compression technique used as well as the compression ratio; the lesser the difference, the closer is the reconstructed image to the original.

- *Compression ratio.* The compression ratio between the original image and the compressed image file is the ratio between computer storage required to store the original image versus that of the compressed data file. Thus a 4:1 compression on a $512 \times 512 \times 8 = 2,097, 152$-bit image requires only 524,288 bits of storage, or 25% of the original image storage space. There is another way to describe the degree of compression by using the term "bpp" (bit per pixel). Thus, if the original image is 8 bit/pixel, or 8 bpp, a 4:1 compression means the compressed image becomes 2 bpp, because the compression ratio computed from pixel-by-pixel or volex-by-volex differences between the original and the compressed image is not necessary an exact number. A 4:1 compression means the compression is approximate 4:1.

6.2 BACKGROUND

Picture archiving and communication systems (PACS) would benefit from image compression for obvious reasons: to speed up the image transmission rate and save on data storage space. The amount of digital medical images captured each year in the United States alone is in many petabytes (i.e., 10^{15}) and is increasing rapidly year by year. Image compression is key to alleviating the storage and communication speed requirements for managing the voluminous digital image data of PACS. First, the bit size required to store and represent the images would be reduced, while maintaining relevant diagnostic information. Second, compressed images would enable fast transmission of large medical image files to image display workstations over networks for review.

Technically, most image data compression methods can be categorized into two types. One is *reversible* or *lossless or error-free compression*, shown in Figure 6.1. A reversible scheme achieves modest compression ratios of the order of 2 to 3 but allows exact recovery of the original image from the compressed file. An irreversible *or lossy* type would not allow the exact recovery after compression but could achieve much higher compression ratios, such as in the range of 10 to 50 or more. Generally, higher compression is obtained at the expense of image quality degradation; that is, image quality declines as the compression ratio increases. Another type of compression used in medical imaging is *clinical image compression*, which stores only a few medically relevant images, as determined by the physicians, out of a series or multiple series of many real-time obtained images, thus reducing the total number of images in an examination file. The stored images may be further compressed by the reversible scheme. In an ultrasound examination, for example, the radiologist may collect data for several seconds, at 25 to 30 images per second, but keep only 4 to 8 relevant frames for documentation in the patient record, and discarding the rest after the diagnostic decision had been made. In multislice CT or a multiple sequence MRI examination, it can accumulate up to 200 to 1000 images, of which only several may be important for the diagnosis.

Image degradation from irreversible compression may or may not be visually apparent. The term "visually lossless" has been used to characterize lossy schemes that result in no visible loss under normal radiological viewing conditions. An image reconstructed from a compression algorithm that is visually lossless under certain viewing conditions (e.g., a 19-in. video monitor with 1024×1024 pixels at a viewing distance of 4 ft) could result in visible degradations under more stringent conditions, such as viewed at a 2000-line LCD monitor or printed on a 14×17in. film.

A related term used by the American College of Radiology, the National Electrical Manufacturing Association (ACR-NEMA), and in Digital Imaging and Communication in Medicine (DICOM) is *information preserving*. The ACR-NEMA standard

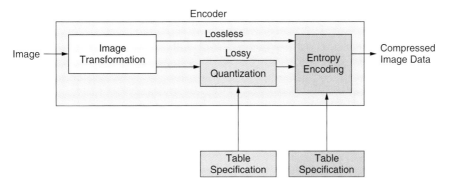

Figure 6.1 General framework for image data compression. Image transformation can be as simple as a shift of a row and a subtraction with the original image, or a more complex mathematical transformation. The quantization determines whether the compression is lossless or lossy. The decoder in image reconstruction is the reverse of the encoder.

report defines the compression scheme as information preserving if the resulting image retains all of the significant information of the original image. However, both "visually lossless" and "information preserving" are subjective terms, and extreme caution must be taken in their interpretation.

Lossy algorithms are not yet used by radiologists in primary diagnoses because physicians and radiologists are concerned with missing the diagnosis and the legal potential implications of an incorrect diagnosis from a lossy compressed image. Lossy compression has also raised legal questions for manufacturers as well as physicians who use images for medical diagnosis, and, the U.S. Food and Drug Administration (FDA) has instituted certain regulatory guidelines to be discussed in Section 6.9.

Currently the original image is still used for primary diagnosis. After the diagnostic result has been documented and appended with the image file, the image can be compressed to reasonably good quality for storage. The Royal College of Radiologists, London, has even recently announced such a protocol to their fellows. This protocol is already followed extensively in the image distribution of the electronic patient record (ePR) as practiced by many academic hospital affiliations. This topic will be revisited in Chapter 22.

6.3   ERROR-FREE COMPRESSION

This section presents three error-free image compression methods. The first method is based on certain inherent properties of the image under consideration; the second and third are standard data compression methods.

6.3.1   Background Removal

Backgrounds can be removed in both sectional and projection images. The idea is to reduce the size of the image file by discarding the background from the image. Figure 6.2A shows a transverse CT body image in which the background around the body is removed by minimizing it to a rectangle containing just the image. Only the information within the rectangle, including the outer boundary of the cross-sectional body CT, is retained. The size and relative location of the rectangle with respect to the original image are then saved in the image header for a later image reconstruction. In Figure 6.2B is a cross-sectional image that is segmented so that only information inside the segmented image is retained for storage (see arrows). In computed and digital radiography (CR and DR), the area outside the anatomical boundary can be discarded through the background removal technique described in Section 3.3.4. Recall that in Figures 3.15A, B the background was removed in the pediatric CR images. Figure 6.3 shows compression of digital mammograms by the background removal technique. Note that, Figure 6.3D achieves a higher compression ratio than does Figure 6.3B. This is because Figure 6.3D has a larger background area. In both cases the removed background images were compressed by discarding background information that has no diagnostic value. The removed background image can be further compressed by using lossless data compression methods to be described in the next two sections.

6.3.2 Run-Length Coding

Run-length coding based on eliminating repeated adjacent pixels can be used to compress rows or columns of images. A run-length code consists of three sequential numbers: the mark, the length, and the pixel value. The compression procedure starts with obtaining a histogram of the image. The histogram of an image is a plot of the frequency of occurrence versus the pixel value of the entire image. The mark is chosen as the pixel value in the image that has the least frequency of occurrence. If more than one pixel value has the same least frequency of occurrence, the higher pixel value will be chosen as the mark. The image is then scanned line by line, and sets of three sequential numbers are encoded.

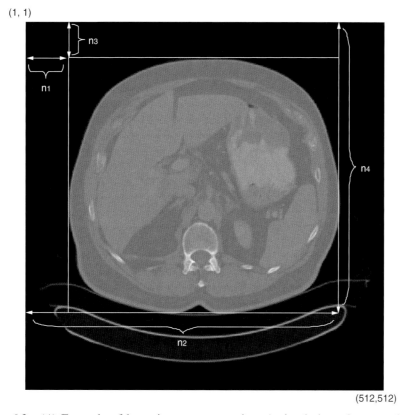

Figure 6.2 (*A*) Example of lossy image compression. A simple boundary search algorithm determines n_1, n_2, n_3, and n_4, the four coordinates required to circumvent the 512×512 CT image by the rectangle with dimensions of $(n_2 - n_1) \times (n_4 - n_3)$. These coordinates also give the relative location of the rectangle with respect to the original image. Each pixel inside this rectangular area can be compressed further by a lossless procedure. (*B*) Segmentation algorithm used to outline the boundary of the abdominal CT image. Pixels outside of the boundary are discarded, and hence the segmentation process reduces the size of the image file.

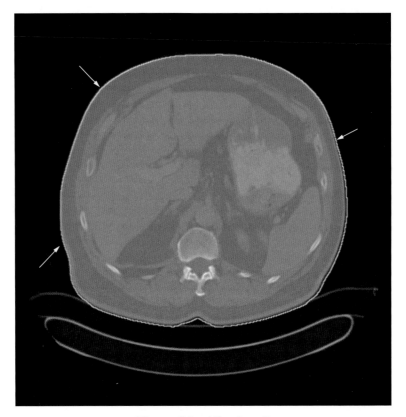

Figure 6.2   *(Continued)*

For example, assume that the lowest frequency of occurrence pixel value in a $512 \times 512 \times 8$ image is 128, then 128 is used as the mark. During the scan, suppose that the scan encounters 25 pixels and all of them have a value of 10, then the run-length code for these sequence of numbers would then be

128   25   10
Mark   Length   Pixel value

If the length is the same as the mark, the three-number set should be split into two sets, for example, the set 128 128 34 should be split into two sets: 128 4 34 and 128 124 34, the length 4 and 124 are arbitrary but should be predetermined before the encoding.

There are two special cases in the run-length code:

1. Since each run-length code set requires three numbers, there is no advantage in compressing adjacent pixels with value repeating less than four times. In this case each of these pixel values is used as the code.

2. The code can consist of only two sequential numbers:

128   128 :   Next pixel value is 128
128   0 :   End of the coding

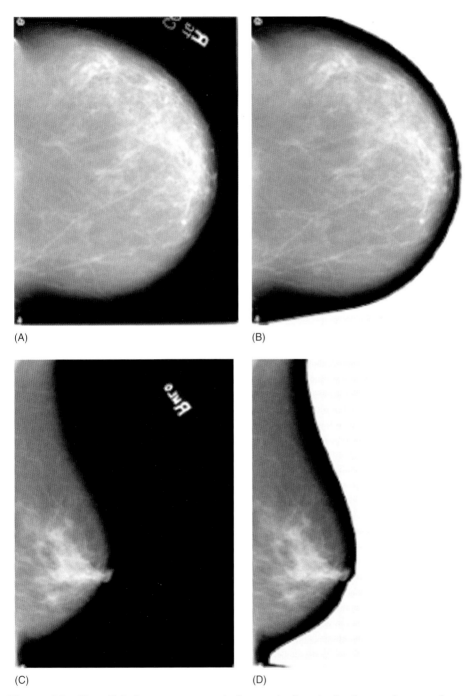

(A)   (B)

(C)   (D)

Figure 6.3 Two digital mammograms before and after the background removal providing immediate image compression. (*A*) A large breast occupies most of the image. (*B*) Background removed image, compression ratio 3.1:1. (*C*) A small breast occupies a small portion of the image. (*D*) Background removed image, compression ratio 6.3:1; (Courtesy of Jun Wang)

To decode the run-length coding, the procedure checks the coded data value sequentially. If a mark is found, the following two codes must be the length and the gray level, except for the two special cases. In the first case, if a mark is not found, the code itself is the gray level. In the second case, a 128 following a 128 means the next pixel value is 128, and a 0 following a 128 means the end of the coding.

A modified run-length coding called **run-zero coding** is sometimes more practical to use. In this case the original image is first shifted one pixel to the right, and a shifted image is formed. A subtracted image between the original and the shifted image is obtained, which is to be coded. A run-length code on the subtracted image requires only the mark and the length because the third code is not necessary: it is either zero or not required because of the two special cases described earlier. The run-zero coding requires that the pixel values of the leftmost column of the original image to be saved for the decoding procedure.

6.3.3 Huffman Coding

Huffman coding based on the probability (or the frequency) of occurrence of pixel values in the shifted-then-subtracted image described in the last section can be used to compress the image. The encoding procedure requires six steps:

1. From the original image (Fig. 6.4*A*), form the shifted-then-subtracted image (Fig. 6.4*C*).
2. Obtain the histograms of the original image (Fig. 6.4*B*) and the shifted-then-subtract image (Fig. 6.4.*D*).
3. Rearrange the histogram in Figure 6.4*D* according to the probability (or frequency) of occurrence of the pixel values and form a new histogram (Fig. 6.4*E*).
4. Form the Huffman tree of Figure 6.4*F*. A Huffman tree with two nodes at each branch is built continuously following rules, described in steps 5 and 6, until all possible pixel values have been exhausted.
5. Assign a "1" to the left and a "0" to the right node throughout all branches of the tree, starting from the highest probability branches (see Fig. 6.4*F* and Table 6.1).
6. The last step is to assign contiguous bits to each pixel value according to its location in the tree. Thus each pixel value has a new assigned code that is the Huffman code of the image.

Table 6.1 shows the Huffman code of the shifted-then-subtracted image (Fig. 6.4*E*). Because of the characteristic of the rearranged histogram, the Huffman coded image always achieves some compression. The compression ratio of Figure 6.4*C* is 2.1:1. To reconstruct the image, the compressed image file is scanned sequentially, bit by bit, to match the Huffman code; and then decoded accordingly.

Figure 6.4 presents an example of an error-free image compression using the Huffman coding on a shifted-then-subtracted digitized chest X-ray image (512 × 512 × 8). To obtain higher error-free compression ratios, the run-length method can be used first, followed by the Huffman coding.

TABLE 6.1 Huffman tree of the chest images: Compression ratio, 2.1:1

Node	Branch Left (1)	Branch Right (0)	Pixel Value of the Node Left	Pixel Value of the Node Right	Histogram[a] Left	Histogram[a] Right	Sum
111	110	109			157947	104197	262144
110	108	107			85399	72548	157947
109	106	56[†]		0[b]	55417	48780	104197
108	105	55		1	46639	38760	85399
107	54	104	−1		38546	34002	72548
106	103	53		−2	29787	25630	55417
105	52	102	2		25493	21146	46639
104	101	51		3	18400	15602	34002
103	50	100	−3		15473	14314	29787
102	99	98			11176	9970	21146
101	49	48	−4	4	9244	9156	18400
100	97	96			7334	6980	14314
99	47	46	−5	5	5618	5558	11176
98	95	94			5173	4797	9970
97	45	93	−6		3692	3642	7334
96	44	92	6		3607	3373	6980
95	91	43		7	2645	2528	5173
94	42	90	−7		2416	2381	4797
93	89	41		8	1937	1705	3642
92	40	88	−8		1699	1674	3373
91	87	86			1434	1211	2645
90	39	38	−9	9	1198	1183	2381
89	85	84			1031	906	1937
88	37	36	−10	10	847	827	1674
87	83	82			769	665	1434
86	35	34	11	−11	613	598	1211
85	81	80			558	473	1031
84	33	32	12	−12	473	433	906
83	79	31		−13	404	365	769
82	78	30		13	337	328	665
81	77	29		14	297	261	558
80	76	28		−14	249	224	473
79	75	27		−15	214	190	404
78	74	26		15	175	162	337
77	25	24	16	−16	150	147	297
76	73	23		−17	131	118	249
75	72	71			110	104	214
74	22	21	17	18	98	77	175
73	70	20		−19	74	57	131
72	69	19		−18	56	54	110
71	18	68	19		53	51	104
70	67	66			42	32	74
69	17	16	−20	20	29	27	56
68	15	65	21		26	25	51
67	14	13	−22	−21	22	20	42

(continued overleaf)

TABLE 6.1 (*Continued*)

| Node | Branch | | Pixel Value of the Node | | Histogram[a] | | |
	Left (1)	Right (0)	Left	Right	Left	Right	Sum
66	64	63			19	13	32
65	12	11	22	24	13	12	25
64	10	62	−24		10	9	19
63	61	9		23	7	6	13
62	8	60	25		5	4	9
61	7	59	−23		4	3	7
60	58	57			2	2	4
59	6	5	−25	−36	2	1	3
58	4	3	−28	−26	1	1	2
57	2	1[b]	26	66	1	1	2

[a]The count of each terminal node is the frequency of occurrences of the corresponding pixel value in the subtracted image. The count of each branch node is the total count of all the nodes initiated from this node. Thus the count in the left column is always greater than or equal to the right column by convention, and the count in each row is always greater than or equal to that of the row below. The total count for the last node "111" is $262144 = 512 \times 512$, which is the size of the image.

[b]Each terminal node (1–56) corresponds to a pixel value in the subtracted image: minus signs are possible because of the subtraction.

6.4 TWO-DIMENSIONAL IRREVERSIBLE (LOSSY) IMAGE COMPRESSION

6.4.1 Background

Irreversible compression is done in the transform domain, and hence it is called transform coding. The procedure of transform coding is to first transform the original image into the transform domain with a two-dimensional transformation—for example, Fourier, Hadamard, Cosine, Karhunen–Loeve, or wavelet. The transform coefficients are then quantized and encoded (see Fig. 6.1). The result is a highly compressed 1-D data file.

The image can be compressed in blocks or in its entirety. In block compression, before image transformation, the entire image is subdivided into equal size blocks (e.g., 8×8), and the transformation is applied to each block. A statistical quantitation method is then used to encode the 8×8 transform coefficients of each block. The advantages of the block compression technique is that all blocks can be compressed in parallel, and it is faster to perform the computation in a small block than for an entire image. However, blocky artifacts can appear in the reconstructed image that in a medical image can compromise the diagnostic value of the image when compression ratios are high. Further image processing on the reconstructed image is sometimes necessary to smooth out such artifacts.

The full-frame compression technique, on the other hand, transforms the entire image into the transform domain. Quantitation is applied to *all* transform coefficients of the entire transformed image. The full-frame technique is computationally tedious, expensive, and time-consuming. However, it does not produce blocky artifacts and hence is more suitable for medical image compression in terms of compressed image quality.

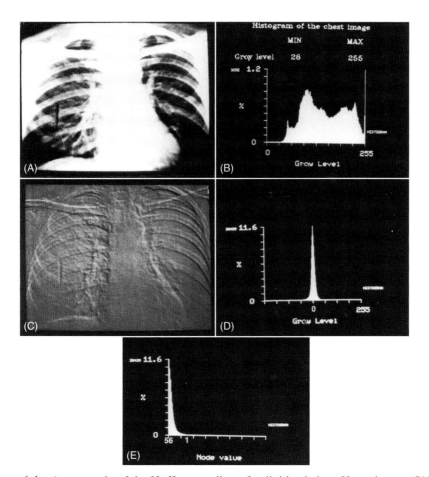

Figure 6.4   An example of the Huffman coding of a digitized chest X-ray image (512 ×
512 × 8). Shifting the image one pixel down and one pixel to the right, produces a
subtracted image between the original and the shifted image. Huffman coding of the
subtracted image yields a higher compression ratio than that of the original image. The
first row and the leftmost column of the original image are retained during the encoding
process and are needed during the decoding process. (A) Original digitized chest image;
(B) histogram of the original image; (C) the shifted-subtracted image; (D) histogram of
the subtracted image; (E) the rearranged histogram. (F) the Huffman tree with codes of
the subtracted image. The histogram of the subtracted image has 56 gray levels: see (E).
Branch node 57 (see last row in Table 6.1) consists of the left node 2 (gray level 26)
and right node 1 (gray level 66), each having a frequency of occurrence equal to 1; the
total frequency of occurrence of node 57 is 2. Branch node 109 consists of left node 106
and right node 56 (gray level 0). The compression ratio of the shifted-subtracted image
is about 2.1:1.

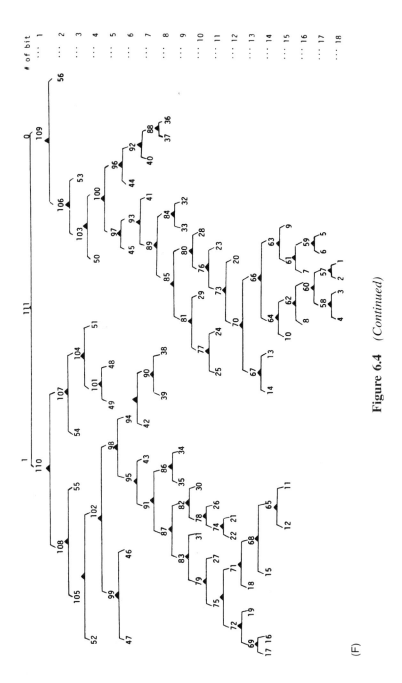

Figure 6.4 *(Continued)*

(F)

186

6.4.2   Block Compression Technique

The most popular block compression technique using forward two-dimensional discrete cosine transform is the JPEG (Joint Photographic Experts Group) standard. Sections 6.4.2.1 through 6.4.2.4 summarize this method, which consists of four steps: (1) two-dimensional forward discrete cosine transform (DCT), (2) bit-allocation table and quantitation, (3) DCT coding, and (4) entropy coding.

6.4.2.1   *Two-dimensional Forward Discrete Cosine Transform*   Forward discrete cosine transform, a special case of discrete Fourier transform discussed in Section 2.4.3, has proved to be an effective method for image compression because the energy in the transform domain is concentrated in a small region. So the forward DCT method can yield larger compression ratios and maintain image quality compared with many other methods. The forward DCT of the original image $f(j, k)$ is given by

$$F(u, v) = \left(\frac{2}{N}\right)^2 C(u)C(v) \left(\sum_{k=0}^{N-1} \sum_{j=0}^{N-1} f(j, k) \cos \frac{u(j + 0.5)}{N} \cos \frac{v(k + 0.5)}{N}\right)$$

(6.1)

The inverse discrete cosine transform of $F(u, v)$ is the original image $f(j, k)$:

$$f(j, k) = \sum_{v=0}^{N-1} \sum_{u=0}^{N-1} F(u, v)C(u)C(v) \cos \frac{u(j + 0.5)}{N} \cos \frac{v(k + 0.5)}{N} \qquad (6.2)$$

where

$$C(O) = \left(\frac{1}{2}\right)^{[1/2]} \qquad \text{for } u, v \neq 0$$
$$= 1 \qquad \text{for } u, v = 0$$

and $N \times N$ is the size of the image.

Thus, for the block transform, $N \times N = 8 \times 8$, whereas for the full-frame compression of a 2048×2048 image, $N = 2{,}048$.

6.4.2.2   *Bit Allocation Table and Quantization*   The 2-D forward DCT of an 8×8 block yields 64 DCT coefficients. The energy of these coefficients is concentrated among the lower frequency components. To achieve a higher compression ratio, these coefficients are quantized to obtain the desired image quality. In doing so, the original values of the coefficients are compromised; hence some information lost. Quantization of the DCT coefficient $F(u, v)$ can be obtained by

$$F_q(u, v) = \text{NINT} \left(\frac{F(u, v)}{Q(u, v)}\right) \qquad (6.3)$$

where $Q(u, v)$ is the quantizer step size, and NINT is the nearest integer function.

One method of determining the quantizer step size is by manipulating a bit allocation table $B(u, v)$, which is defined by

$$B(u, v) = \log 2[|F(u, v)|] + K \qquad \text{if } |F(u, v)| \geq 1 \qquad (6.4)$$

$$= K \qquad\qquad\qquad \text{otherwise}$$

where $|F(u, v)|$ is the absolute value of the cosine transform coefficient, and K is a real number that determines the compression ratio. Notice that each pixel in the transformed image $F(u, v)$ corresponds to one value of the table $B(u, v)$. Each value in this table represents the number of computer memory bits used to save the corresponding pixel value in the transformed image. The value in the bit allocation table can be increased or decreased to adjust for the amount of compression by assigning a certain value to K. Thus, for example, if a pixel located at (p, q) and $F(p, q) = 3822$, then $B(p, q) = 11.905 + K$. If one selects $K = +0.095$, then $B(p, q) = 12$ (i.e., 12 bits are allocated to save the value 3822). On the other hand, if one selects $K = -0.905$, then $B(p, q) = 11$, which means $F(p, q)$ is compressed to 11 bits.

Based on Eq. (6.4), Eq. (6.3) can be rewritten as

$$F_q(u, v) = \text{NINT} \left[(2^{|B(m,n)-1|} - 1) \frac{F(u, v)}{|F(m, n)|} \right] \qquad (6.5)$$

where $F(u, v)$ is the coefficient of the transformed image, $F_q(u, v)$ is the corresponding quantized value, (m, n) is the location of the maximum value of $|F(u, v)|$ for $0 \leq u, v \leq N - 1$, and $B(m, n)$ is the corresponding number of bits in the bit allocation table assigned to save $|F(m, n)|$. By this formula, $F(u, v)$ has been normalized with respect to $(2^{|B(m,n)-1|} - 1)/|F(m, n)|$.

The quantized value $F_q(u, v)$ is an approximate value of $F(u, v)$ because of the value K described in Eq. (6.4). This quantized procedure introduces an approximation to the compressed image file.

6.4.2.3 DCT Coding and Entropy Coding

For block quantization with an 8×8 matrix, the $F(0, 0)$ is the DC coefficient and normally is the maximum value of $|F(u, v)|$. Starting from $F(0, 0)$, the rest of the 63 coefficients can be coded in the zigzag sequence shown in Figure 6.5. This zigzag sequence facilitates entropy coding by placing low-frequency components, which normally have larger coefficients, before high-frequency components.

The last step in block compression is the entropy coding. At this step additional lossless compression is provided by a reversible technique such as run-length coding or Huffman coding, as described in Sections 6.3.2 and 6.3.3.

6.4.2.4 Decoding and Inverse Transform

The block-compressed image file is a sequential file containing the following information: entropy coding, zigzag sequence, bit allocation table, and the quantization. This information can be used to reconstruct the compressed image. The compressed image file is decoded by using the bit-allocation table as a guide to form a two-dimensional array $F_A(u, v)$, which

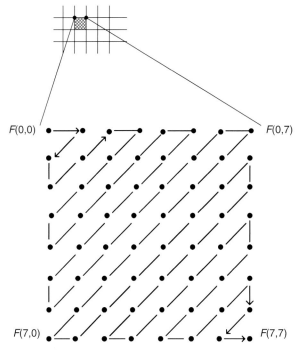

Figure 6.5 Zigzag sequence of an 8×8 matrix used in the cosine transform block quantization.

is the approximate transformed image. The value of $F_A(u, v)$ is computed by

$$F_A(u, v) = \frac{|F(m, n)| \cdot F_q(u, v)}{2^{|B(m,n)-1|} - 1} \tag{6.6}$$

Equation (6.6) is almost the inverse of Eq. (6.5), and $F_A(u, v)$ is the approximation of $F(u, v)$. Inverse cosine transform Eq. (6.2) is then applied to $F_A(u, v)$, which gives $f_A(x, y)$, the reconstructed image. Since $F_A(u, v)$ is an approximation of $F(u, v)$, some differences exist between the original image $f(x, y)$ and the reconstructed image $f_A(x, y)$. The compression ratio is dependent on the amount of quantization and the efficiency of the entropy coding. Figure 6.6 shows the block compression result of a section from a 3-D body CT image volume. The section is compressed using the DICOM JPEG standard (see Chapter 9) with a compression ratio of 20:1. Observe the block artifacts shown in the difference image, Figure 6.6*C*. (See also Figs. 6.19 and 6.20.)

6.4.3 Full-frame Compression

The full-frame bit allocation (FFBA) compression technique in the cosine transform domain was developed primarily for large size radiological images. It is different from the JPEG block method in that the transform is done on the entire image. Applying image compression on blocks of the image gives blocky artifacts that may affect diagnostic accuracy.

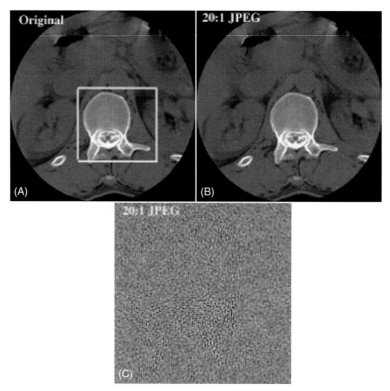

Figure 6.6   One slice of a 3-D CT volume data compressed with a compression ratio of 20:1 using the cosine transform JPEG compression method: (*A*) Original image; (*B*) JPEG reconstructed image; (*C*) the difference image. Observe the block artifact in the difference image due to the cosine transform block quantization (see also Fig. 6.19 and Fig. 6.20).

Basically the FFBA technique is similar to the block compression technique, as can be seen from the following steps: The transformed image of the entire image is first obtained by using the forward DCT (Eq. 6.1). A bit allocation table (Eq. 6.4) designating the number of bits for each pixel in this transformed image is then generated, the value of each pixel is quantized based on a predetermined rule (Eq. 6.5), and the bit allocation table is used to encode the quantized image, forming a one-dimensional sequentially compressed image file. The one-dimensional image file is further compressed by means of lossless entropy coding. The compression ratio between the original image and the compressed image file depends on the information in the bit allocation table, the amount of quantization on the transformed image, and the entropy coding. The compressed image file and the bit allocation table are saved and used to reconstruct the image.

During image reconstruction the bit allocation table is used to decode the one-dimensional compressed image file back to a two-dimensional array. An inverse cosine transform is performed on the two-dimensional array to form the reconstructed image. The reconstructed image does not exactly equal to the original image because approximation is introduced in the bit allocation table and in the quantization procedure.

Despite this similarity, the implementation of the FFBA is quite different from the block compression method for several reasons. First, it is computationally tedious and time-consuming to carry out the 2-D DCT when the image size is large. Second, the bit allocation table given in Eq. (6.4) is large when the image size is large, and therefore it becomes an overhead in the compressed file. In the case of block compression, one 8×8 bit allocation table may be sufficient for all blocks. Third, zig-zag sequencing provides an efficient arrangement for the entropy coding in a small block of data. In the FFBA, zig-zag sequencing is not a good way to rearrange the DCT coefficients because of the large matrix size. The implementation of the FFBA is best accomplished by using a fast DCT method and a compact full-frame bit allocation table along with the consideration of computational precision and implemented in a specially designed hardware module. Figure 6.7*A* shows a chest (CH), a reno-arteriogram (RE), the SMPTE phantom (PH), and a body CT image (CT), and Figure 6.7*B* is the corresponding full-frame cosine transforms of these images. Although the full-frame compression method does not produce blocky artifacts and preserves higher image quality in the compressed image, it is not convenient to use for medical images especially in the DICOM environment (see Chapter 9).

6.5 MEASUREMENT OF THE DIFFERENCE BETWEEN THE ORIGINAL AND THE RECONSTRUCTED IMAGE

A common concern raised in image compression is how much an image can be compressed and still preserve sufficient information required by a given clinical application This section discusses some parameters and methods used to measure the trade-offs between image quality and compression ratios.

6.5.1 Quantitative Parameters

6.5.1.1 *Normalized Mean-Square Error*   The normalized mean-square error (NMSE) between the original $f(x, y)$ and the reconstructed $f_A(x, y)$ image can be used as a quantitative measure of the closeness between the reconstructed and the original image. The formula for the normalized mean-square error of a square $N \times N$ image is given by

$$\text{NMSE} = \frac{\sum_{x=0}^{N-1} \sum_{y=0}^{N-1} (f(x, y) - f_A(x, y))^2}{\sum_{x=0}^{N-1} \sum_{y=0}^{N-1} f(x, y)^2} \tag{6.7}$$

or

$$\text{NMSE} = \frac{\sum_{u=0}^{N-1} \sum_{v=0}^{N-1} (F(u, v) - F_A(u, v))^2}{\sum_{u=0}^{N-1} \sum_{v=0}^{N-1} F(u, v)^2} \tag{6.8}$$

because cosine transform is a unitary transformation, where $F(u, v)$ is the transformed image, and $F_A(u, v)$ is an approximation of $F(u, v)$.

NMSE is a global measurement of the quality of the reconstructed image; it does not provide information on the local measurement. It is obvious that the NMSE is a function of the compression ratio. A high compression ratio will yield a high NMSE value.

6.5.1.2   Peak Signal-to-Noise Ratio   Another quantitative measure is the peak signal-to-noise ratio (PSNR) based on the root mean square error between $f(x, y)$ and $f_A(x, y)$:

$$\text{PSNR} = \frac{20 \log(f(x, y)_{\max}}{\left(\sum_{x=0}^{N-1} \sum_{y=0}^{N-1} (f(x, y) - f_A(x, y))^2)^{1/2} / (N \times N)\right)} \tag{6.9}$$

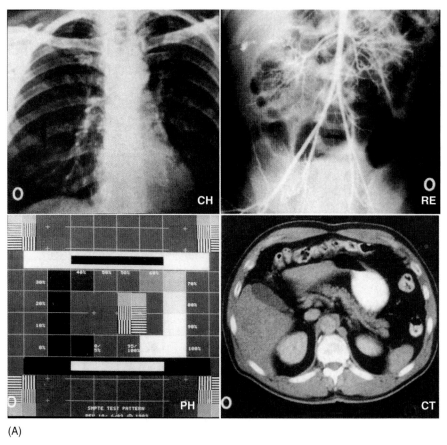

(A)

Figure 6.7   (*A*) Clockwise, the original chest image, an reno-arteriogram, the digital SMPTE phantom, and a body CT image. (*B*) Cosine transforms of the entire chest radiograph (CH), the reno-arteriogram (RE), the SMPTE phantom (PH), and the CT scan (CT) shown in (*A*). The origin is located at the upper left-hand corner of each image. Note that the frequency distribution of the cosine transforms of the chest radiograph and of the renoarteriogram is quite similar; more low frequency components concentrate in the upper left corner, representing the lower frequency components. The frequency distribution of the cosine transform of the CT is also spread toward the higher frequency region, whereas in the case of the SMPTE phantom, the frequency distribution of the cosine transform is all over the transform domain, including higher frequencies, and hence the cosine transform technique is not a good method to compress the digital phantom because of edges are everywhere in the phantom.

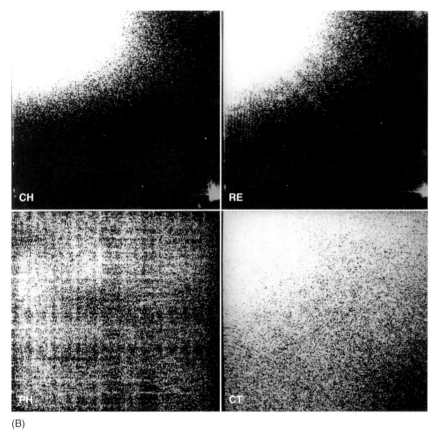

(B)

Figure 6.7   *(Continued)*

where $f(x, y)_{max}$ is the maximum value of the entire image, $N \times N$ is the total number of pixels in the image, and the denominator is the root mean square error between $f(x, y)$ and $f_A(x, y)$.

6.5.2   Qualitative Measurement: Difference Image and Its Histogram

The difference image between the original and the reconstructed image gives a qualitative measurement that compares the quality of the reconstructed image with that of the original image. The corresponding histogram of the difference image provides a global qualitative measurement of the difference between the original and the reconstructed images. A very narrow histogram means a small difference, whereas a broad histogram means a very large difference.

6.5.3   Acceptable Compression Ratio

Consider the following experiment. Compress a $512 \times 512 \times 12$-bit body CT image with compression ratios 4:1, 8:1, 17:1, 26:1, and 37:1. The original image and the five reconstructed images arranged in clockwise are shown in Figure 6.8. It is not difficult to arrange these images in the order of quality. But it is more difficult to answer the question, which compression ratio is acceptable for clinical diagnosis? From the figure it is seen that reconstructed images with compression ratios less than and equal to 8:1 do not exhibit visible deterioration in image quality. In other words, compression ratio 8:1 or less is visually acceptable in this case. But visually unacceptable does not necessary mean that it is not suitable for diagnosis because it depends on which body region and what diseases are under consideration. Receiver operating characteristic (ROC) analysis described in the next section is an acceptable objective method used in diagnostic radiology to address this question.

6.5.4 Receiver Operating Characteristic Analysis

Receiver operating characteristic (ROC) analysis, based on the work of Swets and Pickett, and Metz, is used to measure the difference between the quality of the original and the reconstructed image. This method was originally developed for comparing the image quality between two imaging modalities, such as CT and US body region studies. In the case as above where we want to compare the quality of the reconstructed images using two compression ratios, the method can be briefly summarized as follows:

To begin, a clinical problem is defined; for example, we want to use a hand radiograph to determine evidence of subperiosteal resorption in children. We would like to determine the acceptable compression ratio on the radiograph that can still be used for the diagnosis. So the experiment starts with a panel of experts selecting a set of good quality hand radiographs containing the evidence of subperiosteal resorption and matched by a set of normal radiographs. The selection process includes a method of determination of the "truth" which is the verification of the evidence of subperiosteal resorption in the images selected, the distribution between normal and abnormal images, and any subtle presence of subperiosteal resorption in the images. The images in the set are next compressed to a predetermined compression ratio and reconstructed. The result is two sets of images: the original and the reconstructed, each containing both pathological and normal images.

Experts on the diagnosis of subperiosteal resorption are then invited to participate as observers in the review of all images. For each image an observer is asked to give an ROC confidence rating of 1 to 5 on the likelihood of disease presence. A confidence value of 1 indicates that the disease is definitely not present, and a confidence value of 5 indicates that the disease is present. Confidence values 2 and 4 indicate that the disease process is probably not present or probably present, respectively. A confidence value of 3 indicates that the presence of the disease process is equivocal or indeterminate. Every image is read randomly, and blindly, by every reviewer in a systematic fashion to keep memory retention from affecting the interpretation of the result. The ratings of all images by a single observer are graded. Two plots are generated showing true positive (TP) versus false positive (FP) results. The first plot is an ROC curve representing the observer's performance in diagnosing the selected evidence of subperiosteal resorption from the original images; the second plot indicates the performance on the reconstructed images. The area A_z under the ROC curve is an index of quantitative measurement of the observer's performance on these images. Thus, if the A_z (original) and the A_z (reconstructed) of the two ROC curves are very close to each other, we can say that the diagnosis

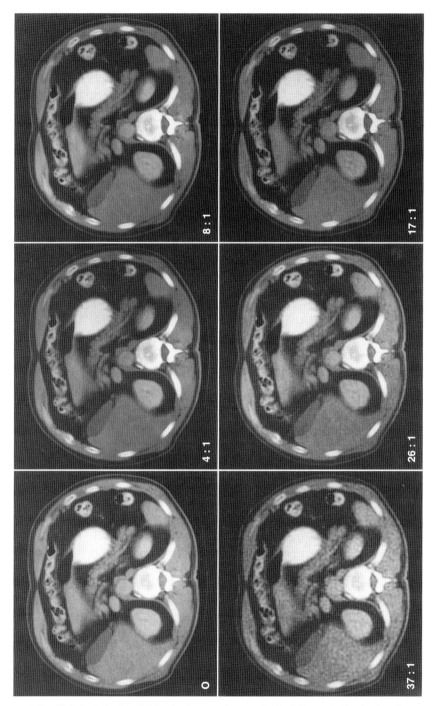

Figure 6.8 Original body CT body image (upper left) followed clockwise, by reconstructed images with compression ratios of 4:1, 8:1, 17:1, 26:1, and 37:1 (the full-frame method was used).

of the evidence of subperiosteal resorption based on the reconstructed images with the predetermined compression ratio will be as good as that made (by this observer) from the original images. In other words, this compression ratio is acceptable for making the diagnosis on hand radiographs with bone re-absorption.

In doing ROC analysis, the statistical "power" of the study is important: the higher the power, the more confidence can be placed in the result. The statistical power is determined by the number of images and the number of observers used in the study. A meaningful ROC analysis often requires many images (100 or more) and five to six observers to determine one type of image with a given disease. Although performing an ROC analysis is tedious, time- consuming, and expensive, this method is acceptable by the radiology community for determination of the quality of the reconstructed image.

For example, we describe a study based on work by Sayre et al. (1992) entailing the analysis of 71 hand radiographs, of which 45 were normal and 26 had subperiosteal resorption. The images were digitized to $2K \times 2K \times 12$-bit resolution and printed on film (14×17in.). The digitized images were compressed to 20:1 using the full-frame cosine transform method and printed on film of the same size. Figures 6.9 and 6.10 show the results from using ROC analysis with five observers. Figure 6.9*A*, *B*, and *C* show an original hand radiograph with evidence of subperiosteal resorption, 20:1 compression ratio reconstructed image, and the difference image, respectively. Figure 6.10 shows the ROC curves of the original and the reconstructed images from the five observers: statistics demonstrate that there is no significant difference between using the original or the reconstructed images with the 20:1 compression ratio for the diagnosis of subperiosteal resorption from hand radiographs.

6.6 THREE-DIMENSIONAL IMAGE COMPRESSION

6.6.1 Background

So far we have discussed two-dimensional image compression. However, acquisition of three- and four-dimensional (3-D, 4-D) medical images is becoming increasingly common in CT, MR, US, and DSA (Chapters 4 and 5). The third dimension considered in this section can be in the spatial domain (e.g., sectional images) or in the time domain (e.g., in an angiographic study with time as the third dimension). The acquisition processes significantly raises the volume of data gathered per study. To compress 3-D data efficiently, one must consider decorrelation images. Some earlier works done on 3-D compression reported by Sun and Goldberg (1988), Lee (1993), and Koo (1992) included correlation between adjacent sections. Chan, Lou, and Huang (1989) reported a full-frame discrete Fourier transform (DCT) method for DSA, CT, and MRI. They found that by grouping four to eight slices as a 3-D volume, compression was twice as efficient as it was with 2-D full-frame DCT for DSA. The 3-D method of compressing CT images was also more efficient than 2-D. However, 3-D compression did not achieve very high efficiency in the case of MR images.

The publication of works by Daubechies (1988) and Mallat (1989) on the use of wavelet transform for image compression attracted a lot of attention. The primary advantage of the wavelet transform compared with the cosine transform is that wavelet transform is localized both in the 3-D spatial domain and the 2-D spatial

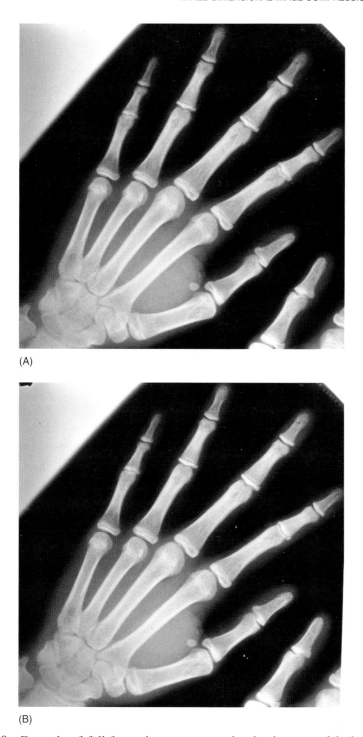

(A)

(B)

Figure 6.9 Example of full-frame image compression hardware used in hand radio-graphs with evidence of subperiosteal resorption (light green highlighter). (*A*) A digitized 2048 × 2048 × 12-bit hand image; (*B*) reconstructed image with a compression ratio of 20:1; (*C*) the difference image (Sayre et al., 1992).

(C)

Figure 6.9 *(Continued)*

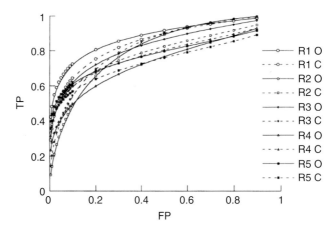

Figure 6.10 Comparison of five observer ROC curves obtained from a hand image compression study: TP = true-positive, FP = false-positive; O = original image, C = compressed image with a 20:1 compression ratio. Five readers (R1, ..., R5) were used in the study.

domains with time as the third dimension. Therefore the transformation of a given signal contains 3-D spatial or 2-D spatial plus time information of that signal. In addition the cosine transform basis extends infinitely, with the result that the 3-D spatial or 2-D spatial plus time information is spread out over the whole transform domain, which is a waste of information energy. Therefore, using wavelet transform for image compression can retain certain local properties of the image that are important in the medical imaging application. Research results obtained in the 1990s demonstrated that wavelet transform compression outperforms cosine transform (Cohen, 1992; Antonini, 1992; Villasenor, 1995; Lightstone, 1994; Albanesi, 1992). The DICOM standard has a wavelet transform supplement for image compression (see Section 6.8 and Chapter 9). Below we present image compression of selected 3-D data sets using JPEG, 2-D, and 3-D wavelet transform and then compare these results (Wang, 1995, 1996, 2008).

6.6.2   Basic Wavelet Theory and Multiresolution Analysis

Image transformation usually relies on a set of basis functions by which the image is decomposed to a combination of functions. In cosine transform, the basis functions are a series of cosine functions, and the resulting domain is the frequency domain. In the case of wavelet transform, the basis functions are derived from a mother wavelet function by dilation and translation operations. In 1-D wavelet transform, the basis functions $\psi_{a,b}(x)$ are formed by mathematical dilation and translation of the mother wavelet $\psi(x)$ such that

$$\psi_{a,b}(x) = \frac{1}{\sqrt{a}}\psi\left(\frac{x-b}{a}\right) \qquad (6.10)$$

where a and b are the dilation and translation factors, respectively. The continuous wavelet transform of a function $f(x)$ can be expressed as

$$F_w(a,b) = \frac{1}{\sqrt{a}}\int_{-\infty}^{\infty} f(x)\psi^*\left(\frac{x-b}{a}\right)\, dx \qquad (6.11)$$

where $*$ is the complex conjugate operator.

The basis functions given in Eq. (6.10) are redundant when a and b are continuous. It is possible, however, to discretize a and b so as to form a mathematical orthonormal basis. One way of discretizing a and b is to let $a = 2^p$ and $b = 2^p q$, so that Eq. (6.10) becomes

$$\psi_{p,q}(x) = 2^{-p/2}\psi(2^{-p}x - q) \qquad (6.12)$$

where p and q are integers. The wavelet transform in Eq. (6.11) then becomes

$$F_w(p,q) = 2^{-p/2}\int_{-\infty}^{+\infty} f(x)\psi(2^{-p}x - q)dx \qquad (6.13)$$

Since p and q are integers, Eq. (6.13) is called a wavelet series. It is seen from this representation that the transform contains both the spatial and frequency information. Equation (6.13) can be converted to a discrete form as in the Fourier transform for image compression applications.

Wavelet transform also relies on the concept of multiresolution analysis, which decomposes a signal into a series of smooth signals and their associated detailed signals at different resolution levels. The smooth signal at level m can be reconstructed from the $m + 1$ level smooth signal and the associated $m + 1$ detailed signals, where $m = 1, 2, \ldots$.

6.6.3   One-, Two-, and Three-dimensional Wavelet Transform

6.6.3.1   One-dimensional (1-D) Wavelet Transform   We use a one-dimensional (1-D) case to explain the concept of multiresolution analysis. Consider the discrete signal f_m at level m, which can be decomposed into the $m + 1$ level by convoluting it with the h (low-pass) filter to form a smooth signal f_{m+1}, and the g (high-pass) filter to form a detailed signal f'_{m+1}, respectively, as shown in Figure 6.11. When $m = 0$, it is the original signal (or in the case of 2-D, it is the original image to be compressed). This can be implemented in the following equations using the pyramidal algorithm suggested by Mallet:

$$f_{m+1}(n) = \sum_k h(2n - k) f_m(k)$$

$$f'_{m+1} = \sum_k g(2n - k) f_m(k)$$

(6.14)

where f_{m+1} is the smooth signal and f'_{m+1} is the detailed signal at the resolution level $m + 1$.

The total number of discrete points in f_m is equal to that of the sum of f_{m+1} and f'_{m+1}. For this reason, both f_{m+1} and f'_{m+1} are needed to be sampled at every other data point after the operation described in Eq. (6.14). The same process can be further applied to f_{m+1}, creating the detailed and smooth signal at the next resolution level, until the desired level is reached. But f'_{m+1} does not need to be processed any further.

Figure 6.12 depicts the components resulting from three levels of decompositions of the 1-D discrete signal f_0. The horizontal axis indicates the total number of discrete points of the original signal, and the vertical axis is the level, m, of the decomposition. At the resolution level $m = 3$, the signal is composed of the detailed

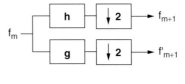

Figure 6.11   Decomposition of a 1-D signal f_m into a smooth f_{m+1} and a detailed signal f'_{m+1} h: low-pass filter; g: high-pass filter.

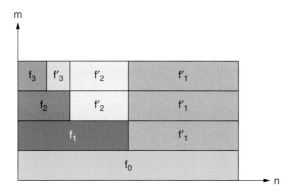

Figure 6.12 Three-level (1, 2, and 3) f_1, f_2, and f_3 wavelet decompositions of the signal f_0. The signals without the primes are the smooth signals, with the primes are the detailed signals. Note that the sum of all pixels n in each level is the same.

signals of the resolution levels f_1', f_2', and f_3' plus one smooth signal f_3. Thus the original signal f_0 can be reconstructed by

$$f_0 = f1' + f_2' + f_3' + f_3 \qquad (6.15)$$

Equation (6.15) is actually a *lossless* reconstruction using the wavelet transform compression of the origin discrete signal. In later sections we will discuss the DICOM 2000 lossless compression standard, which is an extension of Eq. (6.15) to 2-D and 3-D images with high-level decompositions.

Each of f_1', f_2', and f_3', and f^3 can be compressed by different quantization and encoding methods to achieve the required compression ratio. Accumulation of these compressed signals at all levels can be used to reconstruct the original signal f_0 using Eq. (6.15). In this case the compression is lossy since each f_i', $i = 1, 2, 3$, and f_3 have been compromised during the quantization.

6.6.3.2 Two-dimensional (2-D) Wavelet Transform

In the case of two-dimensional (2-D) wavelet transform, the first level results in four components, the x direction and the y direction (see Fig. 6.15, left and middle columns, x direction and y direction only). Figures 6.13 and 6.14 show a two level 2-D wavelet decomposition of a digital mammogram and a sagittal head MR image. Note the different characteristics between the mammogram and MRI at each level. In the mammogram, not much information is visible in the detailed images at levels 2 and 3, whereas in the MRI, detailed images at levels 2 and 3 retain various anatomical properties of the original image.

6.6.3.3 Three-dimensional (3-D) Wavelet Transform

Three-dimensional wavelet transform is a very effective method for compressing 3-D medical image data, and it yields a very good quality image volume set even at very high compression ratios. The 3-D method can be extended from the 1-D and 2-D pyramidal algorithm. Figure 6.15 shows one level of the decomposition process from f_m to f_{m+1}. Each line in the x direction of the 3-D image data set is first convoluted with filters h (low) and g (high), followed by subsampling every other voxel in the x direction to form the smooth and detailed data line. The resulting voxels are

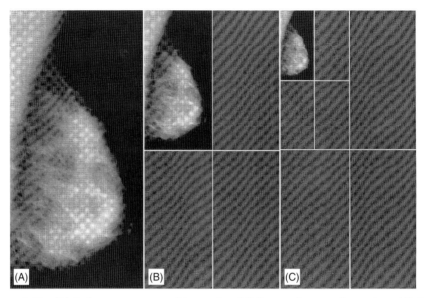

Figure 6.13 Digital mammogram with two-level 2-D wavelet transformation. (*A*) Original image; (*B*) one-level decomposition; (*C*) two-level decomposition. The total number of pixels after two levels of decomposition is the same as the original image. The smooth image is at the upper left-hand corner of each level. There is not much visible information in the detailed images at each level (compared with Fig. 6.14)

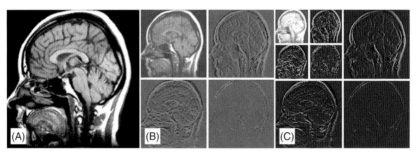

Figure 6.14 Two-level 2-D wavelet decomposition of a MR head sagittal image. (*A*) Original image; (*B*) one-level decomposition, (*C*) two-level decomposition. In each level the left upper corner shows the smooth image, and the other three quadrants are the detailed images. Observe the differences in the characteristics of the detailed images between the mammogram and head MRI. In the MRI all detailed images in each level contain visible anatomical information.

convoluted with h and g in the y direction, followed with subsampling in the y direction. Finally, the same procedure is applied to the z direction.

The resulting signal has eight components, f_{m+1} and f'_{m+1} s. Since h is a low-pass filter, only one component contains all low-frequency information, f_{m+1}. The seven remaining components are convoluted at least once with the high-pass filter g, so they contain some detailed signals f'_{m+1} in three different directions.

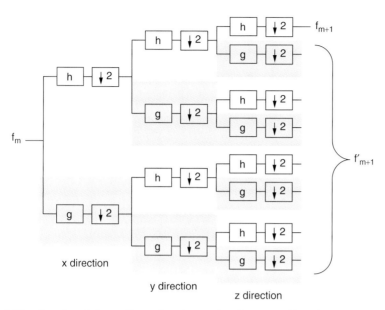

Figure 6.15 One-level three-dimensional wavelet decomposition in x, y, and z directions. Green shading signifies high-pass filters; blue shading signifies low-pass filters. Observe that only one component, f_{m+1}, is filtered by all low-pass filters. The resulting signal has eight components. f_{m+1} is the smooth image; all other seven f'_{m+1} are detailed images. If only x and y directions are decomposed, it is a 2-D wavelet decomposition.

The same process can be repeated for the low-frequency signal f_{m+1}, to form the next level of wavelet transform, and so forth, until the desired level is reached.

6.6.4   Three-dimensional Image Compression with Wavelet Transform

6.6.4.1   The Block Diagram Wavelet transform is a very effective method for compressing a 3-D medical image data set to obtain high compression ratio images with good quality. Figure 6.16 shows the block diagram of 3-D wavelet transform compression and decompression procedures. In the compression process, a 3-D wavelet transform is first applied to the 3-D image data set using the scheme shown in Figure 6.15, resulting in a 3-D multiresolution representation of the image. Then the wavelet coefficients are quantized using scalar quantization. Finally, run-length and then Huffman coding are used to impose entropy coding on the quantized data. The quantization and entropy coding steps are described in Sections 6.6.4.4 and 6.6.4.5.

The decompression process is the inverse of the compression process. The compressed data are first entropy decoded, a de-quantization procedure is applied to the decoded data, and the inverse 3-D wavelet transform is used, yielding the reconstructed 3-D image data.

6.6.4.2   Mathematical Formulation of the Three-dimensional Wavelet Transform For the 3-D case, a scaling Φ function and seven wavelet functions ϕs are chosen such that the 3-D scaling and wavelet functions are mathematically

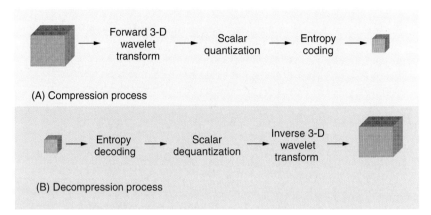

(A) Compression process

(B) Decompression process

Figure 6.16 Compression and decompression procedures of 3-D image block data using the 3-D wavelet transform.

separable. The scaling function (low-pass filter function) has the form

$$\Phi = \phi(x)\phi(y)\phi(z) \tag{6.16}$$

where $\phi(x)$, $\phi(y)$, and $\phi(z)$ contain the low pass filter "h" in the x, y, and z directions, respectively (see Eq. 6.14).

The seven wavelet functions have the forms:

$$\Psi^1(x, y, z) = \phi(x)\phi(y)\Psi(z), \quad \Psi^2(x, y, z) = \phi(x)\Psi(y)\phi(z),$$

$$\Psi^3(x, y, z) = \Psi(x)\phi(y)\phi(z),$$

$$\Psi^4(x, y, z) = \phi(x)\Psi(y)\Psi(z), \quad \Psi^5(x, y, z) = \Psi(x)\phi(y)\Psi(z),$$

$$\Psi^6(x, y, z) = \Psi(x)\Psi(y)\phi(z),$$

$$\Psi^7(x, y, z) = \Psi(x)\Psi(y)\Psi(z) \tag{6.17}$$

where $\Psi(x)$, $\Psi(y)$, and $\Psi(z)$ contain the high-pass filter g in the x, y, and z directions, respectively (see Eq. 6.14). Equations (6.16) and (6.17) describe the eight wavelet transform functions. During each level of the transform, the scalar function and the seven wavelet functions are applied, respectively, to the smooth (or the original) image at that level, forming a total of eight images, one smooth and seven detailed images. The wavelet coefficients are the voxel values of the eight images after the transform.

Figure 6.17 shows two levels of 3-D wavelet transform of an image volume data set. The first level decomposes the data into eight components: f_1 is the low (smooth) resolution portion of the image data, and the remaining seven blocks are high (detailed) resolution components f_1's. As Figure 6.17 shows, f_1 can be further decomposed into eight smaller volumes labeled f_2 (one smooth) and f_2' s (seven detailed). The detailed images f_1' on level 1 contain more level 1 high-frequency components than those f_2' of level 2.

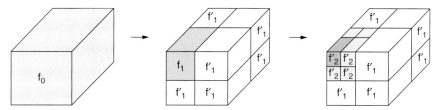

Figure 6.17 Volume data set after two-level decomposition by the 3-D wavelet transform. f_1 and f_2 are the smooth images at each level, respectively. Others are all detailed images.

With properly chosen wavelet functions, the low-resolution component in the m level is $1/(2^3)^m$ of the original image size after the transformation, but contains about 90% of the total energy in the m level, where m is the level of the decomposition. It is clear that the high-resolution components are spread into different decomposition levels. For these reasons the wavelet transform components provide a better representation of the original image for compression purposes. Different levels of representation can be encoded differently to achieve a desired compression ratio.

6.6.4.3 *Wavelet Filter Selection*   Wavelet filter selection is a very important step for high-performance image compression. A good filter bank should have a finite length so that the implementation is reasonably fast and provides a transform with most of the energy packed in the fewest coefficients. Today many filter functions have accumulated in public filter banks, and these have been tested to yield good quality compressed image of different categories. Their different applications are a matter of choice by the user (Strang, 1995).

6.6.4.4 *Quantization*   After the wavelet transformation, the next step is quantization of the wavelet transform coefficients. The purpose of quantization is to map a large number of input values into a smaller set of output values by reducing the precision of the data. This is the step where information may be lost. Wavelet transformed coefficents are floating point numbers and consist of two types: low-resolution image components (smooth image), which contain most of the energy, and high-resolution image components (detailed images), which contain the information on sharp edges.

Since the low-resolution components contain most of the energy, it is better to maintain the integrity of these data. To minimize data loss in this portion, each floating point number can be mapped onto its nearest integer (NINT) neighbor. Among the high-resolution components of the wavelet coefficients, there are many coefficients of small magnitude that correspond to the flat areas in the original image. These coefficients contain very little energy, so they can be eliminated without creating significant distortions in the reconstructed image. A threshold number T_m can be chosen, such that any coefficients less than can be set to zero. Above, a range of floating point numbers is mapped onto a single integer. If the quantization number is Q_m, high-frequency coefficients can be quantized as follows:

$$a_q(i, j, k) = \text{NINT}\left[\frac{a(i, j, k) - T_m}{Q_m}\right], \qquad a(i, j, k) > T_m$$

$$a_q(i, j, k) = 0, \qquad -T_m \leq a(i, j, k) \leq T_m$$

$$a_q(i, j, k) = \text{NINT}\left[\frac{a(i, j, k) + T_m}{Q_m}\right], \qquad a(i, j, k) < -T_m \tag{6.18}$$

where $a(i, j, k)$ is the wavelet coefficient, $a_q(i, j, k)$ is the quantized wavelet coefficient, and m is the number of the level in the wavelet transform; T_m and Q_m are functions of the wavelet transform level. The function T_m can be set as a constant, and $Q_m = Q2^{m-1}$, where Q is a constant.

6.6.4.5 *Entropy Coding* The quantized data are subjected to run-length coding followed by the Huffman coding. Run-length coding is effective when there are pixels with the same gray level in a sequence. Since thresholding of the high-resolution components results in a large number of zeros, run-length coding can be expected to significantly reduce the size of data. Applying Huffman coding after run-length coding can further improve the compression ratio.

6.6.4.6 *Some Results* This section presents two examples to demonstrate 3-D wavelet compression results compared to those obtained by other methods. The first example uses a 3-D MRI data set with 124 images each with $256 \times 256 \times 16$ bits. Both 2-D and 3-D wavelet compressions are used; the 2-D compression method is similar to that of the 3-D compression algorithm except that a two-dimensional wavelet transform is applied to each slice. Figure 6.18 compares the compression ratios using the 3-D and 2-D algorithms for a fixed PSNR; the horizontal axis is the peak signal-to-noise ratio (PSNR) defined in Eq. (6.9), and the vertical axis represents the compression ratio. At the same PSNR, compression ratios of the 3-D method are about 40% to 90% higher than that of the 2-D method.

The second example following the same example shown in Figure 6.6 where the same 3-D body CT image volume was used. Figures 6.19 and 6.20 depict the same section from the body CT image volume with 2-D wavelet comparison. In addition 3-D wavelet was used to compress the 3-D volume, with the reconstructed

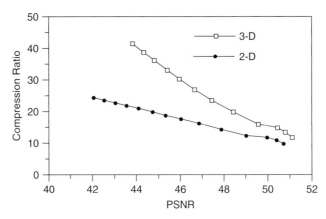

Figure 6.18 Performance comparison using 3-D versus 2-D wavelet compression of a 3-D MR head image set. Note that 3-D wavelet transform is superior to the 2-D transform for the same peak signal-to-noise ratio (PSNR, Eq. 6.9).

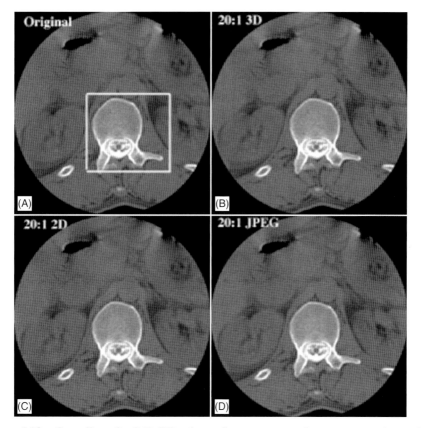

Figure 6.19 One slice of a 3-D CT volume data compressed at a compression ratio of 20:1 with 3-D wavelet, 2-D wavelet, and Cosine transform JPEG compression methods: (*A*) original image; (*B*) 3-D wavelet reconstructed image; (*C*) 2-D wavelet reconstructed image; (*D*) JPEG reconstructed image.

image of the same section as shown. It is observed that the quality of the 3-D wavelet reconstructed image with a compression ratio of 20:1 is nearly the same quality as that of the original image since the difference image contains minimum residual anatomy of the original image (Fig. 6.20*B'*). 3-D wavelet compression is also superior than both results from the 2-D wavelet (Fig. 6.20*C'*) and the 2-D JPEG cosine transform (Fig. 6.20*D'*).

6.6.4.7 *Wavelet Compression in Teleradiology* The reconstructed image from wavelet transform compression has four major characteristic, it:

1. retains both 3-D spatial, and 2-D spatial plus time information of the original image,
2. preserves certain local properties,
3. reconstruction results show good quality even at high compression ratios, and
4. can be implemented by software using the multiresolution scheme.

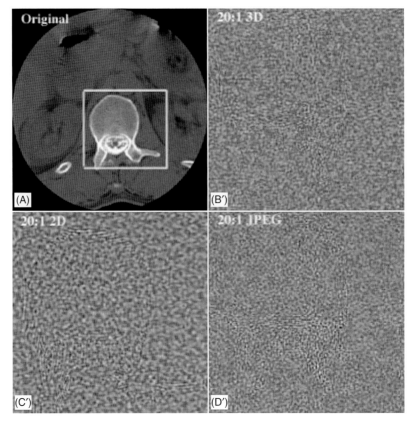

Figure 6.20 Subtracted images in an enlarge square region near the vertebra corresponding to Figure 6.19*B* through *D*: (*B'*) original—20:1 3-D wavelet; (*C'*) original—20:1 2-D wavelet; (*D'*) original—20:1 JPEG. (See also Fig. 6.6.)

For these reasons wavelet transform compression is used extensively in viewing images at workstations (Chapter 12) in teleradiology (Chapter 15). The detailed implementation of the method is discussed in Chapter 12.

6.7 COLOR IMAGE COMPRESSION

6.7.1 Examples of Color Images Used in Radiology

Color images are seldom used in radiology because radiological images do not traditionally use a light source to generate diagnostic images. Color, when used, is mostly for enhancement, namely by a range of gray levels converted to pseudo colors in order to enhance the visual appearance of features within this range. Examples are in nuclear medicine, SPECT, and PET. In these cases, however, compression is seldom used for studies with small image files. Other color images used in some medical applications can have very large image files per examination. An example is Doppler ultrasound (US) (see Fig. 3.27), which can produce image files as large as 225 Mbytes in 10 seconds. Other light imaging like ophthalmoscope (Fig. 3.30A, *B*), microscopy

(Fig. 3.32*A*, *B*), and endoscopy (Fig. 3.34) can also yield large color image files. Recent 3-D rendering of medical images could produce pseudo images that make use of color compression. So color image compression deserves some consideration. Color image compression requires a different approach from gray image compression because a color image is composed of three image planes: red, green, and blue, yielding total 24 bits per pixel. Further the three color planes have certain correlations among them that allow special compression techniques to be used.

6.7.2 The Color Space

A static color image with $512 \times 512 \times 24$ bits is decomposed into a red, a green, and a blue image in the RGB color space, each with $512 \times 512 \times 8$ bits (see Fig. 3.29, Section 3.9.2). In color video, a pixel can be up to 24 bits, methods of compressing color video will be discussed in Section 6.8.1. Each red, green, and blue image is treated independently as an individual 512×512 image. The display system combines three images through a color composite video control and displays them as a color image on the monitor. This scheme is referred to as the color space, and the three-color decomposition is determined by drawing a triangle on a special color chart developed by the Commission Internationale de L'Eclairag (CIE) with each of the base colors as an endpoint. The CIE color chart is characterized by isolating the luminance (or brightness) from the chrominance (or hue). Using these characteristics as guidelines, the National Television System Committee (NTSC) defined a new color space YIQ, representing the color components: the luminance (Y), in-phase chrominance (Cb), and quadrature chrominance (Cr), respectively as the three color coordinater. In digital color imaging a color space called YCbCr is used instead of the conventional RGB space. The conversion between the standard RGB space to YCbCr is given by

$$\begin{bmatrix} Y \\ Cb \\ Cr \end{bmatrix} = \begin{bmatrix} 0.2990 & 0.587 & 0.114 \\ -0.1687 & -0.3313 & 0.5 \\ 0.5 & -0.4187 & -0.0813 \end{bmatrix} \begin{bmatrix} R \\ G \\ B \end{bmatrix} \qquad (6.19)$$

where R, G, B pixel values are between 0 and 255.

There are two advantages of using the YCbCr coordinate system. First, it distributes most of the images information into the luminance component (Y), with less going to chrominance (Cb and Cr). As a result the Y element and the Cb, Cr elements are less correlated, and they therefore can be compressed separately for efficiency. Second, through field experience, the variations in the Cb and Cr planes are known to be less than that in the Y plane. Therefore Cb and Cr can be subsampled in both the horizontal and the vertical direction without losing much of the chrominance. The immediate compression from converting the RGB to YCbCr is 2:1. This can be computed as follows:

Original color image size: $512 \times 512 \times 24$ bits
YCbCr image size: $512 \times 512 \times 8 + 2 \times (0.25 \times 512 \times 512 \times 8)$ bits
(Y)   (Cb and Cr)   Subsampling

That is, after the conversion, each YCbCr pixel is represented by 12 bits: eight bits for the luminance (Y), and four bits for both chrominances (Cb and Cr) combined, which are subsampled in every other pixel and every other line. The Y, Cb, and Cr image can be compressed further as three individual images by using error free compression. This technique is used by JPEG for general color image compression.

6.7.3 Compression of Color Ultrasound Images

A general US Doppler study generates an average of 20 Mbytes per image file. There are studies that can go up to between 80 and 100 Mbytes. To compress a color Doppler image (see Fig. 3.27), the color RGB image is first transformed to the YCbCr space by Eq. (6.19). But instead of subsampling the Cb and the Cr images as described earlier, all three images are subject to a run-length coding independently. Two factors favor this approach. First, an US image possesses information within a sector. Outside the sector, it contains only background information. Discarding the background information can yield a very high compression ratio (Section 6.3.1). Second, the Cb and Cr images contain little information except at the blood flow regions under consideration, which are very small compared with the entire anatomical structures in the image. Thus run-length coding of Cb and Cr can give very high compression ratios, eliminating the need for subsampling. On average, two-dimensional, error-free run-length coding can give a 3.5:1 compression ratio, and in some cases, it can be as high as 6:1. Even higher compression ratios can result if the third dimension (time) of a temporal US study is considered using video compression methods.

6.8 FOUR-DIMENSIONAL IMAGE COMPRESSION AND COMPRESSION OF FUSED IMAGE

6.8.1 Four-dimensional Image Compression

6.8.1.1 *MPEG (Motion Picture Experts Group) Compression Method*
One 4-D image compression method is to first perform 3-D compression in the spatial domain at time $t = 0, 1, \ldots, t_n$ contagiously, where n is the last 3-D volume in the time domain. In this approach, there is no compression in the time domain. The other method is to use the video compression MPEG (Motion Picture Experts Group Compression) technique. A video compression scheme originally conceived as the "moving video" equivalent of the JPEG single-image compression. Because of the demand in the video entertainment business during the past years, MPEG2, announced by the MPEG Committee in 1994, has evolved to include many comprehensive compression techniques for moving pictures and video frames. In MPEG2, each pixel can have a maximum of 32 bits, 8 for the luminance element, and 24 bits for chrominance (Cb and Cr) elements (see Section 6.7).

6.8.1.2 *Paradigm Shift in Video Encoding and Decoding*   Traditional consumer video services have been in the broadcasting mode, from terrestrial cable TV to satellite services, by which a single broadcaster (encoder) is able to serve millions of TVs (decoders). The design principle has been an expensive, comprehensive, and complicated (server) encoder and volumes of simple (TV) decoders. The proliferation of mobile devices with video capture capabilities in the recent years has resulted in a paradigm shift that may require a simpler encoder for the broadcaster but a more complicated decoder for the mobile devices. So the burden of performance has shifted

to the decoder residing in the mobile handheld device or the home desktop computer to process, manipulate, and manage volumetric video captures. This paradigm shift is creating an opportunity for new generations of video encoding/decoding methods, processing algorithms, and system architectures in meeting the challenges of more complicated video environment. The opportunity now exists for medical imaging to take advantage of video encoding and decoding for 4-D medical imaging compression applications.

6.8.1.3 *Basic Concept of Video Compression*   The concept in MPEG 2 video compression can be described as follows:

1. MPEG can be applied to both black and white, and color videos.

2. In video, high-compression ratios come from the time domain compression plus standard compression methods in the spatial domain (as described in this chapter). To obtain high compression ratios and retain reasonable video quality, the change of objects of interest with respect to time should be minimal from one frame to the next. And each video frame should not have too many sharp-edged objects.

3. MPEG compression is accomplished by four steps: preprocessing, temporal predication, motion compensation, and quantization coding. During preprocessing, the smaller subsets (like object movement) in the video frames are determined; other subsets can just duplicate themselves from frame to frame (hence the high compression ratio). Quantization coding could be like the discrete cosine transform described in Section 6.4. Temporal predication and motion compensation (see Items 7, 8, 9) are discussed in following paragraphs.

4. MPEG uses multiple video frames to perform compression in the time domain.

5. Compression is performed by dividing the video into many temporal compression groups, each made up of three types of video frames.

6. There are three types of frame: one intra-coded and two inter-coded frames. The I-frames, or intra-coded frames, are used as reference frames of the original video. One out of 10 to 15 frames on average in each temporal compression group is an I-frame. The P-frames and the B-frames are inter-coded frames. The P-frames are forward predicted from the nearest I-frame or P-frame if available. The B-frames are bi-directional, so they use predicted data from the nearest preceding or following I-frame *and* P–frame (see Fig. 6.21). In each temporal compression group consisting of all three types of frames, one frame is the I-frame.

7. Predications include the pixel (or object) forward and/or backward movement, and the change of pixel value from predicted frames.

8. Trained motion vectors from knowledge derived from the original 4-D image set are used to translate and shift the pixels (objects) after predictions.

9. Iterative prediction error compensation based on knowledge is used to obtain better results.

Figure 6.21 illustrates the MPEG concept. In medical imaging—for example, in 4-D US and 4-D cardiography—knowledge on motion vectors and predication error compensation can be obtained from large clinical samples besides from the current

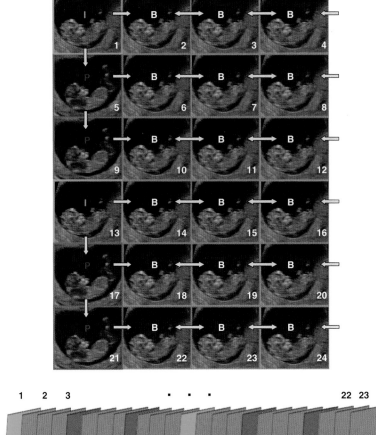

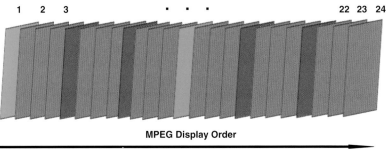

MPEG Display Order

I-frame : Reference for predicting subsequent frames

P-frame: Predicted from information presented in the
nearest preceding 'I' or 'P' frame

B-frame: Bi-directional frames using predicted data
from the nearest preceding I or P frame
AND the nearest following I or P frame

Figure 6.21 MPEG 2 compression technique (Long, Ringl). The example shows two sequential temporal compression groups, each consists of 12 frames, with one I-frame, two P-frames, and nine B-frames. Numerals are the frame number, arrows show the movement direction of predicted data. I-frame: reference for predicting subsequent frames; P-frame: predicted from information presented in the nearest preceding I or P frame; B-frame: bi-directional frames using predicted data from the nearest preceding I or P frame and the nearest following I or P frame.

object case under consideration. The compression ratio obtained after the encoding is completed depends on the object type, amount of the object's movement, repetitive motion, and changes in pixel values, among other factors. The International Standards Organization ISO/IEC MPEG2 has developed an International Standard, ISO/IEC 13818-2 (MPEG2, Part 2), for the video compression of generic coding of moving pictures and associated audio information.

6.8.2 Compression of Fused Image

Compression of the fused image requires following three steps:

1. Defuse the fused image. The result would be two original images before fusing, for example, a CT and a PET. In this case, it is cautioned that the original PET image might have been changed to a different size, for example, from 256×256 to 512×512 in order to fuse with the CT, and/or to a color look-up-table (LUT) for viewing.
2. Compress the two defused CT and PET images. This procedure takes two steps. First, the CT image is compressed using a favorable CT compression algorithm; followed by using a different tailored algorithm for the PET image. The two compressed images are then fused again.
3. Re-adjust the original gray scale and color LUTs Due to different compression algorithms used, unless adjustments are made, the fused image may not be favorable for viewing.

6.9 DICOM STANDARD AND FOOD AND DRUG ADMINISTRATION (FDA) GUIDELINES

Lossless compression provides a modest reduction in image size, with a compression ratio of about 2:1. Lossy compression, on the other hand, can yield very high compression ratios and still retain good image quality, especially when the wavelet transform method is used. However, lossy compression may engender a legal issue because some information in the original image has been discarded.

The use of image compression in clinical practice is influenced by two major organizations: the ACR/NEMA (American College of Radiology/National Electrical Manufacturers Association), which issued the DICOM 3.5 (Digital Imaging and Communication in Medicine) standard (See Chapter 9), and the Center for Devices and Radiological Health (CDRH) of Food and Drug Administration (FDA).

6.9.1 FDA Compression Requirement

The FDA, as the regulator, has chosen to place the use of compression in the hands of the user. The agency, however, has taken steps to ensure that the user has the information needed to make the decision by requiring that the lossy compression statement as well as the approximate compression ratio be attached to lossy images. The manufacturers must provide in their operator's manuals a discussion on the effects of lossy compression in image quality. Data from laboratory tests are to be included in premarket notifications when the medical device uses new technologies and asserts new claims. The PACS guidance document from the FDA (1993), however, allows manufacturers to report the normalized mean-square error (NMSE) of their communication and storage devices using lossy coding techniques. This measure was chosen because it is often used by the manufacturers, so there is some objective basis for comparisons. Nevertheless, as discussed in Section 6.5.1.1, NMSE does not provide any local information regarding the type of data loss (e.g., spatial location or spatial frequency).

6.9.2   DICOM Standard in Image Compression

When DICOM introduced the compression standard (see Chapter 9), it used JPEG based on sequential block DCT followed by Huffman coding for both lossless and lossy (with quantization) compression (see Sections 6.4.2, 6.3.2, and 6.3.3). In 2000 DICOM added JPEG 2000 (ISO/IS 15444) (International Standards Organization) based on wavelet transform (see Section 6.6) for both lossless and lossy compression. Features defined in JPEG 2000 part 1 specify the coding representation of compressed image for both color and gray scale still images. Inclusion of a JPEG 2000 image in the DICOM image file is indicated by transfer syntax in the header of DICOM file. Two DICOM transfer syntaxes are specified for JPEG 2000. One is for lossless only, and the other is for both lossless and lossy.

DICOM 3.5-2008 Part 5 Data Structures and Encoding has an Annex A.4 used for the transfer syntaxes for encapsulation of encoded pixel data as shown in Table 6.2. Annex F gives description of encapsulated compressed images with

TABLE 6.2   DICOM PS 3.5 Data Encoding Specifications

Code	Specification
A.4.1 JPEG image compression	Use JPEG based on sequential block DCT followed by Huffman coding for both lossless and lossy (with quantization) compression (see Sections 6.4.2, 6.3.2, and 6.3.3)
A.4.2 RLE Compression	Use RLE (Run Length Encoding) compression for black-and-white image or graphics (see Section 6.3.2)
A.4.3 JPEG-LS image compression	Use JPEG-LS lossless compression, which is an ISO standard for digital compression for lossless and near-lossless coding of continuous-tone still image
A.4.4 JPEG 2000 image compression	Use wavelet transform method (see Section 6.6) for lossless and lossy compression
A.4.5 MPEG2 image compression	Use International Standard, ISO/IEC 13818-2 (MPEG2 Part 2), for the video compression of generic coding of moving pictures or video and associated audio information.

Source: Extracted and modified from DICOM Standard, 3.5–2008 Part 5, Annex A.4.

methods presented in Table 6.2 as part of a DICOM message, and Annex G gives that for the RLE compression.

References

Albanesi MG, Lotto DI. Image compression by the wavelet decomposition. *Sig Process* 3(3): 265–74; 1992.

Antonini M, Barlaud M, Mathieu P, Daubechies I. Image coding using wavelet transform. *IEEE Trans Image Process* 1: 205–20; 1992.

Cohen A, Daubechies I, Feauveau JC. Biorthogonal bases of compactly supported wavelets. *Comm Pure Appl Math* 45: 485–560; 1992.

Daubechies I. Orthonormal bases of compactly supported wavelets. *Comm Pure Appl Math* 41: 909–96; 1988.

Lightstone M, Majani E. Low bit-rate design considerations for wavelet-based image coding. *Proc SPIE* 2308: 501–12; 1994.

Long, M. Understanding MPEG2 Digital Video Compression. http://www.mlesat.com/ Article7.html, 1996.

Mallat SG. A theory for multiresolution signal decomposition: the wavelet representation. *IEEE Trans Pattern Anal Mach Intell* 11(7): 674–93; 1989.

Ringl H, Schrnthaner R, Sala E, et al. Lossy 3D JPEG2000 compression of abdominal CT images in patients with acute abdominal complaints *Radiology* 248: 476–84; 2008.

Strang G, Nguyen T. *Wavelets and Filter Banks*. Wellesley-Cambridge Press; Boston, MA, 1995.

Villasenor JD, Belzer B, Liao J. Wavelet filter evaluation for image compression. *IEEE Trans Image Process* 4(8): 1053–60; 1995.

Wang J, Huang HK. Three-dimensional medical image compression using wavelet transformation. *IEEE Trans Med Imag* 15(4): 547–54; 1996.

Wang J, Huang HK. Three-dimensional image compression with wavelet transforms. In: Bankman IN, et al., eds. *Handbook of Medical Imaging*. San Diego: Academic Press; 2008, 851–62.

PART II

PACS FUNDAMENTALS

CHAPTER 7

Picture Archiving and Communication System Components and Workflow

This chapter discusses the basic components of PACS, namely the general architecture, requirements, and functions of the system. The chapter shows how the current clinical PACS architectures—stand-alone, client/server, and Web-based—illustrate the three prevailing PACS operation concepts. The chapter ends with consideration of teleradiology with regard to PACS and enterprise PACS. Figure 7.1 shows how the topics of this chapter are positioned with relation to other chapter topics of Part II.

7.1 PACS COMPONENTS

The major components in PACS consist of an image and data acquisition gateway, a PACS server and archive, and several display workstations (WSs) integrated together by digital networks. PACS can be further connected with other healthcare information systems by database gateways and communication networks as shown in Figure 7.2.

7.1.1 Data and Image Acquisition Gateways

PACS acquires images sent from imaging modalities (devices) and related patient data from the hospital information system (HIS) and the radiology information system (RIS). There are two types of gateways (GW) to the PACS server and archive, the database GW (Fig 7.2, green) for textual data, and the image acquisition GW (Fig. 7.2, yellow) for imaging data. A major task in PACS is to acquire images reliably and in a timely manner from each radiological imaging modality via the acquisition GW, and relevant patient data, including study support text information of the patient, description of the study, and parameters relevant to image acquisition and processing through the database GW.

Image acquisition is a major task in PACS. Because the imaging modality is not under the control of a single PACS manager, the imaging modalities supplied by manufacturers each have their own DICOM-compliant statements (see Chapter 9). Worse, some older imaging modalities may not even be DICOM compliant. For the many imaging modalities to connect to a PACS requires many hours of labor-intensive work and the cooperation of modality manufacturers. Next, image acquisition is a slow operation because patients' examinations are the documents involved in the

PACS and Imaging Informatics, Second Edition, by H. K. Huang
Copyright © 2010 John Wiley & Sons, Inc.

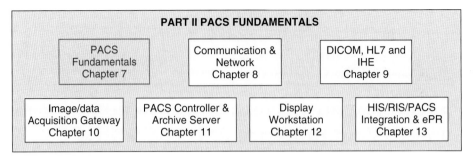

Figure 7.1   Position of Chapter 7 in the organization of this book. Color codes are used to highlight components and workflow in chapters of Part II.

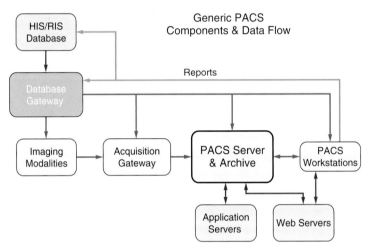

Figure 7.2   PACS basic components (yellow) and data flow (blue: internal; green and red: external between PACS and other information systems); other information systems (light blue). Application servers and Web servers connected to the PACS controller enrich the PACS infrastructure for other clinical, research, and education applications. HIS: hospital information system; RIS: radiology information system.

acquisition process. Inevitably it takes the imaging modality and the radiological technician considerable time to acquire the necessary data for image reconstruction and to compile a complete image file (Section 4.2). Last, images and patient data generated by the modality sometimes contain format information unacceptable for the on-site PACS operation. To address their problem, an acquisition gateway computer, as some manufacturers called it (modality integration unit, MIU), is often placed between the imaging modality(s) and the rest of the PACS network to isolate the host computer in the radiological imaging modality from the PACS. Isolation is necessary because traditional imaging device computers lack the necessary communication and coordination software that is standardized within the PACS infrastructure. If, the host computers do not contain enough intelligence to work with the PACS server to recover various errors, the acquisition gateway computer has three primary tasks: It acquires image data from the radiological imaging device can convert the data from the manufacturer specifications to a PACS standard format (header format, byte ordering, and matrix sizes) that is compliant with the DICOM data formats and then forward the image study to the PACS server or display WSs.

Interfaces of two types connect a general-purpose PACS acquisition gateway computer with a radiological imaging modality. With peer-to-peer network interfaces, which use the TCP/IP (Transmission Control Protocol/Internet Protocol) Ethernet protocol (Chapter 8), image transfers can be initiated either by the radiological imaging modality (a "push" operation) or by the destination PACS acquisition gateway computer (a "pull" operation). The pull mode is advantageous because, if an acquisition gateway computer goes down, images can be queued in the radiological imaging modality computer until the gateway computer becomes operational again, at which time the queued images can be pulled and normal image flow resumed. Provided that sufficient data buffering is available in the imaging modality computer, the pull mode is the preferred mode of operation because an acquisition computer can be programmed to reschedule study transfers if failure occurs (due to itself or the radiological imaging modality). If the designated acquisition gateway computer is down, and a delay in acquisition is not acceptable, images from the examination can be automatically re-routed to another networked designated backup acquisition gateway computer or a WS.

The second interface type is a master-slave device-level connection such as the de facto old industry standard DR-11 W. This parallel-transfer direct-memory access connection is a point-to-point board-level interface. Recovery mechanisms again depend on which machine (acquisition gateway computer or imaging modality) can initiate a study transfer. If the gateway computer is down, data may be lost. An alternative image acquisition method must be used to acquire these images (e.g., the technologist manually sends individual images stored in the imaging modality computer after the gateway computer is up again, or the technologist digitizes the digital hard copy film image). These interface concepts are described in more detail in Chapter 11.

There is a way to speed up the image review process after the image examination is completed. If the imaging modality and the PACS are produced by the same manufacturer, the image file can be transmitted to the PACS WS immediately after the image file is ready for the radiologist to review because PACS will readily accept the same manufacturer's imaging modality. Chapter 10 elaborates more on the concept and structure of the GW.

7.1.2 PACS Server and Archive

Imaging examinations along with pertinent patient information from the acquisition gateway computer, the HIS, and the RIS are sent to the PACS server via the gateways. The PACS server is the engine of the PACS and consists of high-end computers or servers. The PACS server and archive have two major components: a database server and an archive system. Table 7.1 lists some major functions of a PACS server. The archive system can accommodate short-term, long-term, and permanent storage. These components will be explained in details in Chapter 11.

TABLE 7.1 Major functions of the PACS server and archive

- Receives images from examinations (exams) via acquisition gateways
- Extracts text information describing the received exam from the DICOM image header
- Updates the database management system
- Determines the destination workstations to which newly generated exams are to be forwarded
- Automatically retrieves necessary comparison images from historical exams from a cache storage or long term library archive system
- Automatically corrects the orientation of computed or digital radiography images
- Determines optimal contrast and brightness parameters for image display
- Performs image data compression if necessary
- Performs data integrity check if necessary
- Archives new exams onto long-term archive library
- Deletes images that have been archived from the acquisition gateway
- Services query/retrieve requests from WSs and other PACS controllers in the enterprise PACS
- Interfaces with PACS application servers

7.1.3 Display Workstations

A workstation (WS) includes communication network connection, local database, display, resource management, and processing software. High-quality WSs for radiologists to make primary diagnosis are called diagnostic WS, the others are generally called review WS. The fundamental workstation operations are listed in Table 7.2.

Until three years ago there were four types of display workstations categorized by their resolutions: (1) high-resolution (2.5 K $\times$ 2 K or higher resolution) liquid crystal display (LCD) for primary diagnosis at the radiology department, (2) medium-resolution (2000 $\times$ 1600 or 1600 $\times$ 1K) LCD for primary diagnosis of

TABLE 7.2 Major functions of PACS workstations

Function	Description
Case preparation	Accumulation of all relevant images and information belonging to a patient examination
Case selection	Selection of cases for a given subpopulation through DICOM query/retrieve
Image arrangement	Tools for arranging and grouping images for easy review
Interpretation	Measurement tools for facilitating the diagnosis
Documentation	Tools for image annotation, text, and voice reports
Case presentation	Tools for a comprehensive case presentation, including 3-D image display for a large 3-D file, and fusion images
Image reconstruction	Tools for various types of image reconstruction for proper display

sectional images and at the hospital wards, (3) physician desktop WS (1K to 512) LCD, and (4) hard copy/copying WS for copying images on CD or print on film or paper. In a stand-alone primary diagnostic WS (Chapter 12), current and historical images are stored in local high-speed magnetic disks for fast retrieval. WS also has access to the PACS server database for retrieving longer term historical images if needed. Chapter 12 elaborates more on the concept and applications of WS.

Over the past three years, as more affordable WS became available in the market, the aforementioned WS categories are no longer applicable. An average-income consumer can purchase a very good PC (personal computer) with 1K LCD display for less than US$1000. The classical PACS WS model has evolved to the client-server model concept. Network computing is now gradually dominating PACS WS deployment. In this model, the terms thick client, thin client, smart client, and fat client emerge and become popular on manufacturers' PACS WS list. A thick client PACS WS has local storage and many image processing functions and only needs to communicate with the server occasionally; a thin client PACS WS, on the other hand, has no local storage, very minimal image processing functions, and needs the support from the server continuous. In between are the smart client and fat client WSs. We will discuss this model in Chapter 12 in more detail.

7.1.4 Application Servers

Application servers (see Fig. 7.2, light blue) are connected to the PACS server and archive. Through these application servers, PACS data can be filtered to different servers tailored for various applications, for example, Web-based image-viewing server (Chapter 12), radiation therapy ePR server (Chapter 23), image-guided surgery ePR server (Chapter 24), CAD server (Chapters 25, 26), and education server (Chapter 28).

7.1.5 System Networks

A basic function of any computer network is to provide an access path by which end users (e.g., radiologists and clinicians) at one geographic location can access information (e.g., images and reports) from another location. The required networking data for system design include location and function of each network node, frequency of information passed between any two nodes, cost for transmission between nodes with various speed lines, desired reliability of the communication, and required workflow throughput. The variables in the design include the network topology, communication line capacities, and flow assignments.

At the local area network level, digital communication in the PACS infrastructure design can consist of low-speed Internet (10 Mbits/s signaling rate), medium-speed (100 Mbits/s) or fast (1 Gbit/s) Internet, and high-speed asynchronous transfer mode technology (ATM, 155–622 Mbits/s and up). In wide area networks, various digital service (DS) speeds can be used, which range from DS-0 (56 kbits/s) and DS-1 (T1, 1.544 Mbits/s) to DS-3 (45 Mbits/s) and ATM (155–622 Mbits/s). There is a trade-off between transmission speed and cost.

The network protocol used should be standard, for example, the TCP/IP (Transmission Control Protocol/Internet Protocol; Chapter 8) and DICOM communication protocol (a higher level of TCP/IP). A low-speed network is used to connect the imaging modalities (devices) to the acquisition gateway computers because the time-consuming processes of imaging acquisition do not require high-speed connection. Sometimes several segmented local area Internet branches can be used in transferring data from imaging devices to a GW. Medium- and high-speed networks are used on the basis of the balance of data throughput requirements and costs. A faster image network is used between GWs and the PACS server because several GWs may send large image files to the server at the same time. High-speed networks are always used between the PACS server and WSs.

Process coordination between tasks running on different computers connected to the network is an extremely important issue in system networking. The coordination of processes running either on the same computer or on different computers is accomplished by using interprocessor communication methods with socket-level interfaces to TCP/IP. Commands are exchanged as American Standard Code for Information Interchange (ASCII) messages to ensure standard encoding of messages. Various PACS-related job requests are lined up into the disk resident priority queues, which are serviced by various computer system DAEMON (agent) processes. The Queue software can have a built-in job scheduler that is programmed to retry a job several times by using either a default set of resources or alternative resources if a hardware error is detected. This mechanism ensures that no jobs will be lost during the complex negotiation for job priority among processes. Communications and networking will be presented in more detail in Chapter 8.

7.2 PACS INFRASTRUCTURE DESIGN CONCEPT

The four major ingredients in the PACS infrastructure design concept are system standardization, open architecture and connectivity, reliability, and security.

7.2.1 Industry Standards

The first important rule in building a PACS infrastructure is to incorporate as many industry de facto standards as possible that are consistent with the overall PACS design scheme. The idea is to minimize the need of customized software. Furthermore, using industry standard hardware and software increases the portability of the system to other computer platforms. For example, the following industry standards, protocols, computer operating systems, programming languages, workflow profiles should be used in the PACS infrastructure design: (1) UNIX operating system, (2) WINDOWS NT/XP operating system, (3) C and C++ programming languages, (4) Java programming language platform (Just Another Vague Acronym), (5) XML (extensible markup language) for data representation and exchange on the World Wide Web, (6) SQL (structured query language) as the database query language, (7) X WINDOW platform for graphical user interface (GUI), (8) TCP/IP communication protocols, (9) DICOM standard for image data format and communication, (10) HL7 (Health Level 7) for healthcare database information and textual data format exchange, (11) IHE (Integrating the Healthcare Enterprise) for workflow profiles, and (12) ASCII text representation for message passing.

The implications of following these standards and protocols in PACS implementation are several. First, implementation and integration of all future PACS components and modules become standardized. Second, system maintenance is easier because the concept of operation of each module looks logically similar to that of the others. Moreover, defining the PACS primitive operations serves to minimize the amount of redundant computer code within the PACS system, which in turn makes the code easier to debug, understand, and search. It is self-evident that using industrial standard terminology, data format, and communication protocols in PACS design facilitates system understanding and documentation among all levels of PACS developers. Among all standards, HL7 and DICOM are the most important; the former allows interfaces between PACS and HIS/RIS, the latter interfaces images among various manufacturers. Following the IHE workflow profiles allows for smooth PACS components interoperation. These topics will be discussed in more detail in Chapter 9.

7.2.2 Connectivity and Open Architecture

If PACS modules in the same hospital cannot communicate with each other, they become isolated systems, each with its own images and patient information, and it would be difficult to combine these modules to form a total hospital-integrated PACS. That is why packaging a mini-PACS system with the purchase of a modality like CT or MR is not a good idea in a long run.

Open network design is essential, allowing a standardized method for data and message exchange between heterogeneous systems. Because computer and communications technology changes rapidly, a closed architecture would hinder system upgradability. For instance, suppose that an independent imaging WS from a given manufacturer would, at first glance, make a good additional component to an MRI scanner for viewing images. If the WS has a closed proprietary architecture design, then no components except those specified by the same manufacturer can be augmented to the system. Potential overall system upgrading and improvement would be limited. Considerations of connectivity are important even when a small-scale PACS is planned. To be sure that a contemplated PACS is well designed and allows for future connectivity, the following questions should be kept in mind all the time:

Can we transmit images from this PACS module to other modules, and vice versa?

Does this module use HL7 standard for textual data and DICOM for images?

Does the computer in the module use a standard communication protocol?

7.2.3 Reliability

Reliability is a major concern in a PACS for two reasons. First, a PACS has many components; the probability of a failing component is high. Second, because the PACS manages and displays critical patient information, extended periods of downtime cannot be tolerated. In designing a PACS, it is therefore important to use fault tolerant measures, including error detection and logging software, external auditing programs (i.e., network management processes that check network circuits, magnetic disk space, database status, processer status, and queue status), hardware redundancy, and intelligent software recovery blocks. Some fail recovery mechanisms that can be used include automatic retry of failed jobs with alternative resources and algorithms and intelligent bootstrap routines (a software block executed by a computer when it is restarted) that allow a PACS computer to automatically continue operations after a power outage or system failure. Improving reliability is costly; however, it is essential to maintain high reliability of a complex integrated information system. This topic will be considered in depth in Chapter 16.

7.2.4 Security

Security, particularly the need for patient confidentiality, is an important consideration because of medicolegal issues and the HIPAA (Health Insurance Portability and Accountability Act) mandate. There are, in general, three types of data violation: physical intrusion, misuse, and behavioral violations. Physical intrusion relates to facility security, which can be handled by building management. Misuse and behavioral violations can be minimized by account control and privilege control. Most sophisticated database management systems have identification and authorization mechanisms that use accounts and passwords. Application programs may supply additional layers of protection. Privilege control refers to granting and revoking the user's access to specific tables, columns, or views from the database. These security measures provide the PACS infrastructure with a mechanism for controlling access to clinical and research data. With these mechanisms the system designer can enforce policy as to which persons have access to clinical studies. In some hospitals, for example, referring clinicians are granted image study access only after a preliminary radiology reading has been performed and attached to the image data. Examples of using fingerprint identification and facial verification are given in Chapters 24 and 27.

An additional security measure can be implemented in data security and data communication security in which image digital signature can be embedded in the image during its storage and transmission. If implemented, this feature would increase the system software overhead, but data transmission through open communication channels is more secure. Image security is discussed in Chapter 17.

7.3 A GENERIC PACS WORKFLOW

This chapter emphasizes PACS workflow. For this reason, whenever appropriate, a data workflow scenario will accompany the PACS model at its introduction. This section discusses a generic PACS workflow starting from the patient registering in the HIS, RIS ordering examination, technologist performing the exam, image viewing, reporting, to image archiving. Compare this PACS workflow with the PACS components and workflow is depicted in Figure 7.2, and the radiology workflow shown in Figure 3.1. Clearly, PACS has replaced many manual steps in the film-based workflow. Now follow the PACS workflow numerals shown in Figure 7.3:

1. Patient registers in HIS, with radiology exam ordered in RIS, and exam accession number automatically assigned.
2. RIS outputs HL7 messages of HIS and RIS demographic data to PACS broker/interface engine.
3. PACS broker notifies the archive server of the scheduled exam for the patient.

A Generic PACS Workflow

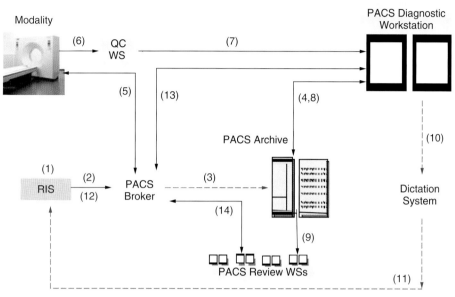

Figure 7.3 Generic PACS workflow. Compare the PACS workflow with the PACS components and workflow shown in Figure 7.2, and radiology workflow depicted in Figure 3.1.

4. Following on prefetching rules, historical PACS exams of the scheduled patient are prefetched from the archive server and sent to the radiologist reading workstation (WS).

5. Patient arrives at modality. Modality queries the PACS broker/interface engine for the DICOM worklist.

6. Technologist acquires images and sends the PACS exam of images acquired by the modality and patient demographic data to quality control (QC) WS in a DICOM format.

7. Technologist prepares the PACS exam and sends to the radiologist the diagnostic WS as the prepared status.

8. On its arrival at the radiologist reading WS, the PACS exam is immediately sent automatically to the archive server. Archive server database is updated with the PACS exam as the prepared status.

9. Archive server automatically distributes the PACS exam to the review WSs in the wards based on patient location as received from the HIS/RIS HL7 message.

10. Reading radiologist dictates a report with the exam accession number on the dictation system. The radiologist signs off on the PACS exam with any changes. The archive database is updated with changes and marks the PACS exam as signed-off.

11. Transcriptionist fetches the dictation and types a report that corresponds to the exam accession number within RIS.

12. RIS outputs HL7 message of results report data along with any previously updated RIS data.

13. Radiologist queries the PACS broker for previous reports of PACS exams on the reading WSs.

14. Referring physicians query the broker for reports of PACS exams on the review WSs.

7.4 CURRENT PACS ARCHITECTURES

There are three basic PACS architectures: (1) stand-alone, (2) client-server, and (3) Web-based. From these three basic PACS architectures, there are variations and hybrid design types.

7.4.1 Stand-alone PACS Model and General Data Flow

The stand-alone model described here is also called thick client model. The three major features of the stand-alone model are as follows:

1. Images are automatically sent to the designated diagnostic and review WSs from the server.

2. WSs can also query/retrieve images from the archive server.

3. WSs have short-term cache storage.

Data workflow of the stand-alone PACS model is shown in Figure 7.4. The numerals indicate the following:

1. RIS notifies the imaging modality and the PACS server of a patient registration.

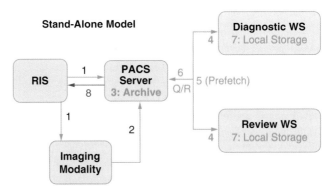

Figure 7.4 Stand-alone PACS model and general data flow. The data flow starts when RIS notifies imaging modality and the PACS server that a patient has registered (1). Images are sent from the modality to the PACS server (2), PACS server archives the images (3) and sends to WSs automatically (single-headed red arrows, 4) along with prefetched images (single-headed red arrows, 5); images can also be query/retrieve by the WSs (double-headed red arrows, 6). All WSs have local storage (7). Diagnostic reports are sent back to the PACS server or directly to RIS (purple arrow, 8).

2. After the examination, the modality sends images to the PACS server.

3. PACS server archives the images.

4. Multiple copies of the images are distributed to selected diagnostic and review WSs. The server performs this image distribution function automatically based on the default setting.

5. Server also prefetches pertinent historical images and sends copies to selected WSs.

6. WSs can also use DICOM query/retrieve function through the server to obtain images for review. In addition, if automatic prefetching fails, a WS can query/retrieve historical images from the server.

7. Each WS contains a local storage to hold a preset number of PACS exams.

8. WS returns the diagnosis to the server then to the RIS.

Advantages

1. If the PACS server goes down, imaging modalities or acquisition GWs have the flexibility to send images directly to designated WSs so that radiologist scan continue reading new cases.

2. Because multiple copies of the PACS exam are distributed throughout the system, there is less risk of losing PACS image data.

3. Some historical PACS exams will still be available in WSs because they have local storages.

4. System is less susceptible to daily variations of network performance because PACS exams are preloaded onto the WS's local storage and available for viewing immediately.

5. Modification to the DICOM header can be performed if necessary during the quality control before archiving.

Disadvantages

1. Users must rely on correct image distribution and prefetching of historical PACS exams based on the preset default table, which is not possible all the time.

2. Because images are sent to designated WSs, each WS may have a different worklist, which makes it inconvenient for radiologists to read/review all examinations assigned to him/her at any WS in one setting.

3. Users sometime need to use query/retrieve function to retrieve pertinent PACS exams from the archive, this task can be a complex function compared to the client/server model.

4. Radiologist may duplicate the reading of the same case from a different WS because the same exam may be sent to several WSs.

7.4.2 Client-Server PACS Model and Data Flow

The client-server model described here is also called thin client model, the three major features of the client/server model are as follows:

1. Images are centrally archive in the PACS server.
2. From a single worklist at the client WS has a sinlge worklist of all examinations where a user selects the patient and images via the PACS server.
3. WSs have no local storage, images are flushed after reading.

Data flow of the client-server PACS model is shown in Figure 7.5. The numerals indicate the following steps:

1. RIS notifies the imaging modality and the PACS server of a patient registration.
2. After the examination, the modality sends images to the PACS server.
3. PACS server archives the images.
4. Client WSs have access to the complete worklist from where images, and exams can be retrieved from the PACS server and archive. For more efficient image retrievals, the worklist can be shortened by a preset filter.
5. Once the exam is selected, images from the PACS archive are loaded directly into the image memory of the client WS for viewing. Prefetched historical exams are loaded to the WS in the same manner.
6. Once the user has completed reading/reviewing the exam, the image data are flushed from memory, leaving no image data in image memory of the client WS.
7. WS returns the diagnosis to the server and then to the RIS.

Advantages

1. Any exams are available on any PACS WS at any time, making it convenient to retrieve and to read/review.

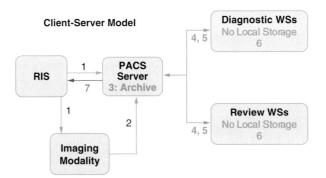

Figure 7.5 Client-server PACS model and general data flow. The first three data flow steps are the same as those of the stand-alone model. Data flow starts when RIS notifies imaging modality and the PACS server that a patient has registered (1). Images are sent from the modality to the PACS server (2), and PACS server archives the images (3). The client WSs has access to the completed current worklist as well as the list of prehistorical exams of the same patient. Current images as well as historical images can be retrieved from the worklist for review and viewing. (4, 5 double-headed red arrows). All reviewed images are discarded from the WS after review (6). Diagnostic reports are sent back to the PACS server or directly to RIS (purple arrow, 7) the same as in the stand-alone model.

2. No prefetching or study distribution is needed.

3. No query/retrieve function is needed. The user just selects the exam from the worklist on the client WS and the images are loaded automatically.

4. Because the main copy of a PACS exam is located in the PACS server archive and is shared by client WSs, radiologists will know immediately if they are reading the same exam and thus avoid duplicate readings.

Disadvantages

1. The PACS server is a single point of failure; if it goes down, the entire PACS is nonfunctional. Users then are not be able to view any exams on the any client WSs. All newly acquired exams must be held back from the archive at the modalities storage until the server is repaired.

2. Because there are more database transactions in the client-server architecture, the system is exposed to more transaction errors, making it less robust compared to the stand-alone architecture.

3. The architecture is dependent on network performance, especially when WAN (wide area network) is being used. Slow WNS performance is problematic for teleradiology operation (see Chapter 15).

4. Modification to the DICOM header in the image for quality control is not possible until the image is archived.

7.4.3 Web-Based Model

The Web-based PACS model has an architecture similar to the client-server model. The main difference is that the client and server software are for Web-based applications. A couple of additional advantages of the Web-based model as compared to the client-server model are:

1. The client workstation hardware can be platform independently as long as the Web browser is supported.

2. The system is a completely portable. The Web-based application can be used on site as well as at home with an Internet connection.

A disadvantages as compared to the client-server model is that the system may be limited in the amount of functionality and performance by the Web-based browser.

For the past three years the client-server model and the web-based model have emerged as the dominant PACS models in clinical operation.

7.5 PACS AND TELERADIOLOGY

This section considers the relationship between teleradiology and PACS. Two topics, the pure teleradiology model and the PACS and teleradiology combined model, are presented. A more detailed treatise on the various models and functionalities is found in Chapter 15.

7.5.1   Pure Teleradiology Model

Teleradiology can be an entirely independent system operated in a pure teleradiology model as shown in Figure 7.6. This model serves better for several imaging centers and smaller hospitals with a radiological examination facility, but no or not enough in-house radiologists to cover the reading. In this model the teleradiology management center serves as the monitor of the operation. It receives images from different imaging centers, $1, \ldots, N$, keeps a record but not the images, and routes images to different expert centers, $1, \ldots, M$, for reading. Reports come back to the management center, it records the reading, and forwards reports to the appropriate imaging centers. The management center is also responsible for the billing and other administrative functions like image distribution and workload balancing. The wide area networks used for connection between various imaging centers, the management center, and expert centers can be of mixed types, with various performances dependent on requirements and costs. This model is used most for night and weekend coverage.

7.5.2   PACS and Teleradiology Combined Model

PACS and teleradiology can be combined to form the unit as shown in Figure 7.7. The two major components are the PACS, shown inside the upper dotted rectangle,

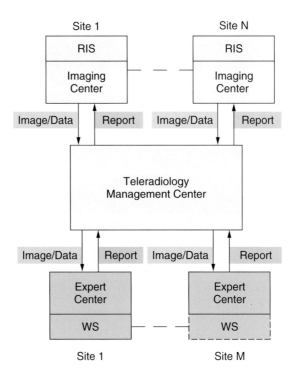

Figure 7.6   Basic teleradiology model. The management center monitors the operation to direct workflow between imaging centers and expert centers.

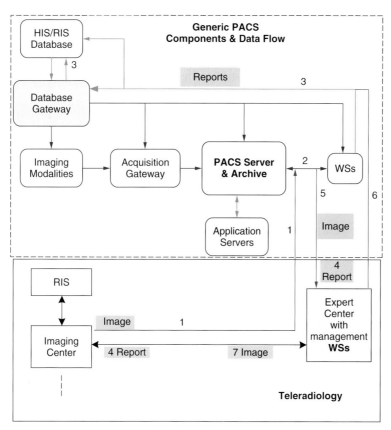

Figure 7.7   PACS and teleradiology combined model. The top rectangle is the PACS components and workflow (detail from Fig. 7.2), and the bottom rectangle is the teradiology model modified from Figure 7.6. Red lines show communication between PACS and teleradiology.

and the pure teleradiology model (see Fig. 7.6), shown in the lower rectangle. The workflow of this combined model is as follows:

- Radiologists at PACS WSs read exams from the outside imaging centers (step 1).
- After reading by PACS radiologists from its own WSs (step 2), reports are sent to the HIS database via the database gateway for its own record (step 3) and to the expert center (steps 4, 5) from where the report (step 4) is also sent back to the imaging center.
- PACS can also send its own exams to the outside expert center for reading (step 5). The expert center returns the report to the PACS database gateway (step 6).
- The image center can send images to the expert center for reading as in the pure teleradiology model (step 7).

The combined teleradiology and PACS model is mostly used in a healthcare center with (1) satellite imaging centers, (2) multiple affiliated hospitals, and (3) with backup radiology coverage between hospitals and imaging centers.

7.6 ENTERPRISE PACS AND ePR SYSTEM WITH IMAGE DISTRIBUTION

Enterprise PACS is for very large scale PAC systems integration. It has become particularly popular in today's enterprise healthcare delivery system. Figure 7.8 shows the generic architecture of an enterprise PACS. In the generic architecture, three major components are PACS at each hospital in the enterprise, the enterprise data center, and the enterprise ePR. The general work flow is as follows:

- The enterprise data center supports all PAC systems in the enterprise.
- Patient images and data from each PACS are sent to the enterprise data center for long-term archive (step 1).
- Filtered patient data and images from the Web server at each site are sent to the electronic patient record system (ePR) in the data center (step 2). The ePR

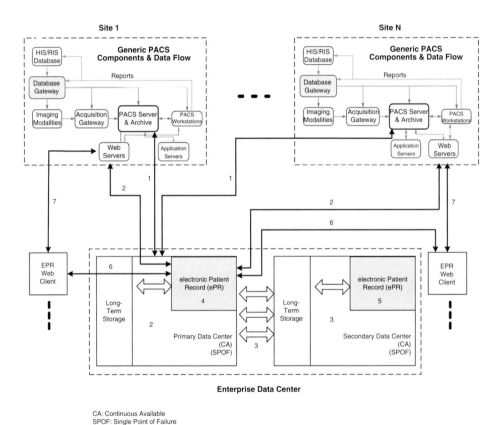

Figure 7.8 Enterprise PACS and ePR with images. The enterprise data center supports all sites in the enterprise. The primary data center has a secondary data center for backup to avoid a single point of failure. The enterprise ePR system is accessible from any ePR Web clients, and allows image distribution of the patient's electronic record within the enterprise.

system is the master Web-based client-server ePR system with filtered data and images.

- The data center has a primary data center, backed by the secondary data center (step 3) avoiding a single point of failure (SPOF) in the enterprise PACS.
- In the data center, the ePR (step 4) is responsible for combining patient electronic records with images from all sites of the enterprise. The ePR has a backup at the secondary data center (step 5). Details of the ePR will be presented in Chapter 16.
- ePR Web clients throughout the enterprise can access patient electronic records with images from any sites in the enterprise through the data center ePR system (step 6) or its own site patient through its own Web server (step 7).

Details and examples of enterprise PACS and ePR with images will be presented in Chapter 16.

7.7 SUMMARY OF PACS COMPONENTS AND WORKFLOW

In this chapter we gave an overall view of PCAS components and workflow. In particular, we discussed PACS major components: acquisition gateways, PACS server and archive, workstation, application servers; and PACS integration with HIS, RIS, and ePR. The PACS infrastructure design concept is given emphasizing the use of industrial standards, system connectivity and open architecture, and system reliability security. The concepts of stand-alone model and client-server model are briefly mentioned as these are the current prevailing models in PACS implementation. The extension of PACS in clinical arena are its connection with teleradiology, and its role in large-scale enterprise PACS.

References

Huang HK. Enterprise PACS and image distribution. *Comp Med Imag Graph* 27(2–3): 241–53; 2003.

Huang HK. *PACS and Imaging Informatics: Principles and Applications*. Hoboken, NJ: Wiley; 2004.

CHAPTER 8

Communications and Networking

This chapter presents three communication and network topics related to PACS. First is provided basic background knowledge on communication architecture and network systems (Sections 8.1, 8.2, and 8.3). The discussion next turns to PACS network design and considers some examples (Sections 8.4 and 8.5). Last covered are the emerging network technologies, Internet 2, wireless, and scalable network, all of which may benefit and change future PACS operations (Sections 8.6, 8.7, and 8.8). Figure 8.1 repeats Figure 1.3 to show the position of this chapter with relation to other chapters of Part II. Figure 8.2 repeats Figure 1.2 to emphasize the importance of communications and networks in PACS components and other healthcare information systems interconnection.

8.1 BACKGROUND

8.1.1 Terminology

Communication by way of media involves the transmission of data and information from one place to another. The media may be bound (cables) or unbound (broadcast, wireless). *Analog* communication systems encode data into some continuum (video) of signal (voltage) levels. *Digital* systems encode the information into two discrete states ("0" and "1") and rely on the collection of these binary states to form meaningful data and information. Wireless communication is the transfer of information over a distance without the use of wires. Advancements in wireless communication (wireless) technology over the past several years have altered the classic conception of PACS as distributing images only through bound media. Wireless applications of PACS will be emphasized whenever appropriate throughout this book.

A communication standard or protocol encompasses detailed specifications of the media, the explicit physical connections, the signal levels and timings, the packaging of the signals, and the high-level software necessary for the transport. A video communication standard describes the characteristics of composite video signals, including interlace or progressive scan, frame rate, line and frame retrace times, number of lines per frame, and number of frames per second. In PACS, soft copy display on the monitor consists of video or digital signals, and depending on the monitor types used, these video/digital signals also follow certain standards.

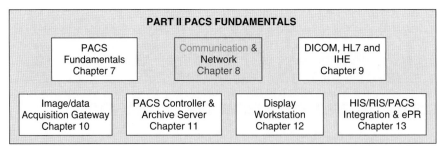

Figure 8.1 Position of Chapter 8 in the organization of this book. Color codes are used to highlight components and workflow in chapters of Part II.

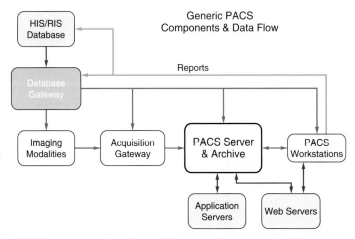

Figure 8.2 PACS components and workflow require communication networks for connectivity. PACS basic components (yellow); data flow (blue: Internal; green and orange: external between PACS and other information systems); and other information systems (light blue) use various networks and protocols for connection. HIS: hospital information system; RIS: radiology information system.

In digital communications, the packaging of the signals to form bytes, words, packets, blocks, and files is usually referred to as a communication protocol. *Serial* data transmission moves digital data, one bit at a time. The transmission of data can be over a single wire or a pair of wires or be wireless. The single bit stream is reassembled into meaningful byte/word/packet/block/file data at the receiving end of a transmission.

Parallel data transmission, on the other hand uses many wires or multiple wireless receivers to transmit bits in parallel. Thus at any moment in time a serial wire, or receiver has only one bit present but a set of parallel wires or receivers may have an entire byte or word present. Consequently parallel transmission provides an n-fold increase in transmission speed, where is the number of wires/receiver used.

In applications that call for maximum speed, *synchronous* communication is used. That is, the two communication nodes share a common clock, and data are transmitted in a strict way according to this clock. *Asynchronous* communication, used when simplicity is desired, relies on start and stop signals to identify the beginning and end of data packets. Accurate timing is still required, but the signal encoding allows wide variance in the timing at the different ends of the communication line. We discuss the asynchronous transfer mode (ATM) technology in Section 8.1.3.2.

In digital communication, the most primitive protocol is the RS-232 asynchronous standard for point-to-point communication, promulgated by the Electrical Industry Association (EIA).This standard specifies the signal and interface mechanical characteristics, gives a functional description of the interchange circuits, and lists application-specific circuits. This protocol is mostly used for peripheral devices (e.g., the trackball and mouse in a display workstation). The RS-232 protocol is still being used in many non-imaging devices, notably in surgical live supported systems in the operation room (see Chapter 24 for an example). Current digital communication methods are mostly communication networks. Table 8.1 lists five popular network topologies, and Figure 8.3 shows their architecture. The bus, ring, and star architectures are most commonly used in PACS applications. A network that is used in a local area (e.g., within a building or a hospital) is called a local area network, or LAN. If it is used outside of a local area, it is called a metropolitan area network (MAN) or wide area network (WAN), depending on the area covered.

8.1.2 Network Standards

Two most commonly used network standards in PACS applications are the DOD standard developed by the U.S. Department of Defense, and the OSI (Open Systems Interconnect) developed by the International Standards Organization (ISO). As shown in Figure 8.4, the former has four-layer protocol stacks and the latter has

TABLE 8.1 Five commonly used cabled network topologies

Topology	PACS Applications	Advantages	Disadvantages
Bus	Ethernet	Simplicity	Difficult to trace problems when a node fails
Tree	Video broadband headend	Simplicity	Bottleneck at the upper level
Ring	Fiber-distributed data interface (FDDI), High speed ATM SONET ring	Simplicity, no bottle neck	In a single ring, the network fails if the channel between two nodes fails
Star (hub)	High-speed Ethernet switch, ATM switch	Simplicity, easy to isolate the fault	Bottleneck at the hub or switch, a single point of failure at switch
Mesh	Used in wide area network applications	Immunity to bottleneck failure	Complicated

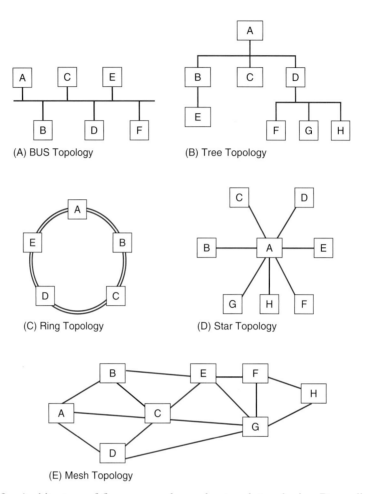

Figure 8.3   Architecture of five commonly used network topologies. Depending on the clinical environment, these topologies can be linked together to provide efficient PACS operation.

seven-layer stacks. In the DOD protocol stacks, the FTP (file transfer protocol) and the TCP/IP (Transport Control Protocol/Internet Protocol) are two popular communication protocols used widely in the medical imaging industry. The seven layers in the OSI protocols are defined in Table 8.2.

We use an example to explain how data are sent between two nodes in a network using the DOD TCP/IP transmission. Figure 8.5 shows the procedure (the steps by which a block of data is transmitted with protocol information listed on the left). First, the block of data is separated into segments (or packets) of data, whereupon each segment is given a TCP header, an IP header, and then a packet header; followed by the application header and packet trailer. The packet of encapsulated data is then sent, and the process is repeated until the entire block of data has been transmitted. The encapsulated procedure of a data packet (single rectangle at the top, Fig. 8.5) is represented by the boxes shown at the bottom of Figure 8.5 with six rectangles, of

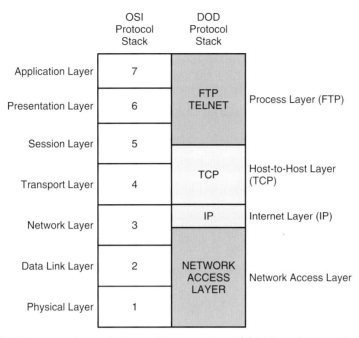

Figure 8.4   Correspondences between the seven-layer OSI (Open Systems Interconnect, yellow) and the four-layer DOD (Department of Defense, blue) communication protocols. TCP/IP (purple) in the DOD is most popular in medical imaging and PACS applications.

TABLE 8.2   Seven-layer open systems interconnect (OSI) protocols

Layer	Protocol	Definition
7	Application Layer	Provide services to users
6	Presentation Layer	Transformation of data (encryption, compression, reformatting)
5	Session Layer	Control applications running on different workstations
4	Transport Layer	Transfer of data between endpoints with error recovery
3	Network Layer	Establish, maintain, and terminate network connections
2	Data link Layer	Medium access control—network access (collision detection, token passing) and network control logical links control—send and receive data messages or packets
1	Physical Layer	Hardware layer

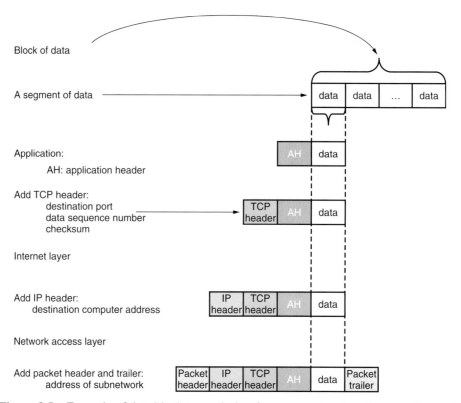

Figure 8.5 Example of data block transmission from one network node to another node with the TCP/IP. The data block is divided into segments. The figure illustrates how a segment of data (yellow) is encapsulated with the application header (blue), the TCP header (purple), IP header (pink), and the packet header and packet trailer (green). All these headers and the trailer (color blocks) are data overhead.

which only one is the data. In TCP/IP there are two types of transmission overhead: the storage and the time. Storage overheads are the application header, TCP header, the IP header, packet header, and the packet trailer; the time overheads are the encoding and decoding processes. While TCP/IP is very reliable, it does add to overhead, which can delay image transmission.

8.1.3 Network Technology

Two commonly used network technologies in PACS applications are the Ethernet and asynchronous transfer mode (ATM) running on TCP/IP communication modes.

8.1.3.1 Ethernet and Gigabit Ethernet

Standard Ethernet The standard Ethernet (luminiferous ether), which is based on IEEE Standard 802.3, Carrier Sense Multiple Access with Collision Detection (CSMA/CD), uses the bus topology or start topology (see Fig. 8.3). It operates from 10 Mbits/s to 1 Gbit/s over half-inch coaxial cables, twisted pair wires, fiberoptic cables, or wireless systems. Data are sent out in packets to facilitate the sharing of the cable. All nodes on the network connect to the backbone cable via Ethernet taps or Ethernet switches or hubs (taps are seldom used now except in older establishments). New taps/switches can be added anywhere along the backbone, and each node possesses a unique node address that allows routing of data packets by hardware. Each packet contains a source address, a destination address, data, and error detection codes. In addition each packet is prefaced with signal detection and transmission codes that ascertain status and establish the use of the cable. For twisted pair cables the Ethernet concentrator acts as the backbone cable.

As with any communication system, the quoted operating speed or signaling rate represents the raw throughput speed of the communication channel—for example, a coaxial cable with a base signal of 10 Mbits/s. The Ethernet protocol calls for extensive packaging of the data (see Fig. 8.5). Because a package may contain as many as 1500 bytes or much more for image transmission, a single file is usually broken up into many packets. This packaging is necessary to allow proper sharing of the communication channel. It is the job of the Ethernet interface hardware to route and present the raw data in each packet to the necessary destination computer. Dependent on the type of computer and communication software used, the performance of a node at a multiple-connection Ethernet can deteriorate from 10 Mbits/s to as slow as 500 Kbits/s.

Fast Ethernet and Gigabit Ethernet   Advances in fast Ethernet (100 Mbit/s) and gigabit Ethernet (1.0 Gbit/s or higher) switches allows nodes to be connected to them with very high speed performance. Fast Ethernet is in the same performance ranges as the ATM OC-3 (155 Mbits/s), and the gigabit Ethernet has better performance than the ATM OC-12 (622 Mbits/s; see Section 8.1.3.2).

High-speed Ethernet technology is a star topology very much like the ATM. Each switch allows for a certain number of connections to the workstations (WSs) through a standard 100 Mbits/s board or an adapter board in the WS for higher speed connection. A gigabit Ethernet switch can be branched out to many 100 Mbit/s WSs; and 100 Mbits/s Ethernet switches can be stepped down to several 10 Mbit/s switches and many 10 Mbit/s WSs connections as shown in Figure 8.6. Because backbone Ethernet is mostly used for LANs, and ATM can be used for both LANs and WANs, it is important to know that the gigabit Ethernet switch can also be used to connect to ATM OC-3 switches, providing an inter-connection for these two network technologies (Fig. 8.6). Currently a two-node connection in a Gbit/s Ethernet switch can achieve 500 Mbit/s, which is sufficient for most medical imaging applications.

8.1.3.2 ATM (Asynchronous Transfer Mode) Technology

Ethernet was originally designed for LAN applications, but radiological image communication should have no physical or logical boundaries between LANs and WANs. ATM can step in as a good technology for both LANs and WANs. ATM is a method for transporting information that splits data into fixed-length cells, each consisting of 5 bytes of ATM transmission protocol header information and 48 bytes of data information. Based on the virtual circuit-oriented packet-switching theory developed for telephone circuit switching applications, ATM systems were designed on the star topology, in which an ATM switch serves as a hub. The basic signaling rate of ATM is 51.84 Mbit/s, called Optical Carrier Level 1 (OC-1). Other rates are multiples of OC-1, for example, OC-3 (155 Mbit/s), OC-12 (622 Mbit/s), OC-48 (2.5 Gbit/s), OC-192

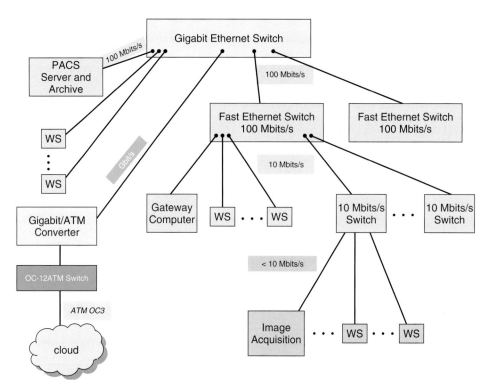

Figure 8.6 Schematic of Gbit Ethernet switch applications in PACS. Blue: Gbit/s; Light green: 100 Mbits/s; Red: 10 Mbits/s; Purple: <10 Mbits/s; Green: OC-12, 622 Mbits/s; Light green: OC-3 155 Mbits/s.

(10 Gbip/s) and up. In imaging applications, TCP/IP and DICOM transmission can be used for both LAN and WAN, and the combination of ATM and Gbit/s Ethernet technologies forms the backbones of the Internet 2 to be discussed in Section 8.6.

8.1.3.3 Ethernet and Internet

Readers who are not in the field of communications and networks may have some confusion about Ethernet and Internet. Ethernet is actually a physical specification for LANs (local area networks) also known as IEEE 802.3. It is the cable (or media) hardware that connects computers to other equipment or to the routers. In olden days, there were many different ways to do this, like the RG-59 cable in a "token ring" configuration. Nowadays, most Ethernets take the form of CAT-5 cables and fiber optics, and lately some are Wi-Fis (or IEEE 802.11, see Section 8.7).

In Ethernet, MAC (media access control) addresses uniquely identify Ethernet network cards (or PCs with built in Ethernet). Although it is true that every computer that uses Ethernet has a unique MAC address, not all Internet connections are made over Ethernet.

The Internet is sometime called a global superhighway. This is a collection of physical machines (servers, hosts, etc.) and software (e.g., World Wide Web) setup in an interconnected global "web" in multitude ways. In later sections of this chapter, the term Internet will be used more often than the term Ethernet as it is identified by physical media including cables and air waves. Put simply, Ethernet is a physical media for connection between computers; Internet is the network of computers.

8.1.4 Network Components for Connection

Communication protocols are used to pass data from one node to another node in a network. To connect different networks, additional hardware and software devices are needed; these are the repeater, bridge, router, and gateway.

A repeater passes data bit by bit in the OSI physical layer. It is used to connect two networks that are similar but use different media; for example, a thinnet and a twisted pair Ethernet (see Section 8.2.1) may be connected by means of hardware in layer 1 of the OSI standard. A bridge connects two similar networks (e.g., Ethernet to Ethernet) by both hardware and software in layer 2. A router directs packets by using a network layer protocol (layer 3); it is used to connect two or more networks, similar or not (e.g., to transmit data between WAN, MAN, and LAN). A gateway, which connects different network architectures (e.g., RIS and PACS), uses an application-level (level 7) protocol. A gateway is usually a computer with dedicated communication software. Table 8.3 compares these four communication devices.

8.2 CABLE PLAN

Even as wireless communications technology is maturing in medical image applications, in the intranet within department, campus, and hospital complexes, cables are still essential for PACS applications. This section describes several types of cables used for networking.

8.2.1 Types of Networking Cables

Although fiber-optic cables have become more popular for PACS applications especially in connection with routers, hubs, switches, and gateways, copper cables have remained basic for medical imaging and PASC use because of copper's lower cost and improved quality for data communication in recent years. The generic cable names have the form "10 BaseX," where 10 means 10 Mbit/s and X represents a medium type specified by IEEE Standard 802.3, because some of these cables were developed for Ethernet use.

10 Base5, also called thicknet or thick Ethernet, is a coaxial cable terminated with *N* series connectors. 10 Base5 is a 10-Mhz, 10 Mbit/s network medium with

TABLE 8.3 Communication devices for inter and intra network connection

Device	Protocol Layer[a]	Network Connections
Repeater	Physical (1)	Similar network but different media
Bridge	Data link (2)	Similar network
Router	Network (3)	Similar or not similar network
Gateway	Application (7)	Different network architecture

[a]The number inside parentheses is the OSI layer defined in Table 8.2.

a distance limitation of 500 m. This cable is typically used as an Ethernet trunk or backbone path of the network. Cable impedance is 50 ohms (W).

10 Base2, also called thinnet or cheaper net, is terminated with BNC connectors. Also used as an Ethernet trunk or backbone path for smaller networks, 10Base2 is a 10-MHz, 10-Mbit/s medium with a distance limitation of 185 m. Cable impedance is 50 W.

10 BaseT, also called UTP (unshielded twisted pair), is terminated with AMP (amplifer) 110, or RJ-45 connectors following the EIA 568 standard. With a distance limitation of 100 m, this low-cost cable is used for point-to-point applications such as Ethernet and the copper-distributed data interface (CDDI), not as a backbone. Categories 3, 4, and 5 UTP can all be used for Ethernet, but Category 5, capable of 100 Mhz and 100 Mbit/s, is recommended for medical imaging applications. *100 BaseT* is used for the fast Ethernet connection to support 100 Mbit/s.

Fiber-optic cables normally come in bundles from 1 to 216, or more fibers. Each fiber can be either multimode (62.5 mm in diameter) or single mode (9 mm). Multimode, normally referred to as 10 BaseF, is used for Ethernet and ATM (see Section 8.1.3.2). The single-mode fiber is used for longer distance communication. 10 BaseF cables are terminated with SC, ST, SMA, or FC connectors, but usually ST. For Ethernet applications, single mode has a distance limitation of 2000 m and can be used as a backbone segment or point to point. 10 BaseF cables are used for networking. Patch cords are used to connect a network with another network or a network with an individual component (e.g., imaging device, image workstation). Patch cords usually are AUI (attachment unit interface—DB 25), UTP, or short fiber-optic cables with the proper connectors.

Air-blown fiber (ABF) is a technology that makes it possible to use compressed nitrogen to "blow" fibers as needed through a tube distribution system (TDS). Tubes come in quantities from 1 to 16. Each tube can accommodate bundles from 1 to 16 fibers, either single mode or multimode. The advantage of this type of system is that fibers can be blown in as needed once the TDS has been installed.

Video cables are used to transmit images to high-resolution monitors. For 2 K monitors, 50-W cables are used: RG 58 for short lengths or RG 214U for distances up to 150 ft. RG 59, a 75-Ω cable used for 1 K monitors, can run distances of 100 ft.

8.2.2 The Hub Room

A hub room contains repeaters, fanouts (one-to-many repeaters), bridges, routers, switches, gateway computers, and other networking equipment for connecting and routing/switching information to and from networks. This room also contains the center for networking infrastructure media such as thicknet, thinnet, UTP, and fiber-optic patch panels. Patch panels, which allow the termination of fiber optics and UTP cables from various rooms in one central location, usually are mounted in a rack. At the patch panel, networks can be patched or connected from one location to another or by installing a jumper from the patch panel to a piece of networking equipment. One of the main features of the hub room is its connectivity to various other networks, rooms, and buildings. Air conditioning and backup power are vital to a hub room to provide a fail-safe environment. If possible, semi–dust-free conditions should be maintained.

Any large network installation needs segmented hub rooms, which may span different rooms and or buildings. Each room should have multiple network connections and patch panels that permit interconnectivity throughout the campus. The center or main hub room is usually called the network distribution center (NDC). The NDC houses concentrators, bridges, main routers, and switches. It should be possible to connect via a computer to every network within the communication infrastructure from this room. From the NDC the networks span to a different building to a room called the building distribution frame (BDF). The BDF routes information from the main subnet to departmental subnets, which may be located on various floors within a building. From the BDF, information can be routed to an intermediate distribution frame (IDF), which will route or switch the network information to the end users.

Each hub room should have a predetermined path for cable entrances and exits. For example, four 3-in. sleeves (two for incoming and two for outgoing cables) should be installed between the room and the area the cables are coming from, to allow for a direct path. Cable laddering is a very convenient way of managing cables throughout the room. The cable ladder is suspended from the ceiling, which allows the cables to be run from the 3-in. sleeves across the ladder and suspends the cables down to their end locations. Cable trays can also be mounted on the ladder for separation of coaxial, UTP, and fiber optics. In addition to backup power, access to emergency power (provided by external generators typically in a hospital environment) is necessary. The room should also have a minimum of two dedicated 20-A, 120-V and 220-V quad power outlets—more may be required, depending on the room size. Figure 8.7 shows the generic configuration of hub room connections.

8.2.3 Cables for Input Devices

Usually an imaging device is already connected to an existing network with one of the four media types: thicknet, thinnet, fiber optics, or twisted pair. A tap or switch of the same media type can be used to connect a gateway computer to this network, or the aid of a repeater may be required, as in the following example. Suppose that a CT scanner is already on a thinnet network, and the acquisition gateway computer has access only to twisted pair cables in its neighborhood. The system designer might select a repeater residing in a hub room that has an input of the thinnet and an output of UTP to connect the network and the computer. When cables must run from a hub room to an image acquisition device area, it is always advisable to lay extra cables with sufficient length to cover the diagonal of the room and from the ceiling to the floor at the time of installation, because it is easier and less expensive than pulling the cables later to clear the way for relocation or upgrade.

When installing cables from the IDF or BDF to areas housing acquisition devices planned for Ethernet use at a distance less than 100 m, a minimum of one category 5 UTP per node, and four strands of multimode fiber per imaging room (CT, MR, US, CR, DR) is recommended. If the fiber-optic broadband video system is also planned for multiple video distribution, additional multimode fiber-optic cables should be allocated for each input device. With this configuration, the current Ethernet technology is fully utilized and the infrastructure still has the capacity to be upgraded to accept any protocols that may be encountered in the future.

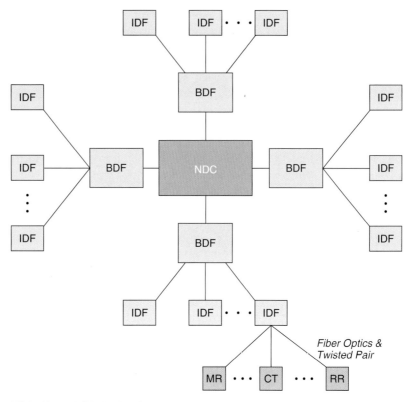

NDC: Network Distribution Center
BDF: Building Distribution Frame
IDF: Intermediate Distribution Frame
MR: Magnetic Resonance Imaging
CT: Computerized Tomography Imaging
RR: Reading Room

— Fiber Optics

Figure 8.7 Generic configuration of hub room connections. IDF is the intermediate distribution frame to which the image acquisition devices and image workstations are connected.

8.2.4 Cables for Image Distribution

Cable planning for input devices and image distribution differs in the sense that the former is ad hoc—that is, most of the time the input device already exists and there is not much flexibility in the cable plan. On the other hand, image distribution requires planning because the destinations usually do not have existing cables. In planning the cables for image distribution, the horizontal runs and the vertical runs should be considered separately. The vertical runs, which determine several strategic risers by taking advantage of existing telecommunication closets in the building, usually are planned first. From these closets vertical cables are run for the connections to various floors. Horizontal cables are then installed from the closets to different hub rooms, to NDC, to BDF, to IDF, and finally to the image workstation areas. All cables at the workstation areas should be terminated with proper connectors and should have enough cable slack for termination and troubleshooting.

Horizontal run cables should be housed in conduits. Because installing conduits is expensive, it is advisable whenever possible to put in a larger conduit than is needed initially, to accommodate future expansion. Very often the installation of conduits calls for drilling holes through floors and building fire walls (core drilling). Drilling holes in a confined environment like a small telephone cable closet in a hospital is a tedious and tricky task. Extreme care must be exercised to check for the presence of any pipes or cables that may be embedded in the concrete. In addition each hole should be at least three times the size of the diameter of the cables being installed, to allow for future expansion and to meet fire code regulations. The following tips will also be useful when planning the installation of cables.

1. Always look for existing conduits and cables, to avoid duplication.
2. If possible, use Plenum cables (fire retardant) for horizontal runs.
3. When installing cables from a BDF to multiple IDFs or from an IDF to various rooms, use optical fiber whenever possible. If the distance is long and if future distribution to other remote sites through this route is anticipated, install at least twice as many fibers as planned for the short term.
4. Label all cables and fibers at both ends with meaningful names that will not change in the near future (e.g., room numbers, building/floor number).

8.3 DIGITAL COMMUNICATION NETWORKS

8.3.1 Background

Within the PACS infrastructure, the digital communication network is responsible for transmission of images from acquisition devices to gateways, the PACS server, and display workstations. Many computers and processors are involved in this image communication chain; some have high-speed processors and communication protocols and some do not. Therefore, in the design of this network, a mixture of communication technologies must be used to accommodate various computers and processors. The ultimate goal is to have an optimal image throughput within a given clinical environment. Remember, in PACS, image communication involves 10 to 100 Mbytes of data per transaction; this is quite different from the conventional healthcare data transmission. Network bottleneck will occur if the network is not designed properly for large files transmission during peak hours.

Table 8.4 describes the image transmission rate requirements of PACS. Transmission from the imaging modality device to the acquisition gateway computer is slower because the imaging modality device is generally slow in generating images. The medium speed requirement from the acquisition computer to the PACS controller depends on the types of acquisition gateway computer used. High-speed communication between the PACS controller and image display workstations is necessary because radiologists and clinicians must access images quickly. In general, 4 Mbytes/s or higher, equivalent to transfer the first $2048 \times 2048 \times 12$-bit conventional digitized X-ray image in an image sequence in 2 seconds, is the average tolerable waiting time for the physician.

TABLE 8.4   Image transmission characteristics among PACS components

	Image Modality Device to Acquisition Gateway Computer	Acquisition Gateway Computer to PACS Controller	PACS Controller to Display Workstations
Speed requirement	Slow 100 kbytes/s	Medium 200–500 Kbytes/s	Fast 4 Mbytes/s
Technology	Ethernet	Ethernet/ATM/Fast or Gigabit Ethernet	ATM/Fast or Gigabit Ethernet
Signaling rate	10 Mbits/s	100 Mbits/s	155, 100,1000 Mbits/s
Cost per connection	1 unit	1–5 units	1–10 units

8.3.2 Design Criteria

The five design criteria for the implementation of digital communication networks for PACS are speed, standardization, fault tolerance, security, and component cost.

8.3.2.1 Speed of Transmission

Table 8.4 shows that the standard Ethernet is adequate between imaging devices and acquisition gateway computers. For image transfer from the acquisition gateway computers to the image archive servers, fast Ethernet or ATM should be used if the acquisition computer supports the technology. For image transfer between the PACS Server to WSs, ATM, fast, or gigabit Ethernet should be used.

8.3.2.2 Standardization

The throughput performance for each of the two networks described above (Ethernet and ATM) can be tuned through the judicious choice of software and operating system parameters. For example, enlarging the TCP send and receive buffer within the UNIX kernel for Ethernet and ATM network circuits can increase the throughput of networks using TCP/IPs. Alternatively, increasing the memory data buffer size in the application program may enhance transmission speed. The altering of standard network protocols to increase network throughput between a client-server pair can be very effective. The same strategy may prove disastrous in a large communication network, however, because it interferes with network standardization, making it difficult to maintain and service the network. All network circuits should use standard TCP/IP network protocols with a standard buffer size (e.g., 8192 bytes).

Still some manufacturers use dedicated or proprietary transmission protocols within their own PACS components to achieve higher speed. Once they are connected, any components not from the same vendor even with standard transmission protocols would render these components inoperable within this vendor's network environment.

8.3.2.3 Fault Tolerance

Communication networks in the PACS infrastructure should have backup. All active fiber-optic cables, twist pairs, Ethernet backbone (thicknet and twisted pair), and switches should have spares. Because standard

TCP/IP transmission are used for all networks, if any higher speed network fails, the socket-based communications software immediately switches over to the next fastest network, and so forth, until all network circuits have been exhausted. The global Ethernet backbone, through which every computer on the PACS network is connected, is the ultimate backup for the entire PACS network.

8.3.2.4 Security There are normally two network systems in a PACS network. The first comprises networks leased from or shared with the campus or hospital, managed by the central network authority (CNA). In this case users should abide by the rules established by the CNA. Once these cables are connected, the CAN enforces its own security measures and provides service and maintenance.

The second network system consists of the PACS network; its cables are confined inside conduits with terminations at the hub rooms. The hub rooms should be locked, and no one should be allowed to enter without authorization from PACS officials.

The global Ethernet should be monitored around the clock with a LAN analyzer. The ATM is a closed system and cannot be tapped in except at ATM switches. Security should be set up such that authorized hospital personnel can access the network to view patients' images at workstations, similar to the setup at a film library or film light boxes. Only authorized users are allowed to copy images and deposit information into the PACS database through the network.

8.3.2.5 Costs PACS communication networks are designed for clinical use and should be built as a robust system with redundancy. Cost, although of utmost importance, should not be compromised in the selection of network components and the fault tolerance backup plan.

8.4 PACS NETWORK DESIGN

PACS networks should be designed as an internal network (within the PACS) with connections to external networks such as the manufacturer's imaging network, radiology information network, hospital information networks, or the enterprise networks. All network connections in blue shown in Figure 8.2 are PACS network except those going outside of the PACS domain like the HIS/RIS application servers and Web servers, which are in orange. The security of external networks is the responsibility of the hospital and the enterprise network authority, the security of the imaging modalities network is the responsibility of the manufacturer's imaging network manager, and PACS internal network security is the responsibility of the PACS administration. The PACS internal network should only be accessible through layers of security measures assigned by the PACS manager.

8.4.1 External Networks

This section describes types of external networks that can be connected to the PACS network.

8.4.1.1 Manufacturer's Image Acquisition Device Network Major imaging manufacturers have their own networks for connecting several imaging devices like CT and MR scanners in the radiology department for better image management. These networks are treated as external networks in the PACS design. Most of these networks are Ethernet based; some use TCP/IP transmission, and others use proprietary protocols for better network throughput. If such a network is already in existence in the radiology department, acquisition gateway computers must be used to connect to this external network first before CT and MR images can be transmitted to the PACS server. This external network has no security with respect to the PACS infrastructure because any user with a password can have access to the external network and retrieve all information passing through it.

8.4.1.2 Hospital and Radiology Information Networks

A hospital or university campus usually has a campus CNA that administers institutional networks. Among the information systems that go through these networks are the HIS and RIS. PACS requires data from both HIS and RIS, but these networks with connection to the PACS network are maintained by the campus CNA, over which the PACS network has no control. For this reason, the PACS infrastructure design considers the hospital or institutional network to be an external network with respect to the PACS domain.

8.4.1.3 Research and Other Networks

One major function of PACS is to allow users to access the wealth of the PACS database. A research network can be set up for connecting research equipment to the PACS. Research equipment should be allowed access to the PACS database for information query and retrieval but not to deposit information. In the PACS infrastructure design, a research network is considered an external network.

8.4.1.4 The Internet

Any network carrying information from outside the hospital or the campus through the Internet is considered an external network in the PACS infrastructure design. Such a network carries supplementary information for the PACS, ranging from electronic mail and library information systems to data files available through FTP. But data received from this network should not be allowed to deposit in the PACS server.

8.4.1.5 Imaging Workstation (WS) Networks

Sometimes it is advantageous to have PACS WSs of similar nature to form a subnetwork for sharing of information. For example, WSs in the intensive care units of a hospital can form an ICU network and neuro WSs can form a neuro network. Networks connecting these display workstations are open to all healthcare personnel needing to view images, and therefore only a minimum security should be imposed. Too many restrictions would deter the users from logging on. However, certain layers of priority can be imposed; for example, some users may be permitted access to a certain level. But at no time are users of these networks allowed to deposit information to the PACS archive. These types of networks are sometimes maintained by the special users' respective departments.

8.4.2 Internal Networks

A PACS internal network (see blue lines, Fig. 8.2), on the other hand, has the maximum security. Data inside the internal network constitute the uncompromised clinical archive. Both image and textual data from acquisition devices and other information systems coming from different external networks just described, except those of display WSs, have gone through gateway computers, where data were checked and scrutinized for authenticity before being deposited in the internal network. Fire wall machines are sometimes incorporated into the gateway computer for this purpose. Only the PACS manager is authorized to allow data to be deposited to the archive through the internal network.

8.5 EXAMPLES OF PACS NETWORKS

8.5.1 An Earlier PACS Network at UCSF

The concept of external and internal PACS networks was conceived in the mid-1990s. For historical purposes, the PACS network developed by the author and colleagues at the University of California at San Francisco (UCSF) as is shown in Figure 8.8 (1995–1999). In this architecture there are several external networks: WAN, campus network, departmental network, the Laboratory for Radiological Informatics (LRI) research network, the Internet, the PACS external network, and workstation networks.

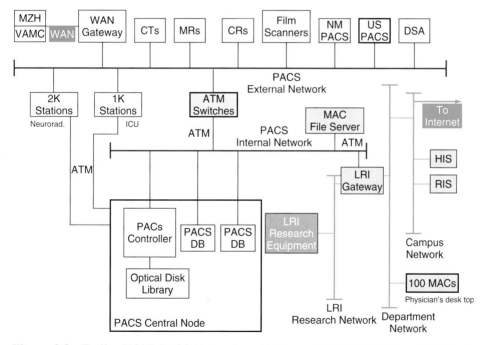

Figure 8.8 Earlier UCSF PACS Network architecture (1995–1999). Blue: PACS networks; Orange: connections to other information systems; Green: Internet and WAN. ATM is the backbone of the networks. Orange: The research network connected to LRI. LRI: Laboratory for Radiological Informatics; MZH: Mount Zion Hospital; VAMC: VA Medical Center.

8.5.2 Network Architecture at IPILab, USC

Since the authors relocated from UCSF, and relocated at USC in 2000, high-speed networks have become readily available including international Internet 2 connections, and the PACS internal and external networks have evolved considerably as well. Figures 8.9 and 8.10 depict the international and connectivity and the IPI-Lab internal network architecture. Some components in the IPILab are described as follows:

USC HCC2 (Healthcare Consultation Center) Building Data Center (Green)
The components in Figure 8.10 are (see numerals in the figure):

1. File Server: A Solaris server with 900 GB tapes, runs Solaris operating system for Data Grid applications.
2. IBM SAN. An IBM serve with 11 TB SAN running the IBM operating system for Data Grid applications.
3. EMC SAN: A SAN archive system, running the Linux RedHat OS with 4.5 TB storage housing the Data Grid GAP components.
4. Fiber Channel (1 Gb/s) with two switches, bridges the two Cisco switches at IPILab and HCC2 server room.

IPILab

5. Firewall at IPILab: Protects network inside IPILab
6. File server: RAID 5 with 1.5 TB capacity. Used for IPILab researchers to store images, code, downloaded software, papers, and the like.
7. SMT server: An aka PDA (personal digital assistant) project server is a SUN PC running Solaris OS.
8. RT ePR: A radiation therapy ePR running Linux OS on a VM (Virtual Machine) server.
9. Web + FTP server: A basic PC running Linux with a public static IP address to enable the IPILab Web site and allow external users to send data into IPILab via FTP (file transfer protocol).
10. OpenVPN server: Allows IPILab researchers to VPN (virtual private network) into the IPILab network from the outside to access resources such as the file server. It uses Windows XP operating system running on a VM server.
11. VM server: It enables a high-powered Server to run multiple operating systems at one time. Where each operating system can basically function as a separate computer.
12. Domain server: A Windows server operating system used to provide user/password authentication for many of our other Windows-based servers: file server, OpenVPN, PACS workstations, and so forth. All user profiles and privileges can be controlled from this one server.

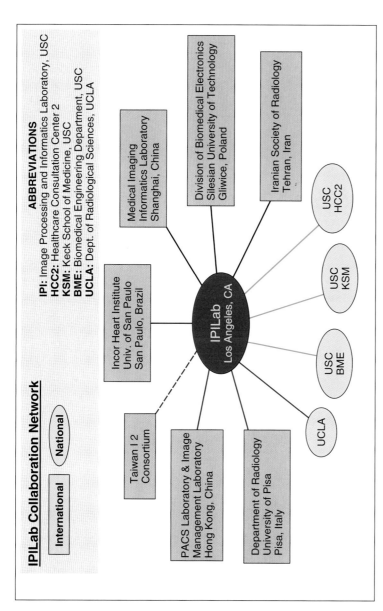

Figure 8.9 IPILab collaboration networks. The IPILab collaboration networks consists of International and national networks. The International networks (blue) are based on Internet 2 and slower speed Internet. The dotted line is in preparation of connection. The national networks (green) are based on high-speed Internet and Intranet. Other International connections (black) were standard available Internet speed.

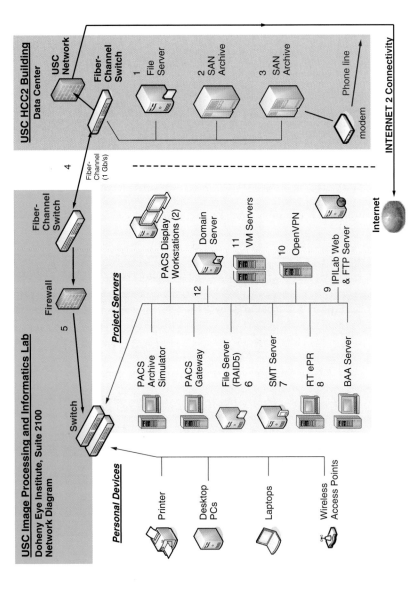

Figure 8.10 IPILab research networks consist of three major networks: (*A*, right; light purple) Connection between IPILab research facility with the USC PACS internal networks (to be described in Chapter 16: Enterprise PACS), data from outside the USC passes the USC network firewall through two fiber-channel switches (upper green and upper purple). The switch in the upper green connects to a second set of switches protected by the IPILab firewall; data transmits to a second set of switches, which distribute it to the light blue and light yellow columns. (*B*, middle column; light blue) projects servers, and (*C*, left; light yellow) personal devices in the laboratory.

8.6 INTERNET 2

In this section we discuss a federal government initiative's WAN communication technology, Internet 2, which is easy to use as the standard Internet and low in cost to operate once the institution is connected to the Internet 2 backbones. It was introduced in the early 2000s and has evolved since then. Most university campuses, academic research laboratories, and some private industrial research laboratory are now equipped with this network connection.

8.6.1 Image Data Communication

PACS requires high-speed networks to transmit large image files between components. In the case of intranet, that is, PACS within a medical center, Gbits/s switches and Mbits/s connections to WSs are almost standard in most network infrastructures. Their transmission rates, even for large image files, are acceptable for clinical operation. However, in the case of the Internet, this is not the case. Table 8.5 shows the transmission rate of current WAN technologies.

Among these technologies, DSL (digital subscriber lines) has emerged as a solid one used my many home office connections, including in small-scale lower speed teleradiology application. DSL is a broadband delivery method using standard copper telephone wires but many times faster than modem dial-up services. DSL is a system that provides subscribers with continuous, uninterrupted connections to the Internet over existing telephone lines, offering a choice of speeds ranging from 32 kbps (kilobits per second) to more than 50 Mbps (megabits per second).

Telemedical imaging applications require low-cost and high-speed backbone WANs to carry large amounts of imaging related data for rapid-turnaround interpretation. Current low-cost commercial WAN is too slow for medical imaging application, whereas the high-speed WAN (T1 and up) is too expensive for cost-effective use. Internet 2 technology is a potential candidate for low-cost and high-speed networks for large-scale image data transmission, especially for those medical centers already equipped with Internet 2 technology.

8.6.2 What Is Internet 2 (I2)?

Internet 2 is a federal government initiative for the integration of higher speed backbone communication networks (up to 10 Gbits/s) as a means to replace the current

TABLE 8.5 **Transmission rate of current wide area network technology**

Technology	Transmission Rate
DS-0	56 kbits/s
DS-1	56 to (24×56) kbits/s
DSL	32 kbits/s to 50 Mbits/s
DS-1 (T1)	1.5 Mbits/s
ISDN	56 kbits/s to 1.5 Mbits/s
DS-3	28 DS-1 = 45 Mbits/s
ATM (OC-3)	155 Mbits/s and up
Internet 2	100 Mbits/s and up

Internet for many applications including medical imaging related data. The nonprofit I2 organization known as the UCAID (University Corporation for Advanced Internet Development) consortium was founded in the summer of 1996 and is supported by the National Science Foundation. It is the network infrastructure backbone in the United States for high-speed data transmission. Members of the consortium, consisting of more than 1000 research universities and nonacademic institutes, are now connecting to the I2 backbones. I2 has evolved from several backbones: vBNS (very high-speed backbone network service, Abilene, and CalREN (California Research and Education Network; and is now consolidated to the current Abilene shown in Figure 8.11. Some segments can go up from 5.6 Gbps (Gegabits per second), to 6.25 Gbps, to 9 Gbps performance. We should distinguish I2 from NGI (next generation Internet); the former refers to the network infrastructure, whereas the latter refers to various I2 applications.

8.6.3 An Example of I2 Performance

8.6.3.1 Connections of Three International Sites
In the early 2000s, the IPI Lab, University of Southern California (United States); Polytechnic University (Hong Kong), and InCor (Brazil) were connected with I2 and ISP (Internet service provider) vendors (when the I2 link was missing). IPI and USC counted as two U.S. sites since performances data could be measured at both sites. Performance values were collected utilizing the FTP (file transfer prototcol), and DICOM transmission protocol to measure real-world clinical applications of medical images studies. In addition a repeatable Web 100 tuning protocol was applied to the three sites, effectively improving the performance by nearly three to eight times in comparison to the standard configuration. Figure 8.12 shows the network configurations. Tables 8.6, 8.7, and 8.8 show some of the results.

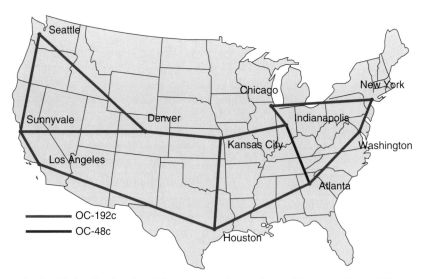

Figure 8.11 Major International interconnection points of Internet 2 at Abilene backbone. Most early International connections to I2 were from a hub near Chicago. OC-48 (2.5 gbps), OC-192 (10 Gbps). (Courtesy of Abilene Network, abiline.internet2.edu.)

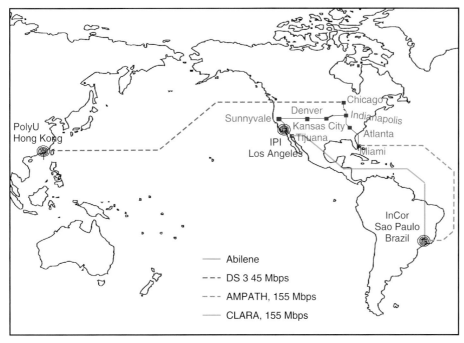

Figure 8.12 Topology of the International Internet 2 connectivity between three test sites on three continents linking IPI/USC, Los Angeles, North America; InCo, Sao Paulo, Brazil, South America; and Polytechnic University, Hong Kong, Asia. Flagtel (DS3) was the ISP vendor connecting IPI to Hong Kong with points of presence (PoPs) in Tokyo and Hong Kong. The routing path from InCor to PolyU utilized AMPATH, and the path between IPI and InCor used CLARA. Both AMPATH and CLARA are ISP providers.

TABLE 8.6. Performance data for different sites connected with International Internet 2

To	From	IPI	USC/HSC	PolyU	InCor
IPI	FTP (Mbps)		28.00*	1.60*	—
	RTT (ms)		—	292*	—
USC/HSC	FTP (Mbps)	10.00*		1.78	2.65
	RTT (ms)	—		253	171
PolyU	FTP (Mbps)	1.60*	2.80		1.12
	RTT (ms)	292*	254		425
InCor	FTP (Mbps)	—	1.50	0.63	
	RTT (ms)	—	172	424	

Note: Round trip times (RTT) in milliseconds and FTP performance times in megabits per second were collected. All sites were running standard Linux. The file size used was 7.8 MBytes. Asterisks show data collected from a different data collection period. A blank line means no data were collected.

TABLE 8.7   Comparison of performance data between sites that utilized the Web 100 tuning protocol (last column) and the same sites utilizing standard linux (STD Linux) without tuning

From	To	Protocol	STD Linux (Mbps)	Tuned (Mbps)
PolyU	InCor	FTP	0.63	4.40
		DICOM	0.62	9.44
InCor	PolyU	FTP	1.12	3.10
		DICOM	1.50	2.97
PolyU	IPI Lab	FTP	1.63*	9.79*
		DICOM	1.36*	3.06*
IPI Lab	PolyU	FTP	1.60*	9.79*
		DICOM	1.36*	3.06*

Note: Performance data were gathered for both FTP and DICOM file transmissions. Asterisks show data collected from a different data collection period. A blank line means no data were collected. With the tuning protocol, the performance was 3 to 4 times better.

TABLE 8.8   Performance data for IPI connectivity to both PolyU and InCor using a commercial high-speed ISP vendor

From	To	RTT (ms)	CT (29 imgs, 15.5MBytes) Untuned (Mbps)	CT Tuned (Mbps)	CR (2 imgs, 16 MBytes) Untuned (Mbps)	CR Tuned (Mbps)
IPI	PolyU	187	3.09	12.24	3.16	6.61
PolyU	IPI	187	2.3	17.9	2.23	17.67
IPI	InCor	805	0.957	10.78	0.928	13.84
InCor	IPI	831	1.36	2.6	1.7	3.04

Note: Round trip times (RTT) were gathered between sites. One CT study of 29 images with 15.5 Mbytes, and one CR study of 2 images with 16 Mbytes were used to evaluate the DICOM transmission protocol performance between the sites.

8.6.3.2 Some Observations   Results gathered from these measurements showed that even without the Web 100 tuning, performance numbers were comparable to that of a T1 connection (e.g., 1.5 Mbps) linking two such geographically distant sites as Brazil and Hong Kong. In addition, these performance numbers were comparable to commercially available high-speed ISPs that require a costly monthly service fee and are subject to fluctuations of performance due to e-commerce traffic—both of which are not characteristics of International Internet 2 connectivity. The performance evaluation showed how three international sites can utilize the International Internet 2 connectivity as well as other non—U.S. research networks as adequate and acceptable solution for almost real-time medical imaging transmission.

8.6.4 Enterprise Teleradiology

I2 is an ideal tool for two types of applications teleradiology and distance learning using PACS image data. Its operation cost is low once the institution is connected to the I2 backbones. Also I2 uses standard Internet technology that most healthcare personnel are familiar with. In enterprise-level teleradiology applications, if each site in the enterprise is already connected to the I2 through its own institution, images can be transmitted very rapidly among the sites in the enterprise, as shown in Tables 8.6, 8.7, and 8.8. Because no T1 or other expensive WAN technologies are needed, teleradiology operation is low cost and efficient.

8.6.5 Current Status

The current I2 technology is a very fast network compared with the commonly used T1 for teleradiology. I2 requires a high initial capital investment for connecting to the backbones, which is generally absorbed by the institution. Once the site is connected to the backbones, the network runs at minimal cost, and its operation is identical to that of using the standard Internet. These characteristics make I2 an ideal technology for developing enterprise-level PACS/teleradiology applications. Table 8.9 summarizes the current status of I2. We discuss I2 again in Chapter 15 with regard to telemedicine and teleradiology.

8.7 WIRELESS NETWORKS

Wireless networks are other emerging technologies for PACS applications. We discuss both the wireless LAN (WLAN) and wireless WAN (WWAN) in this section.

8.7.1 Wireless LAN (WLAN)

8.7.1.1 The Technology
A wireless LAN (WLAN) is a type of LAN that uses high-frequency radio waves rather than wires to communicate between nodes. WLANs are based on IEEE Standard 802.11 also known as wireless fidelity (Wi-Fi). IEEE Standard 802.11 was introduced as a standard for wireless LANs in 1997 and is updated now to IEEE 802.11-1999.The current standard is also accepted by ANSI/ISO. Table 8.10 shows the different standards available in this technology.

IEEE 802.11b is probably the most widely implemented and routinely used wireless LAN today. It operates in the 2.4-GHz band and uses direct sequence spread spectrum (DSSS) modulation. The 802.11b-compliant devices can operate at 1, 2, 5.5, and 11 Mbps. The next improvement of 802.11b is 802.11 g; it can increase the bandwidth to 54 Mbps within the 2.4-GHz band. Standard 802.11a is another high-speed wireless LAN operating in the 5-GHz band, which uses orthogonal frequency

TABLE 8.9   Current status of Internet 2

- Very fast, and will be faster
- Expensive during initial investment
- Relative low cost to use
- Not enough know how personnel for connectivity
- Not enough Internet 2 sites
- Lack communication between IT and Healthcare IT personnel
- Internet Security Issue

TABLE 8.10 Currently available wireless LAN technology

Name	Frequency	Maximum Bandwidth
802.11a	5 GHz	54 Mbps
802.11b	2.4 GHz	11 Mbps
802.11g	2.4 GHz	54 Mbps

division multiplexing (OFDM). The data rates it supports include 6, 9, 12, 18, 24, 36, 48, and 54 Mbps. Standard 802.11a has a range similar to 802.11b in a typical office environment of up to 225 ft. Twelve separate nonoverlapping channels are available for 802.11a; therefore data rates higher than 54 Mbps can be reached by combining channels. Most laptop computers used in clinical environments are equipped with 54-Mbps ports for wireless communication.

In wireless communication technology the term Wi-Fi is often seen. Wi-Fi is a trademark of the Wi-Fi Alliance, founded in 1999 as Wireless Ethernet Compatibility Alliance (WECA), comprising more than 300 companies, whose products are certified by the Wi-Fi Alliance, based on the IEEE 802.11 standards (also called Wireless LAN [WLAN] and Wi-Fi). This certification warrants interoperability between different wireless devices. The alliance was founded because many products did not correctly implement IEEE 802.11 and some included proprietary extensions. This led to incompatibilities between products from different manufacturers.

Another new wireless communication technology, Bluetooth™[1], is emerging in which the Bluetooth Special Interest Group (SIG) has produced a specification for Bluetooth wireless communication devices that is publicly available for the standardization of the technology. Bluetooth devices are characterized by wireless communication using radio waves to transmit and receive data. This technology is specifically designed for short-range (10 m) communication, thus consuming very low power, and is tailored for small, portable personal devices, like a PDA. This technology will be revisited in Chapter 14 when we present the PDA for image management.

8.7.1.2 WLAN Security, Mobility, Data Throughput, and Site Materials

Considerations of security, mobility, data throughput, and site materials are relevant to making adequate decisions when implementing a WLAN. It should be noted that applications using 802.11b and 802.11a wireless LANs require security measures. Current approaches to improve the security of WLANs include allowing connectivity to the access points from valid media access control (MAC) addresses on the wireless interfaces and activating the wired equivalent privacy (WEP) feature. Both approaches have been proved to be insufficient to provide security. In Chapter 17 we will discuss data security further in wireless network environment.

Mobility permits users to switch from one access point to another without modifying any configuration and in a transparent manner. This is critical to users who have to keep connections active for long periods of time. In a clinical environment there could be a need to transfer high volumes of data to a mobile device, for example, laptop, personal digital assistant (PDA), or tablet PC. Thus a permanent connection

TABLE 8.11   Current wireless LAN performance

Type of Space	Maximum Coverage Radius
Closed office	Up to 50–60 feet
Open office (cubicles)	Up to 90 feet
Hallways and other large rooms	Up to 150 feet
Outdoors	Up to 300 feet

Note: "Rule-of-thumb" coverage radius for different types of space.

must be assured regardless of the location of the user. Data throughput is closely related to the number of expected users attached to an access point: the greater the number of users, the slower is the throughput per user.

Building materials, other signals in the same frequency range, and the location and type of the antennas affect signal quality. Table 8.11 shows the maximum coverage radius depending on the type of space to cover.

8.7.1.3 Performance   Some preliminary performance results with the IEEE 802.11a-compliant consumer-quality product in assessment of potential medical imaging are available as shown in Figure 8.13. Two parameters of interest are signal strength and transfer rate. Figure 8.14 shows results obtained with 32-Kbyte data transfers. At 175 ft between two test nodes in an open environment (i.e., no obstruction between nodes), a transfer rate of 18 Mbits/s with 20% signal strength was achieved. This translates to approximately more than 10-MR images per second. In a closed environment, where lead walls and heavy doors are in the transmission path, the performance is far less reliable. Results are shown in Table 8.12 which demonstrates that for over 120 ft the performance became erratic and with a long response time. Data shown in Table 8.12 is difficult to plot because measured data are extremely variable. The signal strength, data rate, and response time flicker from one extreme to the other. Research on the use of WLAN in closed environments is in progress at various laboratories.

8.7.2 Wireless WAN (WWAN)

8.7.2.1 The Technology   For WWAN, the current available technologies are GSM (global system for mobile communication), GPRS (general packet radio

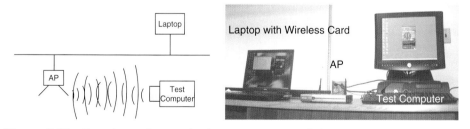

Figure 8.13   Experimental setup in the measurement of the IEEE 802.11a compliant WLAN performance. ☐: 802.11a compliant cardbus; (AP) access point (in this case it is a Dlink Access Point DWL-5000AP).

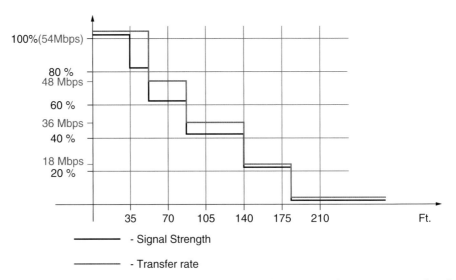

Figure 8.14 Performance of IEEE 802.11a compliant WLAN between two nodes (in feet) in an open environment.

TABLE 8.12 Measured performance of IEEE 802.11a-compliant WLAN between two nodes in a closed environment

Distance (ft)	Signal Strength (%)	Transfer rate (Mbps)	Response Time (ms)
0–35	60–80	36–48	81–101
35–120	60–80	36–48	90–120
120–140	20–40	18–36	Weak response
140–200	20	18–36	No response
200–225	20–0	0–18	No response

service), EDGE (enhanced data rates for GSM evolution), and UMTS (Universal Mobile Telecommunications Service). WWAN devices are much slower than the previously introduced WLAN but are available almost everywhere in the United States. GSM uses the circuit-switched mode can achieve 14.4 Kbits/s and GPRS with 4 slots can achieve 56 Kbits/s download, 28.8 Kbits/s upload. All these technologies are readily available in the market now.

8.7.2.2 Performance The WWAN communication class using GSM 9.6 Kbits/s and 14.4 Kbits/s circuit-switched data transfer rates by sending a 12 MB single file package of 50 functional MRI brain volumes (64 × 64 × 30 matrix, 2 bytes/voxel) between a workstation and an ftp server on the Internet were measured. The average transfer rates were 8.043 Kbits/s (9.6 Kbits/s connection) and 12.14 Kbits/s (14.4 Kbits/s connection), respectively. The current performance of WWAN is still under 1.0 Mbits/s, it may be several years before it becomes available for medical imaging applications.

8.8 SELF-SCALING WIDE AREA NETWORKS

8.8.1 Concept of Self-scaling Wide Area Networks

In this section we discuss the potential of using the three emerging network technologies—Internet 2, WLAN, and WWAN—as an integrated image self-scaling network (ISSN) for medical image management during a local disaster such as an earthquake or a data center failure, during which time many communication networks would be out of service. The selection of Internet 2 for broadband communication is based on flexibility, widespread availability in academic and research environments, as well as cost-benefit factors once the backbone has been installed in the local center. High speeds are achievable at a very low cost for operation once it is installed, representing a very likely and appropriate means of future broadband medical networking for many sites. A network self-scalar can be designed to automatically scale the three networks based on the local environment for a given clinical application. Network self-scaling is defined in this context as a mechanism for selecting the proper networking technology for an application. A disparate grouping of technologies, including image compression, image security, image content indexing, and display, will be variously applied to augment the ISSN with the goal to identify and deliver "just enough" information to the user during a disaster. The full self-scaling mechanism is therefore defined as the combination of network self-scaling and information self-scaling. Figure 8.15 shows the three network technologies and their respective performance, and Figure 8.16 depicts the design concept of the network self-scalar.

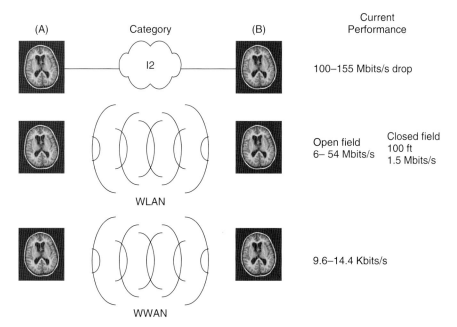

Figure 8.15   Three emerging network technologies used for the design of a self-scaling network: Internet2, WLAN, and WWAN.

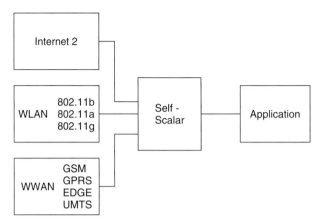

Figure 8.16 Design of an Image Self-scaling network (ISSN) using the Concept of a Self-scalar.

8.8.2 Design of Self-scaling WAN in Healthcare Environment

8.8.2.1 Healthcare Application   The ISSN utilizes three different communication classes, Internet 2, WLAN and WWAN. Figure 8.17 shows the integration of the three classes of network using the concept of a self-scalar for healthcare application. A tandem system is used to provide transparent and fault-tolerant communications between healthcare providers. The self-scalar schematic shown in Figure 8.16 is used as the self-scaling mechanism. Using the Internet Control Message Protocol (ICMP), the ISSN can automatically determine the fastest available network connection between the medical image application site (see Fig. 8.17, left) and the DICOM image server (Fig. 8.17, right). Permanent network monitoring and transfer speed measurements provide the best available service. In addition, each self-scalar can be modified to initially evaluate any one specific path (e.g., Internet 2 first) in each network availability test cycle, before the final selection is made.

8.8.2.2 The Self-Scalar   The key component of the ISSN is the self-scalar (see Fig. 8.17). The DICOM-compliant self-scalar determines automatically which communication classes are available and automatically routes to the fastest available

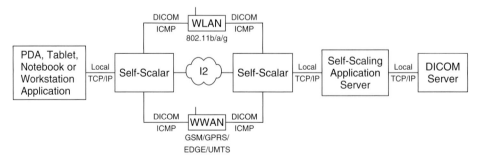

Figure 8.17 Setup of the Self-scaling Network (ISSN) for healthcare applications. ICMP: Internet Control Message Protocol.

connection. As the self-scalar itself is based on a modular concept, new communication classes or devices can be added seamlessly when new technology emerges. Additional WLAN or WWAN ports can be added to increase the transmission rates. ISSN has a broad base of applications in healthcare delivery, especially in mission critical environments.

References

Abilene Network. http://abilene.internet2.edu/.

Arbaugh WA, Shankar, Wan. Your 802.11 wireless network has No clothes. March 30, 2001. http://www.cs.umd.edu/~waa/wireless.pdf.

Borisov N, Goldberg, and Wagner. Intercepting mobile communications: the insecurity of 802.11. Published in the proceedings of the Seventh Annual International Conference on Mobile Computing And Networking, July 16–21, 2001. http://www.isaac.cs.berkeley.edu/isaac/mobicom.pdf.

California Research and Education Network, CalREN2. http://www.calren2.net.

Chan LWC, Cao F, Zhou M, Hau SK. Connectivity issues and performance monitoring of international Internet-2 in tele-imaging consultation. Education Exhibit, RSNA 2003.

Chan LWC, Zhou MZ, Hau SK, Law, MYY, Tang FH. Documet J, international Internet-2 performance and automatic tuning protocol for medical imaging applications. *Computer Med Imag Graph*. 29: 103–14; 2005.

Digital Imaging and Communications in Medicine (DICOM). National electrical Manufacturers' Association. Rosslyn, VA: NEMA, 1996.

Flagtelecom. http://www.flagtelecom.com.

Gast. *802.11 Wireless Networks: The Definitive Guide*. O'Reilly; 2002.

Globalcrossing. http://www.globalcrossing.com.

http://apps.internet2.edu/rsna2003-demos.html#RemoteTreatmentPlanning.

http://networks.internet2.edu/rons.html.

http://www.freesoft.org/CIE/RFC/792/index.htm.

http://www.interne2.edu.

http://www.novatelwireless.com/pcproducts/g100.html.

http://www.siemenscordless.com/mobile_phones/s46.html.

Huang C. Changing learning with new interactive and media-rich learning environments: Virtual Labs Case Study Report, *Comp Med Imag Graph* 27(2–3): 157–64; 2003.

Huang HK. Enterprise PACS and image distribution, *Comp Med Imag Graph* 27(2–3): 241–53.

Huang HK. *PACS and Imaging Informatics: Basic Principles and Applications*. Hoboken, NJ: Wiley; 2004.

Huntoon W, Ferguson J. Internet2 Presentation—May 2002, in I2 members meeting. http://www.web100.org/docs/Web100_I2MM.ppt.

International Exchange Point in Miami, Florida International University, AMPATH. http://www.ampath.fiu.edu.

Internet2 Consortium, UCAID. http://www.internet2.edu.

Latina American Cooperation of Advanced Networks, redCLARA. http://www.redclara.net.

Liu, BJ, Zhou Z, Gutierrez MA, Documet J, Chan L, Huang HK. International Internet2 connectivity and performance in medical imaging applications: bridging the Americas to Asia. *J High Speed Networks* 16(1), 5–20, 2007.

Making the Choice: 802.11a or 802.11g. http://www.80211-planet.com/tutorials/article/0,,10724_1009431,00.html.

Mogel G, Cao F, Huang HK, Zhou M, et al, Internet2 Performance for Medical Imaging Applications, RSNA 2002 Fall Meeting. http://apps.internet2.edu/rsna2002-demos.html.

Mogel GT, Cao F, Huang, HK, Zhou M, Liu, BJ, Huang C. Internet 2 performance for medical imaging applications: in Internet 2 RSNA Demos. *Radiology* 225: 752; 2002.

Rede Nacional de Ensino e Pesquisa, RNP. http://www.rnp.br.

Remote Treatment Planning for Radiation Therapy. Internet2/NLM infoRAD exhibit. RSNA 2003.

Shanmugam R, Padmini R, Nivedita S. *Special Edition Using TCP/IP*, 2nd ed. Indianapolis: Que Pubublishing, 2002.

Stahl JN, Zhang J, Zellner C, Pomerantsev EV, Chou TM, Huang HK. Teleconferencing with dynamic medical images. *IEEE Trans Info Tech Biomed* 4(1): 88–96, 2000.

StarLight. http://www.startap.net/starlight/.

Summerhill R. Internet2 Internet2 Network infrastructure: Abilene current status and future plans. GNEW 2004 Meeting, CERN, Geneva, March 15, 2004.

Tierney BL. TCP tuning guide for distributed application on wide area networks. *Proc. Network Comput* February 2001.

Verio. http://www.verio.com.

Web100 project. http://www.web100.org/.

Wi-Fi Alliance home page. http://www.weca.net/.

Yu F, Hwang K, Gill M, Huang HK. Some connectivity and security issues of NGI in medical imaging applications. *J High Speed Networks* 9: 3–13; 2000.

Zhang J, Stahl JN, Huang HK. Real-time teleconsultation with high-resolution and large-volume medical images for collaborative healthcare. *IEEE Trans Info Tech Biomed.* 4, no. 2, June 2000.

Zhou Z, Gutierrez M, Documet J, Chan L, Huang HK, Liu BJ, The role of a Data Grid in worldwide imaging-based clinical trials. *J High Speed Networks*; 16(1), 21–33, 2007.

CHAPTER 9

Industrial Standards (HL7 and DICOM) and Integrating the Healthcare Enterprise (IHE)

9.1 INDUSTRIAL STANDARDS AND WORKFLOW PROFILES

Transmission of images and textual information between healthcare information systems has always been difficult for two reasons. First, information systems use different computer platforms, and second, images and data are generated from various imaging modalities by different manufacturers. With the emergent healthcare industry standards, Health level 7 (HL7) and Digital Imaging and Communications in Medicine (DICOM), it has become feasible to integrate all these heterogeneous, disparate medical images and textual data into an organized system. Interfacing two healthcare components requires two ingredients: a common data format and a communication protocol. HL7 is a standard textual data format, whereas DICOM includes data format and communication protocols. In conforming to the HL7 standard, it is possible to share healthcare information between the hospital information systems (HIS), the radiology information systems (RIS), and PACS. By adapting the DICOM standard, medical images generated from a variety of modalities and manufacturers can be interfaced as an integrated healthcare system. These two standards are topics to be discussed first. The third topic to be covered is integrating the healthcare enterprise (IHE) model used for driving the adoption of standards. With all the good standards available, it takes a champion IHE to persuade the users to adopt and to use one standard model. The last topic discussed is the computer operating systems and programming languages commonly used in medical imaging and healthcare information technology. Figure 9.1 shows how this chapter corresponds: to other chapters of Part II (as a detail of Fig. 1.3). Figure 9.2 (a reprise of Fig. 2.1) shows topics and concepts covered in Part II and their interrelationships.

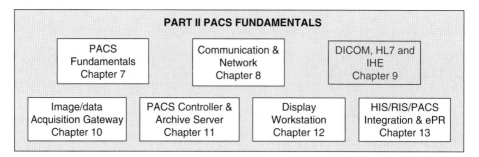

Figure 9.1   Position of Chapter 9 in the organization of this book. Color codes are used to highlight components and workflow in chapters of Part II.

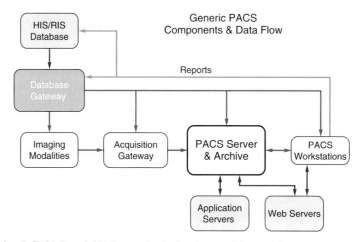

Figure 9.2   DCIOM and HL7 standards in the PACS workflow in which all images and pertinent data needed to be first converted to DICOM and HL7, respectively. PACS basic components (yellow) and data flow (blue: Internal; green and orange: external between PACS and other information systems); other information systems (light blue). HIS: hospital information system; RIS: radiology information system.

9.2   THE HEALTH LEVEL 7 (HL7) STANDARD

9.2.1   Health Level 7

Health Level 7 (HL7), established in March 1987, was organized by a user-vendor committee to develop a standard for electronic data exchange in healthcare environments, particularly for hospital applications. The HL7 standard refers to the highest level, the application level, in the seven communication levels model of Open Systems Interconnection (OSI; see Chapter 8). The common goal is to simplify the interface implementation between computer applications from multiple vendors. This standard emphasizes data format and protocol for exchanging certain key textual data among health care information systems, such as HIS, RIS, and PACS.

Although HL7 addresses the highest level (level 7) of the OSI model of the International Standards Organization (ISO), it does not conform specifically to the defined elements of the OSI's seventh level (see Section 8.1.2). It conforms to the conceptual definitions of an application-to-application interface placed in the seventh layer of the OSI model. These definitions were developed to facilitate data communication in a healthcare setting by providing rules to convert abstract messages associated with real-world events into strings of characters comprising an actual message.

9.2.2 An Example

Consider the three popular computer platforms used in HIS, RIS, and PACS, namely the IBM mainframe computer running the VM operating system, the PC Windows operating system, and the Sun workstation (WS) running UNIX. Interfacing involves the establishment of data links between these three operating systems via TCP/IP transmission (Section 8.1.2) with HL7 data format at the application layer.

When an event occurs, such as patient admission, discharge, or transfer (ADT), the IBM computer in the HIS responsible for tracking this event would initiate an unsolicited message to the remote UNIX or Windows server in the RIS that takes charge of the next event. If the message is in HL7 format, UNIX or Windows parses the message, updates its local database automatically, and sends a confirmation to the IBM. Otherwise, a "rejected" message would be sent instead.

In the HL7 standard, the basic data unit is a message. Each message is composed of multiple segments in a defined sequence. Each segment contains multiple data fields and is identified by a unique, predefined three-character code. The first segment is the message header segment with the three-letter code MSH, which defines the intent, source, destination, and some other relevant information such as message control identification and time stamp. The other segments are event dependent. Within each segment, related information is bundled together based on the HL7 protocol. A typical message, such as patient admission, may contain the following segments:

MSH—Message header segment
EVN—Event type segment
PID—Patient identification segment
NK1—Next of kin segment
PV1—Patient visit segment

In this patient admission message, the patient identification segment may contain the segment header and other demographic information, such as patient identification, name, birth date, and gender. The separators between fields and within a field are defined in the message header segment. Here is an example of transactions of admitting a patient for surgery in HL7:

```
(1) Message header segment
MSH||STORE|HOLLYWOOD|MIME|VERMONT|200305181007|security|
ADT|MSG00201|||<CR>
(2) Event type segment
EVN|01|200305181005||<CR>
(3) Patient identification segment
PID|||PATID1234567||Doe^John^B^II||19470701|M||C|
```

```
3976 Sunset Blvd^Los Angeles ^CA^90027||323-681-2888|||||||<CR>
(4) Next of kin segment
NK1|Doe^Linda^E||wife|<CR>
(5) Patient visit segment
PV1|1|I|100^345^01||||00135^SMITH^WILLIAM^K|||SUR|ADM|
<CR>
```

Combining these five segments, these messages translate to:"Patient John B. Doe, II, male, Caucasian, born on July 1, 1947, lives in Los Angeles, was admitted on May18, 2003 at 10:05 a.m. by Doctor William K. Smith (#00135) for surgery. The patient has been assigned to Room 345, bed 01 on nursing unit 100.The next of kin is Linda E. Doe, wife. The ADT (admission, discharge, and transfer) message 201 was sent from system STORE at the Hollywood site to system MIME at the Vermont site on the same date two minutes after the admit."

The "|" is the data file separator. If no data are entered in a field, a blank will be used, followed by another "|."

The data communication between a HIS and a RIS is event driven. When an ADT event occurs, the HIS would automatically send a broadcast message, conformed to HL7 format, to the RIS. The RIS would then parse this message and insert, update, and organize patient demographic data in its database according to the event. Similarly the RIS would send an HL7-formatted ADT message, the examination reports, and the procedural descriptions to the PACS. When the PACS had acknowledged and verified the data, it would update the appropriate databases and initiate any required follow-up actions.

9.2.3 New Trend in HL7

The most commonly used HL7 today is Version 2.X, which has many options and thus is flexible. Over the past few years Version 2.X has been developed continuously, and it is widely and successfully implemented in healthcare environment. Version 2.X and other older versions use a "bottom-up" approach, beginning with very general concepts and adding new features as needed. These new features become options to the implementers so that the standard is very flexible and easy to adapt to different sites. However, these options and flexibility also make it impossible to have reliable conformance tests of any vendor's implementation. This forces vendors to spend more time in analyzing and planning their interfaces to ensure that the same optional features are used in both interfacing parties. There is also no consistent view of the data when HL7 moves to a new version or that data's relationship to other data. Therefore, a consistently defined and object-oriented version of HL7 is needed, which is Version 3.

The initial release of HL7 Version 3 was in December 2001. The primary goal of HL7 Version 3 is to offer a standard that is definite and testable. Version 3 uses an object-oriented methodology and a reference information model (RIM) to create HL7 messages. The object-oriented method is a "top-down" method. The RIM is an all-encompassing, open architecture design at the entire scope of health care IT, containing more than 100 classes and more than 800 attributes. RIM defines the relationships of each class. RIM is the backbone of HL7 Version 3, as it provides an explicit representation of the semantic and lexical connections between the information in the fields of HL7 messages. Because each aspect of the RIM is well defined, very few options exist in Version 3. Through object-oriented method and RIM, HL7 Version 3 will improve many of the shortcomings of previous 2.X versions. Version 3 uses XML (extensible markup language; Section 7.2.1) for message encoding to increase interoperability between systems. This version has developed the Patient Record Architecture (PRA), an XML-based clinical document architecture. It can also certify vendor systems through HL7 Message Development Framework (MDF). This testable criterion will verify vendors' conformance to Version 3. In addition Version 3 will include new data interchange formats beyond ASCII and support of component-based technology such as ActiveX and CORBA. As the industry moves to Version 3, providers and vendors will face some impact now or in the future, such as:

Benefits

1. It will be less complicated and less expensive to build and maintain the HL7 interfaces.
2. HL7 messages will be less complex, and therefore analysts and programmers will require less training.
3. HL7 compliance testing will become enabled.
4. It will be easier to integrate different HL7 software interfaces from different vendors.

Challenges

1. Adoption of Version 3 will be more expensive than the previous version.
2. Adoption of Version 3 will take time to replace the existing version.
3. Retraining and retooling will be necessary.
4. Vendors will eventually be forced to adopt Version 3.
5. Vendors will have to support both Versions 2.X and 3 for some time.

HL7 Version 3 will offer tremendous benefits to providers and vendors as well as analysts and programmers, but complete adoption of the new standard will take time and effort.

9.3   FROM ACR-NEMA TO DICOM AND DICOM DOCUMENT

9.3.1   ACR-NEMA and DICOM

ACR-NEMA, formally known as the American College of Radiology and the National Electrical Manufacturers Association, created a committee to develop a set of standards to serve as the common ground for various medical imaging equipment vendors. The goal was that newly developed instruments be able to communicate and participate in sharing medical image information, in particular, within the PACS environment. The committee, which focused chiefly on issues concerning information exchange, interconnectivity, and communications among medical systems, began work in 1982. The first version, which emerged in 1985, specified standards in point-to-point message transmission, data formatting, and presentation and included a preliminary set of communication commands and a data format dictionary. The second version, ACR-NEMA 2.0, published in 1988, was an enhancement to the first release. It included both hardware definitions and software protocols, as well as a standard data dictionary. Networking issues were not addressed adequately in either version. For this reason a new version aiming to include network protocols was released in 1992. Because of the magnitude of changes and additions, it was given a new name: Digital Imaging and Communications in Medicine (DICOM 3.0). In 1996 a new version was released consisting of 13 published parts that form the basis of future DICOM new versions and parts. Manufacturers readily adopted this version to their imaging products.

Each DICOM document is identified by title and standard number in the form: PS 3.X-YYYY where "X" is the part number and "YYYY" is the year of publication. Thus PS 3.1-1996 means DICOM 3.0 document part 1 (Introduction and Overview) released in 1996. Although the complexity and involvement of the standards were increased by many fold, DICOM remains compatible with the previous ACR-NEMA versions. The two most distinguished new features in DICOM are adaptation of the object-oriented data model for message exchange and utilization of existing standard network communication protocols.

For a brief summary of the ACR-NEMA 2.0, refer to the first edition of this book. This chapter discusses DICOM 3.0.

9.3.2 DICOM Document

The current DICOM standard PS 3.1–2008 includes 18 related but independent parts following the ISO (International Standardization Organization) directives and are referred to as:

Part 1: Introduction and Overview
Part 2: Conformance
Part 3: Information Object Definitions
Part 4: Service Class Specifications
Part 5: Data Structures and Encoding
Part 6: Data Dictionary
Part 7: Message Exchange
Part 8: Network Communication Support for Message Exchange
Part 9: Point-to-Point Communication Support for Message Exchange *(Retired)*
Part 10: Media Storage and File Format for Media Interchange
Part 11: Media Storage Application Profiles
Part 12: Media Formats and Physical Media-for-Media Interchange
Part 13: Print Management Point-to-Point Communication Support *(Retired)*
Part 14: Gray Scale Standard Display Function
Part 15: Security and System Management Profiles
Part 16: Content Mapping Resource
Part 17: Explanatory Information
Part 18: Web Access to DICOM Persistent Objects (WADO)

Parts 17 and 18 were added to the DICOM standard in 2004. These two additional parts are used to facilitate the linkage of images with structured reporting, other types of report format and languages, and information annexes. Since these two new standards are useful in the imaging informatics to be discussed in Part IV of this book, for convenience, the following three paragraphs are excerpted from the DICOM document.

Part 17: Explanatory Information

This DICOM part contains explanatory information in the form of Normative and Informative Annexes. Some of these Annexes include the following: Explanation of Patient Orientation; SR Encoding Example; Mammography CAD; Clinical Trial Identification Workflow Examples; Ultrasound Templates; Echocardiography Procedure Reports; and Configuration Use Cases.

Part 18: Web Access to DICOM Persistent Objects (WADO)

This standard specified a web-based service for accessing and presenting DICOM persistent objects such as images and reports through a simple mechanism from HTML (Hypertext Markup Language) pages or XML (Extensible Markup Language, see Section 9.6.5) documents, through HTTP/HTTPs (Hypertext Transfer Protocol) using DICOM UID's (Unique Identifiers). Data may be retrieved as specified by the requester in a presentation-ready format, e.g., JPEG (Joint Photographic Experts Group), GIF(Graphic interchange format), or in native DICOM. It does not support facilities for web searching of DICOM images.

DICOM Supplements In addition to the base standard of 18 parts, DICOM has final supplements that enhance the existing base standard. Some of the areas include handling PET Image Fusion data storage, Pathology-related and specimen imaging data storage, breast tomosynthesis data storage, cardiac stress testing data storage, surface segmentation and presentation data, MPEG2 Main Profile/High Level (MP@HL) transfer syntax for high-definition video.

Figure 9.3*A* summarizes the various parts of the DICOM document. There are two routes of communications between parts: network exchange on-line communication (left) and media storage interchange off-line communication (right).

9.4 THE DICOM 3.0 STANDARD

Two fundamental components of DICOM are the information object class and the service class. Information objects define the contents of a set of images and their relationship, and the service classes describe what to do with these objects. Tables 9.1 and 9.2 list some service classes and object classes. The service classes and information object classes are combined to form the fundamental units of DICOM, called service-object pairs (SOPs). This section describes these fundamental concepts and provides some examples.

9.4.1 DICOM Data Format

In this section we discuss two topics in DICOM data format: the DICOM model of the real world and the DICOM file format. The former is used to define the hierarchical

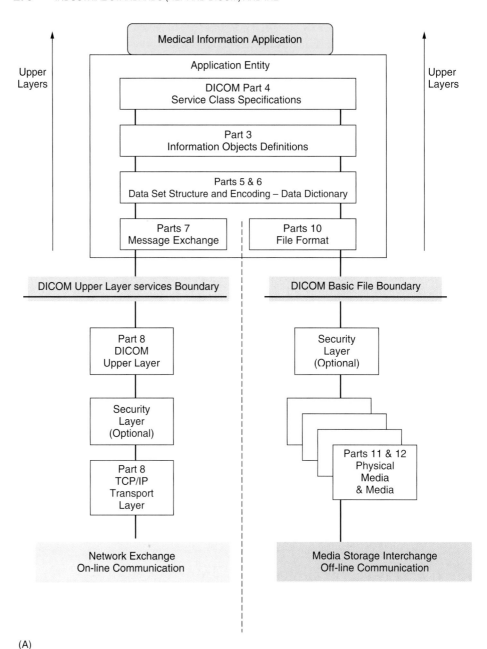

(A)

Figure 9.3 (*A*) Architecture of the DICOM data communication model, and DICOM parts (Section 9.3.2). There are two communication models: the network layers model (left) and the media storage interchange model (right). Both models share the upper-level data structure described in DICOM parts 3, 4, 5, 6. In part 7, message exchange is used for communication only, whereas in part 10, file format is used for media exchange. Below the upper levels, the two models are completely different. (*B*) The simplified DICOM data model of the real world with four levels: patient, study, series, and images. This simplified model can be extended to more complicated data models for various applications, including ePR, radiation therapy, and surgery.

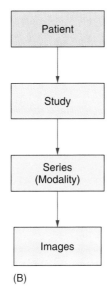

(B)

Figure 9.3   (*Continued*)

TABLE 9.1   DICOM service classes

Service Class	Description
Image storage	Provides storage service for data sets
Image query	Supports queries about data sets
Image retrieval	Supports retrieval of images from storage
Image print	Provides hard copy generation support
Examination	Supports management of examinations (which may consist of several series of management images)
Storage resource	Supports management of the network data storage resource(s)

TABLE 9.2   DICOM information object classes

Normalized	Composite
Patient	Computed radiograph
Study	Computed tomogram
Results	Digitized film image
Storage resource	Digital subtraction image
Image annotation	MR image
	Nuclear medicine image
	Ultrasound image
	Displayable image
	Graphics
	Curve

data structure from patient, to studies, to series, and to images and waveforms. The latter describes how to encapsulate a DICOM file ready for a DICOM SOP service.

9.4.1.1 *DICOM Model of the Real World*

9.4.1.1 DICOM Model of the Real World The DICOM model of the real world defines several real-world objects in the clinical image arena (patient, study, series, image, etc.) and their interrelationships within the scope of the DICOM standard. It provides a framework for various DICOM information object definitions (IOD). The DICOM model documents four object levels: patient; study; series and equipment; and image, waveform, and SR (structured report). Each of these levels can contain several ($1-n$ or $0-n$) sublevels.

A patient is a person receiving, or registering to receive, healthcare services. This person could have had several previous ($1-n$) studies already, and may visit the healthcare faculty and register to have more ($1-n$) studies. For example, a patient has one historical CT chest study and two historical MR brain studies. The patient is also visiting the hospital to have a new CR chest study.

A study can be a historical study, a currently performed study, or a study to be performed in the future. A study can contain a few ($1-n$) series or several study components ($1-n$), each of which can include another few ($1-n$) series. For example, an MR brain study may include three series: transaxial, sagittal, and coronal. A study or several ($1-n$) studies can also have several scheduled procedural steps to be performed in different modalities. For example, an MRI brain study is scheduled in the MRI machine, or one MRI study and one CT study are scheduled in an MRI and a CT scanner, respectively. A study can thus include additional results. The results may be in the form of a report or an amendment.

A series or several series can be created by equipment. Equipment is a modality (e.g., MRI scanner) used in the healthcare environment. A series can include several ($0-n$) images or waveforms, SR (structured report), documents, or radiotherapy objects (see Chapter 23), and so forth. For example, an MR transaxial brain series includes 40 MR brain Images.

An image can be any image from all sorts of modalities, for example, a CT image, MR image, CR image, DR image, US image, NM image, or light image. A waveform is from the modality generating waveform output, for example, an ECG waveform from an ECG device. A SR document is a new type of document for structured reporting. DICOM defines many SR templates to be used in the healthcare environment, for example, a mammography CAD SR template. These topics are discussed in more detail in Section 9.4.6. Contents of this data model are encoded with necessary header information and tags in specified format to form a DICOM file. Figure 9.3*B* shows the simplified DICOM data model of the real model. There are several extended DCIOM data models for various applications, for example, ePR (electronic patient record, Chapters 13, 14, and 22), radiation therapy ePR (Chapter 23), and image-guided surgery ePR (Chapter 24).

9.4.1.2 *DICOM File Format*

9.4.1.2 DICOM File Format DICOM file format defines how to encapsulate the DICOM data set of a SOP instance in a DICOM file. Each file usually contains one SOP instance. The DICOM file starts with the DICOM file meta information (optional), followed by the bit stream of data set, and ends with the image pixel data if it is a DICOM image file. The DICOM file meta information includes file identification information. The meta information uses Explicit VR (value representations) transfer syntax for encoding. Therefore the meta information does not exist in the Implicit VR-encoded DICOM File. Explicit VR and Implicit VR are two coding methods in DICOM. Vendors or implementers have the option of choosing either one for encoding. DICOM files encoded by both coding methods can be processed by most of the DICOM compliant software. The difference between Explicit VR and Implicit VR is that the former has VR encoding, whereas the latter has no VR encoding. For example, an encoding for the element "modality" of CT value in Implicit VR and Explicit VR would be (the first 4 bytes, 08 00 60 00, is a tag):

$$08\ 00\ 60\ 00\ 02\ 00\ 00\ 00\ 43\ 54 \qquad \text{Implicit VR}$$

$$08\ 00\ 60\ 00\ \mathbf{43\ 53}\ 02\ 00\ 43\ 54 \qquad \text{Explicit VR}$$

In the encodings above, the first 4 bytes (08 00 60 00) is a tag. In Implicit VR, the next 4 bytes (02 00 00 00) are for the length of the value field of the data element and the last 2 bytes (43 54) are element value (CT). In Explicit VR, the first 4 bytes are also a tag, the next 2 bytes (**43 53**) are for VR representing CS (code string), one type of VR in DICOM, the next 2 bytes (02 00) are for length of element value, and the last 2 bytes (43 54) are element value.

One data set represents a single SOP Instance. A data set is constructed of data elements. Data elements contain the encoded values of the attributes of the DICOM object. (See DICOM Parts 3 and 5 on the construction and encoding of a data element and a data set.) If the SOP instance is an image, the last part of the DICOM file is the image pixel data. The tag for image pixel data is 7FE0 0010. Figure 9.4 shows an example of Implicit VR little-endian (byte swapping) encoded CT DICOM file.

9.4.2   Object Class and Service Class

9.4.2.1   Object Class   The DICOM object class consists of normalized objects and composite objects. Normalized information object classes include those attributes inherent in the real-world entity represented. The left side of Table 9.2 show some normalized object classes. Let us consider two normalized object classes: study information and patient information. In the study information object class, the study date and image time are attributes of this object because these attributes are inherent whenever a study is performed. On the other hand, patient name is not an attribute in the study information object class but an attribute in the patient object class. This is because the patient's name is inherent in the patient information object class on which the study was performed and not the study itself. The use of information object classes can identify objects encountered in medical imaging applications more precisely and without ambiguity. For this reason the objects defined in DICOM 3.0 are very precise.

However, sometimes it is advantageous to combine normalized object classes together to form composite information object classes for facilitating operations. For example, the computed radiography image information object class is a composite object because it contains attributes from the study information object class (image

INDUSTRIAL STANDARDS (HL7 AND DICOM) AND IHE
Element Tag and Value	Binary Coding
0008,0000, 726	08 00 00 00 04 00 00 00 D6 02 00 00
0008,0005, ISO.IR 100	08 00 05 00 0A 00 00 00 49 53 4F 5F 49 52 20 31 30 30
0008,0016, 1.2.840.10008.5.1.4.1.1.2.	08 00 16 00 1A 00 00 00 31 2E 32 2E 38 34 30 2E 31 30 30 30 38 2E 35 2E 31 2E 34 2E 31 2E 31 2E 32 00
0008,0060, CT	08 00 60 00 02 00 00 00 **43 54**
0008,1030, Abdomen.1abdpelvis	08 00 30 10 12 00 00 00 41 62 64 6F 6D 65 6E 5E 31 61 62 64 70 65 6C 76 69 73
...	...

E0 7F 10 00 00 00 00 00 00 00 00 00 00 00 00 00

....

....

....

20 00 25 00 1° 00 19 00 1C 00 14 00 2D 00

....

....

....

....

....

....

....

Figure 9.4 "0008,0000" in the "element tag and value" column is the tag for the 0008 Group. "726" is the value for the Group length, and it means there are 726 bytes in this Group. The corresponding binary coding of this tag and value are in the same line in "binary coding" column. The next few lines are the tags and values as well as the corresponding coding for "specific character set," "SOP class UID," "modality," and "study description." The image pixel data is not in the 0008 Group. Its tag is "7FE0 0010," and following the tag are the coding for the pixel data. The element tag and value "0008 . . ." becomes "08 00 . . . " in binary coding because of the little-endian "byte swapping."

date, time, etc.) and patient information object class (patient's name, etc.). Table 9.2 (right) show some composite information object classes

DICOM uses a unique identifier (UID), 1.2.840.10008.X.Y.Z, to identify a specific part of an object, where the numerals are called the organizational root and X, Y, Z are additional fields to identify the parts. Thus, for example, the UID for the DICOM explicit values representing little-endian transfer syntax is 1.2.840.10008.1.2.1. Note that the UID is used to identify a part of an object; it does not carry information.

9.4.2.2 DICOM Services DICOM services are used for communication of imaging information objects within a device and for the device to perform a service for the object, for example, to store the object or to display the object. A service is built on top of a set of "DICOM message service elements" (DIMSEs). These DIMSEs are computer software programs written to perform specific functions. There are two types of DIMSEs, one for the normalized objects and the other for the composite objects as given in Tables 9.3 and 9.4, respectively. DIMSEs are paired in the sense that a device issues a command request and the receiver responds

TABLE 9.3   **Normalized DICOM message service element (DIMSE)**

Command	Function
N-EVENT-REPORT	Notification of information object-related event
N-GET	Retrieval of information object attribute value
N-SET	Specification of information object attribute value
N-ACTION	Specification of information object-related action
N-CREATE	Creation of an information object
N-DELETE	Deletion of an information object

TABLE 9.4   **Composite DICOM message service element (DIMSE)**

Command	Function
C-ECHO	Verification of connection
C-STORE	Transmission of an information object instance
C-FIND	Inquiries about information object instances
C-GET	Transmission of an information object instance via third-party application processes
C-MOVE	Similar to GET, but end receiver is usually not the command initiator

to the command accordingly. The composite commands are generalized, whereas the normalized commands are more specific.

DICOM services are referred to as "service classes" because of the object-oriented nature of its information structure model. If a device provides a service, it is called a service class provider; if it uses a service, it is a service class user. Thus, for example, a magnetic disk in the PACS server is a service class provider for the server to store images. On the other hand, a CT scanner is the service class user of the magnetic disk in the PACS server to store images. Note that a device can be either a service class provider or a service class user or both, depending on how it is used. For example, in its routing process that receives images from the scanners and distributes these images to the workstations, the PACS server assumes the roles of both a storage service class provider and a storage service class user. As a service class provider, it accepts images from the scanners by providing a storage service for these images. On the other hand, the PACS server is a service class user when it sends images to the workstation by issuing service requests to the WS for storing the images.

9.4.3   DICOM Communication

DICOM uses existing network communication standards based on the International Standards Organization Open Systems Interconnection (ISO-OSI; see Section 8.1 for details) for imaging information transmission. The ISO-OSI consists of seven layers from the lowest physical (cables) layer to the highest application layer. When imaging information objects are sent between layers in the same device, the process is called a service. When objects are sent between two devices, it is called a protocol. When a protocol is involved, several steps are invoked in two devices; we say that

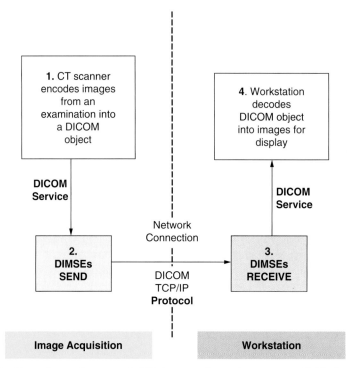

Figure 9.5 Data flow of a set of CT images from the scanner (left) is sent to the workstation (right). Within a device the data flow is called a service; between devices it is called a protocol.

two devices are in "association" using DICOM. Figure 9.5 illustrates the data flow of the CT images from the scanner to the workstation (WS) using DICOM. The numerals represent the steps as follows:

1. CT scanner encodes all images into a DICOM object.
2. Scanner invokes a set of DIMSEs to move the image object from a certain level down to the physical layer in the ISO-OSI model.
3. WS uses a counterset of DIMSEs to receive the image object through the physical layer and move it up to a certain level.
4. WS decodes the DICOM image object.

If an imaging device transmits an image object with a DICOM command, the receiver must use a DICOM command to receive the information. DICOM uses TCP/IP for file transmission. On the other hand, if a device transmits a DICOM object with a TCP/IP communication protocol through a network without invoking the DICOM communication, any device connected to the network can receive the data with the TCP/IP protocol. However, a decoder is still needed to convert the DICOM object for proper use. The TCP/IP method is used to send a full resolution DICOM image from the PACS server to the Web server without invoking DICOM service, as will be discussed in Chapter 14.

9.4.4 DICOM Conformance

DICOM conformance PS 3.2–1996 is Part 2 of the DICOM document instructing manufacturers how to conform their devices to the DICOM standard. In a conformance statement the manufacturer describes exactly how the device or its associate software conforms to the standard. A conformance statement does not mean that this device follows every detail required by DICOM; it only means that this device follows a certain subset of DICOM. The extent of the subset is described in the conformance statement. For example, a laser film digitizer needs only to conform to the minimum requirements for the digitized images to be in the DICOM format, but the digitizer should be a service class user to send the formatted images to a second device like a magnetic disk, which is a DICOM service class provider. Thus, if a manufacturer claims that its imaging device is DICOM conformant, it means that any system integrator who follows this manufacturer's conformance document will be able to interface this device with his/her DICOM-compliant components. In general, the contents of the conformance statement include (quoted from DICOM 2003):

1. The implementation model of the application entities (AEs) in the implementation and how these AEs relate to both local and remote real-world activities.
2. The proposed (for association initiation) and acceptable (for association acceptance) presentation contexts used by each AE.
3. The SOP classes and their options supported by each AE, and the policies with which an AE initiates or accepts associations.
4. The communication protocols to be used in the implementation and
5. A description of any extensions, specializations, and publicly disclosed privatizations to be used in the implementation.
6. A description of any implementation details which may be related to DICOM conformance or interoperability. (DICOM PS3.2 1996)

9.4.5 Examples of Using DICOM

To an end user, the two most important DICOM services are "send and receive" Images, and "query and retrieve") images. In this section we use two examples to explain how DICOM accomplishes these services. Note that the query and retrieve services are built on top of the send and receive services.

9.4.5.1 Send and Receive   Let us consider the steps involved in sending a CT examination with multiple images from the scanner to the DICOM gateway (see Fig. 9.2) using the DICOM protocol. Each individual image is transmitted from the CT scanner to the gateway by utilizing DICOM's C-STORE service. In this transmission procedure, the scanner takes on the role of a client as the C-STORE service class user (SCU) and gateway assumes the role of the C-STORE service class provider (SCP). The following steps illustrate the transmission of a CT examination with multiple images from the scanner to the gateway (Figure 9.6). The CT scanner and the PACS acquisition gateway first establish the connection through DICOM communication "association request and response" commands.

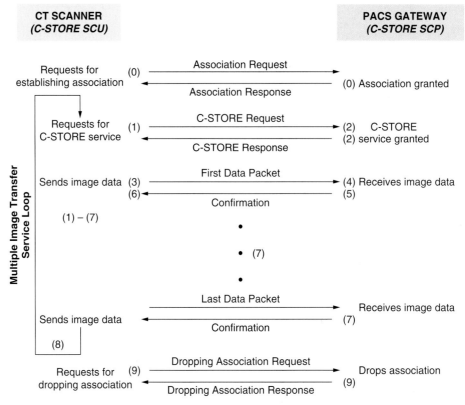

Figure 9.6 DICOM send and receive operations. The example shows the steps involved in sending a set of CT images from the scanner to the acquisition gateway (see Fig. 9.2 for the PACS components involved).

1. The invoking scanner (SCU) issues a C-STORE service request to the PACS gateway (SCP).
2. The gateway receives the C-STORE request and issues a C-STORE response to the invoking scanner.
3. The CT scanner sends the first data packet of the first image to the gateway.
4. The gateway performs the requested C-STORE service to store the packet.
5. On completion of the service, the gateway issues a confirmation to the scanner.
6. After receiving the confirmation from the gateway on the completion of storing the packet, the scanner sends the next packet to the PACS controller.
7. Processes 4 to 6 repeat until all packets of the first image have been transmitted from the scanner to the gateway.
8. The scanner issues a second C-STORE service request to the PACS gateway for transmission of the second image. Steps 1 to 7 repeat until all images from the study have been transmitted.
9. The scanner and the PACS gateway issue DICOM communication command "dropping association request and response" to disconnect.

9.4.5.2 Query and Retrieve The send and receive service class using the C-STORE is relatively simple compared with the query and retrieve service class. Let us consider a more complicated example in which the PACS workstation (WS) queries the PACS server (Server) to retrieve a historical CT examination to compare with a current study already available at the WS. This composite service class involves three DIMSEs: C-FIND and C-MOVE (Table 9.4), and C-STORE described in the last section. In performing the query/retrieve (Q/R) SOP service, both the WS and the Server each have one user and one provider.

	WS	Server
Query/retrieve (Q/R)	User	Provider
C-STORE	Provider	User

Thus in Q/R, the WS takes on the role of user (SCU) and the Server functions as the provider (SCP), whereas in C-STORE, the WS has the role of SCP and the Server has the function of CSU. Referring to Figure 9.7, after the association between the WS and the Server has been established, then:

1. The PACS WS's Q/R application entity (AE) issues a C-FIND service (Table 9.4) request to the Server.
2. The Server's Q/R AE receives the C-FIND request from the querying WS (Fig. 9.7, 2a); performs the C-FIND service (Fig. 9.7, 2b) to look for studies, series, and images from the PACS database; and issues a C-FIND response to the WS (2c).
3. The workstation's Q/R AE receives the C-FIND response from the PACS server. The response is a table with all the requests shown at the WS.
4. The user at the WS selects interesting images from the table (Fig. 9.7, 4a) and issues a C-MOVE service (Table 9.4) request for each individual selected image to the PACS Server (Fig. 9.7, 4b).
5. The Server's Q/R AE receives the C-MOVE (Table 9.4) request from the WS (Fig. 9.7, 5a) and issues an indication to the Server's C-STORE SCU (Fig. 9.7, 5b).
6. The Server's C-STORE SCU retrieves the requested images from the archive device.
7. The Server issues a C-STORE service request to the WS's C-STORE SCP.
8. The workstation receives the C-STORE request and issues a C-STORE response to the Server. From this point on, the C-STORE SOP service is identical to the example given in Figure 9.6.
9. After the WS retrieves the last image, it issues a "dropping association request" and terminates the association.

9.4.6 New Features in DICOM

Several new features and two new Parts 17 and 18 have been added to DICOM that are important for system integration with other inputs not in the realm of conventional

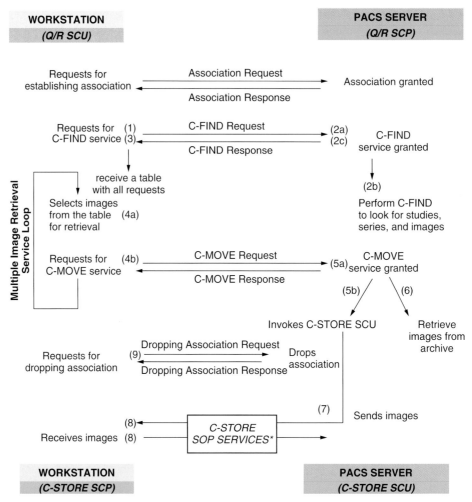

Figure 9.7 DICOM query and retrieve operation. The example shows the steps involved in a workstation Q/R a set of images from the server (see Fig. 9.2 for the PACS components involved).

radiological images. These are visible light image (Section 3.9), structured reporting object, content mapping resource, mammography CAD, JPEG 2000 compression (Section 6.4.2), waveform Information object definition (IOD) (e.g., ECG IOD (information object definition) and cardiac electrophysiology IOD), and security profiles (Chapter 17).

9.4.6.1 Visible Light (VL) Image The visible light (VL) image information object definition (IOD) for endoscopy, microscopy, and photography has become available. It includes definitions of VL endoscopic image IOD, VL microscopic image IOD, VL slide-coordinates microscopic image IOD, VL photographic image IOD, and VL image module. An example is provided in Chapter 24 that utilizes the DICOM endoscopic image format in the minimally invasive spinal surgery.

9.4.6.2   *Mammography CAD (Computer-Aided Detection)* One application of the DICOM structured reporting is in mammography computer-aided detection. It uses the mammography CAD output for analysis of mammographic findings. The output is in DICOM structured report format.

9.4.6.3   *Waveform IOD* The DICOM waveform IOD (information object definition) was mainly developed for imaging cardiac waveforms, for example, ECG and cardiac electrophysiology (EP).The ECG IOD defines the digitized electrical signals acquired by an ECG modality or an ECG acquisition function within an imaging modality. Cardiac EP IOD defines the digitized electrical signals acquired by an EP modality.

9.4.6.4   *Structured Reporting (SR) Object* Structured reporting is for radiologists to shorten their reporting time. SOP classes are defined for transmission and storage of documents that describe or refer to the images or waveforms or the features they contain. SR SOP classes provide the capability to record the structured information to enhance the precision and value of clinical documents and enable users to link the text data to particular images or waveforms. Chapters 25 and 26 provide examples of using SR to link CAD results in the CAD WS with DICOM images in the PACS Server.

9.4.6.5   *Content Mapping Resource* This defines the templates and context groups used in other DICOM parts. The templates are used to define or constrain the content of structured reporting (SR) documents or the acquisition context. Context groups specify value set restrictions for given functional or operational contexts. For example, Context Group 82 is defined to include all units of measurement used in DICOM IODs.

The features described in Sections 9.4.6.4 and 9.4.6.5 together with the new features in Part 17 (explanatory information described in Section 9.3.2) lead to the possibility of linking the CAD SR from the CAD WS with the PACS image data in the PACS archive server. These linkages allow radiologists at PACS WSs to read and review CAD results from the CAD server or WSs along with PACS images. Examples of linking CAD results from its WS to DICOM images and be display by a PACS WS will be given in Chapters 25 and 26.

9.5   IHE (INTEGRATING THE HEALTHCARE ENTERPRISE)

This section is excerpted from *IHE: A Primer from Radiographics 2001* (Siegel and Channin, 2001; Channin, 2001; Channin et al., 2001a; Henderson et al., 2001; Channin, (2001b); Carr and Moore, 2003; Integrating the Healthcare Enterprise (IHE) Overview in IHE Workshop 2006 by D. Russler; IHE Image-Sharing Demonstration at RSNA 2008). During the 2008 Ninth Annual Integrating the Healthcare Enterprise (IHE) Connectathon, representatives from 70 leading companies gathered to test 136 healthcare information technology (IT) systems. More information can be obtained from *IHE@*rsna.org(www.rsna,*org/IHE* and www.himss.org).

9.5.1 What Is IHE?

Even with the DICOM and HL7 standards available, there is still a need of common consensus on how to use these standards for integrating heterogeneous healthcare information systems smoothly. IHE is not a standard nor a certifying authority; instead it is a high-level information model for driving adoption of HL7 and DICOM standards. IHE is a joint initiative of RSNA (Radiological Society of North America) and HIMSS (Healthcare Information and Management Systems Society) started in 1998. The mission was to define and stimulate manufacturers to use DICOM- and HL-7-compliant equipment and information systems to facilitate daily clinical operation. The IHE technical framework defines a common information model and vocabulary for using DICOM and HL7 to complete a set of well-defined radiological and clinical transactions for a certain task. These common vocabulary and model would then facilitate health care providers and technical personnel in understanding each other better, which then would lead to smoother system integration.

The first large-scale demonstration was held at the RSNA annual meeting in 1999, and thereafter at RSNA in 2000 and 2001, at HIMSS in 2001and 2002, and annually since at RSNA. In these demonstrations manufacturers came together to show how their products could be integrated together according to IHE protocols. It is the belief of RSNA and HIMSS that with successful adoption of IHE, life would become more pleasant in healthcare systems integration for both the users and the providers.

9.5.2 IHE Technical Framework and Integration Profiles

There are three key concepts in the IHE technical framework: data model, actors, and integration profiles.

Data Model The data model is adapted from HL-7 and DICOM and shows the relationships between the key frames of reference, for example, patient, visit, order, and study defined in the framework.

IHE Actor An actor is one that exchanges messages with other actors to achieve specific tasks or transactions. An actor, not necessarily a person, is defined at the enterprise level in generic, product-neutral terms.

Integration Profile An integration profile is the organization of functions segmented into discrete units. It includes actors and transactions required to address a particular clinical task or need. An example is the scheduled workflow profiles, which incorporate all the process steps in a typical scheduled patient encounter from registration, ordering, image acquisition, and examination to viewing.

IHE integration profiles provide a common language, vocabulary, and platform for healthcare providers and manufacturers to discuss integration needs and the integration capabilities of products. IHE integration profiles started first in the domain of radiology. During the 2003 implementation there were 12 radiology integration profiles. Since then IHE has branched out and grown rapidly to different domains, including anatomic pathology, cardiology, eye care, IT infrastructure, laboratory, patient care coordination, patient care devices, radiation oncology, and radiology. These domains are briefly presented in the following subsections.

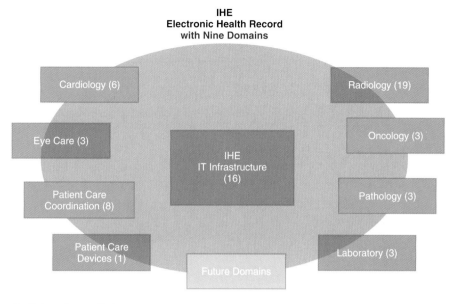

Figure 9.8 IHE framework Infrastructure with nine domains. The IT Infrastructure domain in the center is the major support of the framework. (Modified by courtesy of IHE)

9.5.3 IHE Profiles

The development of IHE profiles are organized across an increasing number of clinical and operational domains. These domains are independent and produce its own set of technical framework documents in close coordination with other IHE domains. Many of these domains have only the framework document, and workflow profiles may not yet be available. The following is a list of the current domains and their corresponding profiles as of today. These numbers of domain and profile will continue to grow, readers should not limited themselves by this list, and should follow the most up-to-day document provided by IHE. Figure 9.8 depicts the organization of the IHE technical framework as of today.

9.5.3.1 *Domain: Anatomic Pathology* Anatomic Pathology Workflow (PWF): Establishes the continuity and integrity of basic pathology data acquired for examinations being ordered for an identified inpatient or outpatient.

9.5.3.2 *Domain: Cardiology*

1. Cardiac Cath Workflow (CATH): Integrates ordering, scheduling, imaging acquisition, storage and viewing for cardiac catheterization procedures.
2. Echocardiography Workflow (ECHO): Integrates ordering, scheduling, imaging acquisition, storage, and viewing for digital echocardiography; retrieves ECG for display; provides access throughout the enterprise to electrocardiogram (ECG) documents for review purposes.
3. Evidence Documents (ED): Adds cardiology-specific options to the radiology ED profile.

4. Implantable Device Cardiac Observation (IDCO): Specifies the creation, transmission, and processing of discrete data elements and report attachments associated with cardiac device interrogations (observations) or messages.

5. Stress Testing Workflow (STRESS): Provides ordering and collecting multimodality data during diagnostic stress testing procedures.

6. Displayable Reports (DRPT): Distributes "display ready" (in PDF format) cardiology clinical reports from the department to the enterprise.

9.5.3.3 Domain: Eye Care

1. Eye Care Workflow (EYECARE): Manages eye care workflow including ordering, scheduling, imaging acquisition, storage and viewing.

2. Eye Care Evidence Document (ECED): Creates, stores, retrieves and uses objects to record eye care evidence.

3. Eye Care Displayable Report (ECDR): Creates, stores and retrieves displayable (in PDF format) clinical professional reports.

9.5.3.4 Domain: IT Infrastructure

1. Consistent Time (CT): Ensures system clocks and time stamps of computers in a network are well synchronized (median error less than 1 second).

2. Audit Trail and Node Authentication (ATNA): Describes authenticating systems using certificates and transmitting PHI (Protected Health Information) related audit events to a repository. This helps sites implement confidentiality policies.

3. Request Information for Display (RID): Provides simple (browser-based) read-only access to clinical information (e.g., allergies or lab results) located outside the user's current application.

4. Enterprise User Authentication (EUA): Enables single sign-on by facilitating one name per user for participating devices and software.

5. Patient Identifier Cross Referencing (PIX): Cross-references patient identifiers between hospitals, care sites, health information exchanges, and so forth.

6. Patient Synchronized Application (PSA): Allows selection of a patient in one application to cause other applications on a workstation to tune to that same patient.

7. Patient Demographics Query (PDQ): Lets applications query a central patient information server and retrieve a patient's demographic and visit information.

8. Cross-enterprise Document Sharing (XDS): Registers and shares electronic health record documents between healthcare enterprises, ranging from physician offices to clinics to acute care in-patient facilities.

9. Personnel White Pages (PWP): Provides basic directory information on human workforce members to other workforce members and applications.

10. Cross-enterprise Document Media Interchange (XDM): Transfers XDS documents and metadata over CD-R and USB memory devices, and over email using a ZIP attachment.

11. Cross-enterprise Document Reliable Interchange (XDR): Provides a standards-based specification for managing the interchange of documents that

healthcare enterprises have decided to explicitly exchange using a reliable point-to-point network communication.

12. Cross-Enterprise Sharing of Scanned Documents (XDS-SD): Defines how to couple legacy paper, film, electronic and scanner outputted formats, represented within a structured HL7 CDA R2 (Clinical Document Architecture Release 2) header, with a PDF or plaintext formatted document containing clinical information.

13. Patient Identifier Cross-reference and Patient Demographics Query for HL7v3: Extends the Patient Identifier Cross-reference and Patient Demographics Query profiles leveraging HL7 version 3.

14. Registry Stored Query Transaction for Cross-enterprise Document Sharing Profile: Adds a single transaction, Stored Query, to the XDS Profile.

15. Stored Query: A large improvement over the existing Query Registry transaction since it removes the use of SQL.

16. Retrieve Form for Data Capture (RFD): Enables EHR applications to directly request forms from clinical trial sponsors and public health reporting.

9.5.3.5 Domain: Laboratory

1. Laboratory Scheduled Workflow (LSWF): Establishes the continuity and integrity of clinical laboratory testing and observation data throughout the healthcare enterprise.

2. Sharing Laboratory Reports (XD*-LAB): Describes a clinical laboratory report as an electronic document.

3. LOINC Test Codes Subset (LTCS): No information available yet.

9.5.3.6 Domain: Patient Care Coordination

1. Medical Summaries (MS): Defines the content and format of discharge summaries and referral notes.

2. Exchange of Personal Health Record Content (XPHR): Describes the content and format of summary information extracted from a PHR system for import into an EHR system, and vice versa.

3. Emergency Department Referral (EDR): Allows clinicians to create electronic referrals to the emergency room including the nature of the current problem, past medical history, and medications. Upon arrival of the patient to the emergency department, the patient is identified as a referral, and the transfer document is incorporated into the EDIS. This profile builds on medical summaries by adding structures to pass data specific for ED referrals such as the estimated time of arrival and method of transport.

4. Basic Patient Privacy Consents (BPPC): Enables XDS Affinity Domains to be more flexible in the privacy policies that they support by providing mechanisms to record patient privacy consents, enforce these consents, and create Affinity Domain defined consent vocabularies that identify information sharing policies. Pre-procedural History and Physical (PPHP) describes the content and format of an electronic Preprocedural History and Physical document.

5. Antepartum Care Summary (APS): Describes the content and format of summary documents used during antepartum (before childbirth) care.

6. Functional Status Assessments (FSA): Describes the content and format of Functional Status Assessments that appear within summary documents.

7. Emergency Department Encounter Record (EDER): Describes the content and format of records created during an emergency department visit.

8. Query for Existing Data (QED): Allows information systems to query data repositories for clinical information on vital signs, problems, medications, immunizations, and diagnostic results.

9.5.3.7 Domain: Patient Care Devices

Device Enterprise Communication (DEC): Communicates PCD data to enterprise applications, such as CDS (Clinical Decision Support), CDRs (Central Data Repository), and EMRs, and so forth.

9.5.3.8 Domain: Radiation Oncology

1. Normal Treatment Planning-Simple (NTPL-S): Illustrates flow of treatment planning data from CT to Dose Review.

2. Multimodality Registration for Radiation Oncology (MMR-RO): Shows how radiation oncology treatment planning systems integrate PET and MRI data into the contouring and dose review process.

3. Treatment Workflow (TRWF): Integrates daily imaging with radiation therapy treatments using workflow.

9.5.3.9 Domain: Radiology

1. Scheduled Workflow (SWF): Integrates ordering, scheduling, imaging acquisition, storage, and viewing for radiology exams.

2. Patient Information Reconciliation (PIR): Coordinates reconciliation of the patient record when images are acquired for unidentified (e.g., trauma), or misidentified, patients.

3. Postprocessing Workflow (PWF): Provides worklists, status and result tracking for post-acquisition tasks, such as computer-aided detection or image processing.

4. Reporting Workflow (RWF): Provides worklists, status and result tracking for reporting tasks, such as dictation, transcription, and verification.

5. Import Reconciliation Workflow (IRWF): Manages importing images from CDs, hardcopy, for example, and reconciling identifiers to match local values.

6. Portable Data for Imaging (PDI): Provides reliable interchange of image data and diagnostic reports on CDs for importing, printing, or optionally, displaying in a browser.

7. Nuclear Medicine Image (NM): Specifies how nuclear medicine images and result screens are created, exchanged, used, and displayed.

8. Mammography Image (MAMMO): Specifies how mammography images and evidence objects are created, exchanged, used, and displayed.

9. Evidence Documents (ED): Specifies how data objects such as digital measurements are created, exchanged, and used.

10. Simple Image and Numeric Report (SINR): Specifies how diagnostic radiology reports (including images and numeric data) are created, exchanged, and used.

11. Key Image Note (KIN): Lets users flag images as significant (for referring, for surgery, etc.) and add notes.

12. Consistent Presentation of Images (CPI): Maintains consistent intensity and image transformations between different hardcopy and softcopy devices.

13. Presentation of Grouped Procedures (PGP): Facilitates viewing and reporting on images for individual requested procedures (e.g., head, chest, abdomen) that an operator has grouped into a single scan.

14. Image Fusion (FUS): Specifies how systems creating and registering image sets and systems displaying fused images create, exchange and use the image, registration, and blended presentation objects.

15. Cross-enterprise Document Sharing for Imaging (XDS-I): Extends XDS to share images, diagnostic reports, and related information across a group of care sites.

16. Teaching File and Clinical Trial Export (TCE): Lets users flag images and related information for automatic routing to teaching file authoring or clinical trials management systems.

17. Access to Radiology Information (ARI): Shares images, diagnostic reports, and related information inside a single network.

18. Audit Trail and Node Authentication (ATNA): Radiology option defines radiology-specific audit trail messages.

19. Charge Posting (CHG): Provides timely procedure details from modalities to billing systems.

Of the nine domains, the most well developed is the radiology domain. Of the 19 current workflow profiles, 11 of them were already available in 2003 (see black in the above list); the 8 new profiles in blue have been developed since 2003. Compared this list with the 12 workflow profiles available in 2003, only one: basic security, had been absorbed by other DICOM protocols and IHE workflow profiles. Note that the orders of these profiles have been rearranged from the original IHE profiles in 2003.

9.5.4 Some Examples of IHE Workflow Profiles

In this section we first present a sample IHE use case where the four actors and their roles are given as shown in Figure 9.9. Three examples follow. Example 1 is the Scheduled Workflow Profile within the radiology domain, which provides healthcare information that supports efficient patient care workflow in a typical imaging examination, as is depicted in Figure 9.10 (Carr and Moore, 2003). Two more examples in the radiology domain that are important for post-processing workflow (PWF) such as 3D reformats and handling key images (KIN) from imaging studies are shown in Figures 9.11 and 9.12.

9.5.5 The Future of IHE

9.5.5.1 *Multidisciplinary Effort* So far the main concentration of the IHE initiative has been mainly in radiology. The IHE Strategic Development Committee

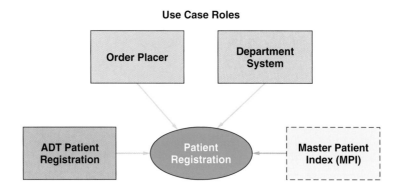

Use Case Roles

Actor: ADT (admission, discharge, transfer)
Role: Adds and modifies patient demographic and encounter information.
Actor: Order Placer
Role: Receives patient and encounter information for use in order entry.
Actor: Department System
Role: Receives and stores patient and encounter information for use in fulfilling orders by the Department System Scheduler.
Actor: MPI
Role: Receives patient and encounter information from multiple ADT systems. Maintains unique enterprise-wide identifier for a patient.

Figure 9.9 Sample IHE use case. The four actors and their respective roles are described.

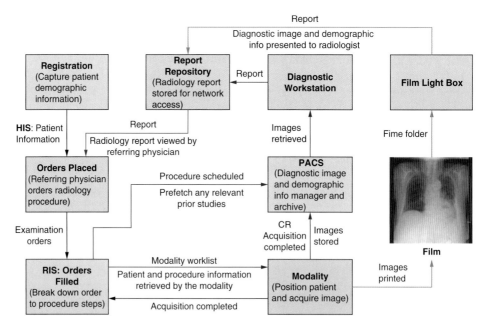

Figure 9.10 IHE scheduled workflow profile including three systems—HIS, RIS, and PACS—and two acquisition devices—conventional films with a digitizer and a CR.

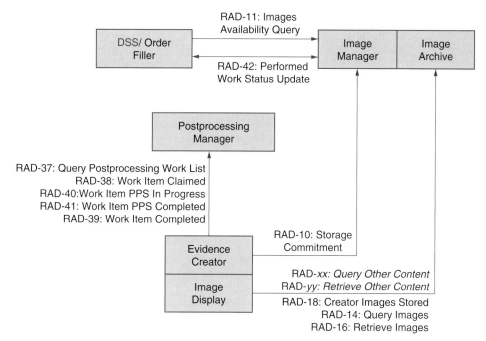

Figure 9.11   IHE Postprocessing workflow profile (PWF) for a radiology imaging study. This profile is used often in the integration of images from a third-party workstation (see Chapter 12) or in the integration of CAD with PACS (see Chapters 25 and 26). (Source: IHE)

was formed in September 2001; its members include representatives from multiple clinical and operational personnel, like cardiology, laboratory, pharmacy, medication administration, and interdepartmental information sharing. Work to identify key problems and expertise in these fields has progressed well. The eight new domains and the expanded domain radiology were presented earlier in Section 9.5.3.

9.5.5.2   *International Expansion*   IHE has expanded internationally. Demonstrations held in Europe and Japan have received the enthusiastic support of healthcare providers and vendors. Three additional goals have emerged: (1) develop a process to enable U.S.-based IHE initiative technology to be distributed globally, (2) document nationally based differences in healthcare policies and practices, and (3) seek the highest possible level of uniformity in medical information exchange. Figure 9.13 shows a scene from an IHE world workshop demonstration in 2006.

9.6   OTHER STANDARDS AND SOFTWARE

In Section 7.2.1 we listed some industry standards, protocols, computer operating systems, programming languages, workflow profiles that should be included in the PACS infrastructure design. Here we give more details on the five industrial software standards used commonly in PACS operation.

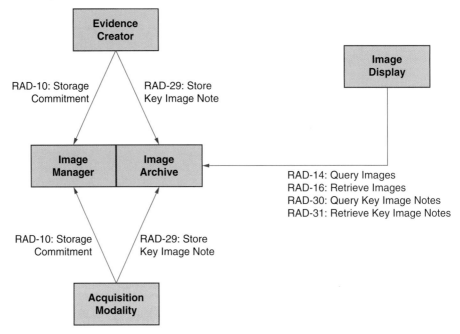

Figure 9.12   IHE key image note (KIN) workflow profile for a radiology imaging study. This profile is used often in the integration of CAD with PACS (see Chapters 25 and 26). (Source: IHE)

9.6.1 UNIX Operating System

The first UNIX operating system (System V) was developed by AT&T and released in 1983. Other versions of UNIX from different computer vendors include BSD (Berkeley Software Distribution by the University of California at Berkeley), Solaris (Sun Microsystems), HP-UX (Hewlett-Packard), Xenix (Microsoft), Ultrix (Digital Equipment Corporation), AIX (International Business Machines), and A/UX (Apple Computers).

Despite its many varieties the UNIX operating system provides an open system architecture for computer systems to facilitate the integration of complex software systems within individual systems and among different systems. UNIX offers great capability and high flexibility in networking, interprocess communication, multitasking, and security, which are essential to medical imaging applications. UNIX is mostly used in the server, PACS server, gateway, and specialized high-end workstations (WSs).

9.6.2 Windows NT/XP Operating Systems

Microsoft Windows NT and XP operating systems run on desktop personal computers (PCs) and are a derivative of the University of California at Berkeley's BSD UNIX. Windows NT and XP, like UNIX, support TCP/IP communications and multitasking, and therefore provide a low-cost software development platform for medical imaging applications in the PC environment. Windows NT is mostly used in WSs and low-end servers.

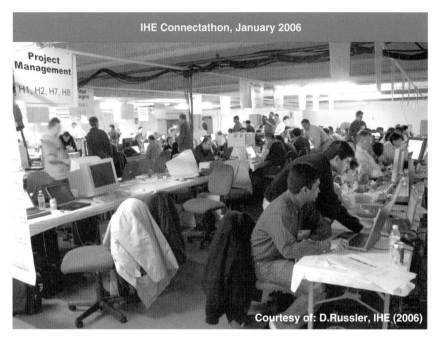

Figure 9.13   A demonstration scene during an IHE Integration Workshop in 2006. Over 100 vendors were involved in this worldwide connectathon, and during that year tested 5 technical frameworks with 37 integration profiles at major conferences world-wide, where 15 active national chapters from 4 continents participated.

9.6.3   C and C++ Programming Languages

The C programming language was simple and flexible, and it became one of the most popular programming languages in computing. C++, added to the C programming language, C++ is an object-oriented language that allows programmers to organize their software and process the information more effectively than most other programming languages. These two programming languages are used extensively in PACS application software packages.

9.6.4   SQL (Structural Query Language)

SQL (structured query language) is a standard interactive and programming language for querying, updating, and managing relational databases. SQL is developed from SEQUEL (structured English query language), developed by IBM. The first commercially available implementation of SQL was from Relational Software, Inc. (now Oracle Corporation).

   SQL is an interface to a relational database such as Oracle and Sybase. All SQL statements are instructions to operate on the database. Hence SQL is different from general programming languages such as C and C++. SQL provides a logical way to work with data for all types of users, including programmers, database administrators, and end users. For example, to query a set of rows from a table, the user defines a condition used to search the rows. All rows matching the condition are retrieved in a single step and can be passed as a unit to the user, to another SQL statement, or to a database application. The user does not need to deal with the rows one by one, or to worry about how the data are physically stored or retrieved. The following are the commands SQL provides for a wide variety of database tasks:

- Querying and retrieving data
- Inserting, updating, and deleting rows in a table
- Creating, replacing, altering, and dropping tables or other objects
- Controlling access to the database and its objects
- Guaranteeing database consistency and integrity

SQL is adopted by both ANSI (American National Standards Institute, 1986) and ISO (International Standards Organization, 1987), and many relational database management systems, such as IBM DB2 and ORACLE, support SQL. Therefore users can transfer all skills they have gained with SQL from one database to another. In addition all programs written in SQL are portable among many database systems. These database products have their proprietary extensions to the standard SQL, so very little modification usually is needed for the SQL program to be moved from one database to another. SQL is used most often in the DICOM query/retrieve operation.

9.6.5 XML (Extensible Markup Language)

XML, a system-independent markup language, is becoming the industry standard for data representation and exchange on World Wide Web, Intranet, and elsewhere. As a simple, flexible, extensible text format language, XML can describe information data in a standard or common format so that it makes data portable.

Although like HTML (hypertext markup language), which was used extensively over the past 10 years for easy data representation and display) XML uses tags to describe the data, it is significantly different from HTML. First, HTML mainly specifies how to display the data, whereas XML describes both the structure and the content of the data. This means that XML can be processed as data by programs, exchanged among computers as a data file, or displayed as Web pages, as HTML does. Second, there is a limit in HTML, where only those predefined tags can be used. However, XML is extensible, as mentioned above. The following are some advantages of XML:

1. Plain Text Format: Because since XML is a plain text, both programs and users can read and edit it.
2. Data Identification: XML describes the content of data, but not how to display it. It can be used in different ways by different applications
3. Reusability: XML entities can be included in an XML document as well as linked to other documents.
4. Easily Processed: Like HTML, XML also identifies the data with tags (identifiers enclosed < ... >), which are treated as "markup tags." Because of these tags, it is easy to build programs to parse and process XML files.
5. Extensibility: XML uses the concept of DTD (document type definition) to describe the structure of data and thus has the ability to define an entire database

schema. DTD can be used to translate between different database schema such as from Oracle schema to Sybase schema. Users can define their own tags to describe a particular type of document and can even define a schema, a file to define the structure for the XML document. The schema specifies what kinds of tags are used and how they are used in XML document. The best-known schema now is DTD, which is already integrated into XML1.0.

Because of these advantages, XML is increasingly popular among enterprises for the integration of data to be shared among departments within the enterprise and with those outside the enterprise.

For example, PACS includes different kinds of data, such as images, waveforms, and reports. A recently approved supplement, "Structured Reporting Object" (Section 9.4.6.4), is used for the transmission and storage of documents that describe or refer to the images, waveforms, or features they contain. XML is almost naturally fit for building this structure report because of its already structured text format, portability, and data identification mode. With a traditional file format, it is almost impossible to include an image and a waveform in one file because this is very hard for applications to parse and process. However, the XML-built structured report can easily link images, waveforms, and other type of reports together by simply including their link address. Therefore most application programs can parse and process it, making the XML-built structured report portable. XML is also good for storage of electronic patient record (ePR) (Section 7.6) and content mapping resource (Section 9.4.6) applications, which are similar to the structured report in that they require multiple forms of data and structured organization of data.

9.7 SUMMARY OF HL7, DICOM, AND IHE

In this chapter we presented two important industrial standards, HL7 for healthcare textual data and DICOM for medical imaging data and communications. HL7 has been a very stable standard for many years and is used widely. DICOM has been stabilized and readily accepted by the imaging industry. However, DICOM is still evolving to include other medical specialties, among these, radiation therapy, surgery, cardiology, and pathology.

IHE, on the other hand, is not a standard, but IHE workflow profiles have been developed to promote the use of DICOM and HL7. IHE is also evolving and has been expanded to over nine domains to include IT and other medical specialties such as radiology, radiation therapy, and surgery.

References

American Medical Association. *Current Procedural Terminology*. Chicago: AMA, 2001.

Carr C, Moore SM. IHE: a model for driving adoption of standards. *Comp Med Imag Graph* 27 (2–3): 137–46; 2003.

Channin DS. Integrating the healthcare enterprise: a primer. II. Seven brides for seven brothers: the IHE Integration Profiles *RadioGraphics* 21: 1343–50; 2001.

Channin D, Parisot C, Wanchoo V, Leontiew A, Siegel EL. Integrating the healthcare enterprise: a primer. III. What does IHE do for me? *RadioGraphics* 21: 1351–58; 2001a.

Channin DS, Siegel EL, Carr C, et al. Integrating the healthcare enterprise: a primer. V. The future of IHE *RadioGraphics* 21: 1605–8; 2001b.

DICOM Standard 2008. http://medical.nema.org/medical/dicom/2008.

DICOM Standard 2003. http://www.dclunie.com/dicom-status/status.html#BaseStandard 2001.

Health Level 7. http://www.hl7.org/.

Health Level 7—HL7 Version 3.0: Preview for CIOs, Managers and Programmers. http://www.neotool.com/company/press/199912_v3.htm#V3.0_preview.

Henderson M, Behel FM, Parisot C, Siegel EL, Channin DS. Integrating the healthcare enterprise: a primer. IV.The role of existing standards in IHE *RadioGraphics* 21: 1597–1603; 2001.

Huff SM, Rocha RA, McDonald CJ, et al. Development of the logical observation identifier: names and codes (LOINC) vocabulary. *J Am Med Info Assoc* 5: 276–92; 1998.

International Classification of Diseases, 9th revision. Washington, DC: U.S. Department of Health and Human Services, 2001. Publication 91–1260.

Internet Engineering Task Force. http://www.ietf.org.

Java web service tutorial. http://java.sun.com/webservices/docs/1.1/tutorial/doc/JavaWS Tutorial.pdf.

Oracle8 SQL Reference Release 8.0. Oracle 8 Documentation CD.

Radiological Society of North America Healthcare Information and Management Systems Society. IHE technical framework, year 3, version 4.6. Oak Brook, IL:RSNA, March 2001.

Recently Approved Supplements. http://medical.nema.org/.

Russler D. Integrating the healthcare enterprise (IHE). Overview in IHE Workshop, 2006.

Siegel EL, Channin DS. Integrating the healthcare enterprise: a primer—Part 1. Introduction *RadioGraphics* 21: 1339–41; 2001.

SQL. http://searchdatabase.techtarget.com/sDefinition/0,,sid13_gci214230,00.html.

XML. http://searchwebservices.techtarget.com/sDefinition/0,,sid26_gci213404,00.html.

CHAPTER 10

Image Acquisition Gateway

The image acquisition gateway computer (gateway) with a set of software programs is used as a buffer between image acquisition and the PACS server. Figure 10.1 shows how this chapter corresponds to the PACS fundamentals content of Part II. Figure 10.2 depicts the gateway in the PACS data flow. In this chapter the terms acquisition gateway computer, gateway computer, acquisition gateway, and gateway have the same meaning.

10.1 BACKGROUND

Several acquisition devices (modalities) can share one gateway. The gateway has three primary tasks: (1) it acquires image data from the radiological imaging device, (2) it converts the data from manufacturer data format specifications to the PACS image data standard format (header format, byte-ordering, matrix sizes) that is compliant with the DICOM data formats, and (3) it forwards the image study to the PACS server or directly to the PACA workstations (WSs). Additional tasks in the gateway are some image pre-processing, compression, and data security. An acquisition gateway has the following characteristics:

1. It preserves the image data integrity transmitted from the imaging device.
2. Its operation is transparent to the users and totally or highly automatic.
3. It delivers images timely to the PACS server and WSs.
4. It performs some image preprocessing functions to facilitate image display.

Among all PACS major components, establishing a reliable gateway in PACS is the most difficult task for a number of reasons. First, a gateway must interface with many imaging modalities and PACS modules made by different imaging manufacturers. These modalities and modules have their own image format and communication protocols that sometime can make the interface task difficult. Even most imaging equipment now follows the DICOM standard; the PACS integrator must negotiate several DICOM conformance statements (see Chapter 9) for a successful interface. Second, performing radiological examinations with an imaging device requires the operator's input, such as entering the patient's name, identification, accession number; and then forwarding images to WSs and server. During this process the potential

PACS and Imaging Informatics, Second Edition, by H. K. Huang
Copyright © 2010 John Wiley & Sons, Inc.

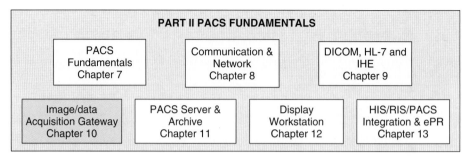

Figure 10.1   Position of Chapter 10 in the organization of this book. Color codes are used to highlight components and workflow in chapters of Part II.

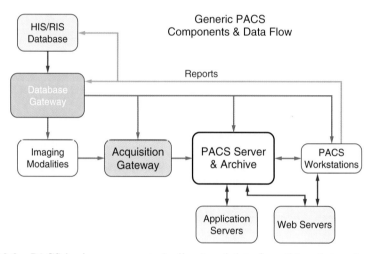

Figure 10.2   PACS basic components (yellow) and data flow (blue: Internal; green and red: external between PACS and other information systems); other information systems (light blue); the color of the gateway (red). HIS: hospital information system; RIS: radiology information system.

for human error is unavoidable. A very minor error from input may have a severe impact on the integrity of the PACS data. We discuss this issue in later sections and in Chapter 19 on PACS pitfalls and bottlenecks. Third, ideally the gateway should be 100% automatic for efficiency and minimizing system errors. However, to achieve a totally automatic component without much human interaction and with equipment from varied manufacturers is very challenging. The degree of difficulty and the cost necessary to achieve this have been focal issues in PACS design.

Automated image acquisition from imaging devices to the PACS controller plays an important role in a PACS infrastructure. The word "automatic" is important here, since relying on labor-intensive manual acquisition methods would defeat the purpose of the PACS. An important measure of the success of an automatic acquisition is its effectiveness in ensuring the integrity and availability of patient images in a PACS system. Because most imaging devices are now DCIOM compliant, this chapter only discusses methods related to the DICOM gateway. For imaging devices that still use an older interface method like light imaging, a DICOM converter has to be available in the gateway to comply with DCIOM image format standard. This chapter first discusses a group of topics related to DICOM interface: the DICOM compliant gateway, the automatic image recovery scheme for DICOM conformance imaging devices, interface with other existing PACS modules, and the DICOM broker.

Because an imaging gateway also performs certain image preprocessing functions to facilitate image archive and display, the second group of topics considers some image preprocessing functions commonly used in PACS. The third topic is the concept of multilevel adaptive processing control in the gateway, which ensures reliability of the gateway as well as the image integrity. This is important because, when the acquisition gateway has to deal with DICOM formatting, communication, and many image preprocessing functions, multiple-level processing with a queuing mechanism is necessary. The last topic is on clinical experience with the acquisition gateway.

10.2   DICOM-COMPLIANT IMAGE ACQUISITION GATEWAY

10.2.1   DICOM Compliance

DICOM conformance (compliance) by manufacturers is a major factor contributing to the interoperability of different medical imaging systems in clinical environment. We describe the DICOM standard in Chapter 9, in which it defines the basis of the interface mechanism allowing image communication between different manufacturers' systems. With the standardized interface mechanism, the task of acquiring images from the DICOM-compliant imaging systems becomes simpler. Figure 10.3 shows the connection between the imaging device and the acquisition gateway computer.

The DICOM-compliant imaging device on the left is the C-Store Client, and the image acquisition gateway on the right is the C-Store Server (see Fig. 9.6). They are connected by a network running the DICOM TCP/IP transmissions (see Section

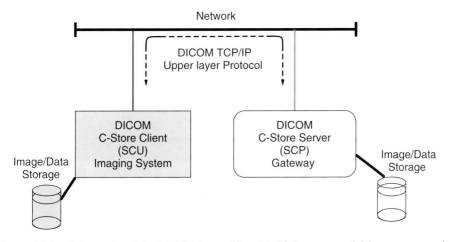

Figure 10.3   Schematic of the DICOM compliant PACS image acquisition gateway with the DICOM C-STORE SOP connecting the imaging device (SCU) to the gateway (SCP).

8.1.2, Fig. 8.4). Regardless of whether a "push" from the scanner or a "pull" operation from the gateway should be used (see Section 7.1.1), one image is transmitted at one time, and the order of transmission depends on the database architecture of the scanner. After these images have been received, the gateway must know how to organize them to form series and studies according to the DICOM data model so that image data integrity is not compromised.

In the gateway a database management system serves three functions. First, it supports the transaction of each individual image transmitted by the modality and received by the acquisition. Second, it monitors the status of the patient studies and their associated series during the transmission. Third, it provides the basis for the automatic image recovery scheme to detect unsuccessfully transferred images. Three database tables based on the DICOM data model of the real world (see Fig. 9.3*B*) are used: study, series, and images. Each table contains a group of records, and each record contains a set of useful data elements. For the study and series database tables, the study name and the series name are the primary keys for searching. In addition the following major data elements are recorded:

1. Patient name and hospital identification number.
2. Dates and times when the study and series were created in the imaging. device and acquired in the gateway.
3. The number of acquired images per series.
4. Time stamp of each image when it is acquired by the gateway.
5. Acquisition status.
6. DICOM unique identification (UID) value for the study and series.

By the DICOM standard used to transmit images, one image is transmitted at a time; the order of transmission does not necessarily follow the order of scan, series, or study. The image device's job queue priority dictates what job needs to be processed next in the scanner's computer, and is always in favor of the scanning and image reconstruction rather than the communication. For this reason an image waiting in the queue to be transmitted next can be bumped and can lose its priority and be placed in the lower priority waiting queue for a long period of time without being discovered. The result is a temporary loss of images in a series and in a study. If this is not discovered early enough, the images may be lost permanently because of various system conditions, for example, a system reboot, disk maintenance, or premature closing of the patient image file at the gateway. Neither a temporary nor a permanent loss of images is acceptable in PACS operation. We must consider an error recovery mechanism to regain images that are temporarily lost.

10.2.2 DICOM-Based PACS Image Acquisition Gateway

10.2.2.1 Gateway Computer Components and Database Management

The acquisition gateway shown in Figure 10.4 consists of four elementary software components: database management system (DBMS), local image storage, storage service class provider (SCP), and storage service class user (SCU); and three error handling and image recovery software components: Q/R SCU, Integrity Check, and Acquisition Delete. The elementary components are discussed in this section; error handling and image recovery components will be discussed in Section 10.3.

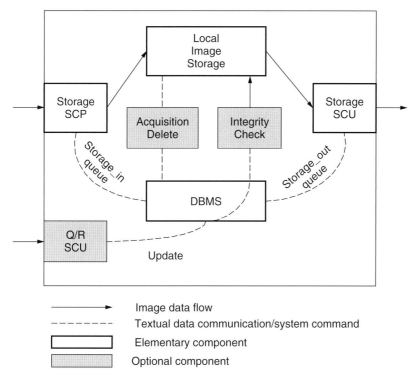

Figure 10.4 Acquisition gateway components and their workflow. The four elementary components are storage SCP, storage SCU, local image storage, and DBMS. The three error-handling and image recovery software components (shaded) are Q/R SCU, integrity check, and acquisition delete.

Database Management System (DBMS)   The local database of the gateway records structurally the textual information about images, problematic images, queues, and imaging devices. It is controlled and managed by DBMS. Because the textual information will be deleted after the archiving is completed, small-scale DBMS, such as Access and MySQL commercial products, is adequate to support normal operation of image acquisition to the gateway. The DBMS mounts extendable database file(s) in which the textual data are actually stored.

The information about image data can be basically stored in four tables: Patient, Study, Series, and Image (see Fig. 9.3*B*). As shown in Figure 10.5, these tables are linked hierarchically with primary and foreign key pairs. Their primary keys uniquely identify each record in these tables. The primary and foreign keys are denoted by (*) and (#), respectively, in Figure 10.5. The Patient table records some demographic data such as patient ID, name, sex, and birth date. The Study and Series tables record infor mation such as the date and time when each study and series are created in the imaging device and acquired in the acquisition gateway and the instance unique identification (UID) of each study and series. The study and series instance UIDs are important for image recovery as discussed in Section 10.3. The Image table records generic image information such as orientation, offset, window, and level values of the images stored before and after image preprocessing. The file name and path are

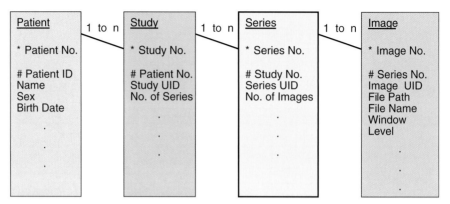

Figure 10.5   Gateway computer database management hierarchies for Patient, Study, Series, and Image tables. (*) denotes primary key and (#), foreign key.

defined for each record in the Image table, providing a link to the local image storage, which can be used to check the integrity of image stored. The records of problematic images are stored in a set of wrong-image tables, which can be displayed to alert the system administrator through a graphical interface.

A set of queue tables is used to record the details of each transaction, such as status (executing, pending, fail, or succeed), date in, time in, date out, and time out. Transactions including storage/routing and query/retrieve can be traced with these tables. The records of the modalities are defined in a set of imaging device tables that provide the generic information of the modalities, including AE title, host name, IP address, and physical location.

Local Image Storage   Local image storage is storage space in the hard disk of the gateway computer. It is a folder that is supported by the operating system and allows full access from any background services so that the local storage SCP and SCU (see Section 9.4.5) acting as automatic background services can deposit and fetch images from this folder. Images from imaging devices are accepted and stored one by one into this storage space. However, the images are not necessarily received in the order in the series. During the transmission from imaging devices to the gateway there is the possibility of image loss (as discussed in Section 8.3). The location of the folder is prespecified during the installation of the acquisition gateway and can be changed during the operation. The change of storage space location will not affect the integrity of the image storage because the file path and name of every image is individually defined at each record in the Image table of DBMS.

Configuring the storage SCP to automatically create subfolders under the storage folder is optional. The subfolders can make a clear classification of the images transparent to the file system. Also the records in the Patient, Study, Series, and Image tables of the local database can be easily recovered from DBMS failure without any database backup or decoding of the image files. So it is advantageous for the system administrator to trace the images in the file system during troubleshooting. Figure 10.6 and Figure 10.7 show two examples of folder structures used for image storage in PCs. The folder structure of the first example uses one layer of subfolders named by auto numbers. Image files in the same series accepted within the same time interval will be grouped into the same subfolder. Each subfolder can be considered as a transaction, and thus the system administrator can easily trace the problem images based on the creation date and time of the subfolders. In the second example, a complete folder structure is used that specifies patient ID, modality, accession number, study date, and study time as the names of subfolders. This structure is very useful for database recovery and storage integrity check.

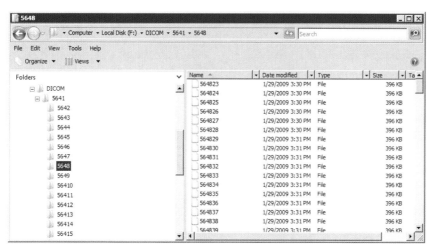

Figure 10.6 "Images" folder (56.48), left, is the storage space and subfolders (right) named by auto-numbers group the images of the same series stored at the same time interval (56.48.23 1/29/2009 3:30 PM), ...

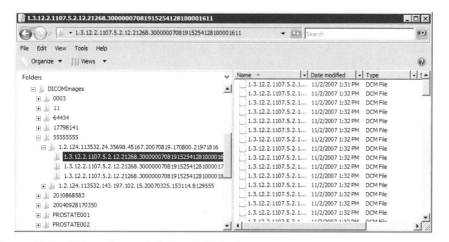

Figure 10.7 "DicomImages" folder (left) is the storage space and the hierarchy of the subfolders according to the order of "Patient ID" (55555555), "Modality" (1.3.12.2 ...) (right), "Accession number_study date_study time" (1.3.12.2 ... 11/2/2007 1:31 PM), and an auto-number. The file names of the images are their image instance UIDs.

The disk storage capacity of the acquisition gateway is expected to be capable of storing images from an imaging device temporarily until these images are archived in the PACS server. Because of the limited capacity, those temporary images in the hard disk must be deleted so as to free up space for new incoming images.

Storage SCP   The purpose of the C-Store server class of the Storage SCP is to receive the C-Store request from the imaging device or the PACS module. The image data will be accepted by the gateway and then temporarily stored in the local image storage. The server class also inserts the corresponding records into the "storage_in" queue table of the local database of the acquisition gateway. The completion of the storing action will update the status of these records to "completed." New records will also be inserted into the "storage_out" queue table to prepare for routing images to the PACS server. The storage SCP is implemented in the system background.

Storage SCU   The purpose of the C-Store client class of the storage SCU is to send the C-Store request to the PACS server when new records are found in the "storage_out" queue table of the local database. The images stored in the local image storage will be routed to the PACS server by this client class. After the routing is completed, the status of the corresponding records in the "storage_out" queue table will be changed to "completed."

10.2.2.2 *Determination of the End of an Image Series*   If DICOM transmits images one by one from the imaging modality like a CT scanner to the gateway, but not necessarily in order, how does the gateway know when a series or a study is completed and when it should close the study file for archive or display? The images of a series and/or a study can only be grouped together by a formatting process when the end of series and/or the end of study is determined, respectively, by the image receiving process. To algorithmically determine the end of a series in a manner both accurate and efficiently is not trivial. We present three algorithms for determining the end of series and discuss the advantages and drawbacks of these algorithms.

Algorithm 1: Presence of the Next Series   The first algorithm for detecting the end of a series is based on the presence of the next series. This algorithm assumes that the total number of images for the current series would have been transmitted to the gateway before the next series began. In this case the presence of the first image of the next series indicates the termination of the previous series. The success of the method depends on the following two premises: (1) the imaging device transmits the images to the gateway in the order of the scan, and (2) no images are lost during the transmission. Note that the first assumption depends on the specific order of image transmission by the imaging system. If the imaging system transmits the image slices in an ordered sequence (e.g., GE Medical Systems MR Signa 5.4 or up), this method can faithfully group the images of a series without errors. On the other hand, if the imaging system transfers the image slices at random (e.g., Siemens MR Vision), this method may conclude the end of a series incorrectly. Even though one could verify the second assumption by checking the order of the image, whether or not the last image has been transmitted remains unknown to the gateway. Another drawback of this method relates to the determination of the last series of a particular study, which is based on the presence of the first image of the next study. The time delay for this determination could be lengthy because the next study may not begin immediately after the first series; for example, there may be a delay of the exam from next patient.

Algorithm 2: Constant Number of Images in a Given Time Interval   The second method for determining the end of a series is based on a time interval criterion. The hypothesis of this method assumes that an image series should be completed within a certain period of time. By this method, the end of a series is determined when the acquisition time of the first image plus a designated time interval has elapsed. This method is obviously straightforward and simple, but a static time interval criterion is not practical in a clinical environment. Thus an alternative recourse uses the concept of the constant number of images in a time interval.

This method requires recording the number of acquired images for a given series at two different times, time t_1 and time $t_2 = t_1 + \Delta t$, for some predetermined constant Δt. By comparing the number of images acquired at time t_1 versus the number of images acquired at time t_2, a premise is constructed for determining whether or not the series is completed. If, for example, the number of images is a constant, we conclude that the series is completed; otherwise, the series is not yet completed. This process (Δt with number of images verification) is iterated until a constant number of images has been reached. Next, let us consider how to select Δt: Should it be a static number or dynamic? A short Δt may result in missing images, whereas a long Δt may result in lengthy and inefficient image acquisition. Usually the first Δt chosen for this method is empirical, depending on the imaging protocols used by the imaging system. For example, if the imaging protocol frequently used in a scanner generates many images per series, then Δt should be long; otherwise, a shorter Δt is preferred. However, it is possible that for a shorter Δt this method may conclude a series prematurely. This is because in some rare cases the technologist or clinician may interrupt the scanning process in the middle of a series to adjust alignment of the patient or to inject a contrast agent. If the time it takes to conduct such procedures is longer than Δt, then images obtained after the procedure would not be grouped into the current series. In a poorly designed PACS, this could result in a severe problem—missing images in a series.

Should Δt be dynamic during the iteration? One thought is that the number of images transmitted from the imaging device to the gateway decreases while the iteration cycle increases. Therefore it seems reasonable that Δt may be reduced proportionally to the number iterations. On the other hand, the number of images transmitted to the gateway may vary with time depending on the design of the imaging device. For example, an imaging device may be designed to transmit images according to the imaging system workload and priority schedule. If the image transmission process has a low priority, then the number of images transmitted during a period when the system workload is heavy will be lower compared with when the workload is light. In this case Δt is a variable.

Algorithm 3: Combination of Algorithm 1 and Algorithm 2   Given the previous discussions, a combination of both methods seems to be preferable. Algorithm 3 can be implemented in three steps:

1. Identify and count the acquired images for a particular series.
2. Record the time stamp whenever the number of acquired images has changed.

3. Update the acquisition status of the series.

The acquired images can be tracked by using a transaction table designed in association with the series database table discussed in Section 10.2.2.1. We first start with the time interval method.

Whenever an image is acquired from the imaging device, a record of the image is created in the transaction table identified by the modality type, the imaging system identification, the study number, the series number, the image number, and the acquisition time stamp. A tracking system can be developed based on these records. Three major events during the current iteration are recorded in the transaction table:

1. The number of acquired images.
2. The t_2 value.
3. The acquisition status declaring the series as standby, ongoing, completed, or image missing.

Here the information regarding the number of acquired images and acquisition status is useful for the maintenance of the image-receiving process. If the series is ongoing, the comparison time is updated for the verification of the number of images during the next iteration.

After the interval method detects the end of a series, it can be further verified by the "presence of the next series" method. If the next series exists in the series database table or the next study exists in the study table, the image series is determined as complete. Otherwise, one more iteration is executed, and the series remains in standby status. In this case the end of the series will be concluded in the next iteration regardless of the existence of the next series or study. In general, Δt can be set at 10 minutes. This way the completeness of an image series is verified by both methods and the potential lengthy time delay problem of the first method is minimized.

10.3 AUTOMATIC IMAGE RECOVERY SCHEME FOR DICOM CONFORMANCE DEVICE

10.3.1 Missing Images

Images can be missing at the gateway computer when they are transmitted from the imaging device. For example, consider an MRI scanner using the DICOM C-Store client to transfer images with one of the following three modes: auto-transfer, auto-queue, or manual-transfer. Only one transfer mode can be in operation at a time. The auto-transfer mode transmits an image whenever it is available, the auto-queue mode transfers images only when the entire study has been completed, and the manual-transfer mode allows the transfer of multiple images, series, or studies. Under normal operation the auto-transfer mode is routinely used and the manual transfer mode is used only when a retransmission is required. Once the DICOM communication between the scanner and the gateway has been established, if the technologist changes the transfer mode for certain clinical reasons in the middle of the transmission, some images could be temporarily lost. In the next section we discuss an automatic recovery method for these images.

10.3.2 Automatic Image Recovery Scheme

10.3.2.1 Basis for the Image Recovery Scheme   The automatic image recovery scheme includes two tasks: identifying the missing studies, series, or images; and recovering them accordingly. This scheme requires that the gateway can access the scanner image database. These two tasks can be accomplished by using the DICOM query/retrieve service class (Section 9.4.5.2) in conjunction with the gateway database described in Section 10.2.2.1. The operation mechanism of the Query-Retrieve service involves three other DICOM service classes: C-Find, C-Move, and C-Store. The task of identifying missing studies is through the C-Find by matching one of the image grouping hierarchies, such as study level or series level, between the gateway database and the scanner database. The missing image(s) can be *recovered* by the C-Move and C-Store service classes. The query/retrieve (Q/R) operation is executed via a client process at the gateway computer and the MRI scanner computer (as an example) as the server.

10.3.2.2 The Image Recovery Algorithm   Figure 10.8 shows the steps of the automatic image recovery algorithm. There are two steps: recover studies and recover series or images.

Recovery of Missing Study   In this step the Q/R client encodes a C-Find query object containing the major information elements such as image study level and a zero-length UID value (unique identification value) defined by the DICOM standard. The zero-length UID prompts the Q/R server to return every single UID for the queried level. Then the query/retrieve server responds with all the matching objects in the scanner database according to the requested image study level. The content of each responded object mainly includes information such as a study number and the corresponding study UID. The information of each responded object is then compared with the records in the gateway database. Those study numbers that are in the responded objects but not recorded in the PACS gateway database are considered missing studies. Each of the missing studies can be retrieved by issuing a C-Move object from the gateway, which is equivalent to an image retrieval request. Because the retrieval is study specific, the study UID must be included in the C-Move object explicitly. In the scanner, after the C-Move object is received by the query/retrieve server, it relays the retrieval request to the C-Store client. As a result the study transfer is actually conducted by the C-Store client and server processes.

Recovery of Missing Series/Image   Recovering missing series or images can be performed with the same recovery mechanism as for the study/image level. The difference between the study level and the series level in the recovery scheme is that a specific study UID must be encoded in the C-Find query object for the series level or the image level as opposed to a zero-length UID for the study level.

The records of available images in the scanner database and the gateway database may not synchronize. This situation can happen during a current study when its associated series and images are being generated in the scanner but not yet transferred to the gateway. This asynchronization can result in incorrect identification because the image recovery process may mistake the current study listed in the scanner database for a missing one because it has not been transferred to the gateway. To avoid this, the responded objects from the Q/R server are first sorted in chronological

GATEWAY COMPUTER   **COMPUTER AT THE SCANNER**

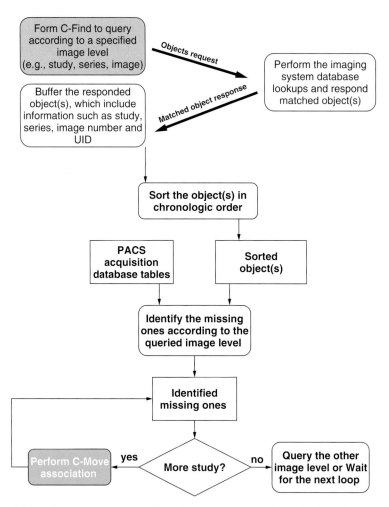

Figure 10.8 General processing flow diagram of the automatic DICOM query-retrieve image recovery scheme. The scheme starts by the acquisition computer issuing a C-Find command (purple, upper left). The recovery starts by a C-Move command (lower left, green). Both commands are received by the imaging device's query/retrieve computer.

order by study creation date and time. If the creation date and time of the most recent study is less than a predefined time interval compared with the current time, it is considered to be the study being generated by the scanner. Thus the image recovery process will not identify the most recent study as a missing study.

Algorithms of determination of the end of an image series and automatic image recovery schemes discussed in Sections 10.2.2.2 and 10.3, had been implemented by most manufacturers in their 3-D or 4-D imaging acquisition schemes. The image acquisition gateway performance was improved dramatically over the past four years. But certain human errors may still exist. Should any recovery errors occur, the contents of these sections should provide some clues for solutions.

10.4 INTERFACE OF A PACS MODULE WITH THE GATEWAY COMPUTER

10.4.1 PACS Modality Gateway and HI-PACS (Hospital Integrated) Gateway

In Section 10.2 we discussed the DICOM image acquisition gateway. This gateway can also be used to interface with a PACS module. A *PACS module* is loosely defined as a self-contained mini PACS comprised of some imaging devices, a short-term archive, a database, some display workstations, and a communication network linking these components together. In practice, the module can function alone as a self-contained integrated imaging unit in which the workstations can show images from the imaging devices. However, without the integration with the general PACS, it will remain as an isolated system, images from this PACS module would not be able to communicate with the PACS database, and vice versa. In the following we give two examples of interfacing the gateway with two PACS modules: US module and dedicated 3-D MRI breast imaging module; both are stand-alone modules in their own respective subspecialty areas. Other PACS modules that can be interfaced to the HI-PACS are the nuclear medicine PACS module, the emergency room module, the ambulatory care module, and the teleradiology module. The requirements for interfacing these modules are an individual specialized DICOM gateway (like the US gateway, or the MRI gateway) in the respective module with DICOM commands for communication and DICOM format for the image file. Multiple modules can be connected to the HI-PACS by using several pairs of acquisition gateways as shown in Figures 10.9 and 10.10.

10.4.2 Example 1: Interface the US Module with the PACS Gateway

The first example is to interface the gateway with an ultrasound (US) PACS module. The US module consists of several US scanners, some WSs with tailored software for displaying US images which are connected to an US server with short-term archive (several weeks) of examinations. There are certain advantages in connecting the US module to a hospital integrated PACS (HI-PACS). First, once connected, US images can be appended into the same patient's PACS image folder (or database) and sharing the general PACS worklist and forming a complete file for long-term archiving. Second, US images can be shown with other modality images in the PACS general display workstations for cross modality comparisons. Third, some other modality images can also be shown in the US module's specialized workstations. In this case, care must be taken because the specialized workstation (e.g., US workstation) may not have the full capability for displaying images from other modalities.

A preferred method of interfacing a PACS module with the HI-PACS is to treat the US PACS module as an imaging device. Two gateways would be needed, one for US PACS gateway connected to the US server, and a PACS image acquisition gateway connected to the HI-PACS. These two gateways are connected by using the method

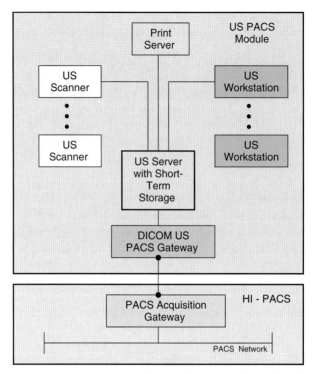

Figure 10.9   Connection of an US PACS module to the HI-PACS. Two gateways are used: US PACS gateway (purple) and HI-PACS gateway (blue).

described in Section 10.2. Figure 10.9 shows the connection of the two gateways. Each patient's image file in the US server contains the full-sized color or black-and-white images (compressed or original), thumbnail (quarter sized) images for indexing, and image header information for DICOM conversion. In the US gateway computer, several processes are running concurrently. The first process is a daemon constantly checking for new US examinations arriving from scanners. When one is found, the gateway uses a second process to convert the file to the DICOM format. Because a color US image file is normally larger (Section 4.6), a third process compresses it to a smaller file, normally with a 3:1 ratio (see Section 6.7.3). The US gateway generates a DICOM send command to transmit the compressed DICOM file to the PACS acquisition gateway computer, by using DICOM TCP/IP transmission. In the PACS acquisition gateway computer, several daemons are running concurrently also. The first is a DICOM command that checks for the DICOM *send* command from the US gateway. Once the *send* command is detected, the second daemon checks the proper DICOM format and saves the information in the PACS gateway computer. The third daemon queues the file to be stored by the PACS server's long-term archive.

To request other modality images from a US workstation, the patient's image file is first Q/R from the PACS long-term archive. The archive transmits the file to the HI-PACS gateway, which sends it to the US PACS gateway. The US gateway computer transmits the file to the US server and then the WS.

10.4.3 Example 2: Interface the 3-D Dedicated Breast MRI Module with the PACS

The second example is to interface the 3-D dedicated breast (DB) MRI module with the PACS through the gateway. The MRI module could have several DB MRI systems forming an enterprise level breast imaging center. The center performs 3-D MRI breast imaging of the patient and compares results with those from historical images of the patient obtained using other breast imaging modalities including US, mammography, and digital mammography. The center also performs breast biopsy and treats the patient.

This example is different from the US images of example 1 in the sense that to integrate US exam results with the total PACS, the US images are reviewed with other exams from the PACS WS. In the breast imaging example, the purpose of integration is to retrieve the patient's other breast-related images from the PACS existing database where the patient has had past breast imaging examinations. The 3-D DB MRI breast images are then integrated with those historical breast images in an electronic patient record (ePR), and reviewed at any WS of the enterprise breast center before the treatment. This section describes the method of integration in the gateway level; the methods of storage of all breast related images, and the treatment process will be discussed in other chapters of the book. Figure 10.10 depicts the connection of breast imaging of the same patient.

10.5 DICOM OR PACS BROKER

10.5.1 Concept of the PACS Broker

The PACS broker is an interface between the radiology information system (RIS) and the PACS (or HIS when RIS is a component of HIS). There are very few direct connections between a RIS and a PACS because most current RIS can only output important patient demographic and exam information in HL7 format (Section 9.2), which is a format that most PACS cannot receive and interpret. A PACS broker acts as an interface by processing the HL7 messages received by different RIS systems and mapping the data into easily customizable database tables. Then it can process requests made by various PACS components and provide them with the proper data format and content.

Figure 10.11 shows the architecture and functions of the PACS broker. It receives HL7 messages from the RIS and maps them into its own customizable database tables. PACS components can then request from the broker specific data and formats. These include the DICOM worklist for an acquisition modality, scheduled exams for prefetching, patient location for automatic distribution of PACS exams to workstations in the hospital ward areas, and radiology reports for PACS viewing workstations.

10.5.2 An Example of Implementation of a PACS Broker

The following is an example of how a PACS broker is implemented, provided that the hospital site has an existing RIS. The hospital plans to implement PACS; however, the PACS needs particular information from the RIS. No interface is available between

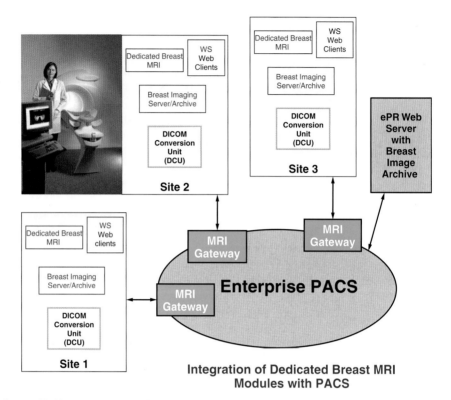

Figure 10.10 Integration of a dedicated breast MRI module with the enterprise PACS. The module has three breast MRI scanners, each connected to the enterprise PACS with a MRI gateway. Each MRI system has a scanner, a server/archive, a DICOM conversion unit (DCU), and a Web-based WS allowing the viewing of 3-D breast MR images as well other breast images from the Web-based ePR of the same patient. Through the gateways, all patients connected to the enterprise PACS can be viewed at any WS of any site. Sections 21.6.3 and 21.6.4 Figure 21.18 present the Data Grid method for ePR Web server archive of 3-D MRI and other breast images from the patient's historical exams. Note that this figure shows the gateway concept of connectivity, whereas Figure 21.18 presents the complete enterprise architecture. (Courtesy of Aurora Imaging Technology, Inc.)

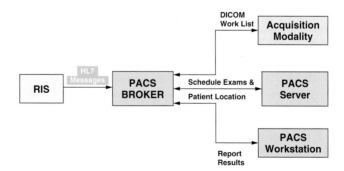

Figure 10.11 Functions of a PACS (DICOM) broker.

the existing RIS and the new PACS to transfer the data. Therefore a commercial broker is purchased and implemented to act as an interface between the two systems. The RIS can output HL7 messages triggered by particular events in the radiology workflow (e.g., exam scheduled, exam dictated, exam completed).

The broker receives the HL7 messages from the RIS. Following the specifications provided by the RIS, the broker has been precon figured to map the incoming HL7 message data into particular fields of its own database tables. The PACS components can now communicate directly with the broker to make requests for information. Some important data that are requested by PACS are as follows:

1. A worklist of scheduled exams for an acquisition modality.
2. Radiology reports and related patient demographic and exam information for PACS viewing workstations.
3. Patient location for automatic distribution of PACS exams to WSs in the wards.
4. Scheduled exam information for prefetching by the PACS server to PACS WSs.

These requests are in addition to general patient demographic data and exam data that are needed to populate a DICOM header of a PACS exam.

10.6 IMAGE PREPROCESSING

In addition to receiving images from imaging devices, the gateway computer performs certain image preprocessing functions before images are sent to the PACS server or WSs. There are two categories of preprocessing functions. The first relates to the image format—for example, a conversion from the manufacturer's format to a DICOM-compliant format of the PACS. This category of preprocessing involves mostly data format conversion, as was described in Section 9.4.1. The second category of preprocessing prepares the image for optimal viewing at the PACS WS. To achieve optimal display, an image should have the proper size, good initial display parameters (a suitable lookup table; see Chapter 12), and proper orientation; any visual distracting background should be removed.

Preprocessing function is modality specific in the sense that each imaging modality has a specific set of preprocessing requirements. Some preprocessing functions may work well for certain modalities but poorly for others. In the remainder of this section we discuss preprocessing functions according to each modality.

10.6.1 Computed Radiography (CR) and Digital Radiography (DR)

10.6.1.1 Reformatting   A CR image have three popular sizes (given here in inches) depending on the type of imaging plates used: $L = 14 \times 17$, $H = 10 \times 12$, or $B = 8 \times 10$ (high-resolution plate). These plates give rise to 1760×2140, 1670×2010, and 2000×2510 matrices, respectively (or similar matrices dependent on manufacturers). There are two methods of mapping a CR image matrix size to a given size LCD monitor. First, because display monitor screens vary in pixel sizes, a reformatting of the image size from these three different plate dimensions may be necessary in order to fit a given monitor. In the reformat preprocessing function, because both the image and the monitor size are known, a mapping between the size of the image and the screen is first established. We use as an example two of the most commonly used screen sizes: 1024×1024 and 2048×2048. If the size of an input image is larger than 2048×2048, the reformatting takes two steps. First, a two-dimensional bilinear interpolation is performed to shrink the image at a 5:4 ratio in both directions; this means that an image size of 2000×2510 is reformatted to 1600×2008. Second, a suitable number of blank lines are added to extend the size to 2048×2048. If a 1024×1024 image is desired, a further subsampling ratio of 2:1 from the 2048 image is performed. For imaging plates that produce pixel matrix sizes smaller than 2048×2048, the image is extended to 2048×2048 by adding blank lines and then subsampling (if necessary) to obtain a 1024×1024 image.

The second method is to center the CR image on the screen without altering its size. For an image size smaller than the screen, the screen is filled with blank (black) pixels and lines. For an image size larger than the screen, only a portion of the image is displayed; a scroll function is used to roam the image (see Chapter 12). Similar methods can be used for DR images.

10.6.1.2 Background Removal

The second CR preprocessing function is to remove the image background due to X-ray collimation. In pediatric, extremity, and other special localized body part images, collimation can result in the inclusion of significant white background that should be removed in order to reduce unwanted background in the image during soft copy display. This topic was extensively discussed in Section 3.3.4, with results shown in Figure 3.15.

After background removal, the image size will be different from the standard L, H, and B sizes. To center an image such that it occupies the full monitor screen, it Is advantageous to automatically zoom and scroll the background removed image in the center of the screen for an optimal display. Zoom and scroll functions are standard image processing functions and are discussed in Chapter 12. Similar methods can be applied to DR images.

10.6.1.3 Automatic Orientation

The third CR preprocessing function is automatic orientation. "Properly oriented" means that when the image displayed on a monitor, it is custom by the radiologist's reading the hard cope from a light box. Depending on the orientation of the imaging plate with respect to the patient, there are eight possible orientations (see Figure 10.12). An image can be oriented correctly by rotating it $90°$ clockwise, $90°$ counterclockwise, or $180°$, or by the y-axis flipped.

AP or PA Chest   The algorithm first determines the body region from the image header. Three common body regions are the chest, abdomen, and extremities. Let us first consider the automatic orientation of the anterior–posterior (AP) or PA chest images. For AP or PA chest images, the algorithm searches for the location of three characteristic objects: spine, abdomen, and neck or upper extremities. To find the spine and abdomen, horizontal and vertical pixel value profiles (or line scans), evenly distributed through the image, are taken. The average density of each profile is calculated and placed in a horizontal or a vertical profile table. The two tables are searched for local maxima to find a candidate location. Before a decision is made regarding which of the two possible (horizontal or vertical) orientations marks the spine, it is necessary to search for the densest area that could belong to either the abdomen or the head. To find this area, an average density value is computed over

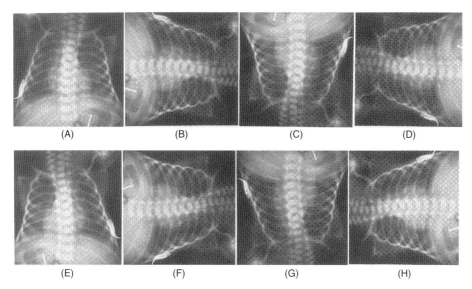

Figure 10.12   Eight possible orientations of an A–P chest radiograph: the automatic orientation program determines the body region shown and adjusts it to the proper orientation for viewing. (Courtesy of Dr. E. Pietka)

two consecutive profiles taken from the top and bottom of both tables. The maximum identifies the area to be searched. From the results of these scans and computations, the orientation of the spine is determined to be either horizontal or vertical.

Neck or Upper Extremities   A threshold image (threshold at the image's average gray value) is used to find the location of the neck or upper extremities along the axis perpendicular to the spine. The threshold marks the external contours of the patient and separates them from the patient background (the area that is exposed but outside the patient). Profiles of the threshold image are scanned in a direction perpendicular to the spine (identified earlier). For each profile, the width of the intersection between the scan line and the contour of the patent is recorded. Then the upper extremities for an AP or PA image are found on the basis of the ratios of minimum and maximum intersections for the threshold image profiles. This ratio also serves as the basis for distinguishing between AP (or PA) and lateral views.

Lateral Chest   The AP and PA images are oriented on the basis of the spine, abdomen, and upper extremity location. For lateral chest images, the orientation is determined by using information about the spine and neck location. This indicates the angle that the image needs to be rotated ($0°$, $90°$ counterclockwise, or $180°$), or by the y-axis flipped.

Abdomen Image   For abdomen images, again there are several stages. First the spine is located by using horizontal and vertical profiles, as before. The average density of each profile is calculated, and the largest local maximum defines the spine location. At the beginning and end of the profile marking the spine, the density is examined. Higher densities indicate the subdiaphragm region. The locations of the spine and abdomen determine the angle at which the image is to be rotated.

Hand Image   For hand images (see also Section 26.7 and Figure 26.15), the rotation is performed on a threshold image: a binary image for which all pixel values are set at zero if they are below the threshold value and at one otherwise. To find the angle (90° clockwise, 90° counterclockwise, or 180°), two horizontal and two vertical profiles are scanned parallel to the borders. The distances from the borders are chosen initially as one-fourth of the width and height of the hand image, respectively. The algorithm then searches for a pair of profiles: one that intersects the forearm and a second that intersects at least three fingers. If no such pair can be found in the first image, the search is repeated. The iterations continue until a pair of profiles (either vertical or horizontal), meeting the abovementioned criteria, is found. On the basis of this profile pair location, it is possible to determine the angle at which the image is to be rotated. DR images do not have the orientation problem because the relative position between the DR receptor and the patient always remains the same.

10.6.1.4 Lookup Table Generation   The fourth preprocessing function for CR images is the generation of a lookup table. The CR system has a built-in automatic brightness and contrast adjustment. Because CR is a 10-bit image (some of them are 12 bit–bit image now), it requires a 10 (or 12)- to 8-bit lookup table for mapping onto the display monitor. The procedure is as follows: After background removal, a histogram of the image is generated. Two numbers, the minimum and the maximum, are obtained from the 5% and 95% points on the cumulative histogram, respectively. From these two values, two parameters in the lookup table: level = (maximum + minimum)/2 and window = (maximum − minimum) can be computed. This is the default linear lookup table for displaying the CR images.

For CR chest images, preprocessing at the imaging device (or the exposure itself) sometimes results in images that are too bright, lack contrast, or both. For these images, several piecewise-linear lookup tables can be created to adjust the brightness and contrast of different tissue densities of the chest image. These lookup tables are created by first analyzing the image gray level histogram to find several key break points. These break points serve to divide the image into three regions: background (outside the patient but still within the radiation field), soft tissue region (skin, muscle, fat, and overpenetrated lung), and dense tissue region (mediastinum, subdiaphragm, and underpenetrated lung).

From these breakpoints, different gains can be applied to increase the contrast (gain, or slope of the lookup table >1) or reduce the contrast (gain, or slope <1) of each region individually. This way the brightness and contrast of each region can be adjusted depending on the application. If necessary, several lookup tables can be created to enhance the radiographic dense and soft tissues, with each having different levels of enhancement. These lookup tables can be easily built in and inserted into the image header and applied at the time of display to enhance different types of tissues. Similar methods can be used for DR images.

10.6.2 Digitized X-ray Images

Digitized X-ray images share some preprocessing functions with the CR: reformatting, background removal, and lookup table generation. However, each of these algorithms requires some modifications. Most X-ray film digitizers are 12 bits and allow a specified subfield in the film to be digitized; as a result the digitized image differs from the CR image in three aspects. First, the size of the digitized image can have various dimensions instead of just three discussed above. Second, there will be no background in the digitized image because the background can be effectively eliminated by positioning the proper window size during digitizing. Third, the image is 12 bits instead of 10 bits. For reformatting, the mapping algorithm therefore should be modified for multiple input dimensions. No background removal is necessary, although the zoom and scroll functions may still be needed to center the image to occupy the full screen size. The lookup table parameters are computed from 12 instead of 10 bits. Note that no automatic orientation is necessary because the user would have oriented the image properly during the digitizing.

10.6.3 Digital Mammography

A digital mammogram size is generally $4K \times 5K \times 12$ bits but with a lot of background outside of the breast contour. For this reason image pre-processing would benefit from an optimization of the spatial presentation and the gray level on the monitor. Three types of pre-processing functions are important. The first function is to perform a background removal of area outside the breast. The background removal process was described in Section 3.3. The background removal in this case is simple because the separation between the breast tissues and the background is distinct. An edge detection algorithm can automatically delineate the boundary of the breast. The background is replaced by an average grey level of the breast tissues (see Fig. 6.3).

The second function is to optimize the default brightness and contrast of the digital mammogram presented on the monitor. A preprocessing algorithm determines the histogram of the image. The 5% and 95% cumulative histogram values are used to generate the initial mean and window for the display of the image.

The third function is to automatically correct the orientation of the mammogram based on the left versus the right side as well as a specific angle mammography projection.

10.6.4 Sectional Images — CT, MR, and US

In sectional imaging the only necessary preprocessing function is the lookup table generation. Two lookup table parameters, window and level, can be computed from each image (either 8 or 12 bits) in a sectional examination similar to that described for the CR image. The disadvantages of using this approach are twofold: inspection of many images in a sectional examination can turn out to be too time-consuming because a lookup table would be needed for each image. The requirement for separate lookup tables will delay the multiple-image display on the screen since the display program must perform a table lookup for each image. A method to circumvent the drawback of many lookup tables is to search the corresponding histograms for the minimum and maximum gray levels of a collection of images in the examination and generate a lookup table for all images.

For US, this method works well because the US signals are quite uniform between images. In CT, several lookup tables can be generated for each region of the body for optimal display of lungs, soft tissues, or bones. This method, in general, works well for CT but not for MR.

In MR, even though a series of images may be generated from the same pulse sequence, the strength of the body or surface coil can vary from section to section, which creates variable histograms for each image. For this reason the automatic lookup table generation method would perform poorly for a set of MR images; the development of an optimal display algorithm remains a challenging topic. In addition in 3-D breast MRI, because positioning of the patient is mostly prone, and because two breasts are normally scanned at the same time, a very carefully planned scanning protocol is needed to label the output 3-D breast images on the display.

10.7 CLINICAL OPERATION AND RELIABILITY OF THE GATEWAY

10.7.1 The Weaknesses of the Gateway as a Single Point of Failure

In clinical hours imaging modalities are continuously sending large amounts of images to the gateway(s), so the workload of the gateway(s) is very heavy, especially when multiple modalities send all images to one gateway or the gateway shares the computer with other PACS processes like image preprocessing. The computer for the gateway may not have enough power to handle the data flow in peak hours. The gateway is a single-point-of-failure component between the modalities and PACS archive server. Even though there are multiple gateways in PACS, each has its own assignment for connection, and switching from one failed gateway to another gateway is mostly manual. Because DICOM communication needs to set up proper DICOM communication parameters, such as AE Title, IP address, and port number, it would require an experienced PACS administrator to set up and switch gateways correctly and quickly. Fixing a failed gateway might take several minutes to half an hour, and hence it affects the data flow of the PACS. Figure 10.13 shows the manual switching (black font) between two gateways in PACS. There are two possible solutions. First, use a built-in fail-safe mechanism in the imaging device to automatically switch a failing gateway to the other (blue font, green switch). The second solution is to develop a fail-safe mechanism in the gateway, as is discussed in the next section.

10.7.2 A Fail-Safe Gateway Design

Because of the possible gateway failure, some PACS manufacturers do not use the term "gateway" any more; they call it DICOM import and export, or multiple integrating unit (MIU). The concept is to bundle several gateways to share the load

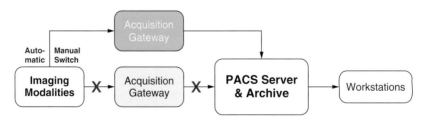

Figure 10.13 Manual switching (right) between two gateways in PACS when one fails. Automatic method (left) is preferred.

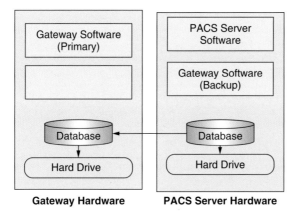

Figure 10.14 The backup gateway uses the PACS server with multiple processors, among them, one is assigned as the backup hardware for the gateway. Two identical gateway software run simultaneously, one in the gateway hardware as the primary and the second in the designated processor of the PACS server as the backup. A tandem database with hard drive for data and metadata archive (see also Fig. 24.17).

balance and possible single-point-of-failure of the gateway. Some manufacturers also combine the PACS server with the gateways by utilizing a very powerful server computer with multiple processors.

In this section we discuss a method in which the gateway is still a separate gateway, and the PACS server is a separate server with multiple processors. Two identical gateway software packages are running simultaneously in both the gateway and one designated processor of the server.

Let us consider the case of the PACS server, which has among many processors one that has a role of backing up a gateway. A dual-system backup mechanism is implemented as follows (see Figure 10.14). First, the PACS processor should have sufficient computation power and configuration as the gateway. Two identical gateway software packages can be implemented: the primary package is in the gateway hardware, and the secondary package is in the selected processor of the PACS server hardware as the backup.

The input data first comes to the gateway hardware, where the gateway software accepts them and put it in the DICOM data model database. In case the gateway hardware fails, the designated processor in the PACS server takes over the role of the gateway hardware and software automatically, and processes the input data accordingly.

Reference

Herrewynen J. Step-by-step integration. *Decisions in Imaging Economics* (December 2002). Also www.imagingeconomics.com/library/200212-13.asp.

CHAPTER 11

PCS Server and Archive

The PACS central node, the engine of the PACS, has two major components: the PACS server and the archive. The former, consisting of the hardware and software architecture, directs the data flow in the entire PACS by using interprocess communication among the major processes. The latter provides a hierarchical image storage management system for short-, medium-, and long-term image archiving. Figure 11.1 shows how this chapter corresponds to the contents of Part II. Figure 11.2 shows the position of the PACS server in the PACS data flow.

Section 11.1 describes the design concept and implementation strategy of the PACS central node, Section 11.2 presents functions of the PACS server and archive, and Section 11.3 discusses the server and archive system operation. Section 11.4 shows the design of the PACS server and archive using DICOM technology, and Section 11.5 shows the server and archive basic hardware and software. Section 11.6 explains the concept of backup archive server and disaster data recovery.

11.1 IMAGE MANAGEMENT DESIGN CONCEPT

Two major aspects should be considered in the design of the PACS image management and storage system: data integrity, which promises no loss of images once they are received by the PACS from the imaging systems, and system efficiency, which minimizes access time of images at the display workstations (WSs). In this chapter we only discuss the DICOM-compliant PACS server and image archive serve (archive).

11.1.1 Local Storage Management via PACS Intercomponent Communication

To ensure data integrity, the PACS always retains at least two copies of an individual image in separate storage devices until the image has been archived successfully to the long-term storage device (e.g., an optical disk or tape library). Figure 11.3 shows the various storage systems used in the PACS. This backup scheme is achieved via the PACS intercomponent communication, which can be broken down as follows (see Fig. 11.2):

- *At the radiological imaging device.* Images are not deleted from the imaging device's local storage until technologists have verified the successful archiving

---

PACS and Imaging Informatics, Second Edition, by H. K. Huang
Copyright © 2010 John Wiley & Sons, Inc.

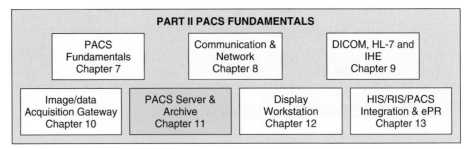

Figure 11.1 Position of Chapter 11 in the organization of this book. Color codes are used to highlight components and workflow in chapters of Part II.

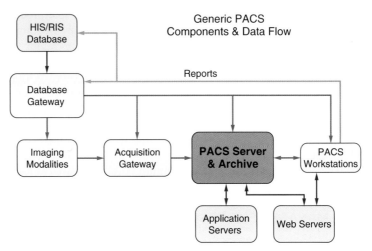

Figure 11.2 PACS basic components (yellow) and data flow (blue: Internal; green and orange: external between PACS and other information systems); other information systems (light blue); the color of the PACS server and archive is orange red. HIS: hospital information system; RIS: radiology information system.

of individual images via the PACS connections. In the event of failure of the acquisition process or of the archive process, images can be re-sent from imaging devices to the PACS.

- *At the acquisition gateway computer.* Images in the acquisition gateway computer acquired from the imaging device remain in its local magnetic disks until the archive system has acknowledged to the gateway that a successful archive has been completed. These images are then deleted from the magnetic disks residing in the gateway so that storage space from these disks can be reclaimed.
- *At the PACS controller and archive server.* Images arriving at the archive server from various acquisition gateways are not deleted until they have been successfully archived to the permanent storage. On the other hand, all archived images are stacked in the archive server's cache magnetic disks and will be deleted based on their aging criteria (e.g., number of days the examination had been performed; or discharge or transfer of the patient).

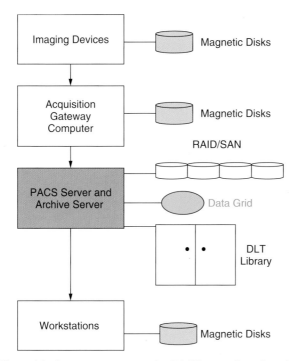

Figure 11.3   Hierarchical storage systems in PACS ensuring data integrity. Until an individual image has been archived in the permanent storage, such as by digital linear tape (DLT) or Data Grid, two copies are retained in separate storage subsystem. DLT can be an archive system within the PACS, Data Grid (green) is mostly external.

- *At the WS.* In general, images stored in the designated WS will remain there until the patient is discharged or transferred. Images in the PACS archive can be retrieved from any WS via the DICOM query/retrieve command. In the thin client architecture (see Section 7.1.3), WS has no storage for images. Once the user has reviewed the images, they are deleted automatically.

11.1.2   PACS Server and Archive System Configuration

The PACS server and the archive server consist of four components: an archive server, a database, a storage system (RAID, SAN, digital linear tape (DLT) library, or connection to the external Data Grid), and a communication network (Fig. 11.4). Attached to the archive system through the communication network are the gateways and WSs. Images acquired by the gateways from various imaging devices are transmitted to the archive server, from which they are archived to the storage system and routed to the appropriate WSs. In the thin client model, Ws has no storage, and all images are resided in the storage system.

11.1.2.1   The Archive Server   The archive server consists of multiple powerful central processing units (CPUs), small computer systems interface (SCSII) data

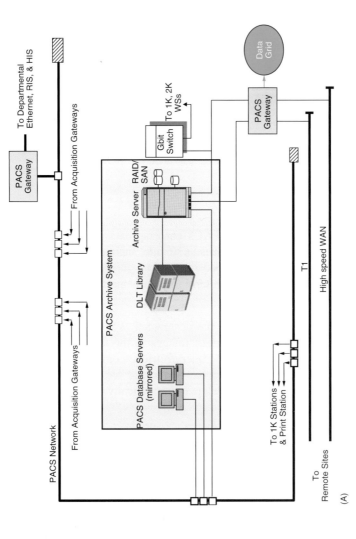

Figure 11.4 (A) Configuration of the archive system and the PACS network. A digital linear tape Library (DLT) for permanent storage or the Data Grid (green, external connection) is used as an example. The archive server is connected to the DLT (light yellow) or the Data Grid (green) and a pair of mirrored database servers. Patient, study, and image directories are stored in the database, images are stored in the DLT or externally in the Data Grid. A local Ethernet network connects all PACS components, and a high-speed Gbit/s switch (as an example) connects the archive server to 1K and 2K WSs, providing fast image display. In addition the archive server is connected to remote sites via T1 and high-speed WAN (bottom), the hospital information system (HIS), and the radiology information system (RIS) via departmental and campus Ethernet (top). (B) Snapshot of RAID/SAN (EMC), cable trays, network switches, patch panels. (Courtesy of UCLA)

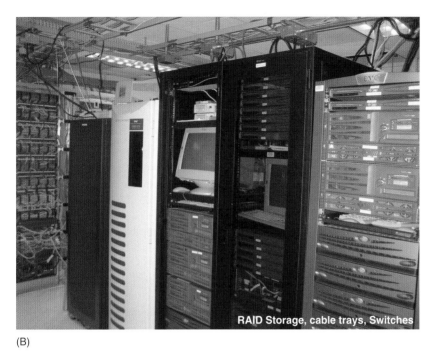

(B)

Figure 11.4 (*Continued*)

buses, and network interfaces (Ethernet and WAN).With its redundant hardware configuration, the archive server can support multiple processes running simultaneously, and image data can be transmitted over different data buses and networks. In addition to its primary function of archiving images, the archive server associated with the PACS server acts as a PACS manager, directing the flow of images within the entire PACS from the gateway to various destinations such as the archive, WSs, and print stations. The archive server uses its large-capacity RAID (redundant array of inexpensive disks) as a data cache, capable of storing several months' worth of images acquired from different imaging devices. For example, four years ago a small 20-Gbyte disk, without using compression, could hold up to 500 computed tomography (CT), 1000 magnetic resonance (MRI), and 500 computed radiography (CR) studies. Each CT or MR study consisted of a sequence of images from one examination with each CR study comprising one exposure. The calculation was based on the average study sizes in the field, in Mbytes: CT, 11.68; MR, 3.47; and CR, 7.46. Nowadays, large RAIDs with several terabytes are being used in the archive server, especially in the client/server model discussed in Section 7.1.3.The magnetic cache disks configured in the archive server should sustain high data throughput for the read operation, which provides fast retrieval of images from the RAID.

11.1.2.2 The Database System The database system consists of redundant database servers running identical reliable commercial database systems (e.g., Sybase, Oracle) with structured query language (SQL) utilities. A mirror database with two identical databases can be used to duplicate the data during every PACS transaction (not images) involving the server. The data can be queried from any PACS computers via the communication networks. The mirroring feature of the system provides the entire PACS database with uninterruptible data transactions that guarantee no loss of data in the event of system failure or a disk crash. Besides its primary role of image indexing to support the retrieval of images, the database system is necessary to interface with the radiology information system (RIS) and the hospital information system (HIS), allowing the PACS database to collect additional patient information from these two healthcare databases (Chapter 13).

11.1.2.3 The Archive Storage The archive storage consists of multiple storage devices, usually large RAID, SAN (storage area network), DLT, and external Data Grid). The archive server allows concurrent storage and retrieval operations on all these devices. The storage must have a large storage capacity of many terabytes and support mixed storage media. Redundant power supply is essential for uninterrupted operation. The average overall throughputs for read and write operations between the magnetic disks of the archive server and the storage devices should be at least several Mbytes/s.

11.1.2.4 Backup Archive To build reliability in the PACS server, a backup archive system should be used. Two copies of identical images can be saved through two different paths in the PACS network to two archive systems. Ideally the two systems would be located in two different buildings to prevent loss in the case of natural disaster. The backup archive has become very important consideration as many healthcare providers are relying on PACS for their daily operation; Section 11.6 discusses a backup archive model.

11.1.2.5 Communication Networks The PACS archive system is connected to both the PACS local area network (LAN) or Intranet, and the wide area network (WAN). The PACS LAN consists of high-speed Ethernet with gigabits/switches and routers. The WAN provides connection to remote sites and can consist of T1 lines and a high-speed WAN-run Internet. The PACS high-speed Intranet transmits large volume image data from the archive server to 1K and 2K WSs. Tens or hundreds Mbits/s of Ethernet can be used for interconnecting slower speed components to the PACS server, including acquisition gateway computers, RIS, and HIS, and as a backup to the Gbit/s Ethernet. Failure of the high-speed network automatically triggers the archive server to reconfigure the communication networks so that images can be transmitted to the 1K and 2K display workstations over slower speed Ethernet without interruption.

11.2 FUNCTIONS OF THE PACS SERVER AND ARCHIVE SERVER

In the PACS server and the archive server, processes of diverse functions run independently and communicate simultaneously with other processes using client-server programming, queuing control mechanisms, and job-prioritizing mechanisms. Figure 11.5 shows the interprocess communications among major processes running on the PACS server and archive, and Table 11.1 describes the functions of these processes. Because the functions of the server and the archive are closely related, we use the term "archive server" to represent both. Major tasks performed by the archive

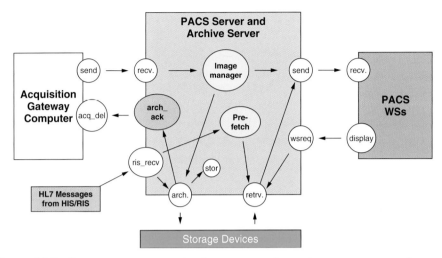

Figure 11.5 Interprocess communications among the major processes running on a PACS archive server. Compare the workflow in a DICOM compliant server shown in Figure 11.9 (see also Fig. 11.6). HL-7: Health Level 7; other symbols are defined in Table 11.1.

server include image receiving, image stacking, image routing, image archiving, studies grouping, platter management, RIS interfacing, PACS database updating, image retrieving, and image prefetching. The following subsections describe the functionality carried out by each of these tasks. Whenever appropriate, the DICOM standard is highlighted in these processes.

11.2.1 Image Receiving

Images acquired from various imaging devices in the gateway computers are converted into DICOM data format if they are not already in DICOM. DICOM images are then transmitted to the archive server via the Ethernet or WAN by using client-server applications over standard TCP/IP transmissions. The archive server can accept concurrent connections for receiving images from multiple acquisition computers. DICOM commands can take care of the send and receive processes.

11.2.2 Image Stacking

Images arrived in the archive server from various gateways are stored in its local magnetic disks or RAID (temporary archive) based on the DICOM data model and managed by the database. The archive server holds as many images in its several large disks as possible and manages them on the basis of aging criteria. For example, images belonging to a given patient during the hospital stay in the server's archive until the patient is discharged or transferred. Thus all recent images that are not already in a display workstation's local storage can be retrieved from the archive server's high-speed short-term archive instead of from the lower speed long-term storage. This feature is particularly convenient for radiologists or referring physicians who must retrieve images from different WSs. In the client-server PACS model, the temporary archive is very large, some in terabytes of capacity.

TABLE 11.1 Major processes and their functions in the archive server

Process	Description
arch	Copy images from magnetic disks to temporary archive and to permanent archive (at patient discharge); update PACS database; notify stor and arch_ack processes for successful archiving (DICOM)
arch_ack	Acknowledge gateway of successful archiving (DICOM)
acq_del	A process at the gateway to delete images from the gateway local magnetic disk
image_manager	Process image information; update PACS database; notify *send* and *arch* processes
prefetch	Select historical images and relevant text data from PACS database; notify *retrv* process
recv	Receive images from the gateway; notify *image_manager* process (DICOM)
ris_recv	Receive HL7 messages (e.g., patient admission, discharge, and transfer; examination scheduling; impression; diagnostic reports) from the RIS; notify *arch* process to group and copy images from temporary archive to permanent archive (at patient discharge, notify *prefetch* process (at scheduling of an examination), or update PACS data base (at receipt of an impression or a diagnostic report) (DICOM Broker)
retrv	Retrieve images from permanent archive; notify *send* process
send	Send images to destined WSs (DICOM)
stor	Manage magnetic storage of the archive server (DICOM)
wsreq	Handle retrieve requests from the display process at the WSs (DICOM)
display	Acknowledge archive server for images received (DICOM)

Note: See Figure 11.5.

11.2.3 Image Routing

In the stand-alone (or peer to peer) PACS model, images that have arrived in the archive server from various gateways are immediately routed to their destination WSs. The routing process is driven by a predefined routing table composed of parameters including examination type, display WS site, radiologist, and referring physician. All images are classified by examination type (one-view chest, CT-head, CT-body, US, etc.) as defined in the DICOM standard. The destination WSs are classified by location (chest, pediatrics, CCU, etc.) as well as by resolution (1K or 2K). The routing algorithm performs table lookup based on the aforementioned parameters and determines an image's destination(s) as the site may have a certain type of WS. Images are transmitted to the 1K and 2K workstations over either intranet and to remote sites over dedicated T1 lines, broadband or high-speed WAN.

11.2.4 Image Archiving

Images arriving in the archive server from gateways are copied from temporary storage to other longer term storage devices. When the copy process is complete, the archive server acknowledges the corresponding gateway, allowing it to delete the images from its local storage and reclaim its disk space. This way the PACS always has two copies of an image on separate magnetic disk systems until the image is archived to the permanent storage. Images that belong to a given patient during a hospital stay with multiple examinations may scatter temporarily into various storage devices. After the patient is discharged or has completed the purposed visit, the entire patient image file is consolidated and moved to reside in the permanent archive device, as discussed in the next section.

11.2.5 Study Grouping

During a hospital stay a patient may have different examinations on different days. Each of these examinations may consist of multiple studies. On discharge or transfer of the patient, images from these studies are regrouped from the temporary storage and copied contiguously to a single permanent storage. Thus the studies grouping function allows all images belonging to the same patient during a hospital stay to be archived contiguously to a single storage device. In addition to saving long-term storage space, logical grouping of consecutive examinations into one volume can reduce time for searching and retrieving them from various storage devices should they be needed again in the future.

11.2.6 RIS and HIS Interfacing

The archive server accesses data from HIS/RIS through a PACS gateway computer. The HIS/RIS relays a patient admission, discharge, and transfer (ADT) message to the PACS only when a patient is scheduled for an examination in the radiology department or when a patient in the radiology department is discharged or trans-ferred. Forwarding ADT messages to PACS not only supplies patient demographic data to the PACS but also provides information the archive server needs to initi-ate the prefetch, image archive, and studies grouping tasks. Exchange of messages among these heterogeneous information systems can use the Health Level Seven (HL7) standard data format running TCP/IP transmissions on a client-server basis as described in Section 9.2.

In addition to receiving ADT messages, PACS retrieves examination data and diag-nostic reports from the RIS. This information is used to update the PACS database, which can be queried and reviewed from any WS. Chapter 13 presents the RIS, HIS, and PACS interface in more detail.

11.2.7 PACS Database Updates

Data transactions performed in the archive server, such as insertion, deletion, selec-tion, and update, are carried out by using SQL utilities in the database. Data in the PACS database are stored in predefined tables, with each table describing only one kind of entity. The design of these tables should follow the DICOM data model for operation efficiency. For example, (1) the patient description table consists of master patient records, which store patient demographics; (2) the study description table consists of study records describing individual radiological procedures; (3) the archive directory table consists of archive records for individual images; and (4) the diagnosis history table consists of diagnostic reports of individual examinations. Individual PACS processes running in the archive server with information extracted from the DICOM image header update these tables and the RIS interface to reflect any changes of the corresponding tables.

11.2.8 Image Retrieving

Image retrieval takes place at the display WSs. The WSs are connected to the archive system through the communication networks. The archive library configured with multiple drives can support concurrent image retrievals from multiple storage devices. The retrieved data are then transmitted from the archive storage to the archive server via the SCSII data buses or fiber-optic channels.

The archive server handles retrieve requests from WSs according to the priority level of these individual requests. Priority is assigned to individual WSs and users based on different levels of needs. For example, the highest priority is always granted to a WS that is used for primary diagnosis, in a conference session, or at an intensive care unit. Thus a WS used exclusively for research and teaching purposes is compromised to allow "fast service" to radiologists and referring physicians in the clinic for immediate patient care area.

The archive system supports image retrieval from 2K WSs for on-line primary diagnosis, 1K stations for ICU and review workstations, and PC desktops for other clinical usage throughout the hospital. To retrieve images from the long-term archive, the user at a WS can activate the retrieval function and request any number of images from the archive system from the WS's worklist. Image query/retrieval is performed with the DICOM commands described in Section 9.4.5. Image retrieval will be discussed in more detail in Chapter 12.

11.2.9 Image Prefetching

The prefetching mechanism is initiated as soon as the archive server detects the arrival of a patient scheduled for an imaging study via the ADT message from HIS/RIS. Selected historical images, patient demographics, and relevant diagnostic reports are retrieved from the archive and the PACS database. Such data are distributed to the destination WSs before the completion of the patient's current examination. The prefetch algorithm is based on predefined parameters such as examination type, disease category, radiologist, referring physician, location of the WS, and the number and the age of the patient's archived images. These parameters determine what historical images should be retrieved, when, and directed to where.

11.3 PACS ARCHIVE SERVER SYSTEM OPERATIONS

The PACS server operates on a 24 hours a day, 7 days a week basis. All operations in a well-designed PACS should be software driven and automatic and should not require any manual operational procedures. The only nonautomatic procedures are removal of old or insertion of new storage media in the off-line archive operation. Even this process was minimized several years ago by the introduction of larger storage devices with periodic preventive maintain service.

A fault-tolerant mechanism in the archive system is used to ensure data integrity and minimize system downtime. Major features of this mechanism include the following:

1. An uninterruptible power supply (UPS) system that protects all archived components, including the archive server, database servers, and archive library from power outages

2. A mirrored database system that guarantees the integrity of the data directory

3. If DLT library is used for long-term archiving, then multiple tape drives and robotic arms that provide uninterrupted image archival and retrieval in the event of failure of a tape drive or robotic arm.

4. A central monitoring system that automatically alerts quality control staff via wireless mobile phone or pagers to remedy any malfunctioning archive components or processes

5. Spare parts for immediate replacement of any malfunctioning computer components, which include network adapter boards and routers, SCSII controllers, and the multi-CPU system board (archive server)

6. A 4-hour turnaround manufacturer's on-site service that minimizes system downtime due to hardware failure of any major archive component.

In Chapter 16 we will discuss the concept of fault-tolerant PACS operation in more detail.

11.4 DICOM-COMPLIANT PACS ARCHIVE SERVER

11.4.1 Advantages of a DICOM-Compliant PACS Archive Server

The purpose of the Digital Imaging and Communications in Medicine (DICOM) standard described in Section 9.4 is to promote a standard communication method for heterogeneous imaging systems, allowing the exchange of images and associated information among them. By using the DICOM standard, a PACS would be able to interconnect its individual components together and allow the acquisition gateways to link to imaging devices. However, imaging equipment vendors often select only a subset of DICOM compliant statements for implementation (Section 9.4.4) for their own convenience, which may lead to difficulties for these imaging systems for interoperation. A well-designed DICOM-compliant PACS server can use two mechanisms to ensure the system integration. One mechanism is to connect to the acquisition gateway computer with DICOM providing reliable and efficient processes of acquiring images from imaging devices. The other mechanism is to develop specialized gateway software allowing interoperability of multivendor imaging systems. Both mechanisms can be incorporated in the DICOM-compliant PACS system.

We have described basic principles of these two mechanisms in Chapters 7, 8, 9, and 10 in the component level. In this section we integrate these mechanisms at the system level based on the knowledge learned in those chapters.

11.4.2   DICOM Communications in PACS Environment

In Section 9.4.5 we discussed two major DICOM communication service-object pair (SOP) classes for image communications: the Storage Service Class and the Query/Retrieve (Q/R) Service Class:

- Storage Service Class: Allows a PACS application running on system A (i.e., a CT scanner) to play the role of a Storage Service Class User (SCU) that initiates storage requests and transmits images to system B (i.e., an acquisition gateway computer), which serves as a Storage Service Class Provider (SCP), accepting images to its local storage device.
- Q/R Service Class: Allows PACS applications running on system A (i.e., a WS) to play the role of a Q/R SCU that queries and retrieves images from system B (i.e., an archive server), which serves as a Q/R SCP, processing query and retrieval requests.

Figure 11.6 illustrates the communication of images utilizing the Storage Service Class and Q/R Service Class in a PACS environment. These two service classes can be used to develop a DICOM-compliant PACS server.

11.4.3   DICOM-Compliant Image Acquisition Gateways

A DICOM-compliant acquisition gateway can be used to provide a reliable and efficient process for acquiring images from imaging devices. The DICOM-compliant

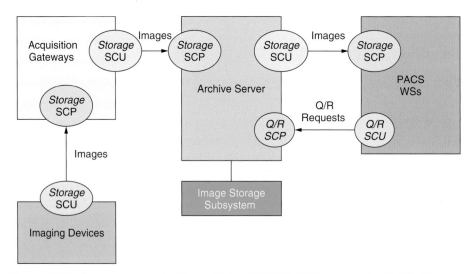

Figure 11.6   Image communication utilizing DICOM SOP services in PACS. The gateway via the storage SOP service acquires images generated from imaging devices. These images are then transmitted to the archive server, where they are routed to the permanent archive subsystem and WSs. The archive server supports query/retrieve (Q/R) SOP service, handling all Q/R requests from WSs (see also Fig. 11.5). SOP: service-object pair; SCU ⬭: service class user; SCP ⬭: service class provider.

software running on a gateway should support two types of image acquisition, the push-mode and the pull-mode operations (see also Section 10.2.1).

11.4.3.1 Push Mode
Push-mode operation utilizes DICOM's storage SOP service. An imaging device such as a CT scanner takes the role of a storage SCU, initiating storage requests. The requesting gateway (storage SCP) accepts these requests and receives the images.

11.4.3.2 Pull Mode
Pull-mode operation utilizes DICOM's Q/R SOP service. The gateway plays the role of a Q/R SCU, initiating query requests, selecting desired images, and retrieving images from an imaging device (Q/R SCP). The pull-mode operation requires the image acquisition process to incorporate with the local database to perform data integrity checks in the gateway computer. This checking mechanism ensures that no images are lost during the acquisition process.

Figure 11.7 summarizes the characteristics of these two modes of operation. In the pull mode, the *ImgTrack* process in the gateway performs data integrity checks by the following procedure:

1. Queries study information from the scanners.
2. Generates acquisition status table.
3. Periodically checks acquisition status of individual image sequences.
4. Invokes *DcmPull* process to retrieve images from the scanners.

The *DcmPull* process, when invoked by the *ImgTrack* process, retrieves the desired images from the scanner and updates the acquisition status table accordingly. Both

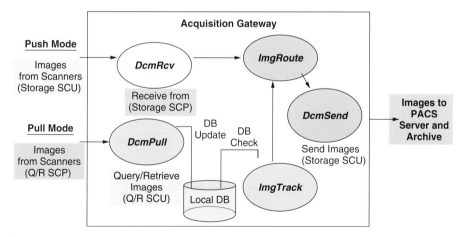

Figure 11.7 Interprocess communication among the major processes running in a DICOM compliant acquisition gateway which supports both push and pull operations for acquiring images from the scanners. The *DcmPull* process (blue) incorporates gateway's local database to perform data integrity check, ensuring no missing images from any image sequences during the acquisition process (see also Fig. 11.6). Dcm : DICOM; SCU ⬭ : service class user; SCP ⬭ : service class provider.

push and pull modes are used in the acquisition gateway; the choice is dependent on the operation condition at the clinical site.

11.5 DICOM PACS ARCHIVE SERVER HARDWARE AND SOFTWARE

This section discusses the system architecture with generic hardware and basic software components of a DICOM PACS server and archive server.

11.5.1 Hardware Components

The PACS server and archive server generic hardware component consists of the PACS server computers, peripheral archive devices, and fast *Ethernet* interface and SCSII and fiber-optics channels. For large PAC systems, the server computers used are mostly UNIX-based machines. The *fast Ethernet* interfaces the PACS archive server to the *high-speed Ethernet networks*, where gateways and WSs are connected. The SCSII and fiber-optic channels integrate peripheral storage devices with the PACS archive server. The main storage devices for PACS server include magnetic disk, RAID, SAN, D LT, and CD/DVD (digital versatile disks). PACS separates its images according to the time it had been acquired; with the current ones relegated to the short-term storage device, and very historical ones to the long-term storage. In-between time image storage depends on the clinical need.

RAID and SAN, because of their fast access speed and reliability, are used for the short-term archive device in PACS, specifically in the client and server architecture. Because of its large data storage capacity and relatively lower cost, DLT is mostly used for long-term and off-site archive. Figure 11.8 provides an example of the server connection to the DLT with the SCSII, and RAID and SAN with the fiber-optic

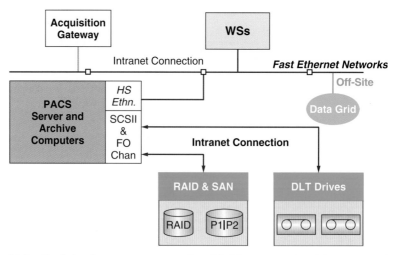

Figure 11.8 Basic hardware components in a PACS server and archive server with high-speed (HS) Ethernet (Ethn.) for broadband Internet, and SCSII and fiber-optic channels (FO Chan) connections. Blue lines: PACS Intranet; SAN: storage area network with multiple partitions, P1, P2, . . . (see also Fig. 11.2).

channels, and to other PACS components with *high-speed Ethernet*. Many different kinds of storage devices are available for PACS application; in the following we describe three of the most popular ones, RAID, SAN, and DLT.

11.5.1.1 RAID RAID is a disk array architecture developed for fast and reliable data storage. A RAID groups several magnetic disks (e.g., 8 disks) as a disk array and connects the array to one or more RAID controllers. The size of RAID is usually from several hundred gigabytes to terabytes. With the size of individual disk increasing for the past several years, the storage size of RAID has increased proportionally. Current RAID can have hundreds of terabytes capacity, which has contributed to one of the reasons why the client-server PACS architecture is so popular. Multiple RAID controllers with multiple interfaces can be used to avoid single points of failure in the RAID device. The RAID controller has SCSII or a fiber-optic channels interface to the PACS server. This topic will be discussed further in Chapter 16.

11.5.1.2 SAN (Storage Area Network) A current data storage trend in large-scale archiving is the storage area network (SAN) technology, and PACS is no exception in this trend. With this new configuration, the PACS server will still have a short-term storage solution in local disks containing unread patient studies. However, for long-term storage, the PACS data is stored in a SAN. The SAN is a stand-alone data storage repository with a single Internet Protocol (IP) address. File management and data backup can be achieved by a combination of digital media (RAID, digital linear tape [DLT], etc.) smoothly and with total transparency to the user. In addition the SAN can be partitioned into several different repositories, each storing different data file types. The storage manager within the SAN is configured to recognize and distribute the different clients' data files and store them to distinct and separate parts of the SAN. The controller software of the SAN manages the partitioning, allocation, I/O, and interfacing with other storage devices.

The SAN example in Figure 11.8 is divided into two partitions, P1 and P2. P1 is used for its own patients' records, and P2 receives backup archives from other sites within the enterprise PACS. Each image in each site has three copies, one in its own SAN P1 and two in SANS P2 of two other sites, each of which has a PACS and a SAN. Note that P2 in each SAN is physically located within the SAN of the site, although logically, once P2 is committed to the enterprise PACS for another site's backup, P2 serves only the enterprise PACS (see Section 21.3.2, and Fig. 21.8).

11.5.1.3 DLT DLT uses a multiple magnetic tape and drive system housed inside a library or jukebox for low cost but large volume and long-term archive. With current tape drive technology, the data storage size can reach 40 to 200 Gbytes per tape. One DLT can hold from 20 to hundreds of tapes. Therefore the storage size of DLT can be from tens to hundreds of terabytes, which can hold PACS images for several years. DLT usually has multiple drives to read and write tapes. The tape drive is connected to the server through SCSI or a fiber-optic connection. The data transmission speed is several megabytes per second for each drive. The tape loading time and data locating time are about several minutes together (e.g., 3.0 min). Hence, in general, it takes several minutes to retrieve one CR image from DLT, but once retrieved the I/O transfer rates are acceptable for off-site clinical retrieval. PACS image data in DLT are usually prefetched to RAID for fast access time.

11.5.2 Archive Server Software

PACS archive server software is DICOM compliant and supports the DICOM Storage Service and Query/Retrieve Service classes. Through DICOM communication the archive server receives DICOM studies/images from the acquisition gateway, appends study information to the database, and stores the images in the archive device, including the RAID, SAN, and DLT. It receives the DICOM query/retrieve request from WSs and sends back the query/retrieve result (patient/study information or images) to WSs. The DICOM services supported by the PACS Server are C-Store, C-Find, and C-Move (see Section 9.4.5). All software implemented in the archive server should be coded in standard programming languages—for example, C and C++ on the UNIX open systems architecture. PACS server software is composed of at least six independent components (processes), including receive, insert, routing, send, Q/R server, and RetrieveSend. It also includes a PACS database. In the following we describe the six most common processes. All these processes run independently and simultaneously and communicate with other processes through Queue control mechanisms. Figure 11.9 shows the PACS archive software components and data flow (compare Fig. 11.5, which shows the general interprocess communications in a PACS server).

11.5.2.1 Image Receiving DICOM studies/images are transmitted from the acquisition gateway to the PACS server *receive* process through DICOM Storage Service Class. The *receive* process acts as a storage SCP. The receive process can simultaneously accept multiple connections from several DICOM storage SCUs at different acquisition gateways. Figure 11.9 shows four images being queued.

11.5.2.2 Data Insert and PACS Database The patient/study information in the DICOM header is extracted and inserted into the PACS database in the *insert*

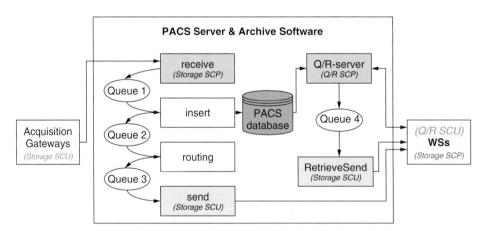

Figure 11.9 DICOM PACS server and archive software components and dataflow. The six components are receive, insert, route, Send, *Q/R-server*, and *RetrieveSend*. Green: SCU; orange red: SCP.

process. The PACS database is a series of relational tables based on the DICOM information object model. The database can be built on a reliable commercial database system such as ORACL or Sybase. The database provides patient/study information management and image index function to support WSs' query/retrieve. In general, after the gateway receives the DCIOM image, it parses the image into two parts: the image header and the image data. The header goes to the database and forms the metadata, and the image data goes to the storage devices. The database manager links the metadata and the image data to form the DICOM image when it is retrieved and transmitted.

11.5.2.3 Image Routing

Images from different modalities are sent to different WSs for radiologists' or physicians' review. The *routing* process is designed to determine where to send. The *routing* process is performed based on a preconfigured routing table. The table includes several parameters, such as modality type, examination body part, WS site, and referring physician. The *routing* process passes the result of routing (destination WS information) to the *send* process for sending images out through a Queue control mechanism.

11.5.2.4 Image Send

Most PACS servers have two ways to distribute images to WSs: auto push to WSs or manual query/retrieve from WSs. In auto-push mode, the images are automatically sent out to WSs based on the preconfigured routing table. The auto-push function is performed by the *send* process, which is acting as the DICOM storage SCU. The client-server PACS architecture uses the query/retrieve from the WSs described in the next two sections.

11.5.2.5 Image Query/Retrieve

The other way to send images to WSs is through query/retrieve from the WSs. The *Q/R-server* process receives the DICOM query/retrieve request from WSs, searches the PACS database, and returns the matching results to the WSs. The *Q/R-server* at the PACS server here acts as query/retrieve SCP, and the process can simultaneously support multiple query/retrieves from different WSs. If the query/retrieve result is the image, the image information is passed to the *RetrieveSend* process through the queue control mechanism, which sends the images to the requested WS.

11.5.2.6 Retrieve/Send

In the DICOM query/retrieve service the images are not sent out by the query/retrieve association; instead, this is performed by a new DICOM storage association. Therefore the images retrieved from the PACS server are not directly sent through *Q/R-server* process. The *RetrieveSend* process performs the transmission function. It receives the image information from *Q/R-server* and sends the images to the WS.

11.5.3 An Example

We use the example shown in Figure 11.10 to illustrate the image data flow involved in sending a CR image from the acquisition gateway through the PACS archive server.

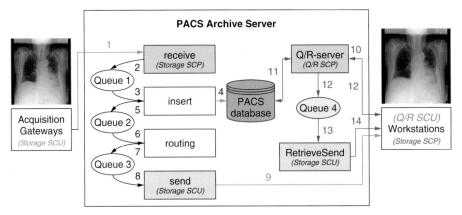

Figure 11.10 Workflow in a DICOM PACS archive server, with CR as an example of data sent from the acquisition gateway, through the server, to the WS. Green and black numerals and lines are the auto-push model; blue are the client and server model with Q/R (refer to Fig. 11.9).

Auto-push Model

1. A CR chest image is sent from the acquisition gateway to the *receive* process through DICOM CR Image Storage Service Class. The *receive* process receives the image and stores the image file on local computer disk.

2. The *receive* process adds the image file information to queue 1 through the Queue control operation.

3. The *insert* process parses the CR image file header information from queue 1, and reads in the image file from local disk.

4. The *insert* process extracts Patient/Study information from the DICOM header of the image and inserts the information into the patient/study tables of the PACS database.

5. The *insert* process adds the new image file information to queue 2 through the Queue control operation.

6. The *routing* process reads the image file information, searches the routing information for this CR image, and finds the destination WS information.

7. The *routing* process adds the image file information and destination WS information to queue 3.

8. The *send* process reads the image file information and destination WS information from queue 3.

9. The *send* process sends the image file to the specified WS through the DICOM CR image Storage Service Class.

Client-Server Model with Q/R

10. The WS can also query/retrieve (Q/R) the same CR image by Q/R Service Class. The *Q/R-server* process receives the Q/R request from the WS.

11. The *Q/R-server* process searches the PACS database and finds the matching results.

12. The *Q/R-server* process sends the query/retrieve result to the WS. If the Q/R results contains the CR image, the *Q/R-server* process adds the image file information and destination WS information to queue 4.

13. The *RetrieveSend* process reads the image file information and destination WS information from queue 4.

14. The *RetrieveSend* process sends the image file to the destination WS.

11.6 BACKUP ARCHIVE SERVER

Two major components in the PACS server and archive are the PACS server and the archive server. When the PACS server fails, a system reboots or a backup server may solve most of the problems; then no data are lost. However, when the archive server fails, data in the storage may be damaged and lead to lose of image data. This section focuses in the discussion of the backup archive server.

11.6.1 Backup Archive Using an Application Service Provider (ASP) Model

The PACS archive server is the most important component in a PACS; even though it may have the fault tolerant feature, chances are it will occasionally fail. A backup archive server is necessary to guarantee its uninterrupted service. The backup archive server can be short term (3 months) or long term. The functions of a backup archive server are twofold: maintaining the PACS continuous operation and preventing loss of image data. Data loss is especially troublesome because if a major disaster occurs, it is possible to lose an entire hospital's PACS data. In addition the scheduled down-times to the main PACS archive could impact the continuity of a filmless institution's operation. Few current PACS archives provides a disaster recovery scheme. Further-more current general disaster recovery solutions vary in the approach toward creating redundant copies of PACS data.

One novel approach is to provide a short-term fault-tolerant backup archive server using the application service provider (ASP) model at an off-site location. The ASP backup archive provides instantaneous, automatic backup of acquired PACS image data and instantaneous recovery of stored PACS image data, all at a low operational cost because it utilizes the ASP business model. In addition, should the downtime event render the network communication inoperable, a portable solution is available with a data migrator. The data migrator is a portable laptop with a large-capacity hard disk that contains DICOM software for exporting and importing PACS exams. The data migrator can populate PACS exams that were stored in the backup archive server directly onto the clinical PACS within a couple of hours to allow the radiologists to continue to read previous PACS exams until new replacement hardware arrives and is installed or until a scheduled downtime event has been completed.

11.6.2 General Architecture

Figure 11.11 shows the general architecture of the ASP backup archive integrated with a clinical PACS. The hospital with a PACS and the ASP site are connected via a T1 line or other broadband WAN. At the hospital site any new exam acquired and

ASP Backup Archive: General Architecture

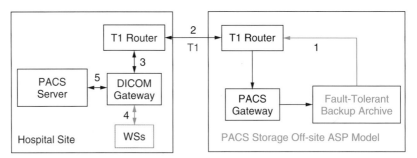

Figure 11.11   General architecture of the ASP backup archive server. One DICOM gateway at the ASP site and one PACS gateway at the hospital site are used as the buffers between the two sites. T1 is used for the broadband WAN. WSs at the hospital site can access PACS images from the ASP, following the route: 1, 2, 3, and 4, should some components in the PACS fail, like the server and the archive. After the PACS components are repaired, the missing images can be recovered via route 5. The image query/retrieve performance is limited only by the network speed, in this example, the T1 at 1.5 Mbit/s.

archived in PACS is also sent to an additional DICOM gateway at the hospital via the clinical PACS server. The DICOM gateway, very much like a PACS acquisition gateway in the PACS system, is crucial in maintaining clinical workflow between the hospital and the ASP site. It provides a buffer and manages the network transfers of the PACS exams by queuing the network transfer jobs to the ASP site. The DICOM gateway transfers an exam through the T1 router across the T1 line to a receiving T1 router at the off-site ASP. At the off-site ASP PACS backup storage site, another gateway receives the PACS exams and queues them for storage in a fault-tolerant backup archive server. The backup archive should be designed as a fault-tolerant storage device (see Chapter 16). All PACS data transmitted throughout this architecture conform to the DICOM protocol standard.

11.6.3   Recovery Procedure

Figure 11.12 shows the recovery procedure of the PACS during a scheduled down-time or an unscheduled downtime such as a disaster. There are two scenarios: network communication still functioning between two sites, and no network connection. If connectivity between the two sites is live, then backup PACS exams can be migrated back to the hospital site and imported directly into the PACS with DICOM com-pliant network protocols. In most disaster scenarios, there is high likelihood that connectivity between the two sites is not functional. In this case the backup PACS exams are imported into the hospital PACS with a portable data migrator. The data migrator exports PACS exams from the backup archive. It is then physically brought on site (this scenario works best if the off site is located in the same metropolitan area as the hospital) to the hospital and the PACS exams are imported directly into a WS or temporary server. The data migrator is DICOM compliant, which means that the PACS exams can be imported without any additional software or translation.

ASP Backup Archive: Recovery Procedure

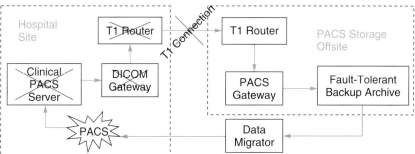

Figure 11.12   Disaster recovery procedures. In a disastrous event the components shown marked can be considered unavailable for use. In this scenario a data migrator can be used physically to export PACS exams and import them directly into PACS using the appropriate DICOM protocols. After the PACS are repaired, the migrator can be used to feed images back to the PACS server via routes 4 and 5.

In addition the data migrator contains up-to- date PACS data because it is always synchronized with the clinical PACS workflow. In either scenario the radiologist will have the previous and current PACS exams to continue with normal clinical work flow reading until replacement hardware is installed, and the hospital PACS archive storage and server are brought back on line.

11.6.4   Key Features

For a backup archive server to be successful in supporting the PACS continuing operation, the following key features at the ASP site are necessary:

- Copy of every PACS exam created must be stored in timely and automatic process.
- Backup archive server must satisfy the CA (continuously available) fault-tolerant condition with 99.999% availability.
- Backup must not be dependent on operator intervention, except in the case where the data are migratory and must be brought from the ASP site to the hospital.
- Backup storage capacity must be easily re-configurable and expandable based on requirements and needs.
- Data recovery and importing data must be back to the hospital PACS within 2 hours if communication network is intact, 1 day if a portable data migrator is needed.
- The ASP archive has to be DICOM compliant.
- The ASP backup system must have no impact on normal clinical workflow.
- Radiologists should read with previous exams until hospital PACS archive is recovered

11.6.5 General Setup Procedures of the ASP Model

The next few paragraphs describe a general step-by-step procedure of deploying this archive backup system. Included are suggestions of potential resources within the hospital as well as any necessary ancillary personnel that should be involved in each of the steps.

1. Determine the configuration that will have the least impact on the hospital clinical workflow. The PACS system administrator and a clinical staff representative should be involved because they are familiar with day-to-day operations of the hospital PACS.

2. Establish communication network connectivity between the two sites. First, the best network connectivity bandwidth and configuration should be determined on the basis of cost and availability. Some connectivity solutions involve a continuous operational fee, whereas others may involve a onetime initial cost for installation. The cost and availability also depend on the distance between the two sites. It is important to include any resource that can provide information on options such as information technology (IT) hospital staff members as well as the radiology administrator, as there will be budget constraints that may factor into the decision-making process.

3. Order hardware and installation. Most likely, a vendor will be responsible for this step, but it is always beneficial to involve IT and telecommunications staff resources at the hospital. Once connectivity has been established, testing should be performed for verification. The vendor performs this step with additional input from both IT and telecommunications staff resources. At this point, the hospital and the off-site locations have connectivity established.

4. Test the clinical PACS workflow and transmission of PACS exams to the backup archive server to verify that the PACS exams are received without any data loss; then observe the impact on the clinical PACS. This crucial step in the procedure is important because the backup archive procedure should appear seamless to the clinical PACS user. The PACS system administrator plays a key role in determining the effects of the system on clinical work flow.

5. Perform trial runs of disaster scenario simulations and PACS data recovery. Coordination between the two sites is key to ensure that results are observed as well as documented. Once all tests are completed and verified, the new workflow is ready for clinical operation.

The ASP system described had been implemented successfully, and PACS exams from S. John's Health Center (Santa Monica, CA) were backed up to an off-site fault-tolerant archive server located within a 30-mile radius of the hospital. The backup storage capacity was short term and configured for two months. The system had been in operation for four years since 2003 until SJHC changed the PACS manufacturer, which provided its own PACS backup archive system. Chapter 19 describes the clinical operation and pitfalls of the ASP backup archive server model.

11.6.6   The Data Grid Model

Advancements in grid computing technology over the past four years promise to offer a more elegant method for PACS data backup using Data Grid, either in an enterprise PACS level or in ASP model. Data Grid technology is presented in Chapter 21 with examples on its use for PACS data backup and disaster recovery.

References

Compaq/Tandem's Non Stop Himalaya. http://www.tandem.com.

HIPAA: http://www.rx2000.org/KnowledgeCenter/hipaa/hipfaq.htm.

Huang HK. PACS: *Basic Principles and Applications*. New York: Wiley; 1999.

Huang HK, Cao F, Liu BJ, Zhang J, Zhou Z, Tsai A, Mogel G. Fault-tolerant PACS server design. *SPIE Med Imag* 4323–14: 83–92; 2001.

Huang HK, Cao F, Liu BJ, Zhang J, Zhou Z, Tsai A, Mogel G. Fault-tolerant PACS server. *SPIE Med Imag* 4685–44: 316–25; 2002.

Huang HK, Liu BJ, Cao F, Zhou MZ, Zhang J, Mogel GT, Zhuang J, Zhang X. PACS simulator: a standalone educational tool. *SPIE Med Imag* 4685–21 (February); 2002.

Liu BJ, Documet L, Sarti DA, Huang HK, Donnelly J. PACS archive upgrade and data migration: clinical experiences. *SPIE Med. Imag* 4685–14: 83–88; 2002a.

Liu BJ, Huang HK, Cao F, Documet L, Sarti DA. A fault-tolerant back-up archive using an ASP model for disaster recovery. *SPIE Med Imag* 4685–15: 89–95; 2002b.

Zhou Z, Cao F, Liu BJ, Huang HK, Zhang J, Zhang X, Mogel G. *A Complete Continuous-Availability PACS Archive Server Solution*. SPIE Med. Imag, Newport Beach, CA; 2003.

CHAPTER 12

Display Workstation

Among all PACS components, PACS display workstation (WS) is the one that all radiologists and clinicians are familiar with. PACS WSs in the radiology department have the highest quality allowing radiologists and clinicians to make primary diagnosis from the images compared with other peripheral workstations not within the radiology department. This section gives details of the WS design, hardware and software, ergonomics, features, utilization, and future development prospective. Figure 12.1 (excerpted from Fig. 1.3) shows how corresponds to the contents of Part II. Figure 12.2 depicts the WS in the PACS data flow.

12.1 BASICS OF A DISPLAY WORKSTATION

The WS is the interactive component in PACS that healthcare providers use for reviewing images and relevant patient information from which patient diagnosis is made. The interpreted result becomes the diagnostic report that feeds back to the hospital and radiology information systems (HIS, RIS) as a permanent patient record along with the images. In this chapter the terms softcopy workstation, display workstation, image workstation, or just workstation (WS) are used interchangeably. The conventional method of viewing radiological images on films relies on a technologist hangs them on an alternator or a light box. Table 12.1 shows the characteristics of a typical alternator.

Because the advantages of an alternator are its large surface area, high luminance, and convenience in use, the design of a soft copy display workstation should incorporate the favorable functions and convenience of the alternator whenever possible.

A WS consists of four major hardware components: a computer, image display boards, display monitors, and local storage devices. A communication network and application software connect these components with the PACS server, as described in Figures 11.5, 11.6, 11.9, and 11.10 before. The computer and image display boards are responsible for transforming the image data for visualization on the monitors. Magnetic disks and RAID are used for local storage devices. The communication network is used for transmitting images into and out of the WS. Figure 12.3 shows the schematic of a typical two monitor WS based on a PC computer. Section 12.1.1 describes the image display board and the display monitor in more detail.

PACS and Imaging Informatics, Second Edition, by H. K. Huang
Copyright © 2010 John Wiley & Sons, Inc.

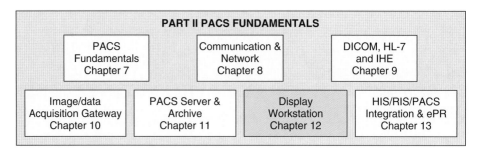

Figure 12.1 Position of Chapter 12 in the organization of this book. Color codes are used to highlight components and workflow in the chapters of Part II.

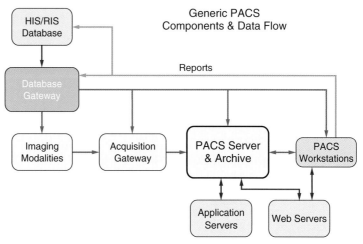

Figure 12.2 PACS basic components (yellow) and data flow (blue: Internal; green and red: external between PACS and other information systems); other information systems (light blue); the color of the PACS workstation is orange red. HIS: hospital Information system; RIS: radiology information system.

12.1.1 Image Display Board

The image display board has two components: a processing unit and image memory. The image memory is used to supplement the computer memory to increase the storage capacity for images and to speed up the image display. There are two types of computer memory, random access memory (RAM) and video RAM (VRAM). RAM usually comes with the computer and is less expensive than VRAM. VRAM has a very high input/output rate and is used to display images or graphics. A WS usually has more RAM than VRAM. In a PACS WS, typical numbers are one Gbyte RAM and 64 Mbyte VRAM, or more.

An image file in the WS coming either from the PACS archive server or from the internal disk is first stored in the RAM. If the RAM is not large enough to store the entire image file, it is split between the RAM and the disk, and disk I/O and RAM swapping is needed. In this case the image display speed would be slower. It

TABLE 12.1   Characteristics of a typical light alternator

Dimension					Viewing Capability			
Width (in.)	Height (in.)	Table Height (in.)	Number of panels	Number of visible panels	Viewing surface per panel height x width (in^2)	Average luminance Ft-L	Viewing height (from table top to top of lower panel) in.	Time required to retrieve a panel seconds
72–100	78	30–32	20–50	2 (upper and lower)	16×56 to 16 × 82	500	32 + 16	6–12

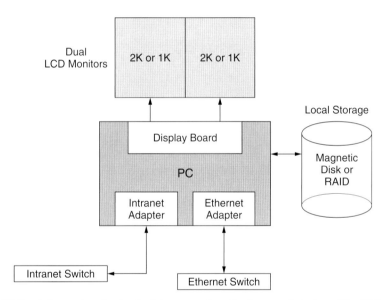

Figure 12.3   Schematic of a typical two-monitor display workstation. The WS is composed of a PC, display boards with image processing capability and image memory (RAM) and video VRAM, dual display LCD monitors (2K or 1K), magnetic or RAID disk, and network connections. No local disk is needed in the client-server model.

is therefore advantageous to have a larger RAM to increase the display speed. After some operations the processed image is moved to the VRAM before it is shown on the monitor. Figure 12.4 shows the data flow of an image from the internal magnetic disk to the display memory. Sometimes we use the term "4 mega pixel" or "5 mega pixel" for a display board, which represent its capability of displaying a full 2K × 2K or 2.5K × 2K" image, respectively. For color images it requires 24 bits/pixel, and for graphic overlay it is 1 extra bit/pixel.

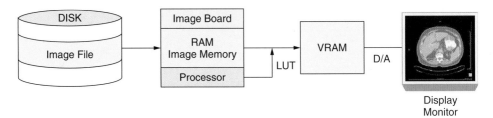

Figure 12.4 WS data flow of an image from the internal magnetic disk to the display monitor. D/A: digital-to-analog conversion; LUT: lookup table.

12.1.2 Display Monitor

The cathode ray tube (CRT) monitor used to be the de facto display in the WS. Over the past several years the quality of gray scale liquid crystal display (LCD) has been improved to the degree that it surpasses the quality of the best CRT video monitor. Most PACS WSs are now changing to LCD display. In locations where physical constraints prevent the use of a CRT, an LCD display allows medical images to be displayed where otherwise impossible. Hallways, rooms with minimal cooling, and very bright rooms are inhospitable to CRT displays. Table 12.2 compares the advantages and disadvantages of CRT and LCD for displaying medical images. The data in Table 12.2 were collected in late 2001; by now, the disadvantages of the LCD have gradually disappeared. In this context we use the word display, monitor, and screen interchangeably.

TABLE 12.2 LCD versus CRT: Advantages and disadvantages

LCD Advantages versus CRT Disadvantage	
LCD Advantage	CRT Disadvantage
Much thninner	Thicker
Light	Heavy
Consumes 4.2A for four-head system	Consumes 7A for four-head system
Maximum luminance 500 cd/m^2 (nice in bright rooms)	Maximum luminance 300–450 cd/m^2
Flat display	Display surface is not flat

LCD Disadvantages versus CRT Advantages	
LCD Disadvantage	CRT Advantage
Contrast only 500:1 (narrow viewing angle)	Contrast 2000:1 (narrow viewing angle)
Contrast only 45:1 (45° viewing angle)	Contrast 1000:1 (45° viewing angle)
Screen artifact due to black between pixels	Smooth transition between pixels
Only 15,000 hours until backlight replacement (although replacement is less than new unit)	30,000 hours until CRT replacement

12.1.3   Resolution

The resolution of a display monitor is specified in terms of the number of lines. For example, the "1K monitor" has 1024 lines; "2K" means 2048 lines. In the strict sense of the definition, however, it is not sufficient to specify spatial resolution simply in terms of the number of lines because the actual resolving power of the monitor may be less. Consider a digitally generated line pair pattern (black and white lines in pairs, see Fig. 2.3). The maximum displayable number of these line pairs on a 1K monitor is 512. However, the monitor may not be able to resolve 1024 alternating black and white lines in both the vertical and horizontal directions because of its instrumentation.

   Several techniques are available for the measurement of resolution. The simplest and most commonly used method employs a test pattern that consists of varying widths of line pair objects in vertical, horizontal, and sometimes radial directions (see Fig. 2.3). It should be noted that this visual approach in measuring the resolution of the total display-perception system, including the visual acuity of the observer, is prone to subjective variations.

   Other techniques include the shrinking raster test, the scanning spot photometer, the slit analyzer, and measurement of the modulation transfer function (MTF; Section 2.5.1.4). One additional factor worthy of attention is that resolution is a function of location on the monitor. Therefore the resolution specification must describe the location of the monitor as well as the luminance uniformity of the monitor. For these reasons the display monitor in PACS requires routine maintenance services using the SMPTE (Society of Motion Picture and Television Engineers) phantom.

12.1.4   Luminance and Contrast

Luminance measures the brightness in candelas per square meter (cd/m^2) or in foot-lambert (ft-L): $1\text{ft-L} = 3.426 \text{ cd/m}^2$. There is more than one definition for contrast and contrast ratio. The one most oftenly used for contrast C is the ratio of the difference between two luminances (L) to one of the larger luminance:

$$C = \frac{L_\text{o} - L_\text{B}}{L_\text{o}} \qquad (12.1)$$

where L_o is the luminance of the object and L_B is the luminance of the background. Contrast ratio C_r is frequently defined as the ratio of the luminance of an object to that of the background. This is expressed by

$$C_\text{r} = \frac{L_\text{max}}{L_\text{min}} \qquad (12.2)$$

where L_max is the luminance emitted by the area of the greatest intensity and L_min is the luminance emitted by the area of least intensity in the image.

   The contrast ratio depends not only on the luminance of the image but also on the intensity of the ambient light. For instance, in bright sunlight the display surface can have an apparent luminance of 3×10^4 cd/m^2. To achieve a contrast of 10, the luminance of the monitor must be 3×10^5 cd/m^2.

12.1.5 Human Perception

The luminance of the monitor affects the physiological response of the eye in perceiving image quality (spatial resolution and subject contrast). Two characteristics of the visual response are acuity, or the ability of the eye to detect fine detail, and the detection of luminance differences (threshold contrast) between the object and its background. Luminance differences can be measured by using an absolute parameter—just-noticeable differences (JNDs)—or a relative parameter—threshold contrast* (TC)—related by

$$TC = \frac{JND}{L_B} \tag{12.3}$$

where L_B is the background luminance.

The relationship between the threshold contrast and the luminance can be described by the Weber–Fechner law. When the luminance is low (1 ft-L), in the double-log plot, the threshold contrast is a linear function of luminance, with a slope of -0.05 sometimes referred to as the Rose model.* When the luminance is high, the threshold contrast is governed by the Weber model, which is a constant function of the luminance, again in the double-log plot.

In the Rose model region, when the object luminance L_O is fixed, the JND and L_B are related by

$$JND = k_1 L_O (L_B)^{1/2} \tag{12.4}$$

In the Weber model region, we write

$$JND = k_2 L_O (L_B) \tag{12.5}$$

where $k1$ and $k2$ are constants.

In general, the detection of small luminance differences by the visual system is dependent on the presence of various noises measurable by their standard deviations, in particular:

- Fluctuations in the light photon flux
- Noise from the display monitor
- Noise in the visual system

Thus the JND depends on L_O and L_B, which are terms affected by the environment, the state of the display monitor, as well as the conditions of the human observer.

12.1.6 Color Display

Although the majority of radiographical images are monochromatic, Doppler US, nuclear medicine, PET, light, molecular, and endoscopc images use colors for enhancement. Further recent developments in image-assisted therapy and minimally

---

*TC $= -0.5L$B in the double-log plot, or TC $= k(L$B$) - 1/2$ in the standard plot, where k is a constant.

invasive surgery use extensive color graphics superimposed on monochromatic images for illustration purposes. To display a color image, three image memories (R, G, B) are needed. As discussed in Section 3.9.2, the composite video controller combines these three memories to form a color display (see Fig. 3.29). Color LCD monitors are today of excellent quality for color medical image display.

12.2   ERGONOMICS OF IMAGE WORKSTATIONS

The human observer at various environments may perceive an image with different qualities on the monitor. Three major factors that may affect the viewing environment are glare, ambient light, and acoustic noise due to hardware. These factors are independent of the workstation design and quality. Therefore we must understand these factors in the ergonomic design of an image workstation.

12.2.1   Glare

Glare, the most frequent complaint among WS users, is the sensation produced within the visual field by luminance that is sufficiently greater than the luminance to which the eyes are adapted to cause annoyance, discomfort, or loss in visual performance and visibility.

Glare can be caused by reflections of electric light sources, windows, and light-colored objects including furniture and clothing. The magnitude of the glare sensation is a function of the size, position, and luminance of a source, the number of sources, and the luminance to which the eyes are adapted at the moment. It may be categorized according to its origin: direct or reflected glare. Direct glare may be caused by bright sources of light in the visual field of view (e.g., sunlight and lightbulbs). Reflected glare is caused by light reflected from the display screen. If the reflections are diffuse, they are referred to as veiling glare.

Image reflections are both distracting and annoying, since the eye is induced to focus alternately between the displayed and reflected images. The reflected glare can be reduced by increasing the display contrast, by wearing dark-colored clothing, by correctly positioning the screen with respect to lights, windows, and other reflective objects, and by adjusting the screen angle.

12.2.2   Ambient Illuminance

An important issue related to the problem of glare is the proper illumination of the WS area. Excessive lighting can increase the readability of documents but can also increase the reflected glare, whereas sufficient illumination can reduce glare but can make reading of source documents at the WS difficult. Ergonomic guidelines for the traditional office environment recommend a high level of lighting: 700 lux (an engineering unit for lighting) or more. A survey of 38 computer-aided design (CAD) operators who were allowed to adjust the ambient lighting indicated that the median illumination level is around 125 lux (125 at keyboard, etc.) with 90% of the readings falling between 15 and 505 lux (Heiden, 1984). These levels are optimized for CRT or LCD viewing but certainly not for reading written documents. An illumination of 200 lux is normally considered inadequate for an office environment. Another study suggests a lower range (150–400 lux) for tasks that do not involve information transfer from paper documents. At these levels lighting is sufficiently subdued to permit good display contrast in most cases. The higher range (400–550 lux) is suggested for tasks that require the reading of paper documents. Increasing ambient lighting above 550 lux reduces display contrast appreciably. If the paper documents contain small, low-contrast print, 550 lux may not provide adequate lighting. Such cases may call for supplementary special task lighting directed only at the document surface. This recommendation is based on the conditions needed to read text, not images, on a screen. Another recommendation specifies the use of a level of ambient illumination equal to the average luminance of an image on the display WS screen.

12.2.3   Acoustic Noise due to Hardware

An imaging workstation often includes components like magnetic disks, RAID, image processors, and other arrays of hardware that produce heat and require electric fans for cooling. These fans often produce an intolerably high noise level. Even for a low-noise computer attached to the WS, it is recommended that the computer be separated from the WS area to isolate the noise that would affect human performance.

As personal computers become more common, the computer, the terminal, and the display monitor become an integrated system insofar as they are connected by very short cables. Most imaging workstations utilize a personal computer as the host, however, and because of the short cabling, the host computer and the image processor wind up in the same room as the terminal, display monitors, and the keyboard. Failure of the image WS designer to consider the consequences of having all these units together creates a very noisy environment at the WS, and it is difficult for the user to sustain concentration during long working hours. Care must be exercised in designing the WS environment to avoid problems due to acoustic noise from the hardware.

12.3   EVOLUTION OF MEDICAL IMAGE DISPLAY TECHNOLOGIES

This section reviews the evolution of medical imaging display technologies. Basically there are three phases: the early period, 1986 to 1994; the 1995 to 1999 period; and the 1999 to 2002 period with a version 2 in the third period. The early period contributions are the Sun workstation with 2K video monitors and ICU (intensive care unit) and pediatric 1K WSs. The 1995–1999 period accomplishments are the production of competitive 2K monitors by several manufacturers, the beginning of the LCD display screen, and PC-based workstations. The 1999–2002 period highlights are DICOM compliant PC-based workstations and several manufacturers' competing shares of the LCD display market. The version 2 of the third period is the domination of LCD in most PACS WS and the post processing WS. Tables 12.3, 12.4, and 12.5 summarize the specifications of these three periods of image technology evolution.

12.4   TYPES OF IMAGE WORKSTATION

Image workstations can be loosely categorized into six types based on their applications: diagnostic, review, analysis, digitizing and printing, interactive teaching, and desktop research workstations.

TABLE 12.3   Display technology evolution phase 1: Early period, 1986 to 1994

Typical applications	Ultrasound acquisition and review Cardio catheterization PACS X ray
Displays and resolutions	10–12 in. 640 × 480 Barco, DataRay RS170 DataRay 1280 × 1024 Siemens 2048 × 2560 MegaScan
Display controllers	Color: VCR (for ultrasound), VGA Custom: Direct from Fluoroscope, etc. Grayscale: VGA, Cemax-Ikon, Dome 256 shades of gray chosen from 1000 now possible
Performance	Image download: 20 MB/s on Sbus Real-time Window and level introduced on Dome RX16
Operating system	Unix, Dos, Macintosh, Windows (starting)
Luminance	100–220 cd/m^2
Reliability	10–15% annual failure rate
Video quality	2–5 ns rise time, 2 ns jitter Focus: Good in center, poor at edges
Calibration	Most equipment calibrated at factory, then some feed-forward correction for common aging mechanisms.

12.4.1   Diagnostic Workstation

A diagnostic WS is used by radiologists for making primary diagnosis. The components in this type of WS are of the best quality and the easiest to use. "Best quality" is used here in the sense of display quality, rapid display time (1–2 seconds for the first image), and the user-friendly display functions. If the WS is used for displaying projection radiographs, multiple 2K monitors are needed. On the other hand, if the workstation is used for CT, M, US images, multiple 1K monitors are sufficient. A diagnostic WS requires a digital dictaphone or voice dictation capability to report the findings. The WS provides software to append the digital voice report to the images. If the radiologist inputs the report himself/herself, the DICOM structured reporting function should be available in the WS. Figure 12.5 shows a generic 2K WS with two LCD monitors showing P–A and lateral views of two CR chest images.

12.4.2   Review Workstation

A review WS is used by radiologists and referring physicians to review cases in the hospital wards or outpatient facilities. The dictation or the transcribed report should already be available with the corresponding images at the workstation. A review workstation may not require 5 mega pixel monitors, because images have already been read by the radiologist from the diagnostic WS. With the report already available, the referring physicians can use the 3 mega pixel or even the 1K monitors

TABLE 12.4   Display technology evolution phase 2: 1995 to 1999

Typical applications	Ultrasound Acquisition and Review Cardio catheterization PACS X ray
Displays and resolutions	12–15 in. 640 × 480 Barco, DataRay, SonQ 1200 × 1600 Image Systems, DataRay, Nortech 1280 × 1024 Siemens, Image Systems 2048 × 2560 MegaScan (declining), Image Systems, DataRay, Siemens, Barco First LCD from dpiX shown, never achieved volume production
Display controllers	Color: VCR (for ultrasound), VGA Grayscale: Dome, Metheus, Cemax 1000 simultaneous shades of gray now possible {Metheus, Astro} First digital controllers shown: Dome, Metheus
Performance	Image Download: 55 MB/s on 2 MP, 90 MB/s on 5 MP
Operating system	Unix, Macintosh (in decline), Windows
Spot size	<2.0 lp/mm
Contrast	CRT contrast ratio 800:1
Luminance	350 cd/m^2 center, 280 cd/m^2 typical
Reliability	5–10% annual failure rate
Video quality	0.7–2.3 ns rise time, 0.5–2 ns jitter Focus: Good all over screen when equipment new
Calibration	Luminance Calibration (Dome), Equalizer (Metheus), MediCal (Barco) Some field sites starting to calibrate displays routinely, most don't

to visualize the pathology from the monitors. Diagnostic and review WSs can be combined as one single WS sharing both diagnostic and review functions like an alternator. Figure 12.6 shows a generic two-monitor 1K (1600 lines × 1024 pixels) video WS used in the intensive care unit.

12.4.3   Analysis Workstation

An analysis workstation differs from the diagnostic and review workstations in that the former is used to extract useful parameters from images. Some parameters are easy to extract from a simple region of interest (ROI) operation, which can be done from a diagnostic or review workstation; others (i.e., blood flow measurements from DSA, 3-D reconstruction from sequential CT images) are computationally intensive and require an analysis workstation with a more powerful image processor and high-performance software (e.g., see Fig. 4.21*B*, an analysis workstation displaying a 3-D rendering of fused MRI and fMRI images).

TABLE 12.5   Display technology evolution phase 3: 1998 to 2002

Typical applications	Ultrasound acquisition and review Cardio and angio PACS X-ray 3D reconstructions Mammography (starting)
Displays and resolutions	640×480 CRT Barco 1200×1600 CRT Barco, Siemens, Image Systems, DataRay 1280×1024 CRT Siemens, Image Systems, Barco 2048×2560 CRT Barco, Siemens, Clinton 1200×1600 Grayscale LCD Totoku, Eizo 1536×2048 Grayscale LCD Dome, Barco 2048×2560 Grayscale LCD Dome
Display controllers	Color: VCR (for ultrasound), VGA Grayscale Analog: Barco(Metheus), Dome, (Astro, Matrox, Wide all starting) Grayscale Digital: Dome 256 shades chosen from 766, Barco 1000 simultaneous shades RealVision 256 shades chosen from 766
Performance	Image download: 100 MB/s on 2 MP (mega pixel), 120 MB/s on 3 MP, 120 MB/s on 5 MP Ability to synchronize image download with vertical refresh added Real-time Window and level operation on 5 MP
Operating system	Unix (in decline), Windows
Spot size	~ 2.1 lp/mm CRT ~ 2.5 lp/mm LCD
Contrast	CRT contrast ratio 2000:1 over wide viewing angle LCD contrast ratio 500:1 over narrow viewing angle
Luminance	CRT 350cd/m2 center, 280 cd/m2 typical Luminance uniformity introduced on Barco CRT—300 cd/m^2 over entire screen Luminance noise of P104 CRT phosphor noted, P45 becomes dominant LCD initially 700 cd/m2, calibrated
Reliability and lifetime	<3% annual failure rate CRT 30,000 hour calibrated life at full luminance LCD 15,000 hour calibrated life for back light, LCD have $\sim 10\%$ cost for backlight replacement
Video quality	Analog 0.5–1.8 ns rise time, 0.2–1 ns jitter Analog focus: Typically good over entire screen Digital bit-errors exist, limited to 1 per billion
Calibration	TQA(Planar-Dome), MediCal Pro (Barco), Smfit (Siemens) Many field sites calibrate displays routinely, many still feel it takes too long Intervention-free front calibration introduced for LCD panels (Barco) Remote network monitoring of conformance introduced (Barco, Dome)

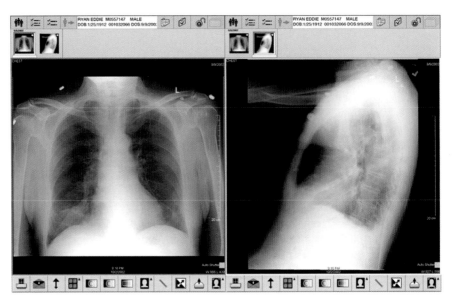

Figure 12.5   A generic 2K display workstation with two LCD monitors showing PA and lateral views of CR chest images.

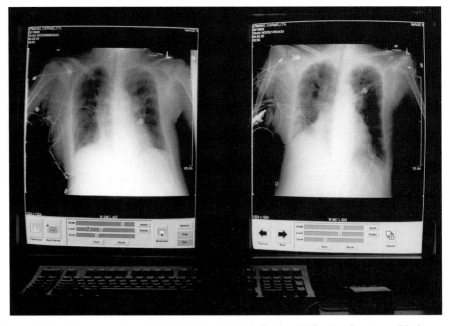

Figure 12.6   Two-monitor 1K (1600 lines) ICU display WS showing two CR images. Left-hand CRT monitor shows the current image; all previous images can be accessed within one second on the right-hand monitor by clicking on the two arrow icons at the bottom (Previous and Next). Simple image processing functions are controlled by the icons located at the bottom of the screens.

12.4.4   Digitizing, Printing, and CD Copying Workstation

The digitizing and printing WS is for radiology department technologists or film librarians who must digitize historical films and films from outside the department. The WS is also used for printing soft copy images to hard copy on film or paper, and for copying images onto a CD for distribution. In addition to the standard WS components already described, the WS requires a laser film scanner (see Section 3.2.3), a laser film imager, a good-quality paper printer, and a CD copier. The paper printer is used for pictorial report generation from the diagnostic, review, and editorial and research workstations. A 1K display monitor for quality control purposes would be sufficient for this type of WS.

12.4.5   Interactive Teaching Workstation

A teaching workstation is used for interactive teaching. It emulates the role of teaching files in the film library but with more interactive features. Figure 12.7 shows a digital mammography teaching workstation for breast imaging.

12.4.6   Desktop Workstation

The desktop WS is for physicians or researchers to generate lecture slides and teaching and research materials from images and related data in the PACS database. The WS uses standard desktop computer equipment to facilitate the user's daily workload. The desktop workstation can also be used as a web client to access images and related information from a Web server connected to the PACS server and archive server.

Image WSs that directly interact with radiologists and physicians are the most important and visible component in a PACS. To design them effectively, a thorough understanding of the clinical operation environment requirements is necessary.

In latter sections and chapters, wherever appropriate, additional image WS types will be presented including post processing workflow and CAD-related WSs, and mobile PDA WS for image management and distribution.

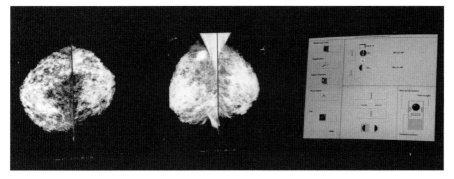

Figure 12.7   Four mammograms shown on a 2K two-monitor digital mammography teaching WS. (left) Left and right craniocaudal views; (middle) left and right mediolateral oblique views; (right) text monitor with icons for image display and manipulation at the WS.

12.5 IMAGE DISPLAY AND MEASUREMENT FUNCTIONS

This section discusses some daily used image display, manipulation, and measurement functions in the display WSs described in Section 12.4.

12.5.1 Zoom and Scroll

Zoom and scroll is an interactive command manipulated via a trackball, mouse, or keyboard to adjust the contrast and brightness of the image displayed on the monitors. The user first uses the trackball to scroll about the image, centering the region of interest (ROI) on the screen. The ROI can then be magnified by pressing a designated button to perform the zoom. The image becomes more blocky as the zoom factor increases, reflecting the greater number of times each pixel is replicated.

Although it is useful to magnify and scroll the image on the screen, the field of view decreases in proportion to the square of the magnification factor. Magnification is commonly performed via pixel replication or interpolation. In the former, one pixel value repeats itself several times in both the horizontal and vertical directions, and in the latter the pixel value is replaced by interpolation of its neighbors. For example, to magnify the image by 2 by replication is to replicate the image 2×2 times.

12.5.2 Window and Level

The window and level feature allows the user to control the grouping and interval of gray levels to be displayed on the monitor. The center of this interval is called the *level value*, and the range is called the *window value*. The selected gray level range will be distributed over the entire dynamic range of the display monitor; thus using a smaller window value will cause the contrast in the resulting image on the screen to increase. Gray levels present in the image outside the defined interval are clipped to either black or white (or both), according to the side of the interval on which they are positioned. This function is also controlled by the user via a trackball, mouse, and keyboard. For example, moving the trackball in the vertical direction typically controls the window value, whereas the horizontal direction controls the level of which gray levels to be displayed on the monitor. Window and level operations can be performed in real time by using an image processor with a fast access memory called a lookup table (LUT). A 256 value LUT inputs an 8-bit (a 4096 value LUT inputs an 12-bit) address whose memory location contains the value of the desired gray level transformation (linear scaling with clipping). The memory address for the LUT is provided by the original pixel value. Figure 12.8 illustrates the concept of the LUT. In the figure the original pixel "5" is mapped to "36" via the LUT.

If the window value is fixed to 1 and the level value is changed by 1 from 0 to 255 continuously, and if the image is displayed during each change, then the monitor is continuously displaying all 256 values of the image, with 1 gray level at a time.

12.5.3 Histogram Modification

A function very useful for enhancing the display image is histogram modification. A histogram of the original image is first obtained and then modified by rescaling each pixel value in the original image. The new enhanced image that is formed will show the desired modification.

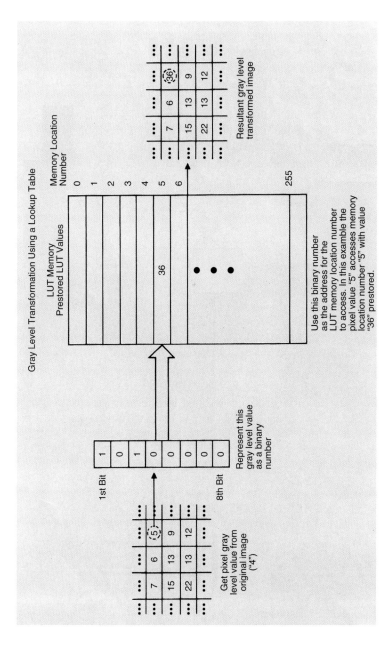

Figure 12.8 Concept of a lookup table (LUT). In this case the pixel value 5 is mapped to 36 through a preset LUT.

363

An example of histogram modification is histogram equalization, in which the shape of the modified histogram is adjusted to be as uniform (i.e., the number of pixels per value) as possible for all gray levels. The rescaling factor (or the histogram equalization transfer function) is given by

$$g = (g_{max} - g_{min})P(f) + g_{min} \tag{12.6}$$

where g is the output (modified) gray level, g_{max} and g_{min} are the maximum and minimum gray level of the modified image, respectively, f is the input (original) gray level, and $P(f)$ is the cumulative distribution function (or integrated histogram) of f.

Figure 12.9 shows an example of modifying an overexposed (too dark) chest X-ray image in the lungs with the histogram equalization method. In this example the frequency of occurrence of some lower gray level values in the modified histogram has been changed to zero to enforce uniformity. It is seen that some details in the lung have been restored.

12.5.4 Image Reverse

An LUT can be used to reverse the dark and light pixels of an image. In this function, the LUT is loaded with a reverse ramp such that for an 8-bit image, the value 255

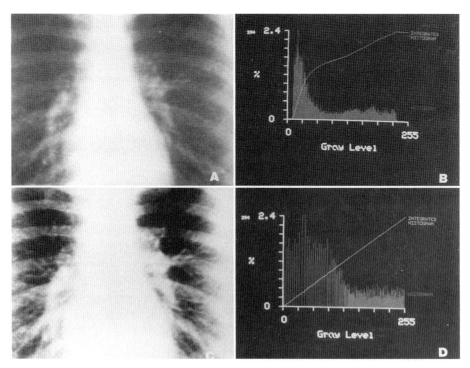

Figure 12.9 Concept of histogram equalization. (*A*) Region in the center of the chest X ray with lung region overexposed, showing relatively low contrast; (*B*) histogram of the chest image. (*C*) lung region in the image enhanced with histogram equalization; (*D*) modified histogram.

becomes 0 and 0 becomes 255. Image reverse is used to locate external objects—for example, intrathoracic tubes in ICU X-ray examinations.

12.5.5   Distance, Area, and Average Gray Level Measurements

Three simple measurement functions are important for immediate interactive quantitative assessment while the radiologist is reading an image because they allow the user to perform physical measurement with the image displayed on the monitor by calibrating the dimensions of each pixel to a pre-assigned physical units or the gray level value to the optical density.

The *distance calibration* procedure is performed by moving the cursor over the image to define the physical distance between two pixels. Best results are obtained when the image contains a calibration ring or other object of known size. To perform *optical density* calibration, the user moves the cursor over many different gray levels and makes queries from a menu to determine the corresponding optical densities. Finally, an interactive procedure allows the user to trace a region of interest from which the *area average and the standard deviation gray level* can be computed.

12.5.6   Optimization of Image Perception in Soft Copy Display

There are three sequential steps to optimize an image for soft copy display: remove the unnecessary background, determine the anatomical region of interest (ROI), and correct for the gamma response of the monitor based on the ROI. These steps can be implemented through properly chosen LUT.

12.5.6.1   *Background Removal*   For display CR or DR, we had discussed the importance of background removal in Section 3.3.4. Figure 12.10*A* and *B* show a CR image with the image background and the corresponding histogram, respectively. After the background of the image in Figure 12.10*A* is removed, the new histogram (Fig. 12.10*D*) has no pixel values above 710.The new LUT based on the new histogram produces Figure 12.10*C*, which has a better visual quality than that in Figure 12.10*A*.

12.5.6.2   *Anatomical Regions of Interest*   It is necessary to adjust for the display based on the anatomical regions of interest because tissue contrast varies in different body regions. For example, in CT chest examinations, there are lung, soft tissue, and bone windows (LUT) to highlight the lungs, heart tissue, and bone, respectively. This method has been used since the dawn of body CT imaging. By the same token, in CR and DR there are also specially designed LUTs for different body regions. Figure 12.11 shows four transfer curves used to adjust for the pixel values in the head, bone, chest, and abdomen regions in CR.

12.5.6.3   *Gamma Curve Correction*   The pixel value versus its corresponding brightness in a monitor (CRT and LCD) is the gamma curve, which is nonlinear and different from monitor to monitor. An adjustment of this gamma curve to a linear curve will improve the visual quality of the image. For a new monitor, a calibration procedure is necessary to determine this gamma curve, which is then used to modify the LUT. Figure 12.12 shows the gamma curve from two different monitors and

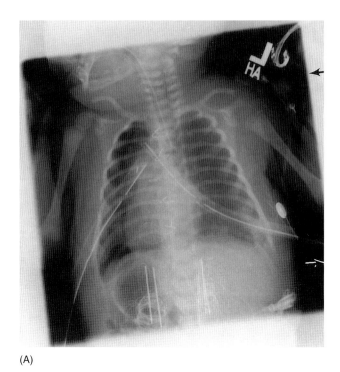

(A)

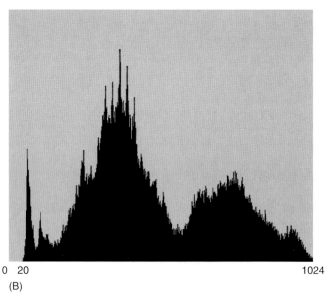

0 20   1024
(B)

Figure 12.10 Results after background removal. (*A*) Original pediatric CR image with background (arrows, white area near the borders); (*B*) corresponding histogram; (*C*) same CR image after background removal, displayed with a different LUT based on the new histogram shown in (*D*). (*D*) The corresponding histogram of the background removed CR image shown in (*C*). All pixels with values greater than 710 in (*D*) have been removed.

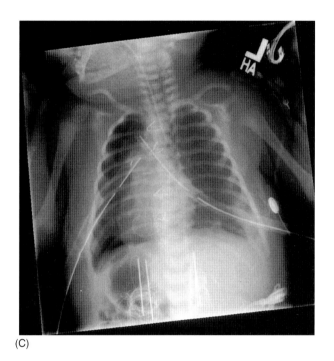

(C)

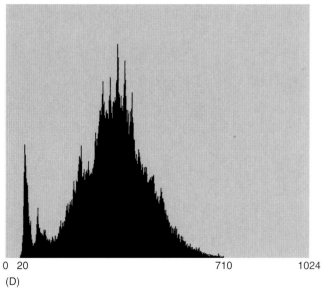

| 0 20 | 710 | 1024 |

(D)

Figure 12.10   (*Continued*)

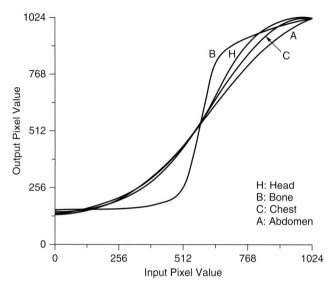

Figure 12.11 Pixel value adjustment for CR images in different body regions: head (H), bone (B), chest (C), and abdomen (A). (Courtesy of Dr. J. Zhang)

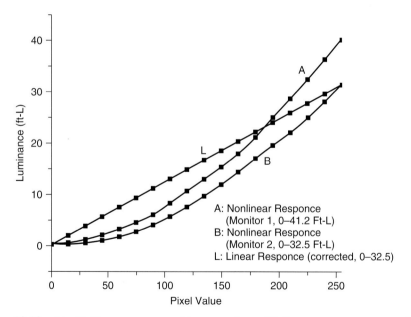

Figure 12.12 (*A, B*) Gamma curves of two monitors; (*L*) linear response curve of both monitors after the gamma correction. (Courtesy of Dr. J. Zhang)

their linear correction. A monitor must be recalibrated periodically to maintain its performance.

12.5.7 Montage

A montage represents a selected set of individual images from a CT, MR, US or any other modality image series for display. Such groupings are useful because only a few images from most series show the particular pathology or features of interest to the referring physicians or radiologists. For example, an average MR examination may contain half a dozen sequences with an average of 30 images per sequence, which gives rise to 180 images in the study. A typical montage would have 20 images, containing the most significant features representing the exam. So typically only 10% of the images taken from an examination are essential and the rest are supplemental. A montage image collection selected by the radiologist would allow the capture of the most important images in a single (or multiple) display screen. Each image selected in the montage can be tagged in its own DICOM header for future quick reference and display.

12.6 WORKSTATION GRAPHIC USER INTERFACE (GUI) AND BASIC DISPLAY FUNCTIONS

12.6.1 Basic Software Functions in a Display Workstation

Some of the basic software functions described in Section 12.5 are necessary in a WS to facilitate its operation. These functions are easy to use with a single click on the mouse at the patient's directory, study list, and image processing icons on the monitors. The keyboard is used or retrieving information not stored in the WS's local disks. In this case the user types in either the patient's name or ID or a disease category as the key for searching information from the archive. Table 12.6 lists some basic software functions required in a WS. Among these functions, the most often used are: select patient, sort patient directory, library search, select image, cine mode, zoom/scroll, and window and level. Results of using some of these functions are shown in Figures 12.13–12.16. Figure 12.13 shows the Patient Directory with the patient list (with fictitious names), ID, date and time of the study, modality, procedure, and the physician's name. The leftmost column is a read icon to delineate whether the study had been read by a radiologist. Figure 12.14*A* shows a single monitor displaying three views of an MRI study, and Figure 12.14*B* a two-monitor workstation displaying a sequence of transverse view on the left and a coronal view on the right monitor. The bottom GUI icons are described in Section 12.6.2. Figure 12.15 shows a two-monitor view of a CT chest exam with the soft tissue window. Figure 12.16 provides a two-monitor view of an obstetrics US exam showing a fetus.

12.6.2 Workstation User Interface

Most PACS manufacturers have implemented the aforementioned display and measurement functions in their WSs in the form of a library. The user can use a pull-down manual to customize his/her preferred interface at the WS. The 12 icons at the bottom

TABLE 12.6   Important software functions in a display workstation

Function	Description
Directory	
Patient directory	Name, ID, age, sex, date of current exam
Study list	Type of exam, anatomical area, date studies taken
Display	
Screen reconfiguration	Reconfigures each screen for the convenience of image display
Monitor selection	Left, right
Display	Displays images according to screen configuration and monitor selected
Image manipulation	
Dials	Brightness, contrast, zoom, and scroll
LUT	Predefined lookup tables (bone, soft tissue, brain, etc.)
Cine	Single or multiple cine on multi-monitors for CT and MR images
Rotation	Rotates an image
Negative	Reverses gray scale
Utilities	
Montage	Selects images to form a montage
Image discharge	Deletes images of discharged patients (a privileged operation)
Library search	Retrieves historical examinations (requires keyboard operation)
Report	Retrieves reports from RIS
Measurements	Linear and region of interest

of each display window in Figures 12.13–12.16 provide examples of customized user interface ICON tool bars designed by the user using a pull-down manual. Figure 12.17 shows these 12 icons, and their descriptions are given in Table 12.7.

12.7   DICOM PC-BASED DISPLAY WORKSTATION

Most PACS WSs nowadays are personal computer (PC) based with either Windows 98 and up or XP operation system. This trend is very natural for the integration of PACS and the electronic patient record (ePR), since the latter is strictly a PC-based system. In this section we give a more precise architecture of the DICOM PC-based display WS in both hardware and software. There may be some duplication of materials from previous sections, but from a system integration point of view, this section becomes a self-contained guideline. The readers may want to treat it as a recipe for developing a PC-based PACS workstation.

12.7.1   Hardware Configuration

The hardware configuration of the workstation is shown in Figure 12.3.

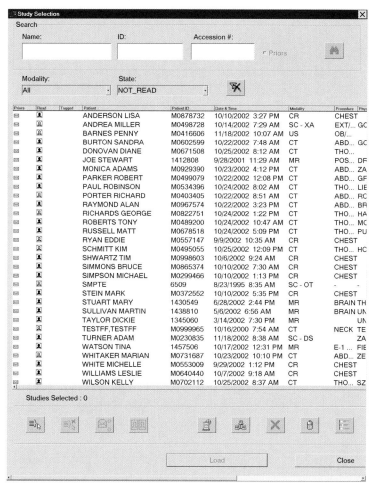

Figure 12.13   Patient directory with the patient list (with fictitious names), ID, date and time of the study, modality, procedure, and physician's name.

12.7.1.1 *Host Computer*   The computer of the WS can be a PC based with a Intel Pentium 4 processor(s) at over 1 GHz, 256–512 Mbytes RAM, PCI bus structure, and 100-GB disks as local storage.

12.7.1.2 *Display Devices*   Display devices include single- or multiple-display CD monitors and video display boards. The display monitor can be from 24-in. 1600 × 1280 to 2.5 K × 1K resolutions in portrait mode. The display board is 4 mega pixels or 5 mega pixels.

12.7.1.3 *Networking Equipment*   In the display WS, high-speed Ethernet, or fiber-optic technology can be used as the primary means of communication, and conventional Ethernet as the backup.

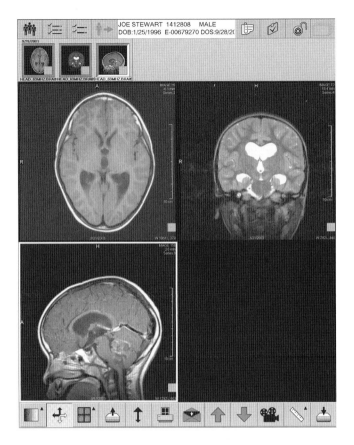

(A)

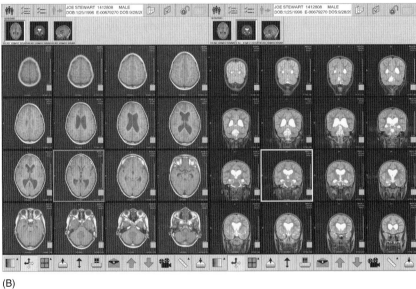

(B)

Figure 12.14 (*A*) Single LCD monitor displaying three views of an MRI study. (*B*) Two- LCD monitor WS displaying transverse view on the left and coronal view on the right monitor.

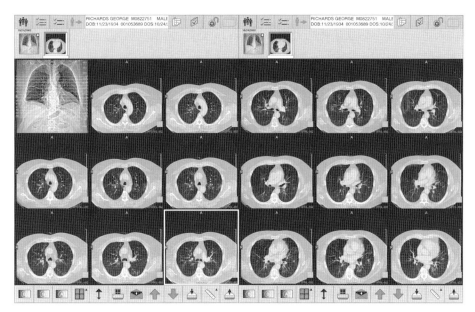

Figure 12.15 Two-LCD monitor WS showing a CT chest exam with the soft tissue window. The first image is the chest scout view of the patient.

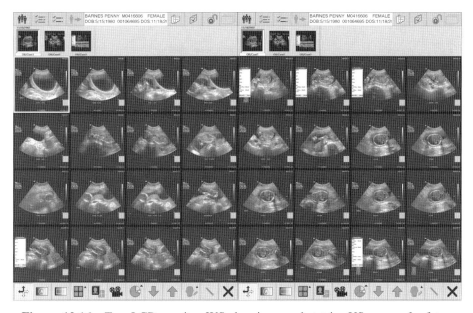

Figure 12.16 Two-LCD monitor WS showing an obstetrics US exam of a fetus.

TABLE 12.7   Description of the user interface Icons and tool bars shown in Figure 12.17

1. Print the selected image
2. Save the selected image
3. Zoom in and out of the image
4. Show a list of display layouts and set the layout
5. Set the bone window/level
6. Set the soft tissue window/level
7. Set the auto display window/level
8. Edge enhancement filter
9. Image Measurement functions
10. Invert the image
11. Reset the image display
12. Select the text level in the image (a lot of text, some, minimum)

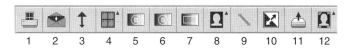

Figure 12.17   Graphical user interface display toolbars and icons.

12.7.2 Software System

The software can be developed based on a Microsoft Windows or XP platform and in the Visual C/C++ programming environment. WinSock communication over TCP/IP, Microsoft Foundation Class (MFC) libraries, standard image processing library, UC Davis DICOM Library, and Windows-based PACS API libraries can be used as development tools. The user interface of the display WS is icon/menu driven with a user-friendly graphical interface.

12.7.2.1 Software Architecture   The architecture of the software system is divided into four layers: application interface layer, application libraries layer, system libraries layer, and operating system (OS) driver layer, which is over the hardware layer. Figure 12.18 shows the software architecture of the WS.

The application interface layer is the top layer of the software system that interfaces with the end user of the display workstation. This layer is composed of four modules: (1) image communication software package, (2) patient folder management, (3) image display program, and (4) DICOM query/retrieve software package. This layer directly supports any application that requires accessing PACS and radiological images.

In the application library layer, the PACS API libraries provide all library functions to support four modules in the application interface layer. Here UC Davis DICOM Network Transport libraries and DIMSE-C libraries ensure DICOM communication protocols and functions, and the specific vendor's image processing library supplies library functions for image display of the workstation.

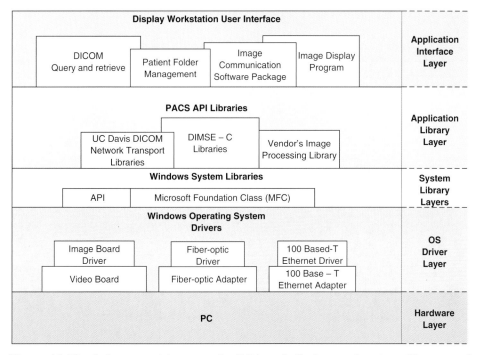

Figure 12.18 Software architecture of a PC-based display workstation. (Courtesy of M. Lei, J. Zhang, and X. Wong)

The system library layer is responsible for providing Windows system libraries, API functions, and MFC (Microsoft foundation class) to serve as a developmental platform. The OS driver layer provides Windows OS and its drivers for connecting with hardware components, which include the vendor's driver for its image board, and optical fiber or high-speed Ethernet communication ports. Software data flow between the layers of the software is shown in Figure 12.19.

12.7.2.2   *Software Modules in the Application Interface Layer*   In the WS the user has access only to the application interface layer, which is composed of the four modules: image communication a patient folder management, image display program, and query and retrieve modules.

Image Communication   The module is responsible for supporting DICOM services with DICOM protocols over TCP/IP to perform two DICOM services: storage service class provider (SCP) and storage service class user (SCU). The DICOM services include C-Echo for verification, C-Store for storage, C-Find for querying, and C-Move for retrieving.

Patient Folder Management   This module manages the local storage with hierarchical, or tree-structure, directories to organize patient folders within the WS. The DICOM decoder is used to extract patient demographic data and examination records from the header of a DICOM image. The reformatter of the module changes the image from DICOM format to the vendor's image board format for display. The extracted

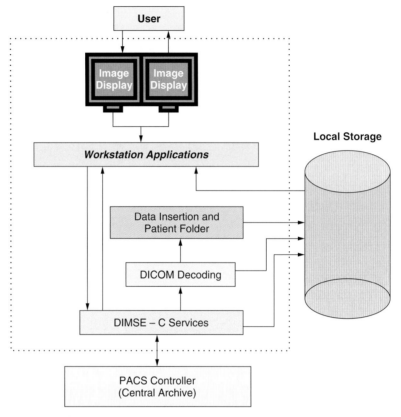

Figure 12.19   Software data flow in the DICOM-compliant PC-based display workstation. Compared this software workflow with the hardware workflow of the WS of Figure 12.3. (Courtesy M. Lei, J. Zhang, and X. Wong)

image data, via the DICOM decoder and the reformatter, is inserted into an individual patient folder. A patient folder follows the DICOM data model, which contains three hierarchical levels: patient, study, and series level. The hierarchy starts with a root directory in the local storage system of the WS. Figure 12.20 is a diagram of the DICOM data model patient folder infrastructure.

A patient's folder is automatically created in the WS on receipt of the first image of the patient. Subsequent images from individual studies and series are inserted into the patient folder accordingly. The patient folder can be automatically deleted from the WS based on certain aging criteria such as the number of days since the folder was created or discharge or transfer of the patient. Figure 12.21 presents the interface of three hierarchical levels of patient folders.

Image Display Program   The image display program supports both single and dual large 1600 × 1280 (up to 2.5K × 2.K) resolution portrait LCD monitors to display patient information and radiological images. Images with the vendor image board header format in a patient folder can be displayed via the image display program. The screen layout of the WS should be user adjustable with one image on one monitor, two on one, four on one, etc. The display program supports multimodality

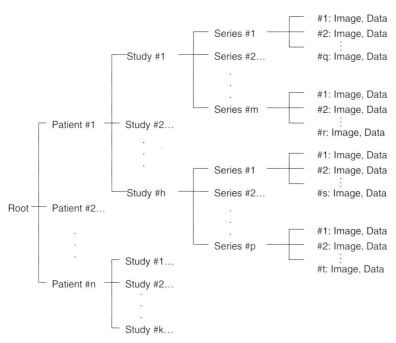

Figure 12.20   Three-level hierarchy of the patient folders based on the DICOM data model managed by the display workstation. (Courtesy of M. Lei, J. Zhang, and X. Wong)

display for CT, MR, US, and CR/DR in the sense that one monitor can display one modality while the second monitor's other modality images.

Image manipulation functions such as zoom, pan, rotation, flip, window and level adjustment, and invert are available. Automatic defaulted window and level preset function is used during imaging loading to minimize the manipulation time. Real-time zoom and contrast adjustment is easily performed by using the mouse.

Query and Retrieve   This module is a DICOM query/retrieve service class user (Q/R SCU) to query and retrieve patient studies from the PACS long-term archive or directly from radiological imaging systems. The query and retrieve module supports DICOM C-Echo, C-Store, C-Find, and C-Move services. With this module, the WS has access capability to Query/Retrieve Service Class Providers, which use the Q/R information models of patient root and study root.

12.8 RECENT DEVELOPMENTS IN PACS WORKSTATIONS

12.8.1 Postprocessing Workflow

During the past several years, the development of multidimensional imaging technology has exploded exponentially, which results in two phenomena. First, hundreds to thousands of images are acquired per examination, which require new approaches and solutions for storage and display technologies. Second, with so many images per exam, radiologists face the time constraint of completing their daily work load.

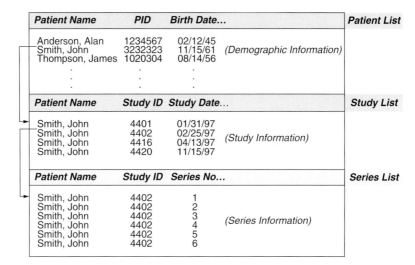

Patient Name	PID	Birth Date...		Patient List
Anderson, Alan	1234567	02/12/45		
Smith, John	3232323	11/15/61	(Demographic Information)	
Thompson, James	1020304	08/14/56		

Patient Name	Study ID	Study Date...		Study List
Smith, John	4401	01/31/97		
Smith, John	4402	02/25/97	(Study Information)	
Smith, John	4416	04/13/97		
Smith, John	4420	11/15/97		

Patient Name	Study ID	Series No...		Series List
Smith, John	4402	1		
Smith, John	4402	2		
Smith, John	4402	3	(Series Information)	
Smith, John	4402	4		
Smith, John	4402	5		
Smith, John	4402	6		

Figure 12.21 Patient folders in the WS. Each folder contains three hierarchical levels: patient, study, and series level. (Courtesy of M. Lei, J. Zhang, and X. Wong)

The trend is to intelligently extract focused qualitative and quantitative results from these images and display them properly and optimally. We have discussed the image storage issue in other chapters. This section presents the image display alternatives compared to traditional viewing methods for everyday's clinical operation.

To circumvent the voluminous images per study, research laboratories around the world have developed new methods for display and productized by manufacturers. The common term used in this development is post-processing workflow (PPW). PPW has two components: a post-processing workstation (WS) to extract information from the images; and a workflow to integrate the input data from PACS and export the output from the WS to PACS for viewing.

The post-processing WS can be a WS to perform multidimensional image display or a CAD (computer-aided diagnosis) WS (see Chapters 20, 25 and 26) with complex algorithms for information retrieval, feature extraction, and computer diagnosis. To integrate CAD results to PACS, Chapter 26 will present a general purpose CAD-PACS integration toolkit. Some post-processing image products may not require the same FDA (Food and Drug Administration) approval as that needed from CAD products because in the former the manufacturer does not change the PACS images and data, only display them differently. Thus, their products can get to the market place faster. Whereas, for a real CAD product, it does require FDA approval, the time from perceiving the concept to the market place may take many years.

The following two subsections focus in PPW of multidimensional image display. The first method is to integrate a software toolkit in the PACS WS, and the second method is to use the vendor provided specific display WS.

12.8.2 Multidimensional Image Display

As multi-Slice CT (128/256 Slices) and 3-D MR imaging modalities are used widely in radiological imaging studies, the image numbers per series are increased from a few of hundreds to more than thousands, and these huge amount of medical image data is generated daily. The traditional 2-D image display modes such as multiple window layout, pan, static stack or dynamic stack are not sufficient for radiologists to handle so many images in one or two display screens at same time. The new three-dimensional (3-D) and four-dimensional (4-D) image display functions have become common diagnostic tools for radiologists to view these images. As many of these studies generate isotropy images in all directions, radiologists can view and analyze image structures and pathology from all directions with different 3-D orientations resulting in methods such as multi-planar reconstruction (MPR), maximum intensity projection (MIP), surface-shaded display (SSD), or volume rendering (VR).

In these types of display, interactive manipulation is essential in obtaining optimal visualization effect. The 3-D image WSs should provide enough and easy to use GUI (graphical user interface) to users when rendering volume and time (fourth dimension) image data. Free and easy to change the visual angle (free-MPR) and to set the rendering pattern are advantageous. Furthermore, in favor of the widespread application of medical image visualization in clinical environment, a small and flexible 3-D display software framework to plug in the existing PACS WS is very suitable for radiologists and physicians to use. It is because there is usually a lack of computing power in the PACS WS's clinical environment. This section provides the concept of a software visualization toolkit (VTK), consisting of the aforementioned functions for displaying multidimensional images, which can be easily applied to medical image WS or Web-based network application. Once the toolkit is installed in the PACS WS, it provides a straightforward PPW between the multidimensional images input data and the PACS WS display. Figures 12.22*A* shows some MPR and MIP display of a cardiac CT study, and Figure 12.22*B*, a head CT MPR, MIP displays and a SSD rendering pattern.

12.8.3 Specialized Postprocessing Workstation

There are at least half a dozen of manufacturers which produce specialized postprocessing (PP) WSs. Each of which has its own specialties and market niche of applications. Since these WSs have more computational power, they can produce faster and usually more comprehensive and better quality of displays, but they pay the penalty of resolving the workflow between the WS and the PACS input and display. As of now, most of these WSs can accept DICOM push function and compute the necessary PP functions at the WSs. But to push back the PP results to PACS WSs for direct display is still not convenient. So currently most of the push back is still manual, requiring the radiologist or clinician based on the worklist at the PACS WS to request the PP results from PP WS to forward to the PACS Ws; from there, the report is dictated. This is "what you see is what you get," as the real PP data are not linked to the PACS WS, and only the screenshot is. Screenshot is a very preliminary technology in DICOM. There is yet a vendor can use the DICOM structured reporting method to link the PP results to the PACS WS (see Chapter 26 for detail). Following are some PP WS results obtained in the radiology department at USC. Figure 12.23 shows the worklist, gallery, viewer, and report of a 3-D display manufacturer's product. Figure 12.24 shows the worklist and PP 3-D MR images for a second manufacturer. Figure 12.25 depicts the

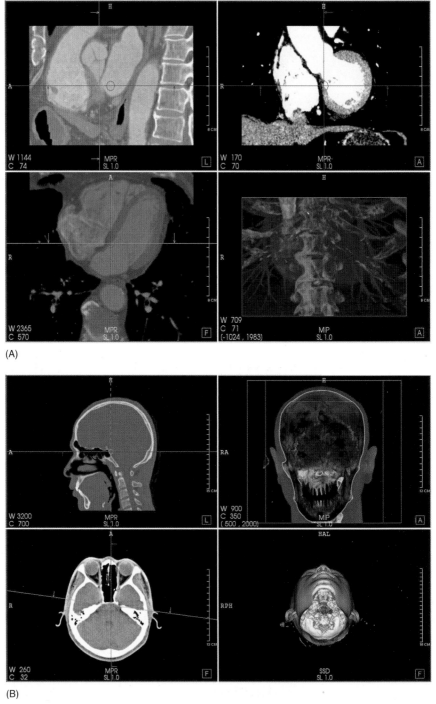

Figure 12.22 (*A*) Screenshot of the visualization of a patient's heart on multislice CT. The upper left window displays the sagittal projecting plane of MPR; the upper right window shows coronal projecting plane of MPR. The bottom left window shows the axial projecting plane of MPR; bottom right window displays a sagittal view of MIP. (*B*) Head CT image series constructed to a 3-D volume dataset and displayed with MPR, MIP, and SSD rendering patterns. (Courtesy of Dr. J. Zhang)

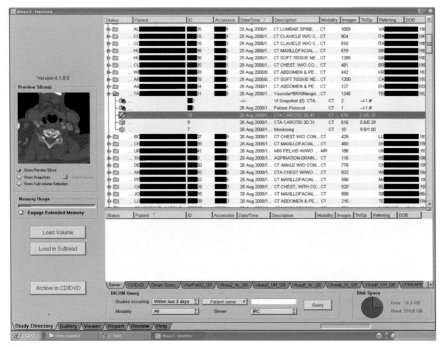

(A)

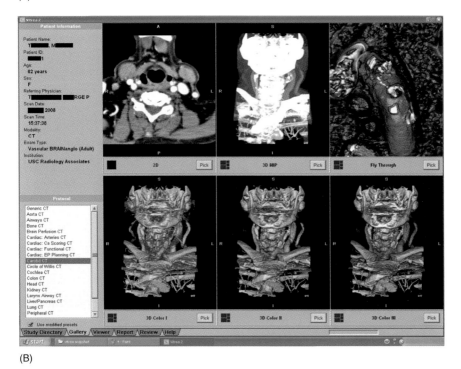

(B)

Figure 12.23   Screen captures of the worklist (*A*), gallery (*B*), viewer (*C*), and report of a 3-D display manufacturer's product (*D*). The middle of (*A*) shows the patient study being reviewed. (Courtesy of Dr. B. Guo)

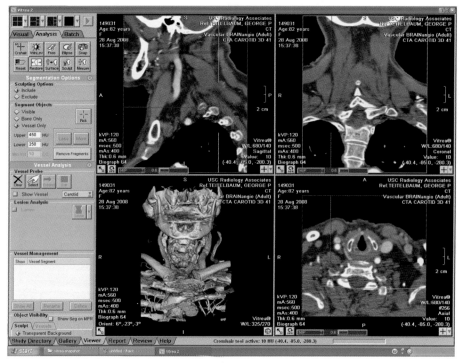

(C)

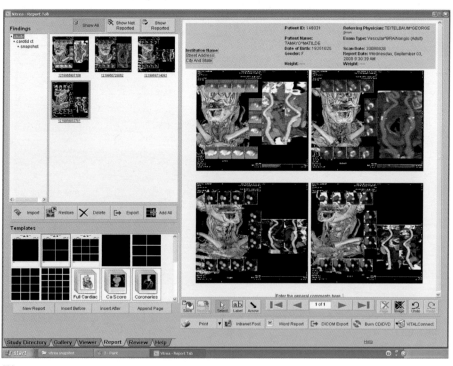

(D)

Figure 12.23 (*Continued*)

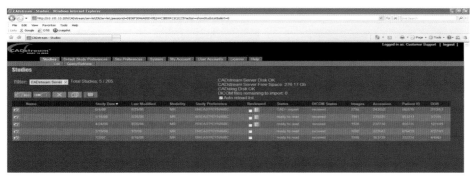

(A)

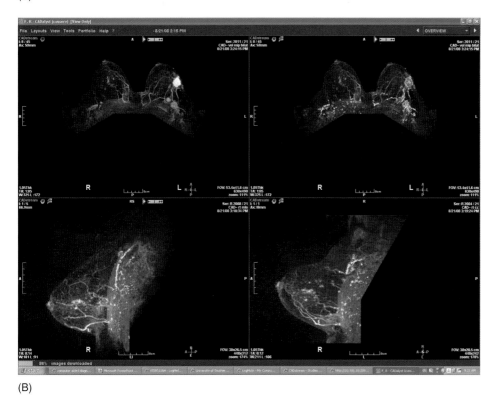

(B)

Figure 12.24   (*A*) Screen capture of the worklist; (*B*) results from the postprocessed 3-D MR images from a manufacturer's workstation. (Courtesy of Dr. B. Guo)

screen capture from a third manufacturer PP WS forwarded to the PACS WS for display.

12.9 SUMMARY OF PACS WORKSTATIONS

PACS display workstation (WS) is used by almost every healthcare provider who has the need to look at patient's image during the diagnostic and treatment processes.

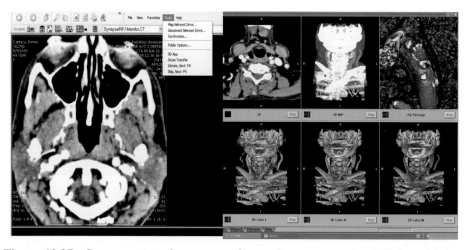

Figure 12.25 Screen capture from a manufacturer's postprocessing WS forwarded to the PACS WS for display. (Courtesy of Dr. B. Guo)

Because many and various background users will encounter with the WS, its design and use has to be simple and easy to use. This chapter discusses the concept of a WS and its design and use both in hardware and software. Different categories of WS and their functions are presented. A recipe book type of manual is given for those who want to build a WS for their own special use. The chapter concludes with a section on R&D trends for the future WS, which will need to handle thousands of images per examination.

References

ISO/IEC 15444-1. JPEG2000 image coding system. Part 1: Core coding system.

Shuai J, Sun J, Zhang J. A Novel multidimensional medical image display framework based on Visualization Toolkit, *SPIE* 6919: 691912–22; 2008.

Junichi H. An implementation of JPEG 2000 interactive image communication system. *Circuits and Systems. IEEE Int Symp* 6: 5922–5; 2005.

Kruglinski DJ, Wingo S, Shepherd G. *Programming Visual C++*, 5th edition. Redmond: Microsoft Press; 1998.

Li M, Wilson D, Wong M, and Xthona A. The evolution of display technologies in PACS applications. *Comp Med Imag Graphics* 27: 175–84; 2003.

Prandolini R, Colyer G, Houchin S. 15444- 9:2004 JPEG 2000image coding system—Part 9: Interactivity tools, APIs and protocols—JPIP. Final Publication Draft Revision 3, ISO/IEC JTC 1/SC29/WG 1N3463. November 2004.

Schroeder W, Avila L, Hoffman W. Visualizing with VTK: A tutorial. *IEEE Computer Graphics and Applications*, 20(5): 20–27, 2000.

Schroeder W, Martin K, Lorensen B. *The Visualization Toolkit, An Object-Oriented Approach To 3D Graphics*, *2nd edition*. Kitware, Inc., Clifton Park, NY; 1997.

Taubman D, Marcellin M. JPEG2000: Image Compression Fundamentals, Standards and Practice. Dordrecht *Kluwer Academic*; 2002.

Taubmana D, Prandolini R. Architecture, philosophy and performance of JPIP: Internet protocol standard for JPEG2000, *Int Symp on Visual Comm Image Process*(VCIP2003); 2003.

The Visualization Toolkit. http://www.vtk.org.

VTK 5.1.0 Documentation. http://www.vtk.org/doc/nightly/html.

Yuan T, Cai W, Sun J, Zhang J. A novel strategy to access high resolution DICOM medical images based on JPEG2000 interactive protocol. *SPIE* in Medical Image; 6919: pp 691912–22, 2008.

CHAPTER 13

Integration of HIS, RIS, PACS, and ePR

PACS is an imaging management system that requires pertinent data from other medical information systems for effective operation. Among these systems, data from the hospital information system (HIS) and the radiology information system (RIS) are the most important. Many functions in the PACS server and archive server described in Chapter 11 (image routing, prefetching, automatic grouping, etc.) rely on data extracted from both HIS and RIS. This chapter presents some HIS and RIS data that are important to the PACS operation and discusses how to interface HIS and RIS with PACS to obtain these data. Another topic of importance related to PACS image distribution is the electronic patient record (ePR), or electronic medical record (eMR), which is discussed in Section 13.5. Figure 13.1 (excerpted from Fig. 1.3) shows how this chapter corresponds to the contents of Part II. Figure 13.2 shows the position of these components (in orange red) in the PACS data flow.

13.1 HOSPITAL INFORMATION SYSTEM

The hospital information system (HIS) is a computerized management system for handling three categories of tasks in a healthcare environment:

1. Support clinical and medical patient care activities in the hospital.
2. Administer the hospital's daily business transactions (financial, personnel, payroll, bed census, etc.).
3. Evaluate hospital performances and costs, and project the long-term forecast.

Most clinical departments in a healthcare center, mainly radiology, pathology, pharmacy, and clinical laboratories, have their own specific operational requirements that differ from the general hospital operations. For this reason special information systems may be needed in these departments. Often these information systems are under the umbrella of the HIS, which supports their operations. However, there are also departments that have different workflow environments that may not be covered by the HIS. So they may need their own separate information systems and must develop mechanisms to integrate data between these systems and the HIS. Such is the story behind RIS, which began as a component of HIS; later an independent RIS was developed because of the limited support from HIS in handling the special data and

---

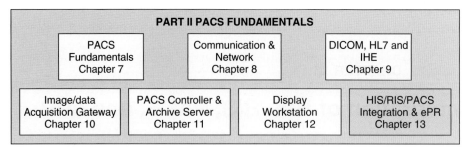

Figure 13.1 Position of Chapter 13 in the organization of this book. Color codes are used to highlight components and workflow discussed in this chapter.

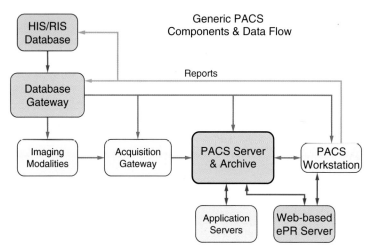

Figure 13.2 PACS basic components (yellow) and data flow (blue: Internal; green and red: external between PACS and other information systems); other information systems (light blue); The four components to be integrated together in this chapter are HIS/RIS, database gateway, PACS server and archive, and ePR in orange.

information required by the radiology operation. However, the integration of these two systems is extremely important for the healthcare center to operate as a total functional entity.

A large-scale HIS consists of mainframe computers and software. The computers are purchased through computer companies offering service and maintenance contracts that include system upgrades. The software can be contracted to a large software company with customized HIS related packages, or it can be home-grown. The software is developed progressively by integrating many commercial products over many years. A home-grown system may contain many reliable legacy hardware and software components, but through years of use their technology may become outdated. Almost all HISs were developed through the integration of many information systems, starting from the days when healthcare data centers were established. While some older components may have since been replaced by newer ones, the older components may still be in operation. Therefore, to interface HIS to PACS, extra care should be taken to understand not only new but also old technologies to circumvent such a legacy problem. Figure 13.3 shows the main components of a typical HIS.

Notice in the figure that in addition to clinical operations, the HIS supports the hospital's and healthcare center's business and administrative functions. It provides automation for such events as patient registration, admissions, discharges, and transfers (ADT), as well as patient accounting. It also provides on-line access to patient clinical results (e.g., laboratory, pathology, microbiology, pharmacy, and radiology). The system broadcasts in real time the patient demographics, and when it encounters

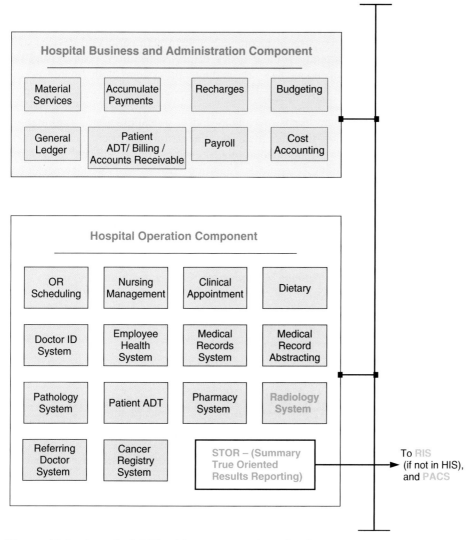

Figure 13.3   A typical HIS with two categories of software packages: business and administration, and clinical operation. Rectangles are major components in each category. The software package STOR (a trade name, other HIS may use different names) provides a path for the HIS to distribute HL7-formatted data to the outside world including PACS.

information with the HL7 standard (see Chapter 9), it moves it to the RIS. By way of this path, ADT and other pertinent data can be transmitted to the RIS and the PACS (see Fig. 13.4*A* and *B*).

13.2   RADIOLOGY INFORMATION SYSTEM

The radiology information system (RIS) is designed to support both the administrative and clinical operation of the radiology department, to reduce administrative overhead, and to improve the quality of radiological examination service. Therefore the RIS manages general radiology patient information, from scheduling to examination to reporting. The RIS configuration is very similar to that of HIS except it is smaller in scale. RIS equipment consists of a computer system with peripheral devices such as RIS workstations (normally without image display capability), printers, and bar code readers. Most independent RIS are autonomous systems with limited access to HIS. Some HIS offers embedded RIS as a subsystem with a higher degree of integration.

The RIS maintains many types of patient- and examination-related information. Patient-related information includes medical, administrative, patient demographics, and billing information. Examination-related information includes procedural descriptions and scheduling, diagnostic reporting, patient arrival documentation, film location, film movement, and examination room scheduling. When integrated with PACS, it includes patient-related PACS data and workflow. The major tasks of the system include:

- Process patient and film (image) folder records.
- Monitor the status of patients, examinations, and examination resources.
- Schedule examinations.
- Create, format, and store diagnostic reports with digital signatures.
- Track film (softcopy) folders.
- Maintain timely billing information.
- Perform profile and statistics analysis.

The RIS interfaces to PACS based on the HL7 standard through TCP/IP over Ethernet on a client-server model using a trigger mechanism (to be described in Section 13.3.7.1). Events such as examination scheduling, patient arrivals, and examination begin and end times trigger the RIS to send previously selected information (patient demographics, examination description, diagnostic report, etc.) associated with the event to the PACS in real time.

13.3   INTERFACING PACS WITH HIS AND RIS

There are three methods of transmitting data between information systems: through workstation emulation, database-to-database transfer, and an interface engine.

13.3.1   Workstation Emulation

This method allows a WS of an information system to emulate a WS of a second system so that data from the second information system can be accessed by the first system. For example, a PACS WS can be connected to the RIS with a simple computer program that emulates a RIS WS.

From the PACS WS, the user can perform any RIS function such as scheduling a new examination, updating patient demographics, recording a film (image) movement, and viewing the diagnostic reports. This method has two disadvantages. First, there is no data exchange between RIS and PACS. Second, the user is required to know how to use both systems. Also a RIS or HIS WS cannot be used to emulate a PACS WS because the latter is too specific for HIS and RIS to emulate. Figure 13.4*A* shows the mechanism of the workstation emulation method.

13.3.2   Database-to-Database Transfer

The database-to-database transfer method allows two or more networked information systems to share a subset of data by storing them in a common local area. For example, the ADT data from the HIS can be reformatted to HL7 standard and broadcasted periodically to a certain local database in the HIS. A TCP/IP transmission can be set up between the HIS and the RIS, allowing the HIS to initiate the local database and broadcast the ADT data to the RIS through either a pull or push operation. This method is most often used to share information between the HIS and the RIS as shown in Figure 13.5.

13.3.3   Interface Engine

The interface engine provides a single interface and language to access distributed data in networked heterogeneous information systems. In operation, it appears that the user is operating on a single integrated database from his/her WS. In the interface engine, a query protocol is responsible for analyzing the requested information, identifying the required databases, fetching the data, assembling the results in a standard format, and presenting them at the requested WS. Ideally, all these processes are done transparent to the user and without affecting the autonomy of each database system. To build a universal interface engine is not a simple task. Most currently available commercial interface engines are tailored to limited specific information systems. Figure 13.6 illustrates the concept of an interface engine for HIS, RIS, and PACS integration.

13.3.4   Reasons for Interfacing PACS with HIS and RIS

In a hospital environment, interfacing the PACS, RIS, and HIS has become necessary to manage data and patient workflow, PACS images, RIS administration, and research and training as described in the following subsections.

13.3.4.1   Diagnostic Process   The diagnostic process at the PACS WS includes the retrieval of not only images of interest but also pertinent textual information describing patient history and studies. Along with the image data and the image description, a PACS also provides all the related textual information acquired and

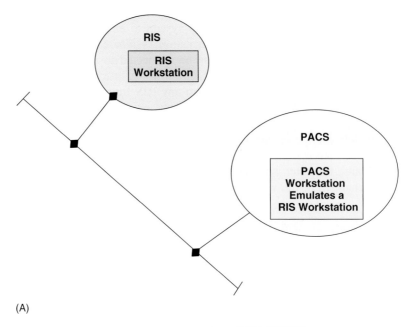

(A)

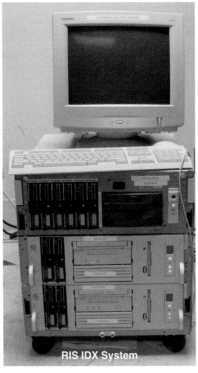

(B)

Figure 13.4 (*A*) PACS workstation emulating a RIS workstation. It can access RIS data but cannot deposit it to PACS; (*B*) vintage RIS system at UCLA.

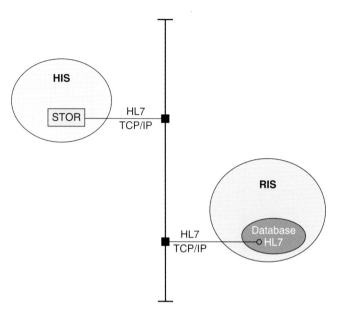

Figure 13.5   Database-to-database transfer using common data format (HL7) and communication protocol (TCP/IP). Data from HIS is accumulated periodically at STOR and broadcast to RIS.

managed by the RIS and the HIS in a way that is useful to the radiologist during the diagnostic process. RIS and HIS information such as clinical diagnosis, radiological reports, and patient history are necessary at the PACS WS to complement the images from the examination under consideration.

13.3.4.2   *PACS Image Management*   Some information provided by the RIS can be integrated into PACS image management algorithms to optimize the grouping and routing of image data via the network to the requesting locations (see Section 11.2). In the PACS database, which archives huge volumes of images, a sophisticated image management system is required to handle the depository and distribution of this image data.

13.3.4.3   *RIS Administration*   Planning of a digital-based radiology department requires the reorganization of some administrative operations carried out by the RIS. For example, the PACS can provide the image archive status and the image data file information to the RIS. RIS administration operations would also benefit from the HIS by gaining knowledge about patient ADT.

13.3.4.4   *Research and Training*   Much research and teaching in radiology involves mass screening of clinical cases and determining what constitutes normal versus abnormal conditions for a given patient population. The corresponding knowledge includes diverse types of information that need to be correlated, such as image data, results from analyzed images, medical diagnosis, patient demographics, study description, and various patient conditions. Some mechanisms are needed to access

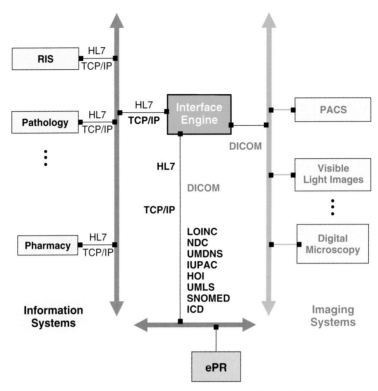

Figure 13.6 The principle of the interface engine. (left) HL7 textual data; (right) DICOM image data; (bottom) Web-based electronic patient record system (ePR, see Section 13.5) showing image and textual data, or messages and images. Message standards depicted are: LOINC: logical observation identifier names and codes; NDC: national drug codes; UMDNS: universal medical device nomenclature system; IUPAC: International Union of Pure and Applied Chemistry; HOI: health outcomes institute; UMLS: unified medical language system; SNOMED: systemized nomenclature of medicine; ICD (ICD-9-CM): the International Classification of Diseases, ninth edition, Clinical Modification.

and to retrieve data from the HIS and the RIS during a search for detailed medical and patient information related to image data. Standardization and data sharing between diverse medical database systems such as HIS, RIS, and PACS are therefore critical to the successful management of research and teaching in radiology. For radiology research and training, see Part IV of this book.

13.3.5 Some Common Guidelines

To interface the HIS, RIS, and PACS, some common guidelines are necessary.

1. Each system (HIS, RIS, PACS) remains unchanged in its configuration, data, and functions.
2. Each system is extended in both hardware and software for allowing communications with other systems.

3. Only data are shared; functions remain local. For example, RIS functions cannot be performed at the PACS or at the HIS WS. Keeping each system specific and autonomous will simplify the interface process, because database updates are not allowed at a global level.

Following these guidelines, successfully interfacing HIS, RIS, and PACS requires the following steps:

1. Identify the subset data that will be shared by other systems. Set up access rights and authorization.
2. Convert the subset data to HL7 standard form. This step, consisting of designing a high-level presentation, solving data inconsistencies, and naming conventions, can be accomplished by using a common data model and data language and by defining rules of correspondence between various data definitions.
3. Define the protocol of data transfer (e.g., TCP/IP or DICOM).

13.3.6 Common Data in HIS, RIS, and PACS

The system software in the PACS server and archive server described in Section 11.2 requires certain data from HIS and RIS that is necessary for it to archive images and associated data in permanent storage and distribute them to workstations properly and timely. Figure 13.7 illustrates data common to the HIS, RIS, and PACS. Table 13.1 describes data definition, the origin and the destination, and the action that triggers the system software functions.

13.3.7 Implementation of RIS–PACS Interface

The RIS–PACS interface can be implemented by either the trigger mechanisms or the query protocol described below.

13.3.7.1 Trigger Mechanism between Two Databases The PACS is notified of the following events in HL7 format when they occur in the RIS: ADT, order received, patient arrived, examination canceled, procedure completed, report approved. The application level of the interface software waits for the occurrence of one of these events and triggers the corresponding data to be sent. The communication level transfers the HL7 file to the PACS server with the processes *send* (to PACS) and *ris_recv*. The PACS server receives this file and archives it in the database tables for subsequent use. Figure 13.8 shows the trigger mechanism interface. The trigger mechanism is used in a systematic and timely fashion when a small amount of predefined information from the RIS is needed from the PACS. In addition to requiring additional storage allocation in both databases, this method is tedious for information updating and is not suitable for user queries.

13.3.7.2 Query Protocol The query protocol allows access to information from the HIS, RIS, and PACS databases by using an application-layer software on top of these heterogeneous database systems. From a PACS WS, users can retrieve information uniformly from any of these systems and automatically integrate them to the

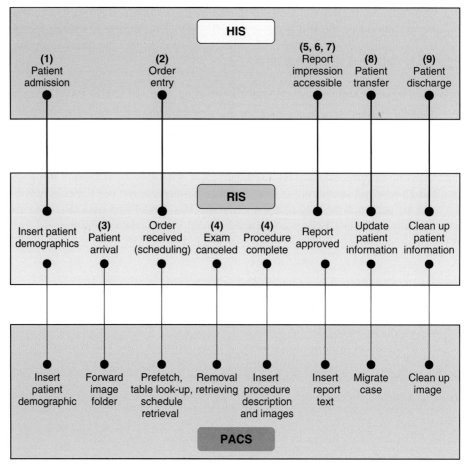

Figure 13.7 Information transfer between the HIS, RIS and PACS. Numerals represent steps of information transfer explained in Table 13.1.

PACS database. Figure 13.9 illustrates the query protocol. The DICOM query/retrieve service class described in Section 9.4.5.2 is one method to implement such a query mechanism. The application-layer software utilizes the following standards:

- SQL as the global query language
- Relational data model as the global data model
- TCP/IP communication protocols
- HL7 data format.

13.3.8 An Example: The IHE Patient Information Reconciliation Profile

We use the IHE patient information reconciliation workflow profile presented by CARR (2003) as an example to explain how the workflow would benefit from the

TABLE 13.1 Information transferred among HIS, RIS, and PACS triggered by the PACS server

Events	Message	From	To	Action	Location
(1) Admission	Previous images/reports	HIS/RIS	PACS server	Preselect images and reports, transfer from permanent archive to workstations	WS at FL, RR
(2) Order entry	Previous images/reports	RIS	PACS server, scanner	Check event (1) for completion	WS at FL, RR
(3) Arrival	PT arrival	RIS	PACS server, scanner	Check events (1) and (2) for completion	WS at FL, RR
(4) Examination complete	New images	Scanner	RIS, PACS server	New images to Folder Manager, WS	Temporary archive; WS at Fl, RR
(5) Dictation	"Wet" reading	RR	Digital dictaph-one	Dictation recorded on DD or VR, digital report to Folder Manager and to WS	DD or VR; WS at FL, RR
(6) Transcript	Preliminary report	RR	RIS, PACS Server	Preliminary report to RIS, temporary archive and to WS, dictation erased from DD	RIS; temporary archive: WS at FL, RR
(7) Signature	Final report	RR	RIS, PACS server	Final report to RIS, to WS, and to temporary archive. Prelim report erased.	RIS: temporary archive; WS at FL, RR
(8) Transfer	Patient transfer	HIS/RIS	PACS server	Transfer image files	WS at new location
(9) Discharge	Images, report	HIS/RIS	PACS server	Patient folder copied from temporary to permanent storage, patient folder erased from WS	WS at FL, RR; temporary and permanent storage

Key: DD: digital dictaphone; VR: voice recognition; FL: floors in the ward; RR: reading rooms in the radiology department; WS: workstations.

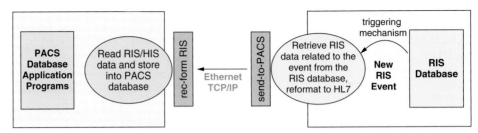

Figure 13.8 RIS-PACS interface architecture implemented with a database-to-database transfer using a trigger mechanism.

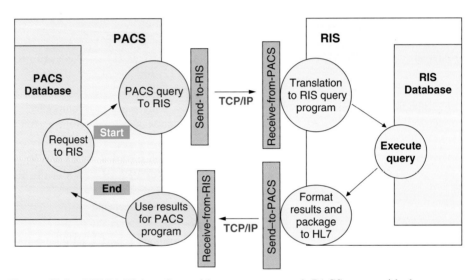

Figure 13.9 RIS-PACS interface with a query protocol. PACS starts with the query to RIS (top), RIS sends the request and received by the PACS (bottom).

integration of HIS, RIS, and PACS (Figure 13.10).This integration profile extends the scheduled workflow profile by providing the means to match images acquired for an unidentified patient (e.g., during a trauma case where the patient ID is not known) with the patient's registration and order history. In the example of the trauma case, this allows subsequent reconciliation of the patient record with images acquired (either without a prior registration or under a generic registration) before the patient's identity could be determined. Enabling this after-the-fact matching greatly simplifies these exception-handling situations. Information systems involved in this integration profile are as follows:

- Enterprise-wide information systems that manage patient registration and services ordering (ADT/registration system, HIS)
- Radiology departmental information systems that manage department scheduling (RIS) and image management/archiving (PACS)
- Acquisition modalities

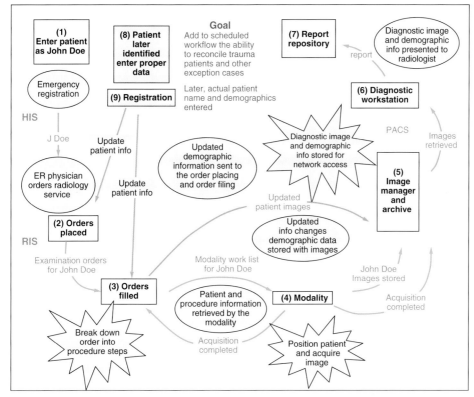

Figure 13.10 IHE patient reconciliation workflow profile used as an example for the HIS-RIS-PACS interface (Carr, 2003). Yellow boxes and green arrows: trauma patient exam without ID; blue boxes and orange arrows: start at step 8, use the IHE workflow profile to reconcile trauma patient ID and demographic data when they become available.

13.4 INTERFACING PACS WITH OTHER MEDICAL DATABASES

13.4.1 Multimedia Medical Data

Among many consultation functions of a radiology specialist in a healthcare center are consulting with primary and referring physicians on prescribing proper radiological examinations for patients, performing procedures, reading images from procedures, dictating and confirming diagnostic reports, and reviewing images with the referring physicians and providing consultation. On the basis of these radiological images, reports, and consultations, the referring physicians prescribe proper treatment plans for their patients. Radiologists also use images from examinations and reports to train fellows, residents, and medical students.

In their practice, radiologists often request necessary patient information (e.g., demographic data, laboratory tests, and consultation reports from other medical specialists) from medical records. Radiologists also review literature from the library information systems and give *formal rounds* to educate colleagues on radiological procedures and new radiological techniques. Thus the practice of radiology requires integrating various types of multimedia information—including voice, text, medical records, images, and video recordings—into proper files/databases for easy and quick retrieval. These various types of information exist on different media and are stored in data systems of different types. Advances in computer and communication technologies allow the possibility of integration of these various types of information to facilitate the practice of radiology. We have already discussed two such information systems, namely HIS and RIS.

13.4.2   Multimedia in the Radiology Environment

"Multimedia" has different meanings depending on the context. In the radiology environment, the term refers to the integration of medical information related to radiology practice. This information is stored in various databases and media in voice form or as text records, images, or video loops. Among these data, patient demographic information, clinical laboratory test results, pharmacy information, and pathological reports are stored in the HIS. The radiological images are stored in the PACS permanent archive system, and the corresponding reports are in the reporting system of the RIS. Electronic mail and files are stored in the personal computer system database. Digital learning files are categorized in the learning laboratory or the library in the department of radiology. Some of these databases may exist in primitive legacy systems; others, for example, PACS, can be very advanced. Thus the challenge of developing multimedia in the radiology environment is to establish infrastructure for the seamless integration of this medical information systems by means of blending different technologies, while providing an acceptable data transmission rate to various parts of the department and to various sites in the healthcare center. Once the multimedia infrastructure is established, different medical information can exist as modules with common standards and be interfaced with this infrastructure. In the multimedia environment, radiologists (or their medical colleagues) can access this information through user-friendly, inexpensive, efficient, and reliable interactive workstations.

RIS, HIS, electronic mail, and files involve textual information requiring from 1 K to 2 K bytes per transaction. For such small data file sizes, although developing interface with each information system is tedious, the technology involved is manageable. On the other hand, PACS contains image files that can be in theneighborhood of 20 to 40 Mbytes. The transmission and storage requirements for PACS are manifold those of text information. For this reason PACS becomes the cente in developing multimedia in the radiology environment.

13.4.3   An Example: The IHE Radiology Information Integration Profile

We use the IHE radiology information integration profile (Carr, 2003) as an example to explain how to use the IHE workflow profiles to access various radiology information. The access to radiology information integration profile (Fig. 13.11) specifies support of a number of query transactions providing access to radiology information, including images and related reports. Such access is useful to the radiology department and to other departments such as pathology, surgery, and oncology. Non-radiology information (e.g., Lab reports) may also be accessed if made available in DICOM format.

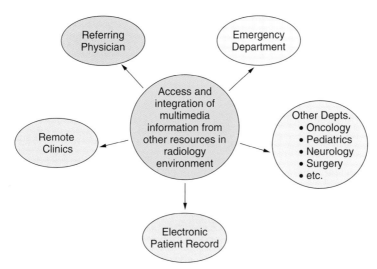

Figure 13.11   Use of IHE access to the radiology information integration profile as an example of multimedia access and integration in the radiology environment.

This profile includes both enterprise-wide and radiology department imaging and reporting systems such as:

- review or diagnostics WSs (stand-alone or integrated with a HIS, RIS, PACS, or modality),
- reporting WSs (stand-alone or integrated with a HIS, RIS, PACS, or modality),
- image archiving and communication system (PACS), and
- report repositories (stand-alone or integrated with a HIS, RIS, or PACS).

13.4.4   Integration of Heterogeneous Databases

For multimedia information to operate effectively in the radiology environment, at least six heterogeneous databases must be integrated, namely the HIS, RIS, PACS, electronic mail and file, digital voice dictation or recognition system, and electronic patient record (ePR). In Section 13.3 we described the HIS/RIS interface. We present the digital voice dictation or recognition system in this section and the ePR system in Section 13.5.

13.4.4.1   *Interfacing Digital Voice Dictation or Recognition System with PACS*   Typically radiological reports are archived and transmitted independently from the image files. They are first dictated by the radiologist and recorded on an audiocassette recorder from which a textual form is transcribed and inserted into the RIS several hours late after the recroding. The interface between the RIS and the PACS allows for sending and inserting these reports into the PACS or RIS database, from which a report corresponding to the images can be displayed on the PACS WS on request by the user. This process is not efficient because the delay imposed by the transcription prevents the textual report from reaching the referring physician in a timely manner.

Figure 13.12 shows a method of interfacing a digital voice system directly to the PACS database. The concept is allowing the referring physician listen to the voice report and review the images simultaneously. Following Figure 13.12:

a) the radiologist views images from the PACS WS and uses the digital dictaphone system to dictate the report, which converts it from analog signals to digital format and stores the result in the voice message server;

b) the voice message server in turn sends a message to the PACS server, which links the voice with the images;

c) referring physicians at the WS, for example, in an intensive care unit, review certain images and at the same time listen to the voice report through the voice message server linked to the images;

d) the transcriber transcribes the voice by using the RIS (the transcribed report is inserted into the RIS database server automatically); and

e) the RIS server sends a message to the PACS database server, links the transcribed report to the PACS image file, and signals the voice message server to delete the voice message.

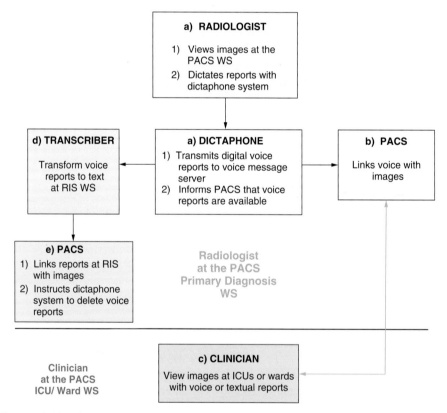

Figure 13.12   Operational procedure of a digital voice system connected with the PACS starts with (top) radiologist at the primary diagnostic WS dictating a report with the digital dictaphone system. Yellow: radiologist uses the digital dictaphone system; green: clinician reviews images with digital voice report; blue: housekeeping steps.

Note that although the interface is between the voice database and the PACS database, the RIS database also plays an active role in this interaction.

13.4.4.2 Impact of the Voice Recognition System and DICOM Structured Reporting to the Dictaphone System
The ideal method of not delaying the report to the referral physicians when the images are ready at the ICUs or wards WSs is to use a voice recognition system that automatically translates voice into text, then links the textual report to PACS images. In the voice recognition system, the dictation is immediately converted to a report form, which is then inserted to the RIS. Although several such voice recognition systems are available in the market, because of the quality of the interpretation and the user inertia, its acceptance rate is still below average.

Another possibility is to request the radiologist to use the DICOM structured reporting (SR) standard (see Chapter 9). In this case the dictation will follow the standard SR format for immediate linking to the image when the physician views the images. When the use of any of these two alternatives become a daily routine, then the benefit of the digital voice dictation system will become limited.

13.5 ELECTRONIC PATIENT RECORD (ePR)

13.5.1 Current Status of ePR

The electronic medical record (eMR) or electronic patient record (ePR) is the ultimate patient centric information system in the healthcare enterprise. In an even broader sense, if the information system includes the health record of an individual, then it is called eHR (electronic health record) system. In this book we concentrate on ePR, the concept of patient centric—the record goes with the patient.

As of now, only small subsets of ePR are actually in clinical operation except two systems (to be discussed in this book). One can consider ePR as the big picture of the future health care information system. Although the development of a universal ePR as a commercial product is still years away, its eventual impact on the health care delivery system should not be underestimated. An ePR consists of five major functions:

1. Accepts direct digital input of patient data.
2. Analyzes across patients and providers.
3. Provides clinical decision support and suggests courses of treatment.
4. Performs outcome analysis and patient and physician profiling.
5. Distributes information across different platforms and health information systems.

HIS and RIS, which deal with patient nonimaging data management and hospital operation, can be considered components of EMR. An integrated HIS–RIS–PACS system, which extends the patient data to include imaging, forms the cornerstone of ePR.

Existing ePRs are mostly Web-based and have certain commonalties. They have large data dictionaries with time stamped in their contents and can query from related healthcare information systems and display the data flexibly. Examples of successfully implemented EMRs (ePRs) are COSTAR (Computer-Stored Ambulatory Record) developed at Massachusetts General Hospital (in the public domain), Regenstrief Medical Record System at Indiana University, HELP (Health Evaluation through Logical Processing) system developed at the University of Utah and Latter-Day Saints (LDS) Hospital, the VAHE (United States Department of Veterans Affairs Healthcare Enterprise Information System), and the Hong Kong Hospital Authority (HKHA) ePR system. Among these systems the VAHE and the HKHA systems are properly the largest and most advanced system in the sense that it is being used daily in many of the VA Medical Centers and Hong Kong public hospitals, respectively, and both systems include image distribution from the ePR. For these reasons both the VAHE and HKHA systems will be discussed extensively in proper sections of this book.

Just like any other medical information system, development of the ePR faces several obstacles:

- Common method to input patient examination and related data to the system.
- Development of an across-the-board data and communication standard.
- Buy-in from manufacturers to adopt the standards.
- Acceptance by healthcare providers.

An integrated HIS–RIS–PACS system provides solutions for some of these obstacles:

- It has adopted DICOM and HL7 standards for imaging and text, respectively.
- Images and patient-related data are entered into the system almost automatically.
- The majority of imaging manufacturers have adopted DICOM and HL7 as de facto industrial standards.

Therefore, in the course of developing an integrated PACS, one should keep in mind of the big picture, the ePR system. Anticipated future connections with the integrated PACS as an input source to the ePR should be considered thoroughly. Figure 13.6 illustrates the concept of using an interface engine as a possible connection of the integrated PACS to ePR.

In addition to present the essentials of the VAHE and the HKHA systems in this book, we also introduce several smaller ePR systems in Part IV, on multimedia ePR system, ePR for spinal surgery, and ePR for radiation therapy.

13.5.2 ePR with Image Distribution

13.5.2.1 The Concept The text-based electronic patient record (ePR) has many advantages over the traditional paper-based medical record, including improved legibility over handwritten notes, easy retrieval and transfer of information, as well as accessibility by multiple parties. However, the full potential of ePR in streamlining patient care cannot be achieved when important information available from images is only available from paper or films outside of the electronic information system. Therefore ePR with image distribution is a natural extension of text-based system.

Alongside with technological advancements that allow economical transfer and storage of the massive amount of data, image distribution in ePR becomes reality. This significantly enhances usability of ePR by filling the missing link of information available in images that is be difficult to be comprehensively and succinctly represented by textual description. The images concerned can be those obtained from radiological examinations, ultrasound, CT, or MRI. Other possible sources include pathology, endoscopy, ophthalmology, dermatology, electrocardiogram or electroencephalogram, diagrams outlining procedures, and so forth. The technological requirements required for handling these very heterogeneous multimedia data of variable formats and sizes can be challenging.

Medical images often involve huge amount of data, especially those associated with modern imaging examinations, such as multislice CT or multiple sequences in MRI examinations, which easily go beyond hundreds to thousands of megabytes in a single examination. This will obviously become burdensome on both storage capacity and network bandwidth. As medical images distributed with ePR are essentially used for review after primary diagnosis has been made. It is rational to employ some form of image selection or compression (e.g., reformat of thick section 2D data from 3D raw data) or selection of representative image data (e.g., photos taken during ultrasound and endoscopic examination).

13.5.2.2 *The Benefits*   Image distribution in ePR brings together information residing in images produced by different sources and other text based data to clinicians in a single platform. Benefits include improvement in diagnosis by allowing:

1. correlation with relevant clinical history (e.g., abnormal FDG [fluorodeoxyglucose] activity shown on PET images can represent infection rather than neoplasm if there is clinical history of sepsis);
2. correlation between different investigations (e.g., a hypervascular tumor shown on contrast enhanced CT together with elevated AFP [Alpha-Fetal Protein, a tumor marker] level on blood test points to hepatocellular carcinoma rather than liver metastasis); and
3. correlation between different imaging examinations (e.g., evaluation of skeletal disease on MRI often requires correlation with prior radiographs, which becomes readily assessable through ePR even if they have been obtained in other imaging facilities).

In addition, other uses of ePR with image distribution include:

1. guidance of procedures with reference to prior imaging findings (e.g., endoscopist can examine images of CT virtual colonoscopy and locate the lesion in question, or urologist can direct biopsy needle to mass detectable on prior ultrasound examination);
2. monitoring disease progression (e.g., an enlarging nodule on CT thorax is highly suspicious of malignancy); and
3. providing basis for clinical decision making (e.g., tumor not regressing at an expected rate, identified on PET images, calls for change in chemotherapeutic regimen).

Last but not least, incorporation of images available to different clinicians enhances communications when visual cues available from images can be readily appreciated by different involved parties. Good communication is essential when collaborative efforts need to be taken.

13.5.2.3 *Some Special Features and Applications in ePR with Image Distribution*   Incorporation of image distribution with ePR is advantageous as discussed before. In addition to incorporating ever more different kinds of images (or multimedia, for that matter), some future developments in ePR with respect to image distribution that are anticipated to improve patient care include technologies in:

1. extracting more useful information from images,
2. decision support, and
3. knowledge discovery.

Information available from images can be obtained by direct visual inspection, direct measurements (distance, volume, signal intensity, etc.), or calculations from imaging parameters (calculations of calcium score, intensity time curve of lesion after contrast injection, serial change over time, etc.). To extract more information, some simple functions like measurements or reformat can be made available to ePR WSs, allowing better evaluation of an abnormality. More sophisticated functions, of course, require a lot more resources, but in most instances, these were already performed by persons making the initial interpretation. Hence capability to include annotations made on the images by prior readers (e.g., radiologist making the primary diagnosis), and to display the annotations as an option, can help highlight some important findings and further enhance communications among clinicians.

To make ePR a more efficient decision support tool, some new tools in imaging informatics (e.g., content-based retrieval of similar images from database and computer aided diagnosis) can be incorporated into ePR. It is also envisaged that automatic assimilation or highlighting of other investigation results, such as tumor marker level from blood tests, can become part of the decision support tools. Another possible development for decision support can be a few links to retrievable clinical management guidelines, selected based on the type of image and region of examination, made available to the viewing clinicians, for example, ACR BIRADS (American College of Radiology Breast Imaging Reporting and Data System Atlas [BI-RADS® Atlas] classification and suggested actions) or alert of follow-up linked to mammogram examination.

With the incorporation of multifaceted information including patient's images with the diagnosis, the ePR database can be an ideal data source for knowledge discovery using data mining.

Some of the aforementioned developments have already been implemented by different research laboratories around the world. The benefits of ePR and those associated with image distribution could become much more far reaching in healthcare delivery than its current state as everyone's medical records and health data become available via some Web-based servers that are accessible by all healthcare providers rather than locked up in isolated information systems in the institutes where the patient is being treated at particular time points. This, of course, means the eHR (electronic health record) must account for entire populations.

References

Huang HK. Towards the digital radiology department. Editorial. *Eur J Radiol* 22: 165; 1996.

Huang HK, Andriole K, Bazzill T, Lou ASL, Wong AWK. Design and implementation of PACS—the second time. *J Digital Imag* 9(2): 47–59; 1996.

Huang HK, Wong AWK, Lou SL, Bazzill TM, et al. Clinical experience with a second generation PACS. *J Digital Imag* 9(4): 151–66; 1996.

Huang HK. PACS, informatics, and the neurosurgery command module. *J Mini Invasive Spinal Techniq* 1: 62–7; 2001.

Huang HK. Enterprise PACS and image distribution, *Comp Med Imag Graph* 27(2–3): 241–53; 2003.

Huang HK. Utilization of medical imaging informatics and biometric technologies in healthcare delivery. *Intern J Comp Asst Rad Surg* 3: 27–39; 2008.

Law M, Huang HK. Concept of a PACS and imaging informatics-based server for radiation therapy. *Comp Med Imag Graph* 27: 1–9; 2003.

PART III

PACS OPERATION

CHAPTER 14

PACS Data Management and Web-Based Image Distribution

In Part II on PACS Fundamentals, we presented the principle concepts of PACS. In Part III, we start our discussion of PACS operation with a look at PACS data management and Web-based image distribution. Figure 14.1 (excerpted from Fig. 1.3) shows the how this corresponds to the contents of Part III. Figure 14.2 (excerpted from Fig. 1.2) shows these PACS components in relation to the workflow.

14.1 PACS DATA MANAGEMENT

In Section 11.2 we considered the PACS server and the archive server functions, including image receiving, stacking, routing, archiving, study grouping, RIS and HIS interfacing, PACS database updates, image retrieving, and prefetching. These software functions are needed for optimal image and information management, distribution, and retrieval at the WS. The availability of IHE has facilitated the integration of these functions into the PACS operation workflow. This section describes methods and essentials of grouping patients' image and data effectively within the patient folder manager concept.

14.1.1 Concept of the Patient Folder Manager

Folder Manager (FM) is a software package residing in the PACS server that manages the PACS by means of event trigger mechanisms. The organizing concept is standardization, modularity, and portability.

The infrastructure of FM includes the following components:

- HIS-RIS-PACS interface (Sections 11.2.6, 13.3)
- Image routing (Section 11.2.3)
- Study grouping (Section 11.2.5)
- On-line radiology reports
- Patient folder management

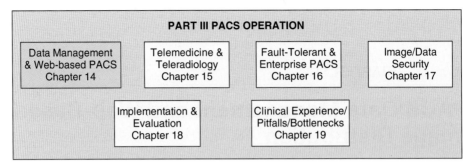

Figure 14.1   Position of Chapter 14 in the organization of this book. Color codes are used to highlight components and workflow in chapters of Part III.

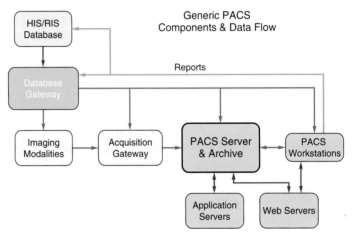

Figure 14.2   PACS data management and Web-based image distribution. PACS data management, patient folder management, Web-based server, and wireless remote control of clinical image workflow are related to the four orange color boxes in the PACS components and workflow.

The first three functions were presented in earlier sections. We discuss the on-line reports and patient folder management functions here, and then supplement them with the concept of IHE integration profiles introduced in Section 9.5.3. For convenience, the radiology domain profiles are excerpted and listed below. Some of these profiles are reviewed here, and others had been or will be reviewed in later sections of the book.

1. Scheduled workflow (SWF)
2. Patient information reconciliation (PIR)
3. Postprocessing workflow (PWF)
4. Reporting workflow (RWF)
5. Import reconciliation workflow (IRWF)
6. Portable data for imaging (PDI)

7. Nuclear medicine image (NM)

8. Mammography image (MAMMO)

9. Evidence documents (ED)

10. Simple image and numeric report (SINR)

11. Key image note (KIN)

12. Consistent presentation of images (CPI)

13. Presentation of grouped procedures (PGP)

14. Image fusion (FUS)

15. Cross-enterprise document sharing for imaging (XDS-I)

16. Teaching file and clinical trial export (TCE)

17. Access to radiology information (ARI)

18. Audit trail and node authentication (ATNA)

19. Charge posting (CHG)

14.1.2 On-line Radiology Reports

The PACS receives radiologist reports and impressions from RIS via the RIS-PACS interface, which is dependent on whether the hospital is using a PACS driven or a RIS driven workflow. The PACS then either stores these text information files in the PACS database or the PACS server has access to it from the RIS. These reports and impressions can be displayed instantaneously at a PACS WS along with corresponding images of a given examination. The PACS also supports on-line queries of reports and impressions from a WS. In Chapter 13 we discussed four methods of on-line radiology reporting mechanism:

- Digital voice dictation as a temporary reporting system for PACS until the written report becomes available (Section 13.4.4.2).
- Voice recognition system as an instantaneous reporting system for PACS (Section 13.4.4.3).
- The DICOM structured reporting standard as a simple reporting mechanism (Section 13.4.4.3).
- Access to the IHE radiology information integration profile, which highlights the reporting stations and the report repositories (Section 13.4.3).

These reporting systems form a component of the patient folder manager, and their implementation can be facilitated by using some of the IHE profiles described in later sections.

14.2 PATIENT FOLDER MANAGEMENT

The PACS server and archive server manage patient studies in folders. Each folder consists of a patient's demographics, examination descriptions, images from current examinations, selected images from previous examinations, and relevant reports and impressions. In the stand-alone PACS model (or thick client model, see Section 7.4), the patient's folder will remain on-line at specific WSs during the patient's entire hospital stay or visit. On discharge or transfer of the patient, the folder is automatically deleted from the WSs. In the client-server model, the patient's folder is always in the PACS server. Readers can perceive the patient folder manager as the prelude of the ePR discussed in Section 13.5, except that the Folder Manager (FM) emphasizes images whereas ePR originally is more textual oriented. Three basic software modules are in the patient's FM:

- Archive management
- Network management
- Display/server management

Table 14.1 describes these three modules and associated submodules, and their essential level for the PACS operation.

14.2.1 Archive Management

The archive manager module provides the following functionalities:

- Manages distribution of images in multiple storage media.
- Optimizes archiving and retrieving operations for PACS.
- Prefetches historical studies and forwards them to display workstations.

Mechanisms supporting these functions include event triggering, image prefetching, job prioritization, and storage allocation.

14.2.1.1 Event Triggering Event triggering can be achieved by means of the following *algorithm*:

TABLE 14.1   Summary of patient folder manager software modules

Module	Submodules	Essential Level
Archive Manager	Image Archive	1
	Image Retrieve	1
	HL7 Message Parsing	2
	Event Trigger	2
	Image Prefetch	2
Network Manager	Image Send (DICOM)	1
	Image Receive (DICOM)	1
	Image Routing	1
	Job Prioritizing and Recover Mechanism	1
Display/Server Manager	Image Selection	2
	Image Sequencing (IHE Profile)	3
	Window/Level Preset	2
	Report/Impression Display	1

Note: Definition of Essential Level (1: Highest, 3: Lowest): (1) minimum requirements to run the PACS; (2) requirements for an efficient PACS; (3) advanced features.

Algorithm Description Event Triggering   Events occurring at the RIS are sent to the PACS in HL7 format over TCP/IP, which then triggers the PACS server to carry out specific tasks such as image retrieval and prefetching, PACS database update, storage allocation, and patient folder cleanup. Events sent from RIS include patient ADT (admission, discharge, and transfer), patient arrival, examination scheduling, cancellation, completion, and report approval.

Essential components for the algorithm to be functional are HIS–RIS–PACS interface, HL7 message parsing, image prefetching, PACS database update, patient folder management, and storage allocation in memory, disk, and tape.

14.2.1.2 Image Prefetching

The PACS server and archive server initiates the prefetch mechanism as soon as it detects the arrival of a patient from the ADT message from the RIS. Selected historical images, patient demographics, and relevant radiology reports are retrieved from the permanent archive and the PACS database based on a predetermined algorithm initiated by the radiology department. These data are distributed to the destination WSs before the patient's current examination.

Prefetch Algorithm Description   The prefetch mechanism is based on predefined parameters such as examination type, section code, radiologist, referring physician, location of WSs, and number and age of the patient's archived images. These parameters determine which historical images should be retrieved. Figure 14.3 shows a four-dimensional prefetching table: the current examination type, disease category, section radiologist, and referring physician. This table determines which historical images should be retrieved from the PACS archive system. For example, for a patient scheduled for a chest examination, the n-tuple entries in the chest column $(2, 1, 0, 2, 0, \ldots)$ represent an image folder consisting of two single-view chest images, one two-view chest image, no CT head scan, two CT body studies, no angiographic image, and so on.

In addition to this lookup table, the prefetch mechanism also utilizes patient origin, referring physician, location of the WSs, number of archived images of this patient, and age of the individual archived images for the determination of the number of images from each examination type to be retrieved.

The prefetch mechanism is carried out by several processes within the archive server (see Section 11.2.9). Each process runs independently and communicates simultaneously with other processes utilizing client-server programming, queuing control mechanisms, and job-prioritizing mechanisms. The prefetch algorithm can be described in the following algorithm:

Execution of the Prefetch Algorithm   The prefetching mechanism is triggered whenever an examination is scheduled or canceled, or when a patient arrival occurs at the RIS. Selected historical images, patient demographics, and relevant radiology reports are retrieved from the long-term archive and the PACS database. These data are distributed to the destination WSs before the patient's current examination starts.

14.2.1.3 Job Prioritization

The PACS server manages its processes by prioritizing job control to optimize the archiving and retrieving activities. For example, a request from a WS to retrieve an image set from the permanent archive will have the highest priority and be processed immediately, and on completion of the retrieval,

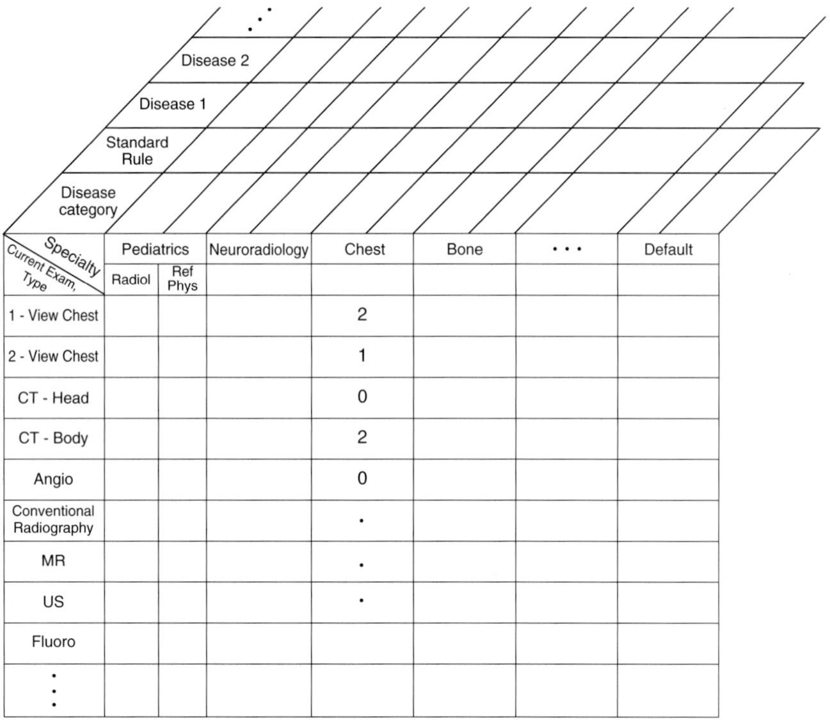

Figure 14.3 Example of a four-dimensional prefetching table with examination type, disease category, section radiologist, and referring physician. Notice the retrieved images are in the patient's "chest" image folder.

the image will be queued for transmission with a priority higher than other images that have just arrived from the image acquisition and are waiting for transmission. By the same token, an archive process must be compromised if there is any retrieval job executing or pending. The use of automatic job prioritizing and compromising between PACS processes will result in a dramatic decrease in the delay in servicing radiologists and referring physicians for their urgent needs.

14.2.1.4 Storage Allocation   In the stand-alone PACS model, during a hospital stay or visit, the patient's current images from different examinations are copied to a temporary disk storage device. On discharge or transfer of the patient, these images are grouped from temporary storage and copied contiguously to permanent storage. In the client server PACS model, all patients' images are in the PACS archive server.

14.2.2 Network Management

The network manager handles the image/data distribution from the PACS server and the archive server. This module, which controls the image traffic across the entire PACS network, is a routing mechanism based on some predefined parameters (see Section 11.2.3). It includes a routing table composed of predefined parameters and a routing algorithm driven by the routing table. The routing table is also designed to facilitate image/data updating as needed. Any change of parameters in the routing table should be possible without modification of the routing algorithm.

In addition to routing image/data to their designated WSs, the network manager performs the following tasks:

- Queue images in the PACS server for future process should the network or WS fail.
- Should the primary network fail, automatically switch the network circuit from the primary Gbit/s network to the secondary network (e.g., conventional Ethernet).
- Distribute image/data based on different priority levels.

The image-sending mechanism can be described in the following algorithm.

Image Distribution Algorithm: Description The send process catches a ready-to-send signal from the routing manager, establishes a TCP/IP connection to the destination host, and transmits the image data to the destination host. On successful transmission, the send process dequeues current job and logs a SUCCESS status. Otherwise, it requeues the job for a later retry and logs a RETRY status. Essential components in the image distribution algorithm are TCP connect, dequeuing, requeuing, and event logging. The DICOM communication standard with the DIMSEs can handle the image send very efficiently.

14.2.3 Display Server Management

Display server management includes four tasks:

- Image sequencing
- Image selection
- Window/level preset
- Coordination with reports and impressions

Window/level preset and coordination with reports and impressions have been described in the IHE profiles. Image sequencing is one of the most difficult tasks in the display server management because it involves users' habits and subjective opinion, and thus it does not have universal rules to govern these preferences. These types of algorithms depend on artificial intelligence, so their implementation is limited to specific applications. Because customization can be grueling work, image selection is handled by the display server management by way of some basic rules that allow user interaction in terms of the algorithm described below:

Image Selection Algorithm: Description The user selects a subset of images from a given image sequence (as in an MR or CT study) on the display monitor(s) of a WS. These selected images are then extracted from the original sequence and grouped into a new sequence (e.g., a montage; see Section 12.5.7), and the command is saved in the DICOM header for future display. The essential components in the image selection algorithm are image display system description, montage function, and PACS database updates (Section 11.2.7).

Some IHE integration profiles that can be used for facilitating display server management are described next. In particular, integration profiles 13 on presentation of grouped procedures, 17, on Access to radiology information (presented in Section 13.4.3), 10 on simple image and numeric report, and 11 on key image note give detailed descriptions on the data flow requirements for display images. For more on integration profiles, refer to Carr (2003).

14.2.3.1 IHE Presentation of Grouped Procedures (PGP) Profile   The grouped procedures (PGP) integration profile presented in Figure 14.4 addresses the complex information management problems entailed when information for multiple procedures is obtained in a single acquisition step (e.g., CTs of the chest, abdomen, and pelvis). During some clinical applications (requested procedures) only subsets of these images in this single acquisition step are needed. In those situations the

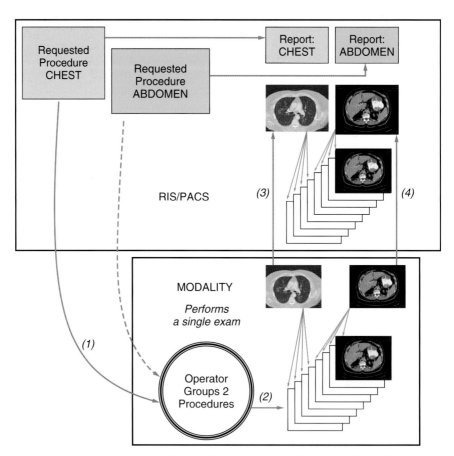

Figure 14.4   IHE (integrating the healthcare enterprise) presentation of the grouped procedures (PGP) profile. (1) A single CT acquisition procedure (solid and dotted lines) is used to acquire both (2) chest and abdominal scans. The IHE scheduled workflow profile provides information for the PGP to split the acquired images into two subsets (orange and green), (3) one for the chest (orange) and (4) the other for the abdomen (green).

PGP provides the ability to view image subsets resulting from a single acquisition and relates each image subset to a different requested procedure. A single acquired image set is produced, but the combined use of scheduled workflow and consistent presentation of images transactions allows separate viewing and interpretation of subsets of images related to each clinical application. Among other benefits, this allows reports to be generated that match the assigned radiologist reading and local billing policies without additional intervention.

The PGP integration profile requires the scheduled workflow integration profile for the selection of image subsets. Subsystems in the PACS involved include:

- image acquisition modalities,
- PACS acquisition gateways,
- radiology information system (RIS), and
- image display WSs.

14.2.3.2 *IHE Key Image Note Profile*   Recall from Section 12.5.7 the montage image function we used to tag images of interest for future review. The key image note integration profile (Figure 14.5) provides a workflow to allow the montage to function by specifying a transaction that enables the user to tag images in a study by referencing them in a note linked with the study.This note includes a title stating the purpose of the tagged images and a user comment field. These notes will be properly stored, archived, and displayed as the images move among systems that support the profile. Physicians may attach key notes to images for a variety of purposes: referring physician access, teaching file selection, consultation with other departments, and image quality issues, to name a few. This integration profile requires the following resources:

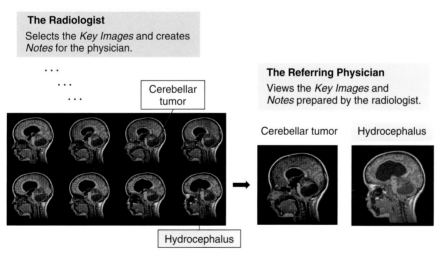

Key Image Note Profile: Improved communication between the radiologist and referring physician

Figure 14.5   IHE key image note profile. A radiologist can use this profile to tag images (red arrows) with notes in the DICOM header for future review or to communicate with the referring physicians (Carr, 2003).

- Review or diagnostics display workstations
- PACS acquisition gateways
- Acquisition modalities

14.2.3.3 IHE Simple Image and Numeric Report Profile   The simple image and numeric report integration profile shown in Figure 14.6 can be used to facilitate the use of digital dictation, voice recognition, and specialized reporting packages by separating the functions of reporting into discrete actors for creation, management, storage, and viewing. Designated numeric codes are used to identify anatomical structures, locations, diseases, and so forth. Separating these functions while defining transactions to exchange reports among them enables the user to include one or more of these functions in an actual system.

The reports exchanged have a simple structure: a title; an observation context; and one or more sections each with a heading, text, image references, and, optionally, coded measurements. Some elements may also be coded to facilitate computer searches. Such reports can be input to the formal radiology report, thus avoiding reentry of information.

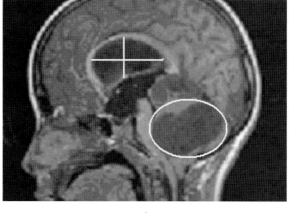

View Section

Diameters and Area
Measurements

Measurement Name	Cellebellar tumor
Measurement Abbreviation	xx
Mean Diameter	XXXXX
Short Axis	XXXXX
Long Axis	XXXXX
Area	XXXXX
Best Illustration of finding	XXXXX
Best Illustration of finding	XXXXX
Measurement Name	XXXXX
Measurement Abbreviation	XXXXX

Figure 14.6   Sample of a page in the display of the PACS WS using the IHE simple image and numeric report profile (Carr, 2003).

This integration profile requires the following resources:

- Review or diagnostics display workstations
- Reporting stations
- RIS with the reporting and repository functions

14.3 DISTRIBUTED IMAGE FILE SERVER

PACS was developed to meet the needs of image management in the radiology department. As the PACS concept evolved, the need for using PACS for other applications increased. For this reason the hospital-integrated PACS design includes distributed image file servers to provide integrated image and textual data for other departments in the medical center and for the entire healthcare enterprise.

The PACS components and data flow diagrammed in Figure 14.2 represent an open architecture design. The display component can accommodate many types of WSs, as described in Section 12.4. However, when the number of WSs (e.g., physician desktop WSs) increases, each with its own special applications and communication protocols, the numerous queries and retrievals generated by the more active WSs will affect the performance of the PACS server (see Section 11.1). Under such circumstances distributed image servers linked to the PACS server should be accounted for in the PACS infrastructure to alleviate the workload of the server. For example, Figure 14.7, an extension of Figure 14.2, shows a multiple-image server design connecting the server to a particular one for physician's desktop computers. For the past several years Web-based image distribution has become very popular and useful in image distribution because of the easy-to-use Web technology, and its potential integration with the ePR infrastructure. In the next section we discuss the Web-based image/data distribution concept, its infrastructure design, and applications.

14.4 WEB SERVER

Section 14.3 described the concept of the distributed image file server, which provides easy access to PACS image/data for different applications. In this section we present an image file server design based on the World Wide Web technology that allows easy access to PACS image/data for both inter- and intrahospital applications.

14.4.1 Web Technology

In Chapter 8 we presented network and communication technology. This section first reviews the Web technology development over the past years and then presents a Web-based image file server for PACS application.

To recap, the Internet was developed by the U.S. government originally for military applications. Through the years its utilization was extended to many other applications. The Internet can be loosely defined as a set of computers connected by various wiring methods that through TCP/IP transmit information to each other (Section 8.1.2) using a public communication network. The Intranet, on the other hand, is a private Internet that transmits information within an administrative entity

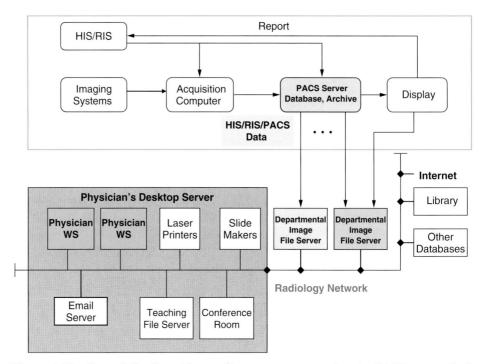

Figure 14.7   Several distributed image file servers connected to the PACS server. Each server provides specific applications for a given cluster of users. The physician desktop server (purple) is used as example for illustration. The concept of the Web server is described in Figure 14.8.

through a secured network environment. The World Wide Web is a collection of Internet protocols that provide easy access to many large databases through Internet connections.

Web is based on the hypertext transfer protocol (HTTP), which supports the transmission of hypertext documents on all computers accessible through the Internet. The two most popular languages used for Web applications that allow for the display of formatted multimedia documents independent of computers used are the hypertext markup language (HTML) and Java language (just another vague acronym; Sun Microsystems, Mountain View, CA). Recently the XML (extensible markup language, Section 9.6.5) has been applied extensively for image and text standard. Nowadays, most Web browsers, such as Microsoft's Internet Explorer and Netscape Navigator, support JPEG (Joint Photo-graphics Experts Group, 24 bits for color images) or GIF (graphics interchange format, 8 bits) for image rendering.

In Web terminology, there are the Web server and clients (or sites, or browsers). The Web site uses trigger processes to access information from the Web server through the HTTP. For the past several years applications of Web technology have been extended to healthcare information applications. Some Web sites now support access to textual information from electronic patient record (ePR) systems. These Web-based ePR systems can be categorized according to their characteristics such as completeness and detail of the information model, methods of coupling between the Web-based and legacy hospital information systems, quality of the data, and the degree of customization.

The use of the Web server as a means to access PACS image/data has been implemented by both academic centers and manufacturers. In the next section, we present the design of a Web-based image file server in the PACS environment as a means for accessing PACS image/data for both intra- and interhospital applications.

14.4.2 Concept of the Web Server in PACS Environment

Consider a Web-based image file server as shown in Figure 14.8. It must:

1. support Web browsers connected through the Internet,
2. interpret queries from the browser written in HTML or Java and convert the queries to DICOM and HL7 standards,
3. support DICOM query/retrieve SOP (service-object pair) to query and retrieve image/data from the PACS server, and
4. provide a translator to convert DICOM images and HL7 text to HTTP.

Figure 14.8 shows the basic architecture of a Web server allowing Web browsers to query and retrieve PACS image/data. Figure 14.9 illustrates eight basic steps involved in a typical query/retrieve session from the Web browser to the Web server for image/data stored in the PACS server and archive system. Note that in step 8, Figure 14.9, the image forwarder can only return 8 bits/pixel, which is not the full resolution of DICOM images. In order to have 12 bits/pixel full DICOM image resolution, we need to use the component-based technology to be described in Section 14.5.

The Web server is a good concept utilizing existing Internet technology available in everybody's desktop computer to access PACS image/data. It works very well in Intranet environments because most Intranets now use well-designed high-speed

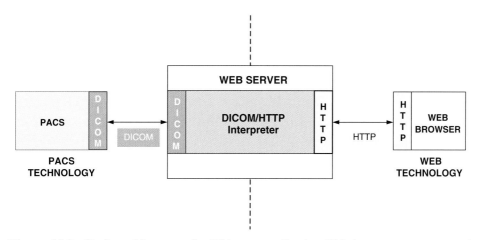

Figure 14.8 Basic architecture of a Web server allowing Web browsers to query and retrieve image/data from PACS through the Web-based server. The DICOM/HTTP interpreter is the key component.

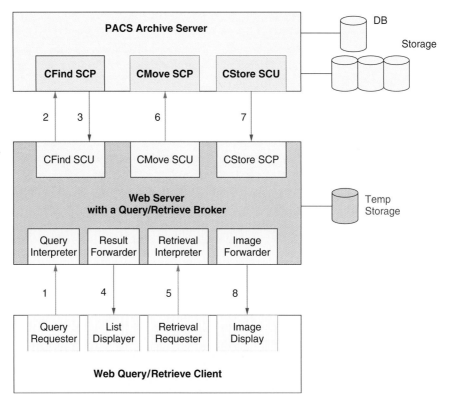

Figure 14.9 Typical query/retrieval session from the Web browser through the Web server requesting images and related data from the PACS server. The session requires eight steps involving both Web (yellow) and PACS (blue) technologies. The resources required in the Web server (Fig. 14.8) for such a session are detailed in the Web broker (middle, orange).

gigabit Ethernet switches or ATM LAN, which has sufficient bandwidth for image transmission. However, there are certain drawbacks in using the current Internet for WAN applications for two reasons. First, the response time for image transmission from the Internet is too slow because of the constraint of the WAN speed (Section 8.6). As a result it is useful only if the number and size of images retrieved are both small. Another problem is that Web technology is not designed for high-resolution gray scale image display, especially when real-time lookup table operation is required. In this case the waiting time for image display and manipulation would be too long to be tolerated. In Section 14.5 we give an example of a Web-based image distribution in the clinical PACS environment.

14.5 COMPONENT-BASED WEB SERVER FOR IMAGE DISTRIBUTION AND DISPLAY

In this section we discuss a method of developing a Web-based distribution of PACS image/data with software component technologies. This method, combining both

Web-based and PACS technologies, can preserve the original 12 bits/pixel image quality and display full-resolution DICOM images in the Web client WS by using a display and processing component.

14.5.1 Component Technologies

Traditional software development requires application executables to be compiled and linked with their dependencies. Every time a developer wants to use different processing logics or new capabilities, it must modify and recompile the primary application to support them. As a result it requires additional resources for software development, which inhibits fast turnaround time of the product and costs more. Component software technologies, which are now widely used in current software engineering, especially in enterprise-level software development, were introduced into software development to alleviate this problem. Component technologies usually consist of two parts: the component software architecture and the component software itself.

Component software architecture is a static framework or skeleton (structure or set of conventions) that provides the foundation for the component software to build on. The architecture defines how the parts relate to each other, including constraints governing how they can relate. The software components are generally any software (or subsystems) that can be factored out and have potential of standardizing or reusable exposed interface. They usually use their interfaces (importing/exporting) to provide special functions and services or to interact with other components or software modules.

Three component software technologies are used widely: CORBA (**C**ommon **O**bject **R**equest **B**roker **A**rchitecture, CORBA@ BASIC); the JavaBeans (JAVA); and COM (Component Object Model), or Active X (www.Microsoft.com/technet). The latter two are best supported and more often used in Microsoft Windows platforms, such as Windows 98, NT, Windows 2000, or XP.

14.5.2 The Architecture of Component-Based Web Server

Let us consider a Web-based PACS image/data distribution server based on the component architecture and the DP (display and processing) component to be described in Section 14.5.4. The XML is used for text messages exchanging between the browsers and web server. Other standard components are the Microsoft Internet Information Server (IIS) as the Web server and Internet Explorer (5.0 or higher) as the default browser supported by the component-based Web server, and Active X Plug-in Pro from Ncompass. Figure 14.10 shows the component-based Web server architecture (see also Fig. 14.8 for the general PACS–Web interface). In this architecture the image processing and manipulation functions are moved to the browser side during the image viewing (Fig. 14.8, right; see Section 14.5.4). The ASP (active server pages) objects, as Web-accessing interfacing objects, bridge the components distributed in the Web server (DICOM services and image database) and the browser display and processing component (DP), and make them interoperate with each other.

14.5.3 The Data Flow of the Component-Based Web Server

The Active X control component of display and processing is first resided in the Web server as a cabinet file. It can be downloaded to any browser to access images

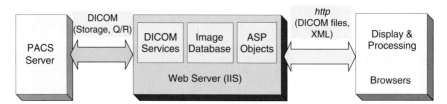

Figure 14.10 Architecture of the component-based Web server for image/data distribution and display (Zhang et al., 2003). IIS: Microsoft Internet information server; ASP: active server pages. The concept is moving the image processing and manipulation objects to the browser during viewing. Blue: DICOM technology; yellow: Web technology.

in the Web server and registered as a plug-in object in the client computer. A client can use a browser the first time to access the web pages containing ASP objects in the Web server. Later on, the user can display and process DICOM images managed by the Web server the same way as in a component-based diagnostic WS (see Section 14.5.4).

14.5.3.1 Query/Retrieve DICOM Image/Data Resided in the Web Server

When the user wants to use the browser to access DICOM images managed by the image database in the Web server (see Fig. 14.10, middle), the browser sends the *http* request to the Web server with MIME (multipurpose internet mail extension) message (XML format, encoded by DP [processing component]). The Web server decodes the XML-formatted message, queries its local database with SQL based on the content of the XML message, compiles the queried results (including patient/study/series/image/files information) to XML format, and sends the *http* response with XML-formatted MIME message to the browser.

Later on, the browser requests the Web server (see Fig. 14.10, right) sending the DICOM files, pointed by URL (uniform resource locator) in the request message, to the browser based on the user selection from the patient list. The Web server decodes the XML message sent from the browser and uploads the DICOM files to the browser through the *http* response, in which the type and content of MIME message are the binary and DICOM files. The browser or DP component receives the DICOM files, decodes the files, and displays the images. Note that the full resolution of the image pixel is preserved and this guarantees that the user can manipulate the images the same way as in a single-monitor diagnostic WS.

14.5.3.2 Query/Retrieve DICOM Image/Data Resided in the PACS Archive Server

Users can also query and retrieve the DICOM images stored in the PACS archiving server by using the browser. The operation and the communications between the browser and Web server for PACS image query and retrieval are similar to that of the Web server image. However, the interoperation between the Web server and PACS server is through *DICOM services*. For example, when the XML formats the query message sent from a client browser and received by the Web server, the message is then posted to the component of the DICOM communication service, and converted to a DICOM query object and sent to the PACS server through DICOM C-FIND service by the DICOM component. When the DICOM component receives the queried result from the PACS server, it converts

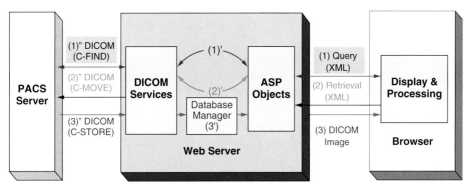

Figure 14.11   Data flow of the query/retrieve operation in the component-based Web server, which preserves the 12 bits/pixel DICOM image in the browser. The DICOM images can be displayed with its full resolution by the display and processing component in the browser, Numerals are the workflow steps. Blue: PACS technology; yellow: Web technology; pink: processing component objects (Zhang et al., 2003). $(1)–(1)'–(1)''$: query; $(2)–(2)'–(2)''–(3)''–(3)'–(3)$: retrieve.

it to a XML message, and sends the XML message to the browser through the Web server.

For the retrieval operation, the data flow is similar to that of the query, but the DICOM communication services between the Web server and the PACS server are C-MOVE and C-STORE. Figure 14.11 shows the data flow of the query/retrieval operation between the browser, the Web server and the PACS server. In Figure 14.11, $(1)–(1)'–(1)''$ denotes the query procedure, and $(2)–(2)'–(2)''–(3)''–(3)'–(3)$ denotes the retrieval procedure.

There is certain similarity in the query/retrieve operation by the browser using the DICOM protocol and format and that using the Web protocol and format. The difference is that in the former discussed in this section, 12 bits/pixel is preserved, whereas in the latter, the Web image format only allows 8 bits/pixel (see Fig. 14.9, where step 8 can only return 8 bits/pixel because of the Web technology used).

14.5.4 Component-Based Architecture of Diagnostic Display Workstation

The purpose of the component-based diagnostic WS is to augment Web-based technologies for displaying and processing full-resolution DICOM images, which the Web-based technology cannot do. The component software architecture of the Web-based WS consists of four components:

1. DICOM communication component,
2. image database component,
3. image processing, and display component, and
4. GUI (graphical user interface) component.

All these components are integrated into one computer with image cache memory and hard disks, as well as a powerful CPU and high-speed network interface. They

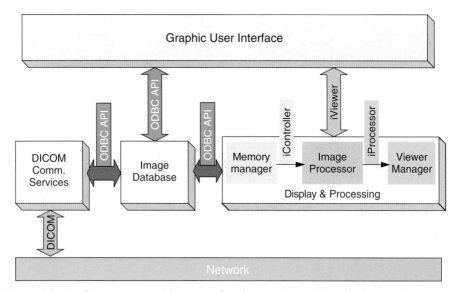

Figure 14.12   Component architecture of a diagnostic WS for display and to process DICOM images in a Web-based server. iViewer, iProcessor, and iController are image processing and display interfaces software (Zhang et al., 2003). API: application program interface; ODBC: open database connectivity.

are interoperated through the standardized or privately defined component interfaces, as shown in Figure 14.12.

We use an example here to show a component-based diagnostic display WS based on the active template library (ATL) to develop the components of DICOM communication services, and image database and Microsoft foundation classes (MFC) to develop the components of GUI and the key component of display and processing. The standardized interfaces used in the WS are DICOM and ODBC (open database connectivity) compliant. Three software programs: iViewer, iProcessor, and iController are for image processing and display interfaces.

There are three kinds of object arrays and one memory bulk object inside the component of display and processing (DP): (1) the array of processing objects, (2) the array of viewing objects, and (3) the array of window objects; the bulk memory storing image objects is managed by the memory manager. The interoperation and data exchanges between these object arrays are done through the interfaces of iController, iProcessor, and iViewer shown in Figure 14.13. There is also a message queue that collects the messages generated from different windows and dispatches them to the proper image processing pipelines, which are formed by the three objects of processing, viewing, and window.

Internally the DP component creates an event-driven window environment to let users use different input devices, such as mouse and keyboard, to manipulate the images displayed and processed through the windows and pipelines in the component with multithreading processing capability. Because the window objects inside the component can be attached to different display devices through the proper software run-time configuration, this component-based display architecture can be implemented in different display systems.

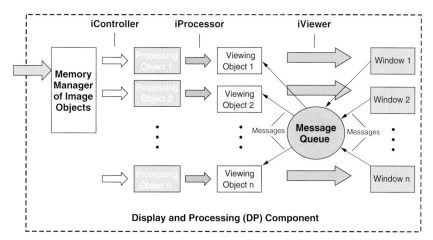

Figure 14.13 Workflow of the display and processing (DP) component in a Web-based server for display and processing of DICOM images (Zhang et al., 2003).

The DP component uses the Active X control component technology. This component can perform all major display functions found in a PACS diagnostic WS and support multimonitor display systems and also can be reused in different Windows platforms and applications, such as Windows- and Web-based applications. The DP component can be plugged in to any Web browser to interact with the component-based Web server described in previous sections to display and manipulate DICOM images.

14.5.5 Performance Evaluation

Because the browser's DP component preserves full-resolution DICOM images and provides most required diagnostic functions, the client WS can be treated as a regular PACS WS for both diagnosis and review except that the query/retrieve images are through the Web-based technology. When this technoclogy was introduced in 2002 and 2003, the question raised was, How would such a DP component in the client's browser built on top of the web-based technology perform in terms of image loading and display time compared with that of a standard web client display? Two experiments were performed (Zhang et al., 2003), with results shown in Figure 14.14*A* and *B*. The experiments used two workstations, one with a standard PACS diagnostic WS and the other a component-based Web display system. Both used the same DP component with 100 Mbits/s Ethernet connected to gigabyte Ethernet switch under a controlled research environment.

Figure 14.14*A* shows the loading and display speed of from one to six CR images to both the web and the PACS diagnostic WSs. Figure 14.14*B* depicts the loading and display speed for the web server to distribute different modality images (CT, MRI, CR) to one to four clients.

From Figure 14.14*A* we see that the speed of image loading and display in the diagnostic WS was reduced from 15 MB/s to 8 MB/s with more CR images selected. On the other hand, the speed of image loading and display from the Web server to the Web clients remained at 4 MB/s, with only a slight decrease. Figure 14.14*B* allows two interesting observations. One is that the shapes of the speed curves,

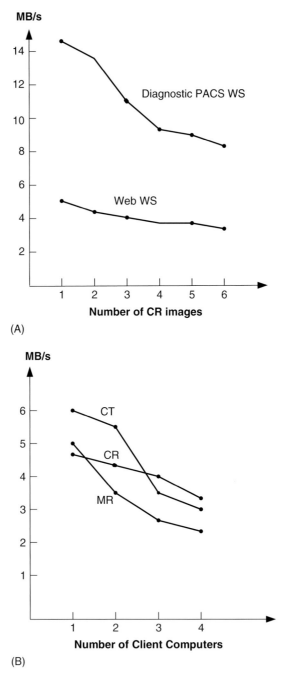

Figure 14.14 (*A*) Comparison of the averaged speeds of image loading and display from one to six CR images between a PACS diagnostic WS and a web server distributing images to one client. (*B*) Averaged speeds of distributing different modality images (CT, MR, CR) from the Web server to one to four clients. All clients requested the web server at the same time. MB/s: megabytes per second (Zhang et al., 2003).

which slope downward in the loading and displaying of different modality images with an increasing number of clients, are almost the same, and that these shapes are somewhat close to those measured from the diagnostic display workstation shown in Figure 14.14*A*. The second observation is that the loading speeds of the CT and MR images drop a little faster than that of the CR images. These results can be used to estimate the performance of image loading and display between the PACS WS and the Web WS with full DICOM viewing capability. For details of the explanation, see (Zhang et al., 2003).

Currently there are two operational models in radiology departments: one is organ based, and the other is modality based. For organ-based radiology departments, the store-forward image delivery method is used quite often, but for modality-based radiology departments, the query-retrieval method is preferred to get images from PACS. As we mentioned in Chapter 12, there are two categories of PACS WSs: one is for primary diagnosis, and the other is for different kinds of medical image applications. Using Web technologies and Web servers to access, view, and manipulate PACS images is a good alternative solution for medical image applications in Intranet and Internet environments, especially when images are to be integrated with ePR. The component-based Web server for image distribution and display can enable users using Web browsers to access, view, and manipulate PACS DICOM images just as in a typical PACS WS.

For the past five years we have witnessed a rising trend of Web-based WS being used for PACS image viewing, even in large-scale enterprise PAC systems for several reasons. The PC-based WS has become very affordable, and Intranet communication technology is very fast and low cost. Additionally Web-based viewing is theoretically much easier to grasp than a dedicated PACS WS because of the wide availability of Web technology.

14.6 WIRELESS REMOTE MANAGEMENT OF CLINICAL IMAGE WORKFLOW

14.6.1 Remote Management of Clinical Image Workflow

This section presents a Web-based PACS management tool that can be used from a PDA (personal digital assistant) that, in conjunction with a wireless network, provides a mobile tool for distributing medical exams. First, we describe the basic ingredients of this tool including design considerations, clinical workflow needs, and the PDA server. The disaster recovery design utilizing this tool based on a particular disaster recovery scenario is presented. Finally, we provide some clinical cases where this tool was used at the Saint John's Health Center (SJHC), Santa Monica, California. Because the tool is a Web-based application, it can be used from any PC (personal computer) or tablet PC as long as these devices have access to the PDA server and a Web-based browser. In this section we introduce several new terminologies. "Destination" is defined as a DICOM node that has been registered at the PDA server and the PACS archive to which the clinical examinations will eventually be sent to. The term "local" is used to refer to the hospital under consideration. Thus "local PACS" means the PACS at the local site, "local PACS archive" means the archive at the local PACS, and "local WS" means the WS connected to the local PACS networks, and so forth.

Although the basic design of the PDA tool is simple, its utilization spreads into a significant range of needs within the clinical environment. In this section we focus on the following two major applications:

- Image Distribution from Local PACS archive This is the most common way to send examinations from the local PACS archive to specific local destinations, which can be any DICOM node, such as diagnostic, review, or physician WS, or a CD burning device connected to the PACS network.
- Disaster Recovery In this application, the local PDA queries and retrieves images from the backup archive located at a remote facility to be sent to the local PACS during a disaster. For example, in an ASP (application service provider) model (documet) using a FT (fault-tolerant) backup archive, the PDA requests examinations from the remote backup archive to be sent to a local PACS WS. The characteristics of this application are that the PDA device, the PDA server, the backup archive, and the final destination could be in different locations. Section 14.6.2.3 describes the design of disaster recovery application in more details.

14.6.2 Design of the Wireless Remote Management of Clinical Image Workflow System

This section describes the clinical need assessment, the design of the PDA server and image query/retrieve operation, and its use for disaster recovery.

14.6.2.1 Clinical Needs Assessment   The practices for delivering healthcare have changed over the years, one of the factors that contributes the most is in technology advancement. However, technology alone cannot solve every need in the clinical environment. It is therefore important to find areas in common where clinical requirements can be improved by modern technology that is capable of offering an effective solution. The PDA server provides some technical features that fulfill the PACS clinical expectations, making it an excellent tool to address the clinical workflow needs. Table 14.2 summarizes the technical features of a PDA device that satisfy certain PACS clinical needs.

14.6.2.2 PDA Server and Graphical User Interface (GUI) Development
A PDA server is the key component of the wireless remote management of clinical image workflow system. We consider here the system being used at the Saint John's Health Center (SJHC) as an example. It serves as a gateway between the users and the DICOM nodes. The PDA server is a Web server (see Section 14.5) combined with a DICOM query/retrieve tool that allows easy and fast translations of Web requests to DICOM commands. The PDA server was implemented in a Red Hat 8.0 server (Pentium 4 CPU 2.8 and 512 MB of RAM) with apache2 as the Web server and perl programming language for server side coding. The server had been secured using the https (hyper text transfer protocol secure) standard, which encrypts the communication between the server and the client. In addition a valid username and password were required to access the application, so only authorized users could use it. The application also provides auditing logs to conform to HIPAA (Health Insurance Portability and Accountability Act of 1996) requirements. Because this application

TABLE 14.2   Clinical requirements and key technical features in designing a wireless PDA server tool

PACS Clinical Requirements	PDA Technical Features
Need ad hoc image and report retrieval	Platform independent (HTTPS and DICOM compliant).
Need secure, flexible, and mobile solution	Fully wireless (IEEE 802.11 locally; Edge/3 G/UMTS nationally).
Need relevant clinical information.	Secure (WEP, SSL)
Easy-to-use all-purpose device	Text and graphics capable
	Scalable implementation/thin client

PDA applications
- Reference/education
- Mobile medical image display
- Workflow/disaster management

Note: HTTPS: secured Hyper Text Transfer Protocol; WEP: wired equivalent privacy; SSL: secured socket layer; UMTS: universal mobile telecommunications system; EDGE: enhanced data for global evolution; IEEE: Institute of Electrical and Electronic Engineers.

utilized wireless infrastructure, special care was needed to avoid vulnerabilities in the security of the application and the hospital's internal network as well. For this reason we utilized the WEP (wired equivalent privacy) protocol to allow the users connect to the wireless network.

Whenever a user depends on the Web client to navigate through the PDA application, the input is passed to the PDA server, which properly converts the query to the DICOM format and communicates it to the designated DICOM node. Because the DICOM standard did not enforce a single manner of implementation, the PDA server was developed to successfully interact with different PAC systems. The current version of the application had been successfully tested against the following DICOM complaint off-the-shelf vendor nodes: Datcard PacsCube, Siemens PACS, Stentor Web application and Cedara I-View 5.0 (see vendor's Web site in the chapter reference list), and IPILab PACS Controller [Liu]. Figure 14.15 shows the system diagram at Saint John's Health Center, Santa Monica, California, for the PDA application.

Because the DICOM query/retrieve application requires easy access from the PDA, one of the key requirements is to keep the GUI as simple as possible. For this reason this application provided only the needed steps to distribute an examination to the destined node. The screenshots from Figure 14.16*A*, *B*, *C*, *D* show the following four steps:

Step A. User submits query.
Step B. PDA shows the queried results.
Step C. User selects studies from query results for retrieval.
Step D. PDA shows the retrieved results.

14.6.2.3 Disaster Recovery Design   In the event of a natural disaster, the need for PACS data may not necessarily be at the local PACS site where the disaster occurred. Therefore a key building block is to establish network connectivity between

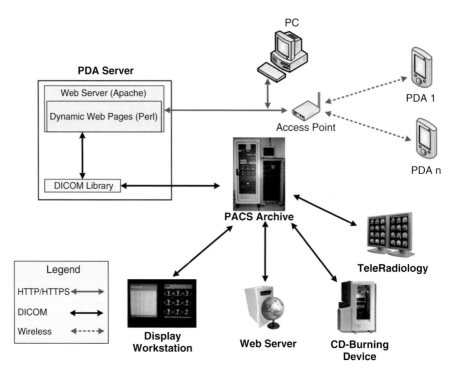

Figure 14.15   Diagram of the PDA server tool used for remote management of the PACS at the Saint John's Health Center.

multiple sites where PACS data can be transferred. Figure 14.17 shows one implementation where three separate sites are connected. The primary site is a community hospital, the secondary site is a nearby academic hospital, and the third site is where the backup clinical images are achieved, IPI (Imaging Processing and Informatics Laboratory at USC). Because the PACS at each site could be different, the types of network connections could vary between sites. Also it is important for each of the three sites to have an internal wireless network (for wireless PDA application) as well as an internal high-speed LAN (local area network) for its own PACS operation.

Once all the key building blocks were implemented, a disaster management tool can be designed and evaluated by creating disaster scenario drills. This is an important step not only to evaluate the success of the overall application but also to fine-tune any components or network connectivity issues. So a disaster scenario is created first and then the drills are designed accordingly. Assuming that all the building blocks are in place, the following is the supposed disaster:

1. Primary site encountered an earthquake that crippled the site's PACS operation.
2. The clinical PACS archive was destroyed.
3. Patients were transferred to the nearby secondary site.
4. Historical PACS exams from the primary site were needed at this secondary site.
5. Physicians and/or radiology needed to view PACS exam immediately at the secondary site.

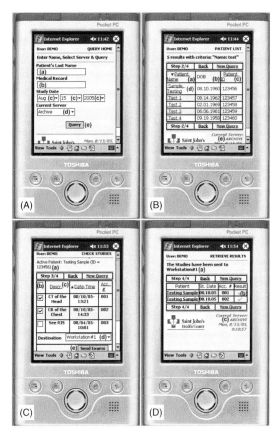

Figure 14.16 (*A*) To query the server, the user can enter the patient's last name in field (a) or enter the medical record in field (b). A logical AND is performed when both inputs are presented. If both are blank, then the study date (c) can be used for the query. The user next uses the current server (d) to select the input server where the query will be performed. Finally the user clicks the "query" button (e) to activate the query request. (In this example, a Toshiba PDA was used; any other brand name with similar capability can be used as well.) (*B*) List of patients that matched the input search criteria from the previous step. The user can sort the result by using either "patient name" (a) or "patient ID" (c). The date of birth (b) is also shown as a reference but is not sortable. To obtain the list of studies for a particular patient, the user can tab the patient name of any of the results. In this example, the patient "testing, sample" (d) is selected. The field (e) shows the current server from where the query was obtained. (*C*) List of studies available for the selected patient. (a) The patient's name and ID are displayed as reference to the user. The checkbox (b) allows the user to select all studies, or each study at the appropriate checkboxes. The user can also sort by study description, study date-time, or accession number; all these columns are shown in (c). The user then selects where to send the selected examinations to by checking the "destination" list (d). Finally clicking the "send exams" button (e) completes the retrieval process. (*D*) Results after the retrieve has been completed. (a) The destination is, in this example, Workstation#1. The check marks at (b) depict that all selected studies from the previous step were successfully sent, the information shown includes "patient," "study date," "accession number." The server from where the studies were retrieved is shown in (c); here the server was chosen in step1 and stayed the same for all other steps. The user can always go back to the previous page to resubmit a query or back to the first page.

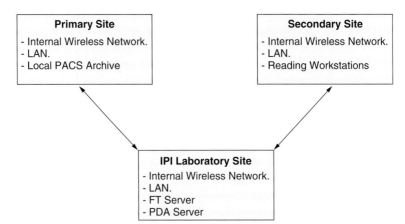

Figure 14.17 Disaster recovery scenario requirements and connectivity for multiple sites. The primary site is a community hospital (upper left), the secondary site is a nearby academic hospital (upper right), and the third site is where the backup clinical images are store at IPI Laboratory, USC (bottom).

6. A second copy of the PACS exams of the primary site had been stored off site in the ASP backup archive, the IPI Laboratory at USC.

Having all the building blocks in place allowed the creation of a real-life scenario for this architecture. It is called a "Mobile Transit Scenario" because the user of the PDA application is in transit in a Metropolitan Area but still capable of performing a remote sending of exams to a chosen destination (in this scenario to secondary site).

The workflow for this scenario is as follows:

1. During normal operations, a copy of the PACS exam is stored off site at the ASP backup archive.
2. The user, while in transit to the secondary site, is connected to the IPI Laboratory network using a VPN connection. It is assumed that the user has access to the Internet from the PDA. So the user is able to connect to a pre-configured PDA server during the disaster recovery scenarios.
3. Once the exam is located, a retrieve is made for the ASP backup archive to forward the exam for viewing when the user teaches the secondary site.

This scenario is challenging to implement because it depends on wireless mobile technologies being integrated at the multiple sites.

14.6.3 Clinical Experience

14.6.3.1 Lessons Learned at Saint John's Health Center (SJHC)   Saint John's Health Center had successfully implemented the PDA server tool to query and retrieve their clinical PACS archive with the flexibility of being mobile and portable for almost two years. From the PDA, studies could be transferred without interrupting the normal workflow functions of SJHC's PACS workstation or the various other DICOM nodes. The 3 most frequently used destinations were CD

distribution, fileroom WS, and ER/outpatients. According to the workflow analysis, this response was expected because most users of the PDA tool were film clerks, file clerks, or imaging managers, who are typically at the center of study workflow management and in charge of these tasks. The emergency room/outpatient DICOM node had the second largest number of retrieves. The PDA tool allowed the staff to send the previous examinations of patients in ER from the remote locations. The highest activities occurred in the transfer of examinations to teleradiology servers for offsite reading and diagnosis. This demonstrated the usefulness of the PDA server in teleradiological applications. For other statistics, the reader is referred to the References.

14.6.3.2 DICOM Transfer of Performance Results in Disaster Recovery Scenarios
In Section 14.6.2.3 we presented a disaster recovery design for three sites that utilized the PDA application. For the sake of comparison and to give an idea of transfer speeds for various medical image types, Table 14.3 and Table 14.4 show the DICOM throughput obtained for a dedicated point to point T1 line and a gigabit fiber connection through a shared network. Notice that the maximum throughputs were 170 Kbytes/s and 2330 Kbytes/s for the T1 line and the gigabit connection, respectively. These differences in the performance numbers were due to the higher performance connectivity between IPI and the USC Health Science Campus.

14.6.4 Summary of Wireless Remote Management of Clinical Image Workflow

The PDA server as a study management tool has proved to be low cost, and to provide fast turn-around time. This tool allows for a flexible distribution of studies to multiple

TABLE 14.3   Throughput from a point to point T1 line for various types of modalities

Modality Type	File Size	Throughput
MRI	130 KB	150 Kbytes/s
CT	512 KB	165 Kbytes/s
CR	7 MB	175 Kbytes/s
Mammography	400 MB	176 Kbytes/s

Note: The measured data were for a 20-mile T1 connection between former location of IPI Laboratory at Childrens Hospital of Los Angeles and Saint John's Health Center.

TABLE 14.4   Throughput for a gigabit connection through a shared network

Modality Type	Average File Size	Average Throughput
MRI	276 KB	179 Kbytes/s
US	358 KB	575 Kbytes/s
CT	512 KB	644 Kbytes/s
CR	6.67 MB	2330 Kbytes/s

Note: The measured data were between former location of IPI Laboratory and Healthcare Consultation Center II (HCCII), USC Health Science Campus both sites located at Los Angeles around 20 miles apart.

DICOM nodes at the fingertips of the user. Based on the workflow analysis results, this tool allows the user to avoid having to query/retrieve the same study at every DICOM node as the study is needed. This is additionally advantageous because these users tend to be mobile and at the center of image workflow management.

At SJHC this tool significantly changed the way studies were sent to a variety of DICOM destinations. It became the first choice for obtaining information on a PACS examination by users who were in charge of the image management workflow. As was shown in previous sections, this tool fits very well for remote distribution of exams both for local or offsite delivery and for disaster recovery measures.

For PACS WSs, in either a stand-alone or client-server architecture, the main function should be reserved for physicians to perform diagnosis and/or review of PACS studies instead of performing study management tasks. Based on the workflow analysis, this tool has greatly freed these resources from performing such tasks as query/retrieve and allows users to maintain multiple PACS study distribution at their fingertips through PDA mobile technology. Also, for some DICOM devices that do not feature DICOM query/retrieve, this tool is even more effective.

Because the PDA tool is Web-based, it can be utilized wherever there is a PC or mobile technology device supporting a Web-based browser, making it particularly useful for the hospital enterprise. With all these features and capabilities, this tool fulfills clinical workflow needs of a low-cost, yet powerful and easy-to-use package.

14.7 SUMMARY OF PACS DATA MANAGEMENT AND WEB-BASED IMAGE DISTRIBUTION

In Part II of this book, we presented the concepts of PACS and its components. In Part III we discuss the software components as well as operation of PACS. In this chapter we started with the PACS data management and Web-based image distribution. Five topics were covered: PACS data management, patient folder management, distributed image file server and Web server, component-based Web server for image distribution and display, and wireless remote management of clinical image workflow.

References

Andrade R, Wangenheim A, Bortoluzzi MK. Wireless and PDA: a novel strategy to access DICOM-compliant medical data on mobile devices. *Int J Med Informat* 71(2–3): 157–63; 2003.

Bosak J. In: XML, Java, and the future of the Web. http://www.ibiblio.org/pub/sun-info/standards/xml/why/xmlapps.htm.

Cao X, Hoo KS, Zhang H, et al. Web-based multimedia information retrieval for clinical application research, *SPIE Proc* 4323: 350–8; 2001.

Cedara I View. http://www.cedara.com/.

Components and Web Application Architecture. http://www.microsoft.com/technet.

CORBA® BASICS. http://www.omg.org/gettingstarted/corbafaq.htm.

Datcard PACScube. http://www.datcard.com.

Huang HK, Wong WK, Lou SL, et al. Clinical experience with second-generation hospital-integrated picture archiving and communication system. *J Digit Imag* 9: 151–66; 1996.

Huang HK. Display workstation In: *PACS Basic Principles and Applications* New York: Wiley–Liss Press; 1999.

Huang HK, Huang C. Internet 2. *Adv Imag Oncol Adm* (October): 52–58; 2003.

Huang HK, Cao F, Liu BJ, Zhang J, Zhou Z, Tsai A, Mogel G. Fault-tolerant PACS server design. *SPIE Med Imag* 4323–14: 83–92; 2001.

Java component architecture. http://java.sun.com/products/javabeans/.

Kim Y, Horii SC. Edited In: *Handbook of Medical Imaging Vol. 3: Display and PACS*. Bellingham, WA: SPIE Press; 2000.

Liu BJ, Huang HK, Cao F, Documet L, Muldoon J. Clinical experiences with an ASP model backup archive for PACS image. *Radiology* 225(P): 313; 2002.

Liu BJ, Huang HK, Cao F, Zhou MZ, Zhang J, Mogel G. A complete continuous-availability (CA) PACS archive server solution. *RadioGraphics* 24: 1203–9; 2004.

Liu BJ, Chao S, Documet J, Lee J, Lee M, Topic I, Williams L. Implementation of an ASP model offsite backup archive for clinical images utilizing Internet 2. *SPIE Med Imag* 5748: 224–31; 2005.

Moore L, Richardson BR, Williams RW. The USU medical PDA initiative: The PDA as an educational tool. *Proc AMIA Symp* 528–532; 2002.

NCompass ActiveX Plugin Proc. http://www.ncompasslabs.com/.

Ratib O, McCoy M, McGill R, Li M, Brown A. Use of personal digital assistants for retrieval of medical images and data on high-resolution flat panel displays. *Radiographics* 23(1): 267–72; 2003.

Sakusabe T, Kimura M, Onogi Y. On-demand server-side image processing for Web-based DICOM image display. *SPIE Proc* 3976: 359–67; 2000.

Siemens PACS. http://www.medical.siemens.com.

Stentor Web Server. http://www.stentor.com/.

Yaghmai V, Salehi SA, Kuppuswami S, Berlin JW. Rapid wireless transmission of head CT images to a personal digital assistant for remote consultation. *Acad Radiol* 11(11): 1291–3; 2004.

Zhang J, Stahl JN, Huang HK, et al. Real-time teleconsultation with high resolution and large volume medical images for collaborative health care. *IEEE Trans Info Techn Biomed* 4: 178–86; 2000.

Zhang J, Zhou Z, Zhuang J, et al. Design and implementation of picture archiving and communication system in Huadong Hospital. *SPIE Proc* 4323: 73–82; 2001.

Zhang J, Sun J, Stahl JN. PACS and Web-based image distribution and display. *CompMed Imag Graph* 27(2–3): 197–206; 2003.

Telemedicine and Teleradiology

Having presented the topics of image data management and Web-based PACS in Chapter 14, we can now logically turn to discussing teleradiology. Web-based PACS leads us from the PACS environment and toward image distribution outside of the enclosed hospital environment. Teleradiology is practicing radiology service outside of the hospital. Figure 15.1 (excerpted from Figure 1.3) shows how this chapter corresponds to the contents of Part III.

15.1 INTRODUCTION

Telemedicine and teleradiology are becoming increasingly important as the U.S. healthcare delivery system gradually changes from fee-for-service to managed capitated care. Over the past ten years we have seen a trend of primary care physicians joining health maintenance organizations (HMOs). HMOs purchase smaller hospitals and form hospital groups under the umbrella of HMOs. Also academic institutions form consortia to compete with other local hospitals and HMOs. This consolidation allows the elimination of duplication and the streamlining of healthcare services among hospitals. As a result costs are reduced, but at the same time because of the downsizing, the number of experts available for service decreases. Utilization of telemedicine and teleradiology is a cost-saving method that also compensates for the loss of expertise.

One of the most comprehensive reviews in assessing telecommunications in healthcare was a study reported by the Institute of Medicine Committee on Evaluating Clinical Applications of Telemedicine in 1996 and its subsequent revisions. Various issues in telemedicine including technical and human context, policy, and methods of evaluation are discussed in detail in this report, so it is an excellent source of reference.

Telemedicine, in terms of applications, can be simply defined as the delivery of healthcare using telecommunications, computer, and information technologies (IT) that include medical images. The well-established consultation by means of telephone conversation alone would not be qualified as telemedicine because it only uses telecommunications, and not the computer or IT. There are two models in telemedicine that involve teleradiology: The referring physician or healthcare provider can, on one hand, consult with specialists at various locations through a

PACS and Imaging Informatics, Second Edition, by H. K. Huang
Copyright © 2010 John Wiley & Sons, Inc.

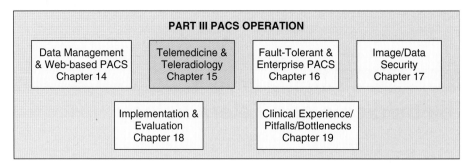

Figure 15.1   Position of Chapter 15 in the organization of this book. Color codes are used to highlight components and workflow in the chapters of Part III.

network or, on the other hand, request opinions from a consolidated expert center where different types of consultation services are provided. In this chapter we concentrate on the expert center model because this is the more dominant trend in the healthcare delivery system.

In the expert center consultation process, three modes of telemedicine are possible: telediagnosis, teleconsultation, and telemanagement. In telediagnosis, the patient's examination results and imaging studies are done at the referring physician's site; then the data and images are transmitted to the expert center for diagnosis. The urgency of this service is nominal, and the turnaround time can take from four hours to a day. In teleconsultation, the patient may be still waiting at the examination site while the referring doctor requests a second opinion or diagnosis from the expert center, the turnaround time can be half an hour. In telemanagement, the patient may still be on the gantry or in the examination room at the remote site and the expert is required to provide immediate management care to the patient. Because of these three different operational modes, technology requirements in telemedicine and teleradiology would be different which would have impacts in the cost of care.

15.2   TELEMEDICINE AND TELERADIOLOGY

Teleradiology is a subset of telemedicine dealing with the transmission, display, and diagnosis from images, in addition to other patient-related information, between a remote examination site and an expert center. The technology requirement for teleradiology is more stringent than that of general telemedicine because the former involves images.

Basically telemedicine without teleradiology requires only very simple technology: a computer gathers all necessary patient information, examination results, and diagnostic reports; arranges them in proper order with or without a standard format at the referring site; and transmits them through telecommunication technology to a second computer at the expert center where the information is displayed as a softcopy on the monitor. One important issue in telemedicine is patient privacy, which has to be considered seriously during the delivery of the telemedicine service. In modern hospitals or clinics, the information gathering and the arrangement of the information in proper order can be handled by the hospital information system

(HIS) or the clinical management system (CMS). In a private practice group or an individual physician's office, these two steps can be contracted out to a computer application vendor. Another requirement of telemedicine is to design communication protocols for sending this prearranged information to the expert center. This requirement needs special hardware and software components.

Hardware and telecommunication choices vary according to the required data throughput. The hardware component includes a pair of communication boards and modems, and a phone line connecting the two computers, one at the referring site and the other at the expert center. The type and cost of such hardware depends on which telecommunication service is selected. Depending on the transmission speed required, the line can be a regular telephone line, a DS-0 (Digital Service, 56 Kbits/s), an ISDN (Integrated Service Digital Network, from 56 Kbits/s to 1.544 Mbits/s), or a DS-1 or Private Line (T-1) with 1.544 Mbits/s. The cost of these lines is related to the transmission speed and the distance between sites. For telemedicine applications without images, a regular telephone line, DS-0, or a single ISDN or DSL line would be sufficient. A local ISDN or DSL line in a large metropolitan area costs $30 to $40 a month.

The software component includes information display with good GUI (graphic user interface) and some quality-assurance and communication protocol programs. All software programs can be supported by either the HIS department or a vendor. Efficient information gathering and selecting proper subsets of information for timely transmission are critical to the success of the telesystem. Once diagnostic results are available from the expert center, they can be transmitted back to the referring site with the same communication chain or through a standard FAX machine. Figure 15.2

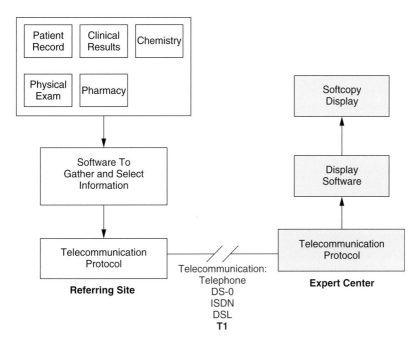

Figure 15.2   Generic telemedicine communication chain. Without images, a T1 line is sufficient for most applications.

shows a generic telemedicine communication chain. During the past several years, web client server model in telemedicine becomes very popular, in this case an Internet service provider (ISP) model can support both hardware and software services. In teleradiology, because it involves images, the technologies required are more demanding. We discuss this topic in more detail in Section 15.3.

15.3 TELERADIOLOGY

15.3.1 Background

As discussed in Section 15.1, the managed, capitated care trend in the healthcare industry creates an opportunity for forming expert centers in radiology practice. In this model, radiological images and related data are transmitted between examination sites and diagnostic centers via telecommunications. This type of radiology practice is loosely called teleradiology. Figure 15.3 shows an expert center model in teleradiology. In this expert model, rural clinics, community hospitals, and HMOs rely on radiologists at the center for consultation. Figure 15.3 clearly shows that in teleradiology, the turnaround time requirement is different depending on the modes of service, which in turn, determine the technology required and cost involved.

15.3.1.1 Why Do We Need Teleradiology? The managed care trend in healthcare delivery is to expedite the report delivery from the teleradiology expert

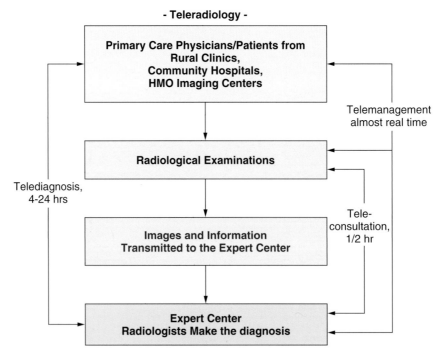

Figure 15.3 Three expert center models in teleradiology: telediagnosis, teleconsultation, and telemanagement.

center. However, even without healthcare reform, teleradiology is an extremely important component in radiology practice for the following reasons:

1. Teleradiology secures images for radiologists to read so that no images will be accidentally lost in transit.
2. Teleradiology reduces the reading cycle time from when the image is formed to when the report is completed.
3. Because radiology is subdivided into many subspecialties, a general radiologist occasionally requires an expert's second opinion. The availability of teleradiology will facilitate the seeking of a second opinion.
4. Teleradiology increases radiologists' income because no images are temporarily lost and subsequently not read.

The healthcare reform adds two more reasons:

1. Healthcare costs are saved because an expert center can serve multiple sites, reducing the number of radiologists required.
2. Healthcare improves in efficiency and effectiveness because the turnaround time is faster and there is no loss of images.

15.3.1.2 *What Is Teleradiology?*

Generally, teleradiology is the process by which images from the patient are sent from the examination site to an expert radiologist for diagnosis and the report is routed to a primary physician for proper treatment. Teleradiology can be very simple or extremely complicated. In the simplest case, an image is sent from a CT scanner, for example, in the evening to the radiologist's home PC workstation (WS) with slow-speed communication technology for a second opinion. During off-hours, evenings and weekends, there may not be a radiologist at the examination site to cover the service. A radiology resident is nominally in charge but requires consultation occasionally from the radiologist at home during off-hours. This type of teleradiology does not require highly sophisticated equipment. A conventional telephone with a modem connected to a PC with display software would be sufficient to perform the teleradiology operation. This type of application originated in the early 1970s, and can range from simple to complex, as shown in the four models of Table 15.1. The complexity is introduced when a current examination requires historical images for comparison, and when the expert needs information from the radiology information system (RIS) to make a diagnosis. Additionally complexity arises when the examination and dictation are required to be

TABLE 15.1 Four models of teleradiology operation according to its complexity

	Historical Images/RIS	Archive
Most simple	No	No
Simple	Yes	No
Complex	No	Yes
Most complex	Yes	Yes

archived and appended to the patient's image data file and record. Teleradiology is relatively simple to operate when no archiving is required. However, when previous information on a patient must be archived and be readily accessible, the operation becomes complicated.

15.3.1.3 Teleradiology and PACS   When the teleradiology service requires a patient's historical images as well as related information, teleradiology and PACS become very similar operationally. Table 15.2 shows the differences between teleradiology and PACS. The biggest difference between them is in the image capture methods. Some current teleradiology operations still use a digitizer as the primary method of converting a film image to digital format, although the trend is moving toward the DICOM standard. In PACS, direct digital image capture is mostly done using DICOM. In networking, teleradiology uses the slower speed wide area networks (WAN) compared with the Intranet, whereas the higher speed local area network (LAN) is used in PACS. In teleradiology, image storage is mostly short term, whereas in PACS it is long term. Teleradiology relies heavily on image compression, whereas PACS may or may not.

Recall Table 2.1. There the second column gives sizes of some common medical images. In clinical applications, one single image is not sufficient for making diagnosis. In general, a typical examination generates between 10 and 20 Mbytes. Notice that the fourth column of Table 2.1 shows an average size of one typical examination in each of these image modalities. The highest extreme is in digital mammography, which requires 160 Mbytes. To transmit 160 Mbytes of information through WAN requires a very high-bandwidth communication technology. One major issue in teleradiology is how to transmit a very large image file through WAN with acceptable speed and cost; an example in telemammography is discussed in more detail in Section 15.4.

15.3.2   Teleradiology Components

Table 15.3 lists some major components of teleradiology, and Figure 15.4 shows a schematic of their connections. Among these components, reporting and billing are common knowledge and are not discussed here. Devices generating images in teleradiology applications include computed tomography (CT), magnetic resonance imaging (MRI), computed and digital radiography (CR, DR), ultrasound imaging (US), nuclear medicine (NM), digital subtraction angiography-digital fluorography (DSA, DF), and film digitizer, which were presented in Chapters 3, 4, and 5. Images

TABLE 15.2   **Differences in technology used between teleradiology and PACS**

Function	Teleradiology	PACS
Image Capture	Digitizer, DICOM	DICOM
Display technology	Similar	Similar
Networking	WAN	LAN
Storage	Hard disk (short term)	Various tech (long term)
Compression	Yes	Maybe

TABLE 15.3   Major teleradiology components

- Imaging acquisition device[a]
- Image capture
- Data reformatting
- Image transmission
- Storage
- Display
- Reporting
- Billing

[a]A necessity for teleradiology operation, but not a teleradiology component

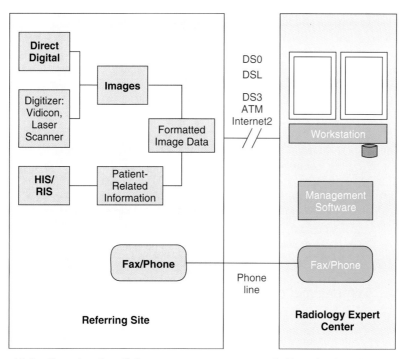

Figure 15.4   Generic teleradiology components set up. (left) Referring site (see top of Fig. 15.6); (right) teleradiology expert center (see bottom of Fig. 15.6).

from these acquisition devices are first generated from the examination site and then sent through the communication network to the expert center if they are already in digital format. Otherwise, if these images are stored on films, they must be digitized first by a film scanner to acceptable quality for diagnosis at the examination site before they are sent.

15.3.2.1   Image Capture   In image capture, if the original image data are on film, then either a video frame grabber or a laser film digitizer is used to convert them to digital format. A video frame grabber produces low-quality digital images but is faster and cheaper. On the other hand, laser film digitizers produce very high quality digital data but take longer and cost more to purchase compared with the video frame grabber. Nowadays teleradiology seldom uses the video frame grabber because of the image quality it produces. For the past several years direct DICOM output images from CR, DR, CT, and MR have been used extensively in teleradiology.

15.3.2.2 Data Reformatting After images are captured, it is advantageous to convert these images and related data to the industry standard because of the multiple vendors' equipment used in the teleradiology chain, such as Digital Imaging and Communication in Medicine (DICOM) for images and Health Level 7 (HL7) for textual data described in Chapter 9. For image data communication, the DICOM and TCP/IP standards described in Chapter 8 should be used.

15.3.2.3 Image Storage At the image receiving end of the teleradiology chain, a local storage device is needed before the image can be displayed. The capacity of this device can range but should be in many gigabytes. At the expert center, a long-term archive, such as a small DLT tape library, is needed for teleradiology applications that require historical images, related patient information, and current examinations and diagnoses archival. The architecture of the long-term storage device is very similar to that used in PACS, as discussed in Chapter 11.

15.3.2.4 Display Workstation For a teleradiology system, a high-end 1K LCD WS is necessary for sectional images, and a 2K WS with multiple monitors for CR/DR and digital mammography primary diagnosis, as described in Chapter 12.

Table 15.4 shows the specifications of high-end 1K and 2K WSs used for teleradiology primary readings. These diagnostic WSs, use two monitors with many gigabytes of local storage, and can display images and reports retrieved from local storage in 1 to 2 seconds. User-friendly image display software (to be presented in a latter subsection) is necessary for easy and convenient use by the radiologist at a workstation.

15.3.2.5 Communication Networks An important component in teleradiology is the communication networks used for the transmission of images and related data from the acquisition site to the expert center for diagnosis. Since most teleradiology applications are not within the same hospital complex, but through inter-healthcare facilities in metropolitan areas or at longer distances, the communication technology involved requires a wide area network (WAN). WAN can be wireless or with cables. Wireless WAN technologies available are microwave transmission and

TABLE 15.4 Specifications of high-end 1K and 2K workstations for teleradiology

- Two LCD monitors
- 1–2 week local storage for current + previous exams
- 1–2 second display of images and reports from local storage
- HL7 and DICOM conformance
- Simple image-processing functions
- Internet communication protocol available

communication satellites. Wireless WAN has not been used extensively in teleradiology due to its higher cost. Table 15.5 (excerpted from Table 8.5, see Section 8.7.1 for more detail) shows cable technology available in WAN from the low communication rate DS-0 with 56 kbits/s; DSL (Digital Subscriber Line, 144 Kbits/s to 24 Mbits/s, depending on data traffic and the subscription); T1 and T3 lines starting from 1.5 Mbits/s; to very high broadband communication DS-3 with 45 Mbits/s. These WAN technologies are available through either a long-distance or a local telephone carrier, or both. The cost of using WAN is a function of transmission speed and the distance between sites. Thus, within a fixed distance, for a DS-0 line with a low transmission rate, the cost is fairly low compared to DS-3, which is much faster but very expensive. Most private lines, for example T1 and T3, are point to point, so the cost depends on the distance between connections. Table 15.6 gives an example showing the relative cost of the DSL and the T1 between University of Southern California and St. John's Health Center about 15 miles apart in the Greater Los Angeles Metropolitan Area.

Table 15.6 demonstrates that the initial investment for the DSL is minimal, since the WAN carrier pays for the DSL modem used for the network connection. The lowest monthly cost is about $40 a month. On the other hand, for T1 service, the up-front investment is $4000 for the two T1 routers and $1000 for installation, and the monthly cost is $600. The up-front investment for the T-1 is much higher than the DSL, and for longer distances its monthly charge is high. For example, the charge

TABLE 15.5 Transmission rate of current wide area network technology

DS-0	56 Kbits/s
DS-1	56 to (24 × 56) Kbits/s
DSL	32 Kbits/s to 50 Mbits/s
DS-1 (T1)	1.5 Mbits/s
ISDN	56 kbits/s to 1.5 Mbits/s
DS-3	28 DS-1 = 45 Mbits/s
ATM (OC-3)	155 Mbits/s and up
Internet-2	100 Mbits/s and up

Note: Excerpted from Table 8.5.

TABLE 15.6 Wide area network cost using DSL (144 Kbits/s–8 Mbits/s) and T-1 (1.5 Mbits/s) between USC and St. John's Hospital 20 miles apart

DSL		T1	
Up front investment	Minimal	Up front investment	$5000
Modems (2)	None	T1 DSU/CSU[a]	
		WAN interface (2)	
		Router (2)	$4000
Installation (2)	Minimal	T1 installation	$1000
Monthly charge (lowest rate)	$40	T1 monthly charge:	$600

[a]DSU/CSU: Data service unit/channel service unit, June 2003 to 2007.

between Los Angeles and Washington, DC, for a T1 line can be as high as $10,000 a month. However, T1 is a point-to-point private line, and it guarantees its 1.5 Mbits/s specification, and provides communication security. The disadvantages of DSL are as follows:

1. Communication is through shared networks, and hence there is no security.
2. Performance depends on the load of the DSL carrier at that moment.
3. DSL is not available everywhere.

Using T1 and DSL for teleradiology is becoming very popular. Some larger IT (information technology) companies lease several T1 lines from telephone carriers and sublease portions of them to smaller companies for teleradiology applications.

Another wide area network listed in Table 15.5, Internet 2 (I2) technology, is ideal for teleradiology application because of its speed of transmission and low cost of operation after the site is connected to the I2 backbone [9]. I2 is a national infrastructure of high-speed communication backbones (over 10 gigabits/s using gigabit switches and asynchronous mode technology [ATM]) supported by the National Science Foundation (NSF). At the local level the users have to obtain permission from the Internet Administration for connection if the organization is involved in education and research and development. Once approved, the users must then learn how to connect the academic hospital and clinic environments to these backbones. For more detail on I2 technology, see Section 8.6 and the results shown in Tables 8.6, 8.7, and 8.8. The disadvantages of using I2 for teleradiology are as follows:

1. The local site has to upgrade its conventional Internet infrastructure to be compatible with the high-speed I2 performance, which is costly.
2. Not enough experts know how to connect from the radiology department to the backbone, and
3. I2 is not yet open for commercial use.

With advances in communications technology, image workstation design, and image compression, teleradiology has become as an integrated diagnostic tool in daily radiology practice.

15.3.2.6 User Friendliness
User friendliness has two measurable parameters: the connection procedure of the teleradiology equipment at both the examination site and the expert center, and the simplicity of using the display workstation at the expert center.

User friendliness means that the complete teleradiology operation should be as simple and automatic as possible, requiring only minimal user intervention. For the WS to be user friendly, it must satisfy three condiions:

1. Automatic image and related data prefetch.
2. Automatic image sequencing and hanging protocol at the monitors.
3. Automatic lookup table, image rotation, and unwanted background removal from the image.

Image and related data prefetch means that all necessary historical images and related data required for comparison by the radiologist should be prefetched from the patient folder at the imaging sites and send to the expert center with the current exam. When the radiologist is ready to review the case, these prefetched images and related data are already available at the expert center.

Automatic image sequencing and hanging protocol at the WS means that all these images and related data are sequentially arranged so that at the touch of the mouse, properly arranged images and sequences are immediately display on the monitors. Pre-arranged data minimizes the time required for the searching and organizing of data by the radiologist at the expert center. This translates to an effective and efficient teleradiology operation.

The third factor, automatic lookup table, rotation, and background removal, is necessary because images acquired at the distant site might not have the proper lookup table set up for optimal visual display, images might not be generated in the proper orientation, and might have some unwanted white background in the image due to radiographic collimation.

All these parameters have an effect on the proper and efficient diagnosis of the images. Figure 15.5 shows an example of automatic splitting of a CT examination of both the chest and the abdomen into a chest and an abdomen sequence for automatic display using the concept of presentation of grouped procedures (PGP) in IHE (Integrating the Healthcare Enterprise, see Chapter 9) profile technology. A good teleradiology display software should be able to split one CT exam into two regions, the chest and the abdomen, and display them properly at the WS with both the chest bone and lung windows for the chest along with the abdominal window.

15.4   TELERADIOLOGY MODELS

In this section we discuss four teleradiology operation models that are common in current practice.

15.4.1   Off-hour Reading

The off-hour reading model is to take care of the off-hour reviewing the images including evenings, weekends, and holidays when most radiologists are not available at the examination sites. In this setup image acquisition devices at different examination sites, including hospitals and clinics, are connected to an off-hour reading center with medium or low-grade transmission speed (like the DSL) because the turnaround time is not as critical as for emergency cases. The connections are mostly direct digital as with the DICOM standard. The reading center is equipped with network switches and various types of workstations compatible with the images generated by imaging devices at examination sites. The staffing includes technical personnel taking care of the communication networks and WSs, and radiologists who come in during the evening, weekend, and holiday shifts and perform on-line digital reading. They provide preliminary accessments of the exams and transmit these to the examination site instantaneously after reading the images. The radiologists at the examination sites verify the readings and sign off the report on the next day. This type

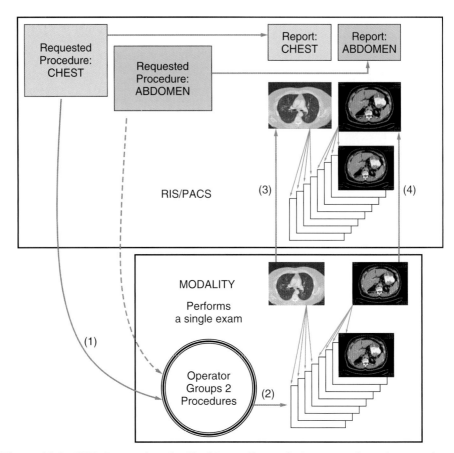

Figure 15.5   IHE (Integrating the Healthcare Enterprise) presentation of grouped procedures profile (PGP). (1) A single CT acquisition procedure (solid and dotted lines) is used to acquire both (2) chest and abdominal scans. The IHE scheduled workflow profile provides information for the PGP to split the acquired images into two subsets (orange and green), (3) one for chest (orange) and (4) the other for abdomen (green).

of teleradiology setup is low technology, but it serves the purpose of compensating for the shortage of radiologists during the off hours. There are many such off-hour reading business establishments throughout the world taking advantage of time zone differences.

15.4.2   ASP Model

ASP (application service provider) model is a business venture taking care of the radiology service where on-site interpretations are not available. This model can be for supplying teleradiology equipment only or for both equipment and radiology reading. In the former, the ASP sets up a technical center housing network equipment, WSs, and reading rooms. It also provides turnkey connectivity for the examination site where images would be transmitted to the center. In the latter, the center provides technical support and radiologists for reading.

15.4.3 Web-Based Teleradiology

Web-based teleradiology is a client-server model (see Chapter 11) mostly used by hospital or larger clinics to distribute images to various parts of the hospitals or clinics, or outside of the hospital. A Web server is designed where filtered images from PAC systems are either pushed from the PACS server to, or pulled by the Web server. Filtered images mean that the Web server has a predetermined directory managing the image distribution based on certain criteria like what types of images to where and to whom. The clients can view these filtered images from the Web server at Web browsers equipped with diagnostic or review WSs. The clients can be referring physicians who just want to take a look at the images, or radiologists who want to make a remote diagnosis. Web-based teleradiology is very convenient and low cost to set up because most of its technologies are readily available, especially within the hospital Intranet environment. The drawback is that since Web is a general technology, the viewing capability and conditions are not as good as that in a regular PACS WS where the setup is geared for radiology diagnosis. In order to have full DCIOM image resolution for visualization and manipulation at the clients' WSs, modifications have to be made at the Web server to receive full 12-bits/pixel data from the PACS server, and at the client to receive additional image display software.

15.4.4 PACS and Teleradiology Combined

This subsection presented in this section was introduced in Section 7.5. For completeness and convenience, we excerpt some materials from the section here. Recall that teleradiology can function as a pure teleradiology operation in (Fig. 15.6, excerpted from Fig 7.6). As we mentioned in Section 7.5.1, the teleradiology management

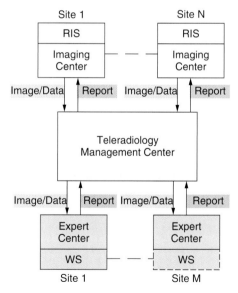

Figure 15.6 Pure teleradiology model. The management center monitors the operation directing workflow between imaging centers and expert centers. (Excerpted from Fig. 7.6, see Section 7.5.1 for workflow steps.)

center acts also as the operation manager. It documents images it receives from different imaging centers, and keeps that record as it routes the images to different expert centers according to diagnostic needs. As the reports come back to the management center, it records them and forwards them to the appropriate imaging centers.

Teleradiology can be combined together with PACS as a healthcare enterprise operation, (Fig. 15.7, excerpted from Fig. 7.7). and the workflow of this combined model is as follows:

- Radiologists at PACS WSs read exams from the outside imaging centers (step 1).
- After reading by PACS radiologists from its own WSs (step 2), reports are sent to the HIS database via the database gateway for its own record (step 3) and to the expert center (steps 4, 5) from where the report (step 4) is also sent back to the imaging center.

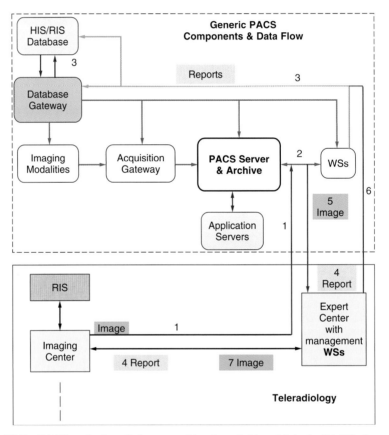

Figure 15.7 PACS and teleradiology combined model in which the PACS also supports imaging centers for teleradiology reading; PACS and teleradiology support each other. The top rectangle is the PACS components and work flow (excerpted from Fig. 7.2), and the bottom rectangle is the teleradiology model modified redrawn from Fig. 15.6. Red lines: Communication between PACS and teleradiology. (excerpted from Fig. 7.7.)

- PACS can also send its own exams to the outside expert center for reading (step 5). The expert center returns the report to the PACS database gateway (step 6).
- The image center send images to the expert center for reading as in the pure teleradiology model (step 7).

Ideally the combined teleradiology and PACS model will be used in a healthcare center with satellite imaging centers, multiple affiliated hospitals, and with backup radiology coverage between hospitals and imaging centers.

15.5   SOME IMPORTANT ISSUES IN TELERADIOLOGY

15.5.1   Image Compression

Teleradiology requires image compression because of the slow speed and high cost of using WAN for image transmission. For lossless image compression, current technology can achieve between 3:1 to 2:1 compression ratios, whereas in lossy compression using cosine transform and wavelet-based MPEG and JPEG hardware or software, 20:1 to 10:1 compression ratios can be obtained with acceptable image quality. Wavelet transform has advantages over cosine transform of a higher compression ratio and better image quality, however, hardware wavelet compression is still being developed. Some Web-based teleradiology systems use a progressive wavelet image compression technique. In this technique the image reconstruction from the compressed file proceeds in a progressively in that a lower resolution image is first reconstructed almost instantaneously and displayed upon requested. The user would immediately recognize that the image was transmitted through the network in real time. Higher quality images would be continuously reconstructed to replace the lower quality ones until the original image in all its details is fully reconstructed and displayed. Another approach would be to only construct a region of interest instead of a full image.

15.5.2   Image Data Privacy, Authenticity, and Integrity

Image transmission in teleradiology is mostly through public networks. For this reason trust in image data has become an important issue. Trust in image data is characterized in terms of privacy, authenticity, and integrity of the data. Privacy refers to denial of access to information by unauthorized individuals. Authenticity refers to validating the source of the image. Integrity refers to the assurance that the image has not been modified accidentally or deliberated during the transmission. Privacy and authenticity are the responsibility of the public network provider based on firewall and password technologies, whereas integrity is the responsibility of the end user.

Imaging integrity is maintained mostly by public and private keys based on a digital signature encrypted with mathematical algorithms during the process of image generation. In general, the public and private keys of the digital signature consists of seven steps:

1. Private and public keys. Set up a system of assigning public and private keys for image transmission between the examination site and the expert center.

2. Image preprocessing. Isolate the object of interest in the image from the background (e.g., the head in a CT image as the object of interest), and extract patient information from the DICOM image header at the examination site while the image is being generated.

3. Image digest. Compute the image digest (digital signature) of the object of interest in the image based on its characteristics using mathematical algorithms.

4. Data encryption. Produce a digital envelope containing the encrypted image digest and the corresponding patient information from the image header.

5. Data embedding. Embed the digital envelope into the background of the image as a further security measure. The background is used because the embedding should not alter the image quality of the object of interest. If the image has no background, like a chest radiograph, then a more complex lossless embedding technique may be used.

6. Digital envelope transmission. Send the image with the embedded digital envelope to the expert site.

7. Image integrity validation by the expert center receiving the image (step 6). Decrypt the image and the signature. Then, to validate the image integrity, compare the two digital signatures, one that comes with the image, and a second one computed from the received image.

Chapter 17 covers image data security in more technical detail.

15.5.3   Teleradiology Trade-off Parameters

There are two sets of trade-off parameters in teleradiology. The first set consists of image quality, turnaround time, and cost, and the second set is the data security, which includes patient confidentiality, image authenticity, and image integrity. Table 15.7 shows the teleradiology trade-off parameters pertaining to image quality, turnaround time, and cost. These three parameters are affected by four factors: the method of image capture, the type of workstation used, the amount of image compressed, and the selected communication technology.

In terms of data security, we must consider patient confidentiality as well as image authenticity. Because teleradiology uses a public communication method to transmit images that has no security, the question arises as to what type of protection one should provide to ensure patient confidentiality and to authenticate the sender. The second issue is image integrity. After the image is created in digital form, can we ensure that the image created has not been altered either intentionally or unintentionally during the transmission? To guarantee patient confidentiality

TABLE 15.7   Teleradiology trade-off parameters

	Image Capture	Workstation	Compression	Communication Technology
Quality	X	X	X	
Turn-around time	X		X	X
Cost	X	X	X	X

and image authenticity, methods such as fire walls can be set up. To protect image integrity, data encryption and digital signatures can be used. These techniques have been in the domain of defense research and development for many years and can be adapted to teleradiology. However, as high security is imposed on image data, it will increase the cost of decryption and decrease easy access because of the many layers of encryption and the required passwords. The trade-offs between cost and performance, confidentiality and reliability, threatens to become a major socioeconomic issue in teleradiology. Figure 15.8 shows a CT image that has been altered digitally by inserting an artificial tumor in the lung (see arrows). Because altering a digital image is fairly easy, developing methods to protect integrity of image data is essential in teleradiology applications. We discuss data integrity and patient confidentiality in more detail in Chapter 17.

15.5.4   Medical-Legal Issues

There are four major medical-legal issues in teleradiology: privacy, licensure, credentialing, and malpractice liability. The ACR (American College of Radiology) Standard for Teleradiology adopted in 1994 defines guidelines for "qualifications of both physician and nonphysician personnel, equipment specifications, quality improvement, licensure, staff credentialing, and liability." Guidelines to these topics, although still being revised from time to time, have been discussed extensively by James, Berger, and Cepelewicz, and Kamp. Readers are encouraged to review the ACR Standard and these authors' publications for current developments regarding these issues.

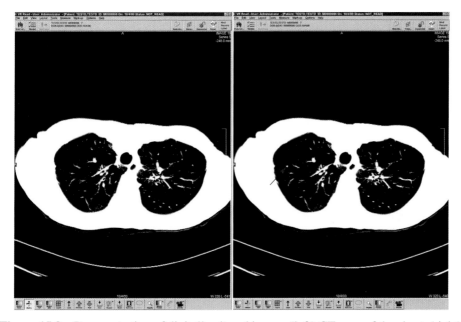

Figure 15.8   Demonstration of digitally altered image. (left) CT scan of the chest; (right) same scan with a digitally inserted artificial tumor (arrow). The insertion process requires minimal image processing effort.

15.6   TELE-BREAST IMAGING

15.6.1   Why Do We Need Tele-breast Imaging?

Breast cancer is the fourth most common cause of death among women in the United States. There is no known means of preventing the disease, and available therapy has been unsuccessful in reducing the national mortality rate over the past 60 years. Current attempts at controlling breast cancer concentrate on early detection by means of mass screening, periodic mammography, and physical examination, because ample evidence and statistics have indicated that screening can lead to early diagnosis and thus lowering the death rate. Massive screening is performed using digital mammography (Section 3.5) and other 3-D breast-imaging technologies (for 3-D US, see Section 4.6, and Section 5.3.1, Fig 5.4; for 3-D MRI, see Section 4.7.4, Fig. 4.20*A* and *B*). Coupling these breast-imaging technologies with teleradiology is called tele-breast imaging. In the case of digital mammography, we use the term telemammography. For an example of tele-breast imaging, the reader is referred to the discussion in Section 21.6 on the dedicated breast MRI enterprise Data Grid and Figure 21.18 for an illustration.

In this chapter, we focus on full-field direct digital mammography (FFDDM; see also Section 3.5.2), which has overcome many of the problems inherent in the screen/film combination detector and at the same time provides better spatial and density resolutions and a higher signal-to-noise ratio in the digital mammogram than that from a digitized mammogram. Real-time telemammography adds the advantage of utilizing expert mammographers (rather than general radiologists) as interpreters of the mammography examinations at the expert center. Setting up a quality tele-mammography service requires the FFDDM at the examination site, a high-speed tele-imaging network connecting the examination site with the mammography expert center (because of the large size of digital mammograms), and high-resolution digital mammogram WSs for interpretation.

15.6.2   Concept of the Expert Center

Telemammography is built on the concept of an expert center. This allows the radiologists with the greatest interpretive expertise to manage and read in real time all mammography examinations. Real time is defined in this context as a very rapid turnaround time between examination and interpretation. Specifically, tele-mammography will increase efficiency, facilitate consultation and a second reading, improve patient compliance, facilitate operation, support computer-aided detection and diagnosis (CAD), allow centralized distributive archives, and enhance education through telemonitoring. In addition mammography screening in mobile units will be made more efficient, and no longer will there be need to transport films from the site of examination to the site of interpretation; rather, image interpretation will be made while patients are still available for repeat or additional exposures. Furthermore telemammography can be used to facilitate a second opinion or interpretation, enabling world-class mammography expertise to be accessible to community practice radiologists.

There are three protocols in telemammography: telediagnosis, teleconsultation, and telemanagement. Telediagnosis uses experts to interpret digital mammograms sent from a remote site. Teleconsultation is used to resolve problem cases.

Telemanagement would replace an on-site general radiologist by remotely located expert mammographers.

15.6.3   Technical Issues

Telemammography services require FFDDM at the examination site, an image compression algorithm, a high-speed tele-imaging WAN connecting the examination site with the mammography expert center, and a high-resolution and efficient digital mammography display workstation for interpretation.

Present technologies available for telemammography applications include the FFDDM with 50-mm spatial resolution with 12 bits/pixel (Section 3.5), ATM or Internet 2 for both LAN and WAN connections, a digital linear tape library for long-term archive, and RAID for rapid image retrieval and display. The telemammograms can be displayed with multiple 2K × 2.5K resolution LCD monitors. Figure 15.9 depicts the schematic of a telemammography WS with possible viewing formats and examples of digital mammograms on the 2K display workstation. Figure 15.10 shows the schematic of a telemammography system used for telediagnosis, teleconsultation, and telemanagement applications.

Telemammography has been used clinically for several years; issues to be considered are the image quality at the expert's workstation, speed of communication, image/data security, and the cost of assembling a high-quality and efficient digital mammography WS, and coupling CAD results as the second reader in clinical workflow.

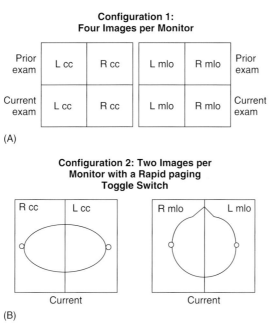

Figure 15.9   Schematic of a 2K two-monitor WS showing the display format of digital mammograms in (*A*) with the four-on-one format and (*B*) with the two-on-one format. (*C*) Eight mammograms display on two monitors with the four-on-one format. (*D*) One-on-one (left) and two-on-one (right) formats with a rapid paging toggle switch.

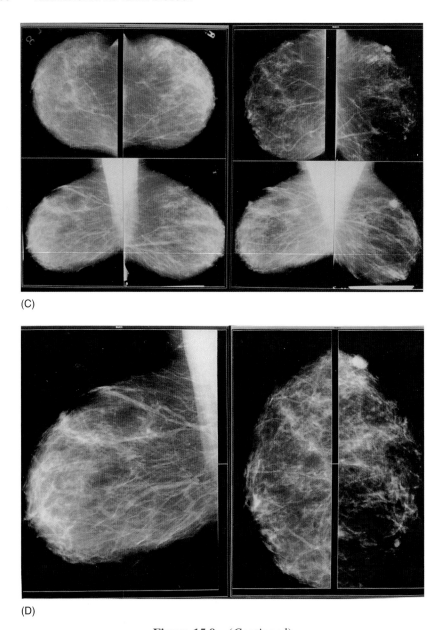

(C)

(D)

Figure 15.9 (*Continued*)

15.6.4 Multimodality Tele-Breast Imaging

We discussed in Section 15.6.1 that there exist breast imaging centers which provide multimodality breast imaging methods including digital mammography, 2-D and 3-D US, and dedicated breast 3-D MRI for both breast screening and biopsy. This results in two new developments in tele-breast imaging. The first is the dedicated breast imaging enterprise for image archive and management. And the second is the development of multimodality image display workstations in order to view these

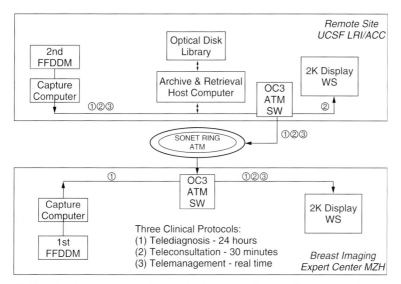

Figure 15.10 A telemammography testbed system for telediagnosis, teleconsultation, and telemanagement (1997–2001) at UCSF. The expert site was located at the breast-imaging center, Mt. Zion Hospital (MZH), and the remote site was at the Ambulatory Care Center (ACC), UCSF. The data center was located at LRI (Laboratory for Radiological Informatics). (1) Telediagnosis: images sent from the FFDDM at MZH or ACC to 2K WS at MZH for interpretation. (2) Teleconsultation: images sent from the FFDDM at ACC to 2K WS at both MZH and ACC. Referring physician at ACC and the expert at MZH used the WS for consultation. (3) Telemanagement: images sent from the FFDDM at ACC to the 2K WS at MZH. The expert at MZH telemanaged the patient, who was still at ACC, based on the reading. Although this testbed was set up almost 10 years ago, the principles of telediagnosis, teleconsultation, and telemanagement are still valid. They can be used for other types of breast-imaging applications in teleradiology. FFDDM: full-field direct digital mammography.

various types of breast images. These topics had been discussed in Section 5.3.1.2 and Figs. 4.20*B* and 5.4; and will be presented in Section 21.6 and Figure 21.18.

15.7 TELEMICROSCOPY

15.7.1 Telemicroscopy and Teleradiology

Telemicroscopy involves the transmission of digital microscopic images (see Sections 3.9 and 4.8) through WANS. Under the umbrella of telemedicine applications, telemicroscopy and teleradiology can be combined into one system. Figure 15.11 provides an example of a generic combined telemicroscopy and teleradiology (low resolution) system; its major components and their functions are described as follows (see Fig. 3.32*A* and *B*):

1. A 1K/2K film scanner for digitization
2. A 512 × 512 display system for quality control
3. A personal computer (PC) with four functions:

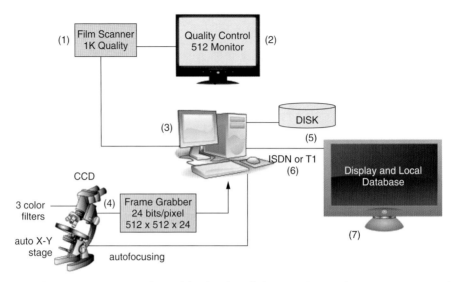

Figure 15.11   A conceptual combined teleradiology and telemicroscopy system for image and textual data transmission. Numerals are the workflow steps.

    a. For teleradiology applications, software for image acquisition, patient data input, and data communication.

    b. For telemicroscopy applications, software control of for (i) automatic focusing, and (ii) automatic x-y stage motion; color filter switching; and frame grabbing. These tools are needed for converting slides to digital images.

    c. A database for managing images and textual data.

    d. A standard communication protocol for LAN and WAN.

4. A light microscope with software control of: automatic focusing, x-y stepping motor controlled stage, RGB color filters, and a CCD camera

5. Standard communication hardware for LAN and WAN

6. Communication networks connection (e.g., T1 or DSL).

7. The WS at the expert site should be able to display 1K x 1K gray level and color images with standard graphical user interface. It needs a database to manage local data. The WS should be able to control microscopic stage motion as well as automatic focusing.

15.7.2   Telemicroscopy Applications

The two main applications of telemicroscopy are in surgical pathology and laboratory medicine. Surgical pathology analyzes surgically obtained tissue specimens, whereas laboratory medicine analyzes samples from peripheral fluids and cell biopsies. Telemicroscopy requires both static and dynamic images. For this reason an automatic x-y moving stage and focusing are necessary during the teleconsultation process when the referring physician and the expert move the microscopic slide during discussion. In Section 3.9.2 we presented the microscopic image acquisition and display components of a digital microscopic system. The telecommunication component in telemicroscopy uses similar technology except that the images are dynamic. Because transmission of dynamic imaging must be rapid, high-bandwidth WAN and/or image compression are necessary. Figure 3.32*A* shows such a a telemicroscopy system. Figure 3.32*B* shows the microscopic image database.

15.8 REAL-TIME TELECONSULTATION SYSTEM

15.8.1 Background

Real-time consultation between referring physicians or general radiologists and an expert is critical for timely and adequate management of problem cases. During consultation, both sides need to:

1. synchronously manipulate high-resolution DR images (over 16 MB/exam), or large-volume MR/CT/US images (over 8–20 MB/exam) in real time,
2. perform interpretation interactively, and
3. converse with audio.

The teleconsultation model becomes even more complex when historical images are required for comparison and when information from the radiology information system (RIS) is needed by the expert. In this situation neither conventional teleconferencing technology nor PACS WSs are sufficient to handle the complex model requirements for two reasons: First, most off-the-shelf teleconferencing technology can only handle "store" and "forward" operations, which have no direct connection to the PACS server for inputting images. Second, PACS WSs do not have the necessary capability for interactive teleconsultation, which requires real-time dual-cursor telecommunication technology.

In this section we present the design and implementation of a real-time teleconsultation system. The teleconsultation system is designed to operate in a DICOM PACS clinical environment with bidirectional remote control technology to meet critical teleconsultation application with high-resolution and large volume medical images in a limited bandwidth network environment. We first give the system design and implementation methods and describe the teleconsultation procedures and protocols. Such a teleconsultation system has been used in a clinical neuroradiology PACS environment (Zhang et al., 2000).

15.8.2 System Requirements

To provide real-time consultation services for serious or difficult cases, real-time teleconsultation systems for high-resolution and large-volume medical images should meet the following requirements:

1. Provide real-time teleconsultation services for high-resolution and large-volume medical images (MR, CT, US, CR, DR, and mammography).
2. Synchronously manipulate images on both local and remote sites, including remote cursor, window/level, zoom, cine mode, overlay, and measurement.
3. Support multimedia including audio and video (option) communications.
4. Interface with PACS through the DICOM standard.

5. Use in Intranet (LAN) and in Internet (WAN) environments with TCP/IP transmission.
6. Operate scalable network connections, including Internet 2, ATM, Ethernet, and modem.
7. Use similar graphical interface and image manipulation functions as the standard PACS WS to minimize user's retraining, and
8. Be cost-effective.

In Section 15.8.3 we describe our teleconsultation system designed to satisfy these conditions.

15.8.3 Teleconsultation System Design

15.8.3.1 Image Display Workflow Real-time teleconsultation relies on the synchronization of the local (referring site) and remote (expert site) WSs. In a clinical PACS environment, images are first acquired by the acquisition computer, sent to the PACS server through a DICOM gateway, and then delivered to different WSs according to some routing schedules. After images arrive at the WS, they are first stored in the local database, accessed by the user through the graphical user interface (GUI), and displayed on the monitors. Most often the image display procedure is a collection of sequential operations, or a pipeline process as shown in Figure 15.12, including loading image data from disk storage to computer memory, processing the data, and rendering the data on the screens. In an event-driven window environment, the user's manipulations of the GUI windows or displayed images by using the input devices (mouse or keyboard) are translated into events. The procedure to display images can be described as a flow of image data through the pipeline that is controlled by these events.

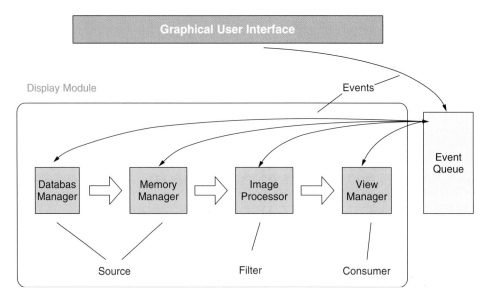

Figure 15.12 Pipeline process showing image display procedure in a PACS WS.

15.8.3.2   *Communication Requirements during Teleconsultation*   Tele-consultation involves a referring site and an expert site. Between the two sites, three kinds of communications are required:

1. Images transmitted from the referring physician or general radiologist site to the expert site.
2. Synchronization of manipulations of displayed images at both sites.
3. Voice conversation between the referring physician and the expert.

Of these three types of communications, image transmitting involves a large amount of data, so the images normally can be preloaded before the consultation session starts unless it is an emergency case (emergency service requires high-speed network connection between two sites). Image preloading can be done with various kinds of network, for example, high-speed ATM network, T1 line, or Internet 2. To synchronize the manipulation operations on displayed images at both sites, the generated events must be exchanged in real time between the two sites. Because the events are usually very short messages, even conventional telephone lines (DS-0 line with 56 Kbits/s) can be used to transmit this kind of message in real time if the maximum message length is less than 2200 bits [$\sim$(56 Kbits/s)/(2200 bits)] and the image repainting rate, after the image is processed, is less than 25/s. Although audio conversation is a real-time on-line procedure, it also can be carried out through the telephone line.

15.8.3.3   *Hardware Configuration of the Teleconsultation System*   Based on the communication analysis the concept of distributed image data storage, and the expert model of teleradiology—a real-time teleconsultation system for the two sites—the expert site, and the general physician or radiologist site can be designed. The hardware configuration of the teleconsultation system at each site includes:

1. one WS linked to the other by an Ethernet, ATM, or modem connection,
2. high-resolution display boards that can be configured to support single or dual monitors,
3. high-resolution gray scale monitor (dual monitors as option), and
4. one telephone for audio communication

Figure 15.13 shows a simplified teleconsultation connection between two sites.

15.8.3.4   *Software Architecture*   Two key software features in the teleconsultation system are the synchronization of user operations and the exchange of messages in real time between local and remote sites. To achieve these features, the consultation WS needs message routing, an interpretation function module, an authoring function, and standard display and manipulation functions similar to a PACS WS. The following are the basic modules:

1. Image display graphic user interface for display and teleconsultation.
2. Database manager for image display and teleconsultation authoring.
3. Memory manager for image data memory management.
4. Image processor for processing image.

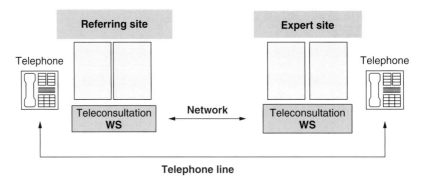

Figure 15.13   Simplified teleconsultation system connecting a referring site and an expert site with one network and a telephone line.

5. Image viewer for image rendering and display.
6. Event interpreter for local and remote message dispatching.
7. Remote control manager for routing messages between local and remote sites.
8. An event/message queue used to transfer the events and remote messages from GUI and remote manager to display module.
9. A queue used to transfer the encoded messages from event interpreter to remote manager.
10. Teleconsultation database used to store the information of selected patients, studies, series, images, as well as expert names, hospitals, and hosts.
11. DICOM communication services for DICOM image receiving and sending between the teleconsultation system, scanners, and PACS server.

Figure 15.14 shows the architecture and data flow of the teleconsultation system. In this design the operation of the WS is very similar to a generic PACS WS, which minimizes the user relearning process. Function modules 1, 2, 3, 4, and 5 are designed for normal display as described in Figure 15.12.

Modules 6 and 7 are specifically designed for bidirectional remote control for teleconsultation. Module 6, the event interpreter, collects the events coming from the display module, encodes them for transmission and puts them into a queue module 9, which transfers the messages to module 7. Module 7, the remote control manager, picks up the encoded messages, sends them to the remote site, and receives the remote messages and posts them to the display module for remote control of the display behavior.

Module 10 is a teleconsultation database for image display and consultation, and module 11 is for the DICOM communication services for transferring DICOM images between teleconsultation workstations and PACS or imaging modalities.

15.8.4   Teleconsultation Procedure and Protocol

A teleconsultation session proceeds as follows: When a case requires a consultation, a general physician or radiologist first reviews the images from the imaging modality or the PACS WSs and sends them with the DICOM protocol to the teleconsultation WS located at the local reading room. At the teleconsultation WS, the referring

Teleconsultation Application

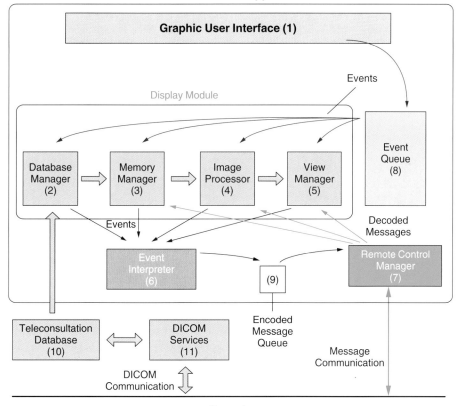

Figure 15.14 Software architecture and data flow in a teleconsultation workstation. Numbers are modules in the software (see also Fig. 15.12).

physician then performs data authoring supplied by the teleconsultation system and sends the images to the teleconsultation WS located at the expert site. This may be done through either the local area network if it is in the same building or campus, or through the wide area network if it is distant. Later either the general physician or an expert can call the other site to start the consultation session. The teleconsultation protocol has three steps:

Data Formatting   The first step is to convert all input images for teleconsultation to the DICOM standard if they are not already DICOM. This is done at the acquisition gateway or at the PACS server.

Data Authoring   The authoring procedure is to prepare the image data for teleconsultation. The authoring module, TeleConApp, is an integrated component in the software package (inside the database manager module) Figure 15.15 shows the data authoring procedure. There are three steps in data authoring:

1. The general physician or radiologist uses the TeleConApp program to create an object called the virtual envelope, which includes information on the selected

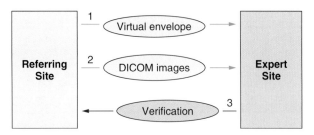

Figure 15.15 Data authoring procedure for teleconsultation.

patients, studies, and series as well as the host name of the expert site and the name of the consultant from the teleconsultation local database. However, the virtual envelope does not yet contain any images. The virtual envelope is sent to the expert site through a network with DICOM communication services.

2. After the expert site receives the envelope, either site can create a consultation session and the general physician site sends the DICOM image objects related to the patient as dictated by the virtual envelope to the expert site.

3. After sending images, the general physician site automatically performs a DICOM query to the expert site, and the expert site verifies the receipt of thevirtual envelope and image object to the general physician site. The consultation session can start once the data are verified.

Data Presentation   Before the data presentation both the expert and the general-physician sites have the virtual envelope and image data. After the consultation session is initiated, the data presentation begins. During data presentation either site can operate the TeleConApp program to display and manipulate images and related information. TeleConApp synchronizes the operations of image display and manipulation at both sites. The challenge is the software synchronization of a dual cursor system at each WS so that both sites can have equal control during the teleconsultation.

Figures 15.16 and 15.17 show the connection of such a teleconsultation system in the PACS environment. Other applications derived from this teleconsultation system are used for teleconferencing with dynamic images (Stahl et al., 2000) and for intravascular US and cardiac angiography (Stahl et al., 2000).

15.9 SUMMARY OF TELERADIOLOGY

The concept of telemedicine and teleradiology originated in the 1970s, but the technology was not ready for real clinical applications for teleradiology until the early 2000s. As teleradiology is integrated into daily clinical service, the associated socioeconomic issues discussed in this chapter will surface. The ongoing research in teleradiology is in how to balance the cost with the requirements of image quality and service turnaround time. Costs are affected by technology used in image capture, workstation, image compression, communication, and image security. We see teleradiology becoming a necessity in medical practices of the twenty-first century, and that teleradiology will be an integral component of telemedicine.

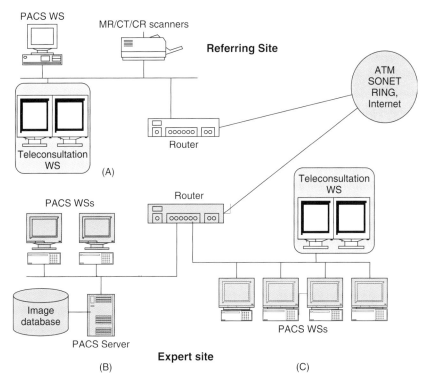

Figure 15.16   WAN network connection of the teleconsultation system with the referring site and the expert site and a PACS WS in PACS environment.

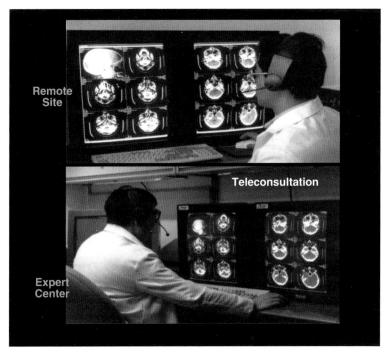

Figure 15.17   Teleconsultation session in neuroradiology showing the remote site and the expert center. (Courtesy of Drs. J Stahl and J. Zhang)

Teleradiology uses the Web and Internet technologies. Issues that must be resolved immediately are how to lower the communication cost and to bundle textual with image information effectively and efficiently to assure efficient operation and for image security. For the former, Internet 2 appears to be an excellent candidate, and for the latter, ePR (electronic Patient Record) with image distribution will evolve as a winner.

References

ACR/NEMA. *Digital Imaging and Communications in Medicine (DICOM): Version 3.0*. Washington, DC: ACR/NEMA Standards Publication; 1993.

Barbakati, N. *X Window System Programming*, 2nd ed. Indianapolis: SAMA Publishing; 1994.

Berger SB, Cepelewicz BB. Medical-legal issues in teleradiology. *Am J Roentgenolo*, 166: 505–10; 1996.

Berlin L. Malpractice issue in radiology-teleradiology. *Am J Roentgenolo* 170: 1417–22; 1998.

Bernman F, Fox G, Hey T. Grid Computing. Hoboken, NJ: Wiley; 2003.

Carr C, Moore SM. IHE: a model for driving adoption of standards. *Comp Med Imag Graph* 27(2–3): 137–46; 2003.

Chatterjee A, Maltz A. Microsoft DirectShow: a new media architecture, *SMPTE J* 106: 865–71; 1997.

DICOM Standard 2003. http://www.dclunie.com/dicom-status/status.html#BaseStandard-2001.

Erickson BJ, Manduca A, Palisson P, Persons KR, Earnest F 4th, Savcenko V, Hangiandreou NJ. Wavelet compression of medical images. *Radiology* 206: 599–607; 1998.

Freier AO, Karlton P, Kocher PC. The SSL Protocol Version 3.0. Internet Draft, http://home.netscape.com/eng/ssl3/draft302.txt, 1996.

GlobusToolkit 3 Core White Paper.

HL7 Version 3.0: Preview for CIOs, Managers and Programmers. http://www.neotool.com/company/press/199912_v3.htm#V3.0_preview http://www-unix.globus.org/toolkit/documentation.html

Huang HK. Towards the digital radiology department. *Eur J Rad* 22: 165; 1996a.

Huang HK. Teleradiology technologies and some service model. *Computer Med Imag Graph* 20: 59–68; 1996b.

Huang HK. Enterprise PACS and Image Distribution, *Comp Med Imag Graph* 27(2–3): 241–53; 2003.

Huang HK, Andriole K, Bazzill T, et al. Design and implementation of a picture archiving and communication system: the second time. *J Digital Imag* 9: 47–59; 1996c.

Huang HK. *PACS and Imaging Informatics: Principles and Applications*. Hoboken, NJ: Wiley; 2004.

Huang HK, Wong A, Lou A, et al. Clinical experience with a second-generation hospital-integrated picture archiving and communication system. *J Digital Imag* 9: 151–66; 1996.

Huang HK, Lou SL, Dillon WP. Neuroradiology workstation reading room in an inter-hospital environment: a nineteen month study. *Comp Med Imag Graph* 21(5); 1997, 309–317.

Huang HK, Lou SL. Telemammography: a technical overview. In Haus AG, Yaffe MJ, eds. *RSNA Categorical Course 1999*. Oak Brook, IL; 1999, 273–81.

Huang HK. Research trends in medical imaging informatics. In: Hwang NHC, Woo SLY, eds. *Frontiers in Biomedical Engineering*. New York: Kluwer Academic; 2003, 269–81.

Huffmann DA. A method for the construction of minimum-redundancy codes. *Proc IRE, IEEE* 40: 1098–1101; 1952.

James AE Jr, James E III, Johnson B, James J. Legal considerations of medical imaging. *Leg Med* 87–113; 1993.

Kamp GH. Medical-legal Issues in teleradiology: a commentary. *Am J Roentgenolo* 166: 511–12; 1996.

Lempel A, Ziv J. Compression of two-dimensional data. *IEEE Trans Info Theory* 32: 2–8; 1986.

Lou SL, Huang HK, Arenson R. Workstation design: image manipulation, image set handling, and display issues. *Radiolog Clin N Am* 34(3): 525–44; 1996.

Mitchell JL, Pennebaker WB, Fogg CE, LeGall DJ. *MPEG Video Compression Standard*. New York: Chapman and Hall; 1997.

Nagle J. Congestion control in IP/TCP Internetworks. *RFC 896*; 1984.

NEMA Standards Publication PS 3.3. Digital imaging and communication in medicine (DICOM). National Electrical Manufacturers Association, Chicago, Ill. 1993.

Nijim YW, Stearns SD, Mikhael WB. Differentiation applied to lossless compression of medical images. *IEEE Trans Med Imag* 15: 555–59; 1996.

Richter J. Window messages and asynchronous input. In: *Advanced Windows*, 3rd ed. Seattle, WA: Microsoft Press; 1997.

Ricke J, Maass P, Lopez Hèanninen E, Liebig T, Amthauer H, Stroszczynski C, Schauer W, Boskamp T, Wolf M. Wavelet versus JPEG (Joint Photographic Expert Group) and fractal compression: impact on the detection of low-contrast details in computed radiographs. *Invest Radiol* 33: 456–63; 1998.

Schroeder W, Martin H, Lorensen B. *The Visualization Toolkit*, 2nd ed. Englewood Cliffs, NJ: Prentice Hall; 1998, 83–96.

Sinha AK. *Network Programming in Windows, N.T.* Reading, MA: Addison-Wesley; 1996, 199–299.

Stahl JN, Tellis W, Huang HK. Network latency and operator performance in teleradiology applications. *J Digital Imag* 13(3): 119–23; 2000.

Stahl JN, Zhang J, Zhou X, Lou A, Pomerantsev EV, Zellner C, Huang HK. Tele-consultation for diagnostic video using Internet technology, *Proc IEEE Multimed Tech Appl Conf* 1998; 210–13.

Stahl JN, Zhang J, Chou TM, Zellner C, Pomerantsev EV, Huang HK. 2000. A new approach to tele-conferencing with intravascular ultrasound and cardiac angiography in a low-bandwidth environment. *RadioGraphics* 20: 1495–1503.

Stahl JN, Zhang J, Zeller C, Pomerantsev EV, Lou SL, Chou TM, Huang HK. Tele-conferencing with dynamic medical images. *IEEE Trans Info Tech Biomed* 4(1): 88–96; 2000.

Stevens WR. Advanced interprocess communication. In: *Advanced Programming in the UNIX Environment*. Reading, MA: Addison-Wesley; 1996.

Tobis J, Aharonian V, Mansukhani P, Kasaoka S, Jhandyala R, Son R, Browning R, Young-blood L, Thompson M. Video networking of cardiac catheterisation laboratories. *Am Heart J* 137: 241–49; 1999.

Wallace GK. The JPEG still picture compression standard. *Comm ACM* 34: 30–40; 1991.

Wendler T, Monnich KJ, Schmidt J. Digital image workstation. In: Huang HK, Ratib O, Babber AR, et al., eds. *Picture Archiving and Communication System in Medicine*. New York: Springer; 1991.

Wang J, Huang HK. Three-dimensional image compression with wavelet transform. In: Rangayyan RM, Woods RP, Robb RA, Huang HK, eds. *Handbook of Medical Imaging*. San Diego: Academic Press; 2000, 851–62.

Wong STC, Huang HK. Networked multimedia for medial imagining. *IEEE Multimedia* 4: 24–35; 1997.

Zhang J, Song K, Huang HK, Stahl JN. Tele-consultation for thoracic imaging. *Radiology* 205(P): 742; 1997.

Zhang J, Stahl JN, Song KS, and Huang HK. Real-time teleconsultation with high resolution and large volume medical imaging. In: Horii SC, Blaine GJ, eds. *PACS Design and Evaluation: Engineering and Clinical Issues*. Vol. 3339. Washington, DC: SPIE; 1998, pp. 185–90, 1998.

Zhang J, Stahl JN, Huang HK, Zhou X, Lou, SL, Song KS. Real-time teleconsultation with high resolution and large volume medical images for collaborative health care. *IEEE Trans Info Tech Biom* 4(1): 178–85; 2000.

Zhou X, Huang HK. Authenticity and Integrity of digital mammography image. *IEEE Trans Med Imag* 20(8): 784–91; 2001.

Ziv J, Lempel A. A universal algorithm for sequential data compression. *IEEETrans Info Theory* 23: 337–43; 1977.

CHAPTER 16

Fault-Tolerant PACS and Enterprise PACS

The PACS system is mission critical because it runs around the clock, 24/7. Operation reliability is vital to its large computer network and system integration of medical images and databases. The purpose of PACS fault-tolerant design is to maintain the continuous available operability of the system. For an enterprise PACS to develop and operate, system fault-tolerance is mandatory.

This chapter focuses on two major components of this system: fault-tolerant PACS and enterprise PACS. In the fault-tolerant PACS, we first review the concepts of system fault tolerance (FT), definitions of high availability (HA) and continuous availability (CA), and possible causes of PACS system failure. No loss of image data and no interruption of PACS data flow are the two main criteria of success in a PACS operation. The chapter presents these criteria and delineates the methods of how to satisfy them with current PACS technology. The topic on fault tolerance concludes with the current concept of a fault-tolerant PACS design. Enterprise PACS is a component whose concept we had briefly introduced in Section 7.6. In this chapter we provide a detailed discussion of the current state of enterprise PACS and image distribution throughout the PACS system.

Since the presentation in this chapter is related to the combined PACS teleradiology model, for convenience we will use some previously defined system diagrams to explain the concept of FT and CA. Figure 16.1 (excerpted from Fig. 1.3) shows how this chapter corresponds to the contents of Part III. Figure 16.2 (excerpted from Fig. 1.2) shows these PACS components within the workflow; and Figure 16.3 (excerpted from Fig 7.7) illustrates the PACS and combined teleradiology model.

16.1 INTRODUCTION

High availability (HA) and continuous availability (CA) are two commonly used terms categorizing the degree of system reliability (IEEE, 1990; Reiner et al., 2000). There is a continuum of HA solutions, ranging from 99% system availability rate (88 hr downtime/yr) achieved by using the simple "hot spare" technology to 99.99% availability (1 hr downtime/yr) achieved with clustered server-based solutions using hardware and fail over software. The fully hardware fault-tolerance (FT) systems

PACS and Imaging Informatics, Second Edition, by H. K. Huang
Copyright © 2010 John Wiley & Sons, Inc.

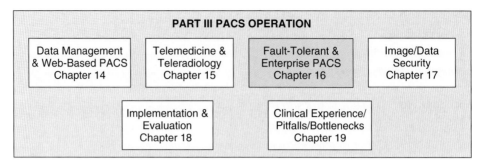

Figure 16.1 Position of Chapter 16 in the organization of this book. Color codes are used to highlight components and workflow in the chapters of Part III.

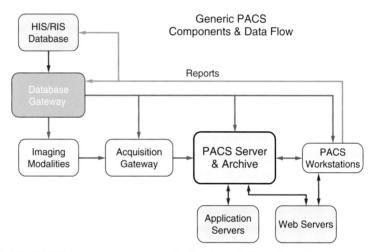

Figure 16.2 PACS basic components (yellow) and data flow (blue: internal; green and orange: external between PACS and other information systems); other information systems (light blue). HIS: Hospital information system; RIS: radiology information system.

are known as CA solutions (we will use these two terms interchangeably), with the highest 99.999% availability rate and a maximum downtime of 5 min/year (http://www.tandem.com, http://IBM.com, http://www.sun.com). PACS is a mission critical operation, continuously running 24 hours a day and seven days a week, and it requires continuous availability. In PACS, four operational criteria are vital to the system's success: no loss of data, continuous availability of the system, acceptable system performance, and user friendliness. Among these four criteria, user friendliness was addressed in Chapters 11 and 12; user friendliness, of course, does not relate to the fault-tolerance nature of the system. So in this chapter we only consider the first three criteria.

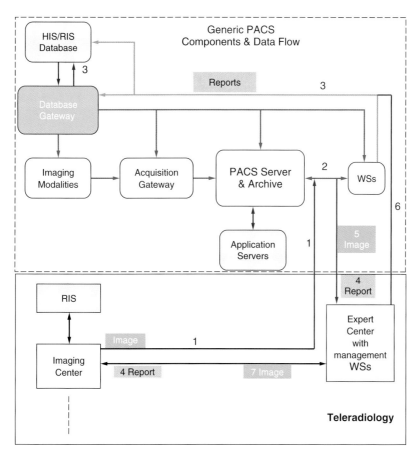

Figure 16.3 PACS and teleradiology combined model in which the PACS supports imaging centers for teleradiology reading, or PACS and teleradiology support one another. The top rectangle is the PACS components and workflow (excerpted from Fig. 7.2), and the bottom rectangle is the teleradiology model modified from Fig. 7.6. Red Lines: Communication between PACS and teleradiology. See Section 7.5.2 for explanation of workflow steps in numerals (excerpted from Fig. 7.7).

PACS's system integration of medical images and patient databases involves additionally many other components: imaging modalities, computers, data storage, display workstations, communication devices, network switches, and computer servers housing healthcare databases. Figure 16.4 shows a generic PACS architecture, and Figure 16.5 depicts the logical connection of some basic components in PACS and teleradiology. All components, including network connection in red, are technically single points of failure (SPOFs) of the system. PACS and teleradiology are mission-critical systems running around the clock and have no tolerance for failure. In Figure 16.4 and 16.5, any component that is a SPOF (compared with Fig 16.2. and Fig. 16.3, respectively) of the system should have the fault-tolerant design built in to ensure CA operation. Section 16.7 will elaborate further on this concept. For

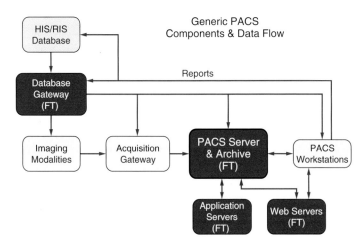

Figure 16.4 Generic PACS components and data flow (modified from Fig. 16.2). All network components and connections are shown in red. The FT/CA (fault-tolerance or continuously available) components should be used to replace the single-point-of-failure (SPOF) components—database gateway, PACS server, application servers, and Web servers. The image acquisition gateway is not a SPOF because there are multiple acquisition gateways in PACS; a failed gateway can be automatic switched to others as a backup.

convenience, we will not distinguish between PACS and teleradiology in this discussion of fault-tolerant design.

16.2 CAUSES OF A SYSTEM FAILURE

Causes of an integrated computer and network system failure can come from human error, natural disaster, software, and component hardware. Table 16.1 shows a survey of the causes of system downtime.

Although no formal data on the causes of PACS downtime have been documented, on the basis of field experience, we can assume that PACS follows the same trend of downtime causes as the general computer and network system shown in Table 16.1 (Resilience Corp., 2000). Among these causes, natural disaster is not predictable and hence cannot be avoided. But it can be minimized for PACS system downtime by choosing proper locations for installation, taking proper natural disaster precautions, and using off-site backup server and archive. Properly chosen locations and special precautions can minimize system shutdown due to natural disaster, and off-site backup can prevent loss of data. In terms of human error and software, the reliability of current PACS software and the refinement of system design to minimize human error have been greatly improved since the last edition of this book in 2004. Redundancy in software architectural design allows the system to be recovered gracefully after a software failure. Minimizing human intervention during PACS operation in the system design can lower the rate of human error. However, hardware failure in the computer, disk, communication processor, or network is unpredictable and hence difficult to avoid.

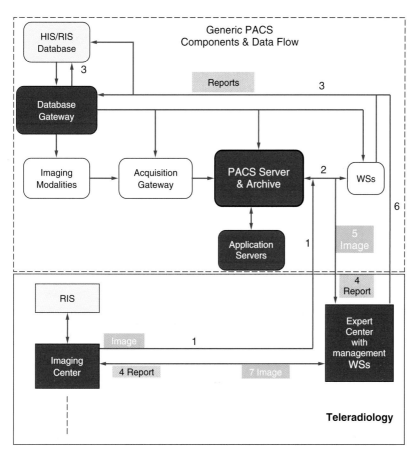

Figure 16.5 Combined PACS and teleradiology model (modified from Fig. 7.7). All network components and connections within PACS, within teleradiolgy, and the connection between PACS and teleradiolgy are shown in red. The FT/CA (fault-tolerance or continuously available) components should be used to replace the single-point-of-failure components—in the PACS database gateway, PACS server, and application servers; in teleradiology: imaging center server and Web server at the expert center.

TABLE 16.1   Causes of computer and network system downtime

Computer hardware	24%
Hard disk drive	26%
Communication processor	11%
Data communication network	10%
Software	22%
Human error	6%
Others	1%
Total	100%

In this chapter we will not discuss natural disaster and human error (see Chapter 19). We first assume that the entire PACS software is fully debugged and is immune to failure. Therefore, in fault-tolerant PACS design, we first address the issue of what would happen if some hardware components fail and how to take care of it so that the PACS operation will not be compromised. We then discuss a fault-tolerant image server design combining both hardware and software for continuously available system operation.

If a hardware component involved is the single point of failure (SPOF) of the system, for example, the PACS server, which is the main server of PACS, its failure can render the entire system inoperable until the problem is diagnosed and resolved. Other critical hardware components that cannot tolerate failure are cluster servers, application servers, Web servers, network switches, imaging acquisition gateways, and database gateways (see Fig 16.4 and 16.5). A failure of one of these components may cripple that branch of operation, which in turn may interrupt the entire system operation. Often a component failure can also result in loss of data. Both interruption of operation and loss of data are not acceptable in a totally digital clinical operation environment. On the other hand, the failure of a display workstation (WS) is not critical because there are duplicate WSs. The failure may cause inconvenience to the user, but it does not cripple the system. Smith et al. (1995) describes a painful experience during a major PACS server failure and the method used to reverse the operation back to film-based operation. The lesson learned by the hospital and the manufacturer has reinforced the importance of constructing a fault-tolerant PACS design.

A software remedy is usually implemented in different PACS components to minimize the impact on system operation of hardware component failure. The software means of rerouting hardware failure calls for an elaborate design that is difficult to implement and full of tedious data. In the following sections, we consider some types of failures and the recovery methods suitable to current PACS technology.

16.3   NO LOSS OF IMAGE DATA

16.3.1   Redundant Storage at Component Levels

To ensure no loss of image data, a PACS always retains at least two copies of an image on separate storage devices until the image has been archived successfully to a long-term storage device (e.g., a RAID farm, optical disk library, a digital tape library, or an ASP model). Recall the various storage subsystems in PACS shown in Figure 11.3. The backup is achieved via a PACS intercomponent communication system. This backup scheme can be broken down as follows:

1. At the imaging device Images are not deleted from the imaging device's local storage until technologists have verified the successful archiving of individual images to other storage devices via the PACS connections. In the event of failure of the acquisition gateway process or of the archive process, images can be re-sent from the imaging device to the PACS.

2. At the acquisition gateway computer Images acquired in the acquisition gateway computer remain in its local magnetic disks until the archive subsystem has acknowledged to the gateway that a successful archive has been completed.

These images are then deleted from the magnetic disks residing in the gateway computer so that storage space from these disks can be reclaimed.

3. At the PACS server Images arriving in the archive server from various image gateways are not deleted until they have been successfully archived to permanent storage. Nevertheless, all archived images are stacked in the archive server's cache magnetic disks or RAID, and they will be deleted based on an aging criteria (e.g., number of days since the examination was performed, or whether patient discharge or transfer occurred).

4. At the display workstation Images stored in the designated WS will remain there until the patient is discharged or transferred. Images in the PACS archive can be retrieved from any WSs via PACS intercomponent communication. In the server-client PACS model, a WS has no local storage, therefore the PACS server has to have built-in backup storage.

16.3.2 The Backup Archive System

The long-term archive has to have redundant components. For example, the digital linear tape (DLT) library consists of multiple input–output drives and controller's housing inside a jukebox that allow concurrent archival and retrieval operations on all of its drives. A redundant power supply is essential for uninterrupted operation. To build a fault-tolerance in the PACS server, a backup archive system can be used. Two copies of identical images can be saved through two different paths in the PACS network to two archive libraries. Ideally, the two libraries should be in two different buildings. In case of natural disaster, the secondary DLT library only requires a computer for control and does not need a PACS controller. Figure 16.6 shows a low-cost backup archive designed for no loss of image data.

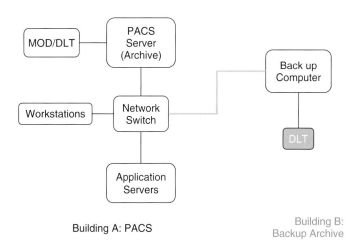

Figure 16.6   Low-cost backup tandem design for no loss of image data using an off-site digital linear tape (DLT, green) backup archive system (right).

16.3.3 The Database System

The database system in PACS records all image transaction, so it is vital to data recovery. The database is comprised of redundant database servers running identical commercial database systems, with structured query language (SQL) utilities. A mirrored database (i.e., two identical databases) can be used to duplicate the data directory during every PACS transaction involving the server. The backup database can reside in a different computer or in a different partition of the same disk of the same computer. The former configuration provides better fault tolerance. The mirroring feature of the database system provides the entire PACS database with uninterrupted data transactions that guarantee the patient record can be retraced in the event of system failure or a disk crash. Although the second method using a different partition of the same disk is not fault tolerant during a disk crash, it guarantees the continuous availability of PACS database during a disk partition failure. The benefits of the latter configuration are lower cost and easier implementation and management of the mirroring database.

16.4 NO INTERRUPTION OF PACS DATA FLOW

In this section we begin with the PACS dataflow in a PACS component, and then show how a hardware component failure can affect the dataflow. Finally we consider methods that ensure dataflow continuity.

16.4.1 PACS Data Flow

PACS is a networked and component-integrated system (see Figs. 16.4 and 16.5). The following summarizes the functions of major components and networks discussed in previous chapters (see Fig. 16.2):

1. Imaging modalities: Generate medical images.
2. Acquisition gateways: Acquire images, process images, and send images to PACS controller. The PACS server has three components—the controller, database server, and archive units
    i. Controller. Receive images from acquisition gateways, intelligently route images to display workstations, access PACS database to update/query image related records, access archive units to store or retrieve images, provide query/retrieve services for display workstations
    ii. PACS database server. Perform PACS image-related information management
    iii. PACS archive units. Store images for the short term and in the long-term archive
3. Display workstations: Display PACS images for diagnosis.
4. PACS networks: Connect PACS components.

An image in a PACS component is usually processed by a sequential processing chain with first-in–first-out (FIFO) model, as shown in Figure 16.7. For example, in a DICOM-compliant CR acquisition gateway computer, process 1 of queue 1 in

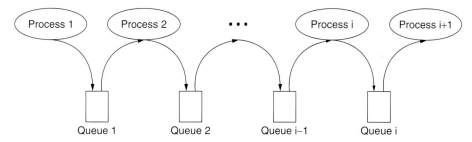

Figure 16.7   First-in–first-out (FIFO) image processing model in a PACS component.

Figure 16.7 is the storage SCP (service class provider) process receiving DICOM CR images from the CR reader; process $i + 1$ is the storage SCU (service class user) process sending the image to the PACS server, which completes the archive task. The processes in between $(2, \ldots, i)$ perform image processing tasks necessary for downstream image archiving to the PACS server and for display on workstations. The queues 1 to i are structured files (if they are located in disk drives) or tables (if they are in database) used for transferring image processing tasks between the processes. In the following, we use the collective term "image processing" to represent these processes.

16.4.2   Possible Failure Situations in PACS Data Flow

The hardware of any component shown in Figure 16.8 can fail, and the failure will interrupt the PACS data flow through that component. If the component is the SPOF, like a PACS server, a network switch, or an application server, it may render the entire system inoperable. The result is the interruption of data flow or even the loss of images.

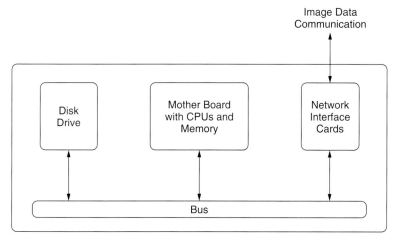

Figure 16.8   Three key components in the computer. The failure of any SPOF component would cause the computer to be inoperable and thus interrupt the PACS dataflow.

16.4.3   Methods to Protect Data Flow Continuity from Hardware Component Failure

16.4.3.1   Hardware Solutions and Drawbacks   There are two possible solutions. The first is hardware redundancy, in which a backup computer or a tandem system is used to replace an on-line failed computer. Figure 16.9 shows the design of a manually activated tandem server in the PACS server. The second solution is to use a cluster controller as the main PACS server which is composed of multiple processors controlled by the cluster manager.

Hardware solutions have two drawbacks. First, they are expensive because of the hardware redundancy and the software involved in designing a fail takeover. Second, it is tedious and labor intensive to recover the current state after a component failure. In the case of hardware redundancy, if the primary component fails, the secondary will take over. After the primary is fixed and on line again, it will attempt to shift the operation from the secondary back to the primary. In the case of cluster server, if one clustered server fails, the recovery process and the return to the original operational state can be a very tedious task.

16.4.3.2   Software Solutions and Drawbacks   Two solutions are possible. The first solution is to design the image data flow in such a way that any image in a transit state has at least two copies in two different identical components. If one hardware component fails, the second component executes the task on the second copy of the image.

The second solution is to utilize the principle that the chance of simultaneous failure of two hardware devices is much less than that of either one of them. This

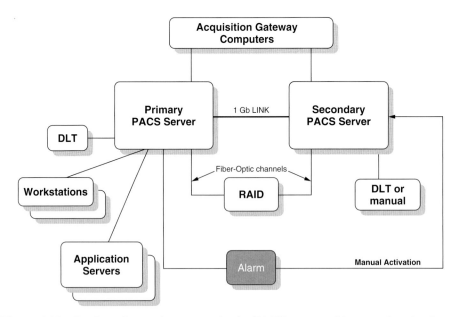

Figure 16.9   Design of a tandem server in the PACS server with manual activation of the secondary server when the primary fails. Manual activation is required (see bottom right).

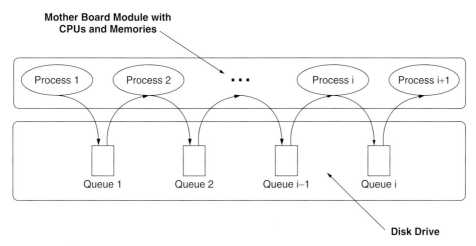

Figure 16.10 Snake road design to minimize interruption of data flow due to hardware failure during an image processing procedure. The snake road passes through different computers (processors) after each process is performed; (top) mother board; (bottom) disk drive.

principle can be used to minimize the loss of image data during an image processing procedure should a device failure occur in a component. A snake road design in the image processing software can be used to partition the FIFO model (described in Fig. 16.7). In this design, data will pass through different hardware devices, for example, between the motherboard (CPU) module (or the network card module if the process is for communication) and the hard disk drive alternately, as shown in Figure 16.10.

The drawback of the first software solution is that it makes the whole PACS software architecture complicated and increases the costs of storage, administration, and software maintenance. The drawback of the second software solution is that it will slow down the execution of the image processing procedure because of too many disk I/O operations for reading and writing of a large image data file. The software architecture is also very weak because any failure in a software process will break down the image processing procedure chain in the snake road. As a result the whole PACS performance decreases and an image stacking effect may be produced in some processing steps that may eventually overflow the capacity of the local disks, leading to loss of image data.

16.5 CURRENT PACS TECHNOLOGY TO ADDRESS FAULT TOLERANCE

Current PACS technology utilizes a mix of software and hardware approaches in addressing PACS fault tolerance. Multiple copies of an image are always in existence in various components at one time until the image is archived in the long-term storage. A second copy of the archived image is stored off line but not necessarily in a library system because of the expense involved.

To ensure that there is no interruption of PACS dataflow, larger PAC systems use distributed server architecture, and almost all systems have a mirrored database design. Most PAC systems have certain software designs to avoid the interruption of data flow due to hardware component failure. However, the most frequent hardware failure is in the hard disk drive (see Table 16.1). In this case the data flow in the branch of the PACS operation related to the disk drive will be interrupted. If the disk is a component in the PACS server, the data flow in the complete system is interrupted; only local functions in the image acquisition computer WSs will remain in operation. No effective method has been derived to circumvent this hardware failure until recently by using the Data Grid method. The technical aspect of Data Grid will be presented in Chapter 21. A PACS and teleradiology combined model schematic using the Data Grid in enterprise PACS will be shown in Section 16.8.5. In Section 16.7, we discuss a fault-tolerant PACS architecture as a means to provide a systemwide solution.

16.6   CLINICAL EXPERIENCES WITH ARCHIVE SERVER DOWNTIME: A CASE STUDY

We use the Saint John's Healthcare Center (St. John's), Santa Monica, CA, as a case study of the possible component failures in the PACS archive server that can cause operation downtime. Methods of remedy are discussed as are implemented in current PACS fault-tolerant technology. For more on the PACS implementation and evaluation experience at St. John's, see Section 18.7.1.

16.6.1   Background

St. John's is a 224-bed community hospital that performs about 120,000 radiology exam procedures each year. Of those exams, approximately 90% are digitally acquired and stored in a PACS archive server. The archive server is also responsible for prefetching and distributing any current and previous exams. It provides patient location information for automatic image distribution to specific review WSs located on the hospital's clinical floors. Like all traditional LAN PACS, the archive server is the command center of St. John's PACS. This case study represents the PACS at St. John's as of 2001. Since that time the PACS has been upgraded to a different server and archive configuration. Although this case study may not reflect the performance of current PAC systems, the types of system failure described could happen even with the state-of-the-art technology.

The hardware configuration for the archive server consisted of a Sun Ultra2 WS, two-mirrored hard disks, a RAID 4 (redundant array of independent disks) storage system, and an optical disk jukebox with two drives and a single robotic arm. The Sun Ultra2 WS had one 4.1-GB hard disk that contained the system software and the application software for the archive server. Attached to the WS was a separate unit that contained two 4.1-GB mirrored hard disks. This mirrored hard disk device contained mirrored data of the patient and image directories of all the exams stored in the RAID and MOD (magnetic optical disk) jukebox. A third copy of the databases was stored on a separate optical disk off line, and backup was performed on a daily basis. The RAID 4 system was connected to the Ultra 2 workstation via the SCSI (small computer system interface) port and was a 90-GB array of hard disks. This RAID system held about two weeks' worth of current exams for fast retrieval. In addition these exams were archived long term in the MOD jukebox. The MOD jukebox contained a single robotic arm that retrieved the platters and inserted them into one of two drives for exam retrievals. The jukebox had the capacity to contain 255 platters for a total of 3.0 TB of data compressed at a ratio of 2.5:1. The SPOF for the archive server were the single system hard disk and one CPU motherboard of the Sun Ultra2 workstation. However, the database, which was a crucial part of the server, was mirrored on two hard disks with a third off-line daily backup.

16.6.2   PACS Server Downtime Experience

For a period of 1.5 years before September 2001, in a 24 hour, 7 days a week operation, the archive server encountered a total of approximately 4 days of downtime spreading across three separate downtime incidents. The first two incidents were due to system hard disk failures, and the third downtime was due to a CPU motherboard failure (see Fig. 16.8). A description of downtime procedures and events and ensuing uptime procedures are presented to give a snapshot of how archive server downtime affects the clinical workplace.

16.6.2.1   Hard Disk Failure   The first two archive server downtimes involved the failure of the server system hard disk. Because the system software and the application software resided on this hard disk, the archive server was considered completely down. The initial diagnosis was made during the early evening hours. A new hard disk was ordered by the service, and the service representative arrived early the next morning to begin bringing the server back up. This was accomplished by replacing the hard disk with a new one and then installing the system software. Once the system software had been installed and properly configured, the next step was to install the server application software. The application setup was complex, especially during the second downtime, because the application software had already just undergone a new software upgrade and only two service personnel within the organization (a very large PACS manufacturer) had complete understanding of the installation procedures of the new software upgrade. In both cases the server was brought up by the end of the day, making a total of 1.5 days of downtime for each incident.

16.6.2.2   Mother Board Failure   The third archive server downtime involved the CPU motherboard. The NVRAM (nonvolatile random access memory) on the motherboard failed and needed replacement. The failure occurred once again during the early evening, and the initial diagnosis was made. A new CPU mother board was ordered, and the service representative arrived early the next morning. The hardware was replaced, and tests were made to ensure that all hardware components within the archive server WS were fully functioning. Because the hard disk was not

corrupted or damaged, the server was brought up around noontime, after a downtime of approximately one day.

16.6.3   Effects of Downtime

16.6.3.1   At the Management Level   During the archive server downtime normal operations and routines that were performed automatically had to be adjusted and then readjusted once the server was brought back up. These adjustments had a major impact on the clinical workflow and will be described further.

Under normal conditions all new exams were automatically routed to the review WSs on the hospital clinical floors based on the location of the patient; the routing information was obtained from the archive server, which in turn obtained it from the radiology information system (RIS) interface. Prefetched exams were distributed to the corresponding WSs along with the current exams for comparison. In addition radiologists and referring physicians handled queries and retrievals on demand for any previous exams that were not located on the local WS. Once the archive server experienced downtime, the workflow changed quite a bit. Communication between all staff personnel was crucial to relay the current downtime status and implement downtime procedures. The technologists had to manually distribute the exams to the specific diagnostic WS along with the corresponding review WS on the floors. Therefore what normally was one mouse click action to begin the auto-routing became a series of manual sending to multiple separate WSs.

For the clerical staff, hard copy reprints for off-site clinics were not possible because most exams that were requested for hard copy reprint did not reside on the local WSs and they could not query and retrieve for them. For the radiologists, any new exams acquired during the downtime did not have prefetched exams at the local diagnostic WS for comparisons. Also neither radiologists nor the referring physicians could query and retrieve any exams from the archive.

16.6.3.2   At the Local Workstation Level   Exam data management procedures on the local WSs were implemented as well during the downtime of the archive server. At the onset of downtime, some WSs had exams that were in the process of being sent to the archive. These sending jobs needed to be cleared from the queue before they started to affect the performance of the WSs. In addition any automatic archiving rules had to be turned off on the local WSs so that no additional exams would be sent to the archive when it was down.

16.6.4   Downtime for over 24 Hours

To prepare for possible downtime of longer than 24 hours, some exams may need to be deleted from the local WS that have already been read and archived to make room for incoming new exams. This process can only be performed manually and thus can be very time-consuming depending on the total number of WSs that receive new exams. Once the archive server is up and running again, the uptime procedures for the reading WSs must be implemented. All automatic archiving rules must be activated. Any new exams that have not been archived must be manually archived. Finally, query and retrieve tests must be performed on the WS to ensure that the PACS system is fully operational again. These final uptime procedures for the WSs consume about two hours of extra time (depending on the number of worksta-tions) in addition to the server downtime to bring the system to full operational status.

16.6.5 Impact of the Downtime on Clinical Operation

In these three downtime experiences, St. John's did not lose any image data. In addi-tion there was no damage to the mirrored database disk system. In fact, with all the downtime procedures implemented, the end users only experienced the inconvenience of not having the query/retrieve functionality or previous exams for comparison stud-ies. The well-trained service PACS team at St. John's was a major reason why these downtime incidents had not cascaded to a major operation catastrophe.

16.7 CONCEPT OF CONTINUOUSLY AVAILABLE PACS DESIGN

The case study given in Section 16.6 describes a fault-tolerant PACS design in clinical practice eight years ago. The concept behind the continuously available (CA) PACS design is to minimize manual intervention and change of management and WS daily operation routines, since these recovery procedures are tedious and labor intensive in clinical operation, not to mention the steps required to bring back PACS operation under the stress of a clinical environment. Therefore an ideal design is to build fault tolerance for each SPOF in the system. Thus the PACS server and each application server are SPOFs of the system (see Fig. 16.4 and Fig. 16.5) and should have fault tolerance built in. The question is how to provide fault tolerance for these SPOFs in the system so that PACS would be CA in operation in the event that any SPOFs occurs. If we use hardware solutions alone, the PACS as a whole will be very expensive and difficult to maintain. If we use software solutions alone, the software development effort will be extensive, and the system performance will suffer, as witnessed in many case studies.

The current concept in CA PACS design is to replace every SPOF in the complete system by a new CA component with the following four conditions:

1. The CA component has an uptime of 99.999% (downtime: 5 min/year) to satisfy the requirement of continuous availability.
2. Should the CA component fails because of a failure in any of its hardware devices, its recovery should be automatic without human intervention, and the recovery time should be within seconds.
3. The CA component is a one-to-one replacement of the corresponding existing PACS component without any modification of the rest of the system.
4. The replacement is easy to install and affordable.

Figure 16.4 and 16.5 (compare with Fig. 16.2 and Fig. 16.3, respectively) are a version of the CA PACS design that is identical to a generic PACS architecture except that all possible SPOFs (PACS server, application servers, database gateway computer; and network switch and connections; see red color) must be replaced by the CA components. Section 16.8 describes such a CA PACS server.

16.8   CA PACS SERVER DESIGN AND IMPLEMENTATION

In this section we present a design of a CA server using both hardware and software for PACS application and use the terms fault tolerance (FT) and CA interchangeably. We first discuss the hardware components in an image server and the CA design criteria. The architecture of the CA image server is then presented with result summary.This CA PACS server was implemented as a 24/7 off-site backup archive server for a clinical PACS from 2002 to 2007.

16.8.1   Hardware Components and CA Design Criteria

16.8.1.1   Hardware Components in an Image Server   Basic hardware components in an image server consist of the CPUs and memory, I/O ports and devices, and storage devices shown in Figure 16.11. Any of these hardware components can fail, and if it is not addressed immediately, operation of the server will be compromised. The design of the CA image server is to develop both hardware and system software redundancy to automatically detect and recover any hardware failure instantaneously. Recall that Table 16.1, shows a current survey of the causes of computer and network system downtime in which computer hardware, hard disk drive, communication processor, and data communication network account for about 71% of the system failure. This design, augmented with software, addresses the issue of the 71% hardware-related failure in the complete image server system, and methods of circumventing that failure with a fail-over mechanism to achieve continuous system availability. PACS application software failure and human errors are not considered in this CA image server.

16.8.1.2   Design Criteria   Fault tolerance (FT) results from the implementation of redundant hardware components with software control in the server such that in the event of a component failure, maximum availability and reliability—without the loss of transactional data can be achieved (Carrasco, 2002; Xu et al., 2002; Bajpai et al., 2002; Some et al., 1995; del Gobbo et al., 1999; Fabre and Perennou, 1998). The requirements for a FT image server are as follows:

1. Highly reliable server system operations
   - No loss of data
   - No workflow interruptions

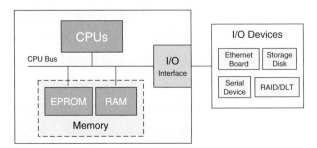

Figure 16.11   General computer system architecture with connection to short-term storage disk (RAID) and long-term (DLT, digital linear tape) library archive. All components in the architecture are SPOF, including the I/O interface and the connection to I/O devices.

Image server reliability refers to server uptime and fault tolerance. In the event of a server hardware component failure, users might notice minimal performance impact during the server fail-over process, since all server functions, such as image archive, retrieval, distribution, and display, remain continuously available. No loss of data and no work interruptions occur, so all current server processes and transactions automatically resume with no interruptions.

2. Acceptable system performance
   - No performance degradation in daily routine operations
   - Occasional glitches in an acceptable amount of time

Performance inclusively measures how well hardware, operating systems, network, and application software perform together. Ultimately the image server's performance affects the end users and the response time of the applications. For FT image servers, the redundant server hardware, once taking over the failed hardware, should be able to handle the same workload in network speed, CPU power, and archive storage as in normal server operations so that the user will not experience a noticeable performance degradation. Normally, server operations and user sessions halt momentarily (about 30 s; see Table 16.2) until the FT image server successfully fails over and resumes in the event of a system glitch. A longer delay (in minutes) is acceptable for noninteractive background processes such as in image archiving.

3. Low cost and easy implementation (Muller et al., 2002)
   - Portable
   - Scalable
   - Affordable

Portability means that existing server software should be able to run on the FT image server without any major changes. Scalability tests how additional hardware and system and application software work with the FT server and impact its ability to handle the workload. High-end million-dollar FT machines such as the Tandem system, which utilizes a sophisticated system design and can recover from system failure in milliseconds, are too expensive for most PACS applications and are often used for short transaction types of applications in the banking, security and stock exchange, and telecommunication industries. The design of the FT server using the concept of the triple modular redundancy (TMR) UNIX server discussed here is affordable; the prototype costs about three times the amount of a comparable UNIX machine but has much longer failover times (in seconds) than the Tandem system.

TABLE 16.2   Average system recovery time for common faults with the Triple Modular Redundant Server

Common Faults	Ethernet	CPU Module	Disks
Range of Recovery Time	3–15	20–40	35–75
Average	5.8	29.8	42.2
Standard Deviation	1.05	4.66	32.86

Total tests: 182 for each of the three scenarios. Times are expressed in seconds.

16.8.2 Architecture of the CA Image Server

16.8.2.1 The Triple Modular Redundant Server

Triple Modular Redundant (TMR) Server Concept and Architecture The CA image server uses TMR to achieve fault tolerance at the CPU/memory level. Figure 16.12*A* and *B* shows the core of the TMR server made up of three identically configured UltraSPARC-based modules (Sun Microsystems). The three modules are tightly synchronized and interconnected through a high-speed backplane for inter-module communications. Each module is a complete, operational computer running Sun's Solaris UNIX OS server, with its own UltraSPARC CPU, memory, I/O interfaces, bridge logic, and power supply. Each module runs all software applications independently and synchronously under the standard Solaris operating environment (Kanoun and Ortalo-Borrel, 2000; http://www.resilience.com).

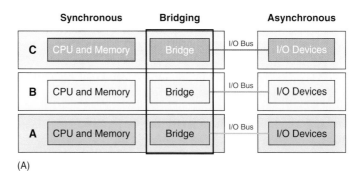

(A)

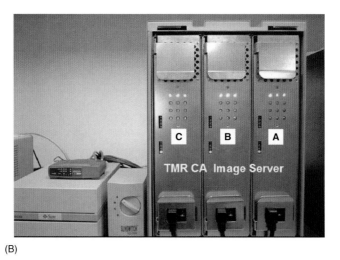

(B)

Figure 16.12 (*A*) Fault-tolerant, continuously available image server with the triple modular redundant (TMR) architecture. Each module contains the basic computer system architecture shown in Figure 16.11. (left) The bridges are used to synchronize the three modules. (*B*) The prototype CA TMR with three modules (resembling Ultra Sparc II architecture) with three separate power supplies (bottom). The console switch (middle) is for managing the three module displays during the debugging stage.

To the UltraSPARC core, a programmable ASIC (application-specific integrated circuit) technology is used to build the TMR bridge logic that keeps the three modules synchronized, continuously monitors and compares their operation, and exchanges I/O data among the three modules. The bridge logic reads Sbus transactions within each module and compares them across the modules. If the logic detects a variation between transactions, it assumes an error. Then the system pauses (typically for 5–30 s depending on memory size) while the diagnostic software determines the faulty module and disables it.

Next, memories of the two remaining modules are synchronized by performing a full memory copy. Once the copy is complete, the system resumes processing by using the remaining two modules.

The Bridge Voting Logic   The hardware in the bridge compares all data that come into, or go out of the synchronous part of the system used to diagnose any problems (Latif-Shabgahi et al., 2001). The hardware voting ASIC built into the bridge unit provides real-time fault detection and masking functions that are transparent to the application program. The TMR voting system uses a simple majority voter shown in Figure 16.13. The data that go in or out of the three modules are correlated and voted on to find the most correct output (Z). A disagreement detector compares a voter's output (Z) with the input (I1, I2, and I3) of each active module. When a disagreement occurs, the detector flags the corresponding module as having failed, and the module is taken off-line automatically. The rationale is that the probability of all systems containing the same error (producing the same bad data given some input) is extremely remote. If only two modules were to be used, the mere fact that the two modules behave differently does not guarantee identification of the faulty module. This is a conceptually simple model because the logic that compares the operation of the three modules need not know what faulty behavior looks like, only that a deviant module should be regarded as faulty.

The fundamental premise of this architecture is that any data that are corrupted will not be a problem until they are sent through the system. The hardware in the bridge compares all data that come into or go out of the synchronous part of the system to

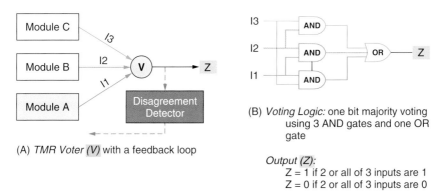

(A) *TMR Voter (V)* with a feedback loop

(B) *Voting Logic:* one bit majority voting using 3 AND gates and one OR gate

Output (Z):
    Z = 1 if 2 or all of 3 inputs are 1
    Z = 0 if 2 or all of 3 inputs are 0

Figure 16.13   TMR majority voting system and logic. (*A*) TMR voter (V) with a feedback loop; (*B*) the voting logic. After the vote the feedback loop will disable the minority module if it exists.

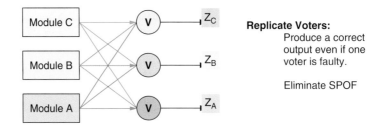

Figure 16.14 TMR system with replicate voters.Three voters (Z) are used to avoid single points of failure (SPOF) in the voter. A replicate voters design is used in the TMR prototype.

diagnose any problems. Because the comparisons occur within the hardware, there is no overhead to the operating system and performance is not affected.

Although using the voting unit in the configuration shown in Figure 16.13*A* provides adequate protection against the hardware faults in a module, it does not allow a fault to occur within the voter itself. To provide total protection, the replicated voters shown in Figure 16.14 were used in the TMR server. Here the voter is triplicated, and the link from each module is passively fanned out through the backplane to each of the voting units. Because each voter built into the bridge unit is logically grouped with the module itself, the voter fault is equivalent to a module fault and will be masked by further voter action at the next stage. Passive fan out of the link connections used in the TMR backplane is necessary to avoid the possible introduction of byzantine (intermittent) faults that could arise from the use of an active fan-out mechanism (Trivedi et al., 1995).

16.8.2.2 The Complete System Architecture

Other Server Components — FT I/O and Storage Subsystem Figure 16.15*A*, *B*, and *C* shows the complete architecture of the TMR and I/O buses and devices (Avizienis, 1997). Other server components in addition to the TMR in the server system are I/O buses and devices. Not only is operating I/O devices such as SCSI or Ethernet interfaces in TMR synchronization extremely difficult, it does not achieve the required systemwide CA. Each I/O subsystem must be regarded individually, with CA implemented in a manner appropriate to each subsystem. The following subsections describe some of these I/O subsystems.

Ethernet Each of the three modules contains its own 100-baseT Ethernet interface, each of which is connected, via independent paths, to the local network backbone. The three interfaces form a single software interface with one IP and MAC (media access control, a unique hardware number) address. One interface acts as the active interface, while the others stand by. Should the module containing the active interface fail, or some element of its connection to the backbone fail, that interface would be disabled and a standby unit would become active in its place. Normal network retry mechanisms hide the failure from applications.

Fault-Tolerant Storage System There are two storage subsystems, RAID for short term and the DLT library for long term. Because the former is mission critical

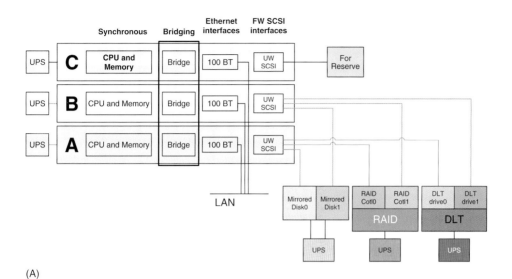

(A)

(B)

Figure 16.15 (*A*) Complete CA image server system architecture. The three Ethernet interfaces from each of the three modules are connected to the LAN, while only one Ethernet interface is active and forms only one IP address for the application. Two mirrored disks (mirrored Disk0 and mirrored Disk1) are connected to module A and module B through the UW (ultrawide) SCSI interface with fail-over mode. Two RAID controllers (RAID Cotl0 and RAID Cotl1) are connected to modules A and B through the UW SCSI interface with fail-over mode. Two DLT controllers (DLT drive0 and DLT drive1) are connected to modules A and B through the UW SCSI interface with fail-over mode. (See the References at the end of the chapter for how this fault-tolerant architecture performs fail over under various conditions.) UPS: uninterruptible power supply, 100 BT: 100 base T Ethernet. (*B*) CA image server connected to the PACS simulator shown during RSNA Scientific Exhibit of 2001 and also at SPIE 2002. The system was demonstrated annually at RSNA until 2005. The simulator consists of the modularity simulator (left) and a gateway (middle), TMR (see Fig. 16.12*B*), and two workstations (right). The RAID and LTD library are not shown in the figure. (*C*) Schematic of the CA image server connected to the PACS simulator system (see Chapter 28) shown during the RSNA Scientific Exhibit of 2001. A similar setup was used as the ASP PACS backup archive and other imaging informatics research and development projects at the IPILab, USC until 2007. It was replaced by the Data Grid discussed in Chapter 21.

CA PACS Simulator Components and Workflow

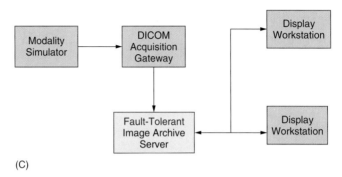

(C)

Figure 16.15   (*Continued*)

in a complete CA image server system, the RAID system needs also an FT design. DLT in the CA image server is used as a peripheral storage subsystem; FT can be designed and implemented up to the connectivity level with the CA image server.

RAID as a short-term storage. Although RAID has its own built-in FT mechanism in handling disk failure, its SPOFs are in the RAID controller and its connection is to the CA image server. In this design a dual-controller RAID is used for short-term storage. TMR modules A and B are connected to each of the two RAID controllers, as shown in Figure 16.16. Disk drive or RAID controller failures are handled by the RAID mechanism. The two redundant connections shown in Figure 16.16 provide a full FT short-term storage solution, which guarantees system survival in an event of failure of one module, one RAID controller, or any combination of both at the same time.

A Hitachi 9200 (325 Gbytes) dual-controller RAID (Hitachi Data Systems, Santa Clara, CA) with Veritas Volume manager software (Mountain View, CA) is

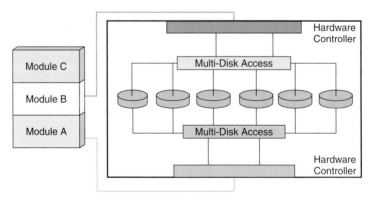

Figure 16.16   A RAID with two hardware (HW) controllers. The module A SCSI port connects to one controller, and the module B SCSI port connects to the other controller, providing redundancy for system reliability. In the early 2000 s, a dual controller for the RAID was a new technology, now it is common to have dual controller for the RAID.

implemented with the CA image server shown in Figure 16.16. The dual hardware controllers connected to modules A and B, respectively, provide the two paths to the TMR server while Veritas software dynamically monitors the two paths and switches automatically from one to another in case one path is disconnected.

DLT library for long-term archive. For long-term archive in the CA image server, a StorageTeK L40 DLT library with 3.2 TB (Storage Technology Corp., Louisville, CO) is used. The library has two drives, each connected to one of the TMR controller modules and providing the redundant paths to the CA image server, and hence the library provides FT connectivity to the server. Meanwhile Veritas Storage Migrator and Netbackup software are installed to automatically migrate and back up the data from short-term RAID to long-term tape library archive. The Veritas Migrator software has a built-in feature to monitor the multiple paths and to fail-over from one to another in case of a failure of any single CPU module or tape driver. But the DLT library itself is not designed as fault tolerant. Its controller and robot arm are still the SPOF. The tape library is used for secondary archive, and the FT can be tolerated. The main purpose is preservation of the data rather than real-time recovery of library system failure.

16.8.3 Applications of the CA Image Server

16.8.3.1 PACS and Teleradiology   The CA image server described in this section can be used to replace SPOFs in the image components of the PACS operation. Figure 16.4 and 16.5 show the generic PACS and teleradiology architecture, where each SPOF marked by "FT" and/or "RED" can be replaced by the CA image server design. The CA image server simulator described in Section 16.8.2 is actually a generic PACS designed for PACS training described in Chapter 28.

16.8.3.2 Off-site Backup Archive—Application Service Provider Model (ASP)

Off-Site Backup Archive—ASP Model for Disaster Recovery   The CA image server can be used as a fault-tolerant solution for disaster recovery of short-term image data by way of an application service provider (ASP) model. The ASP short-term image archive provides instantaneous, off-site automatic backup of acquired image data and instantaneous recovery of stored image data with CA quality and low operational cost. Such an application had been implemented to support an offsite backup archive for the clinical PACS at St. John's Healthcare System, LA, CA from 2002 to 2207 (see Chapter 19). The CA image server with both RAID and DLT Library, as shown in Figure 16.15*A* and *C* located at the Image Processing and Informatics Laboratory (IPI) at USC, served as a short-term off-site backup archive for St. John's. In parallel with the exams being acquired from modalities and archived in the main PACS server from St. John's, 100% of the clinical image data were sent to this ASP CA image server. The connection between the main archive and the ASP storage server was established via a T1 (1.5 Mbits/s) connection.

During the implementation stage a disaster scenario was initiated and the disaster recovery process using the ASP archive server was successful in repopulating the clinical system on site within a short period of time (a function of the data size and data transfer rate).The ASP archive was able to recover two months of image data with no complex operational procedures. Furthermore no image data loss was encountered during the recovery.

16.8.4 Summary of Fault Tolerance and Fail Over

In this section we describe the design and implementation of a CA image server that can achieve 99.999% hardware uptime. The design concept is based on a TMR server with three redundant server modules. The fault tolerance and fail over are based on coupling the TMR with majority vote mechanism and fail-over software architecture. The majority votes detect the faulty component in cycle time, and the software takes care of the automatic fail over. Depending on the types of hardware failure and the state of the execution in the component, the fail over can take from 3 to 75 s (SD = 32.86 s). The longer fail over time and large SD happen in the computer disks, where the SCSI failure can either be captured by the system immediately or by a SCSI ping timeout that yields the large SD. If a mirrored disk fails, the CA image server smoothly continues the runs, but reconstructing the mirrored disk in the background requires more time in accord with the size of the disk under consideration.

16.8.5 The Merit of the CA Image Server

Although the concept of TMR logic has been used in other types of FT design, the TMR CA image server described and implemented is a technology innovation in its handling of fail over. The CA image server connected with the FT storage as a total system for medical image applications has several main advantages over other current FT server designs. It is truly continuously available, lower cost to implement, portable, scalable, affordable, easy to install without extensive change in the application software, and not labor intensive during fail over and system recovery. The TMR CA image server is very suitable for large-scale image database application.

In addition to replacing the SPOF components in an operational PACS, the CA image server can be used as an ASP model for short-term backup archive for disaster recovery and scheduled downtime service. Although the CA server described is based on a UNIX Solaris system, similar concepts can be extended to other computer architecture and software operation systems.

On the continuum of HA solutions are also the full "hot spare" method, ranging from 99% to 99.9% system uptime and being used by many PACS vendors now, and the Data Grid (Chapter 21), which is mostly replacing the TMR system (discussed in Section 16.8). A lesson learned is that in achieving 99.999% or five minutes of downtime once a, the triple modular redundant concept still prevails in any SPOF PACS component.

16.9 ENTERPRISE PACS

16.9.1 Background

Because of the need to improve operational efficiency and to provide more cost-effective healthcare, many large-scale healthcare enterprises have been formed world-wide. Each healthcare enterprise includes hospitals, medical centers, and clinics in its healthcare network. The managers of these enterprises recognize the importance of using PACS and image distribution as a key technology in providing better quality and more cost-effective healthcare delivery at the enterprise level. As a result many large-scale enterprise-level PACS/image distribution pilot studies are under way, concerning full design, and implementation. Some of the larger enterprise PACS currently being designed, developed, and implemented around the world are as follows:

- USA: U.S. Department of Veterans Affairs Medical Centers VistA Project (Sections 22.2), UCLA (Sections 18.7.2, 19.3), USC (Sections 18.7.3, 19.4)
- Europe: The United Kingdom National project and the Italy National and Regional project.
- Asia: The Hong Kong Hospital Authority (Sections 18.7.4, 22.3)

We can learn from their experiences in planning, design, implementation, as well as cost-benefit analysis. The characteristics of these systems can be summarized as:

1. Model: PACS and ePR with image distribution
2. Scale: Large enterprise level, from 39 to 399 hospitals and medical centers
3. Complexity: Total healthcare IT (information technology) integration
4. Ambition: Complete system deployment to the enterprise
5. Costs: Extremely expensive
6. Difficulty of implementation: Culture, resources, timeline, data migration, and overcoming legacy technologies

We briefly introduced the concept of enterprise PACS in Section 7.6. In this section we provide an overview of the current status of enterprise PACS with Web-based ePR image distribution. The concept of enterprise-level PACS/image distribution, its characteristics, and components are discussed. Business models for enterprise-level implementation available from the private medical imaging and system integration industry are highlighted. A case study based on the Hong Kong healthcare environment is used to illustrate possible models of implementation.

16.9.2 Concept of Enterprise-Level PACS

PACS is a workflow-integrated imaging system designed to streamline operations throughout the entire patient care delivery process. One of its major components, image distribution, delivers relevant electronic images and related patient information to healthcare providers in a timely manner, whether the patient care be within a hospital or in a healthcare enterprise.

Enterprise-level health delivery emphasizes sharing of enterprise-integrated resources and streamlining operations. In this regard, if an enterprise consists of several hospitals and clinics, it is not necessary for every hospital and clinics to have similar specialist services. A particular clinical service like radiology can be shared among all entities in the enterprise, resulting in the concept of a radiology expert center relying on the operation of teleradiology. In this setup, all patients are registered in the same enterprise can be referred to the radiology expert center for examinations. So the patient being cared for becomes the focus of the operation. A single index like the patient's name/ID is then sufficient for any healthcare provider in the enterprise to retrieve the patient's comprehensive record. In this scenario, the data management system is not the conventional hospital information system (HIS), radiology information system (RIS), PACS, or other organizational information system. Rather, the electronic patient record (ePR) image distribution concept prevails.

Traditional HIS is hospital operation oriented, so sometimes several separate data information subsystems must be invoked simultaneously before various information of the same patient can be retrieved during a visit. The concept of ePR is that "The patient's record goes with the patient" (Section 13.5). In other words, the ePR server is conceived to have necessary linkages connected to all information systems involved with healthcare. Using the patient's name/ID as the search index, all healthcare providers with the consent of the patient can seamlessly retrieve all relevant information of that patient across different systems in the enterprise ePR system. The majority of current ePR systems are still restricted to the stage of textural information, but to be effective for healthcare delivery, images must be incorporated into the ePR server. Examples were shown in Section 13.5.1.

Enterprise PACS therefore has to have a means of transmitting relevant patient's images and related data to the ePR server, and the ePR server has to have the infrastructure design to distribute images and related data in a timely manner to the healthcare providers at the proper location. Because each healthcare enterprise has its own culture and organization structure, methods of transmitting images/data to the ePR as well as methods of distributing them to the healthcare providers may be different. Figure 16.17A (excerpted from Fig 7.6) shows the ePR-based enterprise PACS with image distribution concept. For the numerals in the figure, see Chapter 21. Figure 16.17B depicts the enterprise PACS and teleradiology integration system (see also Figs. 16.3 and 16.5) using the fault-tolerant Data Grid concept (see Chapter 21). The fault-tolerance Data Grid concept has replaced the TMR concept discussed in Section 16.8.

16.10 DESIGN OF ENTERPRISE-LEVEL PACS

16.10.1 Conceptual Design

Most large-scale healthcare enterprises are organized according to regional clusters (see Sections 22.2 and 22.3). Each cluster operates independently but follows the guidelines of the enterprise. Most often the enterprise provides an overall ITS (information technology service) supporting the enterprise's workstations in the design and implementation of information systems. Its main resources are located in the enterprise data centers. Larger clusters may have their own ITS supporting cluster-related IT requirements. Larger hospitals may also have certain ITS support with a smaller data center. Figure 16.18 depicts a conceptual design of PACS with ePR imaging distribution within a cluster and its connection to the data centers and other clusters (Huang, 2002). The three major components are clinical components, IT supports, and clinical specialties (first column).The clinical components (top row) are flagship, acute, convalescent hospitals, and clinics. Within a hospital, radiology, A&E (ambulatory and emergency), wards, ICU, and other clinical operation are the major units. Clinical specialties (bottom row) include neurosurgery, orthopedic, radiation therapy, and other subspecialties. They can be located within a hospital or within a cluster supporting other entities in the cluster. The IT support (middle row) includes both ITS primary and secondary data centers. Other enterprises or smaller healthcare providers can be connected to the enterprise data centers through a public–private interface, namely the electronic patient record (PPI-ePR) gateway (GW, top right).

16.10.1.1 IT Supports

1. *Networking*: High-speed networks (Gbit/s, or OC-12) should be used for high-volume and high-demand applications. The minimum requirement for image distribution is 100 Mbits/s or OC-3).

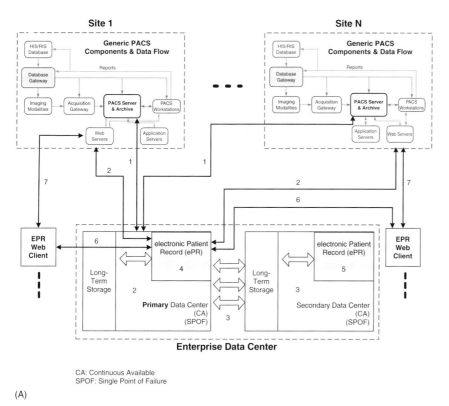

CA: Continuous Available
SPOF: Single Point of Failure

(A)

Figure 16.17 (*A*) Enterprise PACS and ePR with image distribution. The enterprise data center supports all sites in the enterprise. The primary data center has a secondary data center for backup to address any single point of failure. The enterprise ePR system allows the patient's electronic record with images to be accessible to ePR Web clients. (*B*) Combined enterprise level large-scale PACS (blue) and teleradiology (yellow) model using the grid computing technology. The grid computing infrastructure (green) consists of the Data Grid with the DICOM standard (white) and IHE (purple) workflow profiles. Each green box in the PACS represents the contribution of SAN (storage area network) to the grid infrastructure. The Data Grid stores the images and reports, and the other grid computing resources take care of the workflow and management. The top row is the enterprise PACS. The Data Grid's major component is the teleradiology DICOM (bottom green), which directs the image and report workflow. The green boxes represent the data storage contribution of PAC systems and teleradiology to the Data Grid.

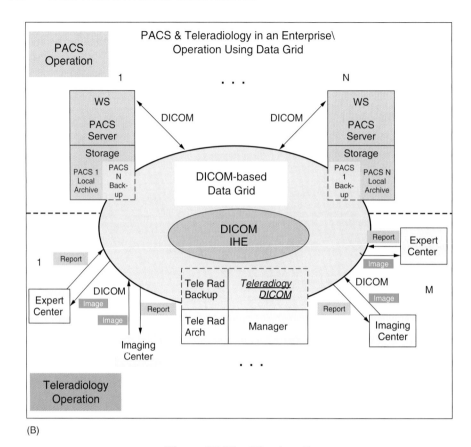

Figure 16.17   (*Continued*)

2. *Standards*: DICOM standards should be used for external communications and image formatting. For Web-based image distribution under the umbrella of ePR, TCP/IP should be used.

3. *Display*: Radiology should use 2 K (2500 × 2000 or 2000 × 1600) or 1 K (1600 × 1200) for sectional image display. A&E, ICUs, wards, and other clinical applications use 1 K; convalescent hospitals and physicians use desktop. In all cases the LCD monitor should be used for better image quality.

4. *Storage*: The storage requirement should be overdesigned. It is more cost-effective to have an overdesign than performing data migration or changing archive architecture at a future point in time.

5. *SPOF*: Single points of failure (SPOFs) should be expected at both the cluster data center and the enterprise ITS data center. Careful design using CA (continuous availability) or HA (high availability) resilience architecture (see earlier sections in this chapter) is essential. Image data backup should include a second copy off site from the primary archive.

6. *Data migration*: A data migration schema should be developed for migrating current image data from existing hospital archives to the enterprise architecture.

7. *Image distribution*: Image distribution should be integrated with ePR, both in archive and in display.

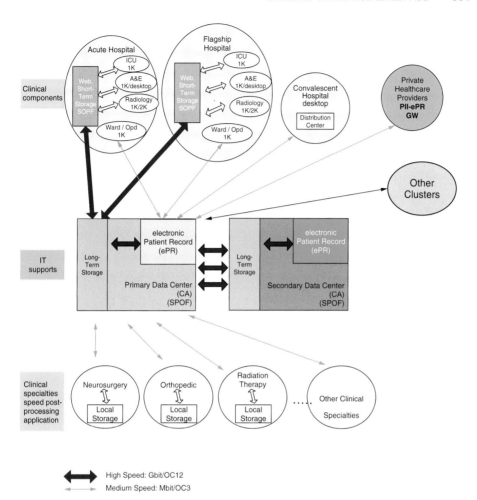

High Speed: Gbit/OC12
Medium Speed: Mbit/OC3

Figure 16.18   Conceptual design of PACS with image distribution within a cluster (light blue and yellow), its connection to the primary data centers (light purple and green), backup in the secondary data center (darker purple and green), and other clusters (pink) in the healthcare enterprise. The left-hand side shows the three components within the cluster (from top down): clinical, IT supports, and clinical specialties. A cluster consists of a flagship hospital, acute hospital, and convalescent hospital (all in blue); clinical specialties include neurosurgery, orthopedic, radiation therapy, and other specialties (all in yellow). Radiology is within the acute and flagship hospitals. The cluster can share patient information with private healthcare providers (orange) through the data center connection using the public–private interface of the electronic patient record (PPI-ePR) gateway (GW).

16.10.1.2 Operation Options

Centralized Data versus Data Distributed from the Hospital   The ePR conceptual design utilizes both centralized and distributed architecture. In the short term (less than three months; this number is adjustable) image data are archived at and distributed from the hospital data center as a distributed operation. The hospital archive distributes images through intra-hospital and inter-hospital networks. Clinical units in the hospital can also query/retrieve images from the database of other hospitals.

When *centralized at the data center*, archived images are sent continuously to the enterprise data center from the hospital for storage in the centralized long-term archive. In the data center, some selected image data are converted to Web-based ePR format for ePR distribution. After three months the image data can be queried/retrieved from the data center with either DICOM or the Web-based ePR.

DICOM versus Web   Images acquired as DICOM from imaging modalities supported with DICOM are archived as DICOM images. In those modalities (e.g., endoscopy images) not supported by DICOM, DICOM headers are inserted and archived as DICOM images. The centralized PACS archive is therefore DICOM based. When images are selected from the DICOM database for ePR distribution, the image format is converted to a Web-based format used by the ePR, preferably preserving the 12 bits/pixel quality. The accumulated Web-based images are archived in the Web-based server either within the ePR database or in an independent Web image database, cross-referenced with the ePR database.

16.10.1.3 Architectural Options

1. The data center should be operationally resilient, that is, designed for 24/7 distribution operations and to accommodate daily peak hours.

2. The cluster data center can be embedded as a subunit in the enterprise data center.

3. The enterprise data center should provide an off-site second copy image. It can either be at a secondary data center or at a cluster data center.

4. A huge storage capability is essential. For example, 300,000 conventional digital radiography procedures showing one view will generate 3TB of data in a year (without compression). A hierarchical archive scheme must be designed, and the capacity of each class of storage must be verified by a pilot implementation study.

5. Local storage for clinical specialties is managed by the specialty and supported by the cluster ITS.

6. Communication and network efficiency are critical for satisfactory system performance. A pilot study should enable data to be obtained on the feasibility of electing either cluster or enterprise-level implementation.

7. System availability is 24/7, and disaster recovery time should be within minutes.

8. Image distribution method can be through both DICOM or Web.

9. A single system integrator contracted by the enterprise has the full responsibility to resolve multiple vendor issues.

10. Image data security is most important. Enterprise ITS has the responsibility of implementing an acceptable scheme balancing ease of use, cost, and security parameters.

16.10.2 Financial and Business Models

Because enterprise PACS is an integrated large-scale image distribution system, the cost of implementation is very high. This section lists some of the financial models available from medical imaging manufacturers and system integration companies (e.g., Philips Medical Systems, Siemens Medical Systems, GE Medical Systems).

Bundled PACS with Image Distribution and Medical Imaging Equipment Purchase   Medical imaging manufacturers provide add-on PACS installation during imaging equipment purchase. The disadvantages of this model are that the add-on PACS normally is limited in scope and not really suitable for enterprise application. The add-on PACS equipment so purchased has three disadvantages. First, most likely the add-on PACS equipment will be obsolete in two to three years. Second, it may be difficult to integrate this equipment to the ePR because the add-on PACS architecture is not flexible. Finally, without a unified DICOM data structure in the enterprise level from the beginning, data compatibility between add-on PACS modules can create confusion in the systemwide worklist, and cause problems with the image distribution roll-out.

Outright Purchase with Maintenance Contract of PACS with Image Distribution Solution   No off-the-shelf enterprise-level PACS/image distribution is offered by any manufacturer, and therefore outright purchase is not possible.

Outsourcing   Outsourcing to maintain the technical components of the PACS with image distribution may be considered after the PACS equipment has been installed, provided that the cost is justifiable. But when planning the PACS with image distribution is de novo, no outsourcing manufacturer is knowledgeable enough about the intricacies of the enterprise-level operation, let alone the cluster or the hospital operation, without embarking on a long learning process. The outsourcing company must further learn the design of the enterprise ePR in order to interface PACS to its architecture. The time required for such a process is too long to be beneficial for the enterprise operation.

ASP Model (Application Service Provider)   Currently the ASP model is an attractive option for smaller subsets of the PACS with image distribution. Supporting off-site archive, long-term image archive/retrieval or second copy archive, DICOM – Web server development, and Web-based image database are some such workable models. But for a large comprehensive enterprise PACS with image distribution, ASP implementation requires investigation by the enterprise on locating a suitable manufacturer. The advantages and disadvantages of the ASP model versus equipment procurement are shown in Table 16.3.

Pay per Procedure   Pay-per-procedure is attractive in a smaller scale operation. This model is popular for smaller clinics where IT support is scarce. This model does not work well in large, multifaceted healthcare operations. The formula for pay per procedure can be complicated. Other disadvantages are similar to those of the outsourcing and ASP models.

TABLE 16.3   ASP model considerations: Some primary ASP benefits and concerns

ASP "Benefits"	ASP "Concerns"
1. Minimizes the initial capital procurement investment.	1. Historically the ASP model has been more expensive over a 2–4 year timeframe (vs. a capital purchase).
2. May accelerate the potential return on investment.	2. Customer relinquishes ownership and management of some/all of the PACS equipment.
3. Reduces the risk of technology obsolescence.	3. Financial equity in solution is minimized.
4. Vendor assumes the equipment costs as image volume increases.	4. Future customizations to meet unique customer needs may be limited.
5. Provides a flexible growth strategy.	
6. Eliminates concerns regarding Required space in data center.	

Software Purchase Only   A new model is software purchase only. The enterprise first designs its own image distribution, architecture, hardware, and workstation distribution. The enterprise then decides what software can be implemented in-house and what must be purchased. In most circumstances all PACS-related software will be purchased. Each such enterprise will negotiate with a manufacturer to procure the necessary software. The procurement will include licensing, installation, upgrade, training, and maintenance, but the enterprise will own the hardware.

The VAHE VisitA imaging component described in Section 22.2 uses this model for VA hospitals that do not purchase a PACS from a manufacturer. They would want the direct support from their internal IT departments. The IT department purchases the software and designs the image distribution for the hospital.

Loosely Coupled Partnership   A loosely coupled partnership is defined as an enterprise and its clusters forming a group partnership with a manufacturer. The partners share some defined responsibility in the planning, design, implementation, and operation. The procurement is similar to an outright purchase but with a favorable discount because of certain contributions from the enterprise. This model is being used by many PACS installations now. However, most partnerships are for one-time installation. The advantage of this model is a lower purchase price, which to many hospitals is attractive. But for an enterprise with many hospitals, this model is not so attractive because it is difficult to achieve a full enterprise-level integration.

Tightly Coupled Partnership   A tightly coupled partnership between the enterprise and a system integrator/manufacturer can be effective for enterprise-level PACS/image distribution implementation. Certain contributions from both partners are necessary:

1. The enterprise must make a long-term commitment with the manufacturer, say five years, to ensure PACS/image distribution support. Technical, personnel, financial, and ethical considerations have a big part in the negotiations.

2. On the technical side, the contracting parties will need to share confidential technical information related to the project's objectives. The manufacturer must guarantee that the equipment and software are up to date by periodic reviews, say every 12 to 18 months. At the end of year 5, the equipment and software should still be state-of-the-art technology.

3. On the personnel side, the parties share responsibility on the completion of the project, as well as for sufficient distribution of human resources dedicated to this objective. The manufacturers must provide adequate training for enterprise personnel to meet a level of engineering and operation sufficiency. "Sufficiency" is defined as the enterprise ITS's ability to install future added-on subsystems alone. Thus daily maintenance and service from the manufacturer should be at a minimum.

4. On the financial side, the enterprise has the responsibility to guarantee a mutually agreeable annual payment to the manufacturer. In return the manufacturer has the responsibility to guarantee that the PACS with image distribution satisfies the cluster workflow requirement and that the equipment is kept up to date for a period beyond, say, five years. Both partners can negotiate a continuing agreement after the five-years period has expired.

5. On the ethical side, the enterprise and the manufacturer must abide by the ethical codes of partnership as recognized by the IT and medical communities.

16.11 THE HONG KONG HOSPITAL AUTHORITY HEALTHCARE ENTERPRISE PACS WITH WEB-BASED ePR IMAGE DISTRIBUTION

16.11.1 Design and Implementation Plan

In this section we present the design and implementation plan of the Hong Kong Hospital Authority (HKHA) enterprise PACS with Web-based ePR image distribution of the Hong Kong Hospital Authority (HKHA) derived from the concept discussed in Sections 16.9 and Section 16.10. We will use HKHA PACS with ePR enterprise system as a case study in several places in this book, including in Sections 18.7.4 and 22.3.

To begin with, Hong Kong, including Kowloon and the new territories, has a population of about 7.0 millions, as shown in Figure 16.19. (This figure is repeated in Fig 22.7A.) Two major healthcare organizations are the HK HA and the Department of Health. The former is in charge of the operation of all public hospitals and clinics, whereas the latter is dedicated to the care of peoples' health. HA was founded in 1990 as the supermanager of all 43 public hospitals, about 93% of the hospital market in Hong Kong. It is organized into seven geographical clusters. Table 16.4 shows the workload of HA.

Ten years ago, HA developed an in-house clinical management system (CMS) supporting all hospitals with about 4000 workstations installed. It beta-tested its in-house ePR system (without images) in 2002 at two hospitals. Several hospitals had partial PACS, and one of them was ready for total filmless operation. In 2002, a consultancy

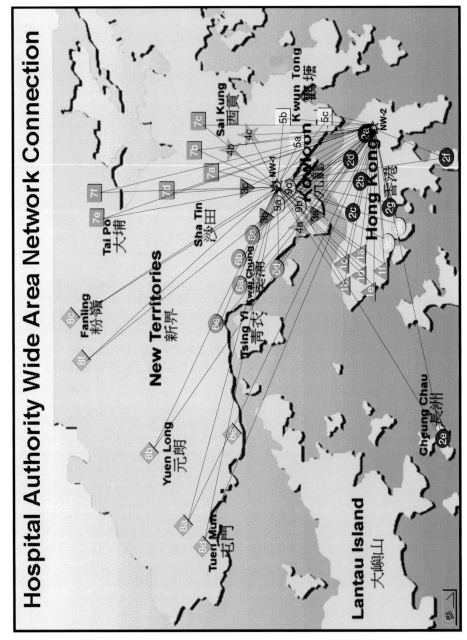

Figure 16.19 Hong Kong Hospital Authority's wide area network supporting 43 hospitals. (Courtesy of HKHA)

TABLE 16.4   The Hong Kong hospital authority estimated annual workload

- In 1999/2000
  - 1,089,330 inpatient discharges
  - 8,216,700 specialist outpatient attendances
  - 2,361,600 accident & emergency attendances
  - About 93% of the Hong Kong hospital market

- In 2000/2001
  - Budget of $28,029 HK Millions (US$3.6 Billions)

- In 2007/2008
  - 27,784 hospital beds
  - 1.2 million in-patient / day-patient discharge episodes
  - 7.4 million patient days (including both in-patient and day-patient)
  - 2.1 million Accident and Emergency (A&E) attendances

TABLE 16.5   Technical versus financial and business models suitable for the HKHA enterprise PACS implementation

	Bundle with Equipment Purchase	Outright Purchase with Maintenance Contract	Application Service Provider	Tightly Coupled Partnership
Generic centralized model			Lock-in	✓
Generic distributed model	Small scale	Small scale		
Generic mixed model			Lock-in	✓
Specific mixed model with ePR			Lock-in	✓

study was commissioned to integrate PACS with the ePR including image distribution (Huang, 2002). Table 16.5 weighed the suitability of various technical, financial, and business models described in Section 16.9.2 for the HKHA enterprise PACS with ePR image distribution development. Figure 16.20 depicts the recommended model, which is a mix of the centralized (in the enterprise level) and distributed (in the hospital level) models with an added ePR feature.

HKHA is composed of seven regional clusters (the organization may change periodically from time to time due to the population shift and service demand) based on locations and population distribution. Each cluster consists of a flagship, and an acute, convalescent hospital where the radiology service is located; the various clinical

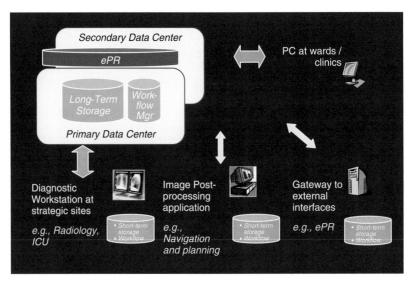

Figure 16.20 Technical option for the Hong Kong Hospital Authority enterprise PACS implementation. (Courtesy of W Chan, HA)

specialties may be shared with other clusters, among these being neurosurgery, orthopedic, and radiation therapy. HKHA has a primary data center backed up by a one-to-one secondary data center, and it has had a home-grown CMS (clinical management system), and ePR system in operation for many years. The operation policy of HKHA has been that each cluster can purchase and select its own PACS, but the PACS has to be connected to the enterprise CMS and the ePR with image distribution at the enterprise level. Figure 16.18, described in Section 16.10.1, shows the architecture of a cluster and its internal and external connections, including to private healthcare providers. This cluster was selected to be the pilot system for the implementation of PACS with ePR image distribution and its operation in this capacity started in 2006. Since then other hospitals have been placed on line for daily clinical use of the system. The last count was 12 PAC systems in other clusters supporting most of the radiological services. Some of PAC systems are new, and others were upgraded from legacy to state-of-the-art systems. The ePR is connected to most large hospitals and clinics, and many have image distribution systems. Some of the materials used in this section, as well as in Section 18.7.4 (on clinical experience) and Section 22.3 (on multimedia ePR), were contributed by a team of consultants and by HKHA personnel.

In the following two sections we will present two selected topics of interest related to the HKHA enterprise PACS with an image distribution system. The first is the process implemented by a flagship hospital in a cluster joining the HKHA enterprise system. The second is the point of view in HKHA of the radiologist utilizing the system.

16.11.2 Hospitals in a Cluster Joining the HKHA Enterprise System

16.11.2.1 Background As each hospital joined the HKHA enterprise PACS with ePR image distribution system, certain procedures had to be devised and followed. We consider here the case of the Tuen Mun Hospital (TMH) and Pok Oi Hospital

(POH) belonging to the Hong Kong New Territories West Cluster (NTWC). In this section we present only the preparation processes regarding the installation. The clinical experience will be discussed in Sections 18.7.4.

The Hong Kong NTWC is a cluster for four hospitals and many clinical facilities that take care of the patients in the West New Territories, northwest of Kowloon, Hong Kong. Tuen Mun (TMH, 1500 beds) and Pok Oi (POH, 1000 beds) are considered the main hospitals, so PACS was selected to be installed in these two hospitals first. One of the NTWC initiatives was to integrate the separate hospital RIS and PACS to provide an infrastructure to support the HA enterprise ePR system with image data distribution.

POH recently had expanded its facilities to 1000 hospital beds from 200, and in the process had a new PACS installed. Integration with TMH required a PACS operation redesign. TMH had already four separate legacy PACS modules from four separate manufacturers. Each PACS module contained specific imaging modality data that were tied to their purchase. TMH further purchased a new PACS from the same manufacturer as had POH, but this PACS has not yet been installed. Before integration with POH, the imaging studies from these disparate PACS modules had to be migrated into a single vendor's PAC system. The processes required integrating the two PAC systems and data migration included configuring the new PACS with the legacy systems installed many years ago.

16.11.2.2 Data Migration Data migration in this context means that data migrates from legacy PACS to a new PACS, and system integration with another PACS as a component of an existing enterprise ePR System with image distribution. The following are the data migration issues that needed to be settled for integrating the two new PACS systems in support of the HKHA enterprise ePR with image distribution:

1. Enterprise level system objectives
2. Parameters to be determined for the PACS to support the Web-based ePR system with image
3. Procedure to be used in divorcing the legacy PAC systems
4. Procedure to be used in integrating two new PAC systems
5. What data would need to be migrated?
6. Schedule for the data migration in coordination with the new PACS installation
7. Method to use in optimizing the migration process
8. How to monitor and check for image integrity
9. How to monitor for retrieval reliability
10. Procedure for checking on demographics
11. Procedure for checking on DICOM image header
12. Procedure for checking on the completion of the patient image record after migration
13. Procedure for checking on DICOM database integrity

In Sections 18.7.4 we will present the current status of the data migration and the two PAC systems integration, with the data migration steps shown in Figure 18.6.

Central Archive, ePR with Image Integration, and Workflow Steps

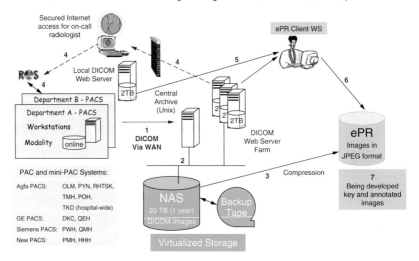

Figure 16.21   Hong Kong Hospital Authority's central archive, ePR with image integration, and workflow steps. The design is based on the existing HKHA clinical information system. See references from this chapter (Modified from Cheung et al. Fig. 3; courtesy of Dr. NT Cheung et al.)

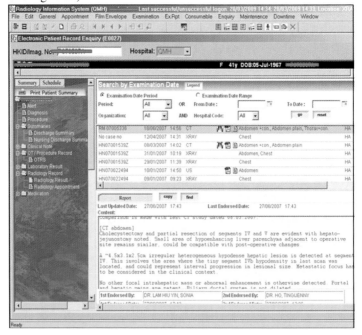

Figure 16.22   Patient A: A screen shot taken from the ePR. The left-hand side window provides a summary of the patient's history by tabs indicating the patient was alert, and the diagnosis, procedure, clinical notes, laboratory results, radiology record, and medication. Clicking on any of these tabs will open the top panel at the right, where from a list of chronologically sorted examinations the results of a particular examination can be selected and displayed in the lower panel. For radiology, the images and their reports are opened using the icons associated with each examination. (Courtesy of Dr. T. Chan)

16.11.3 Case Study of ePR with Image Distribution — The Radiologist's Point of View

HKHA manages in total 43 hospitals and 122 outpatient clinics, with a workforce of 53,000 staff employees. Its enterprisewide ePR with image distribution was implemented in 2004. The basic schema of the ePR with the image distribution architecture was outlined in Figure 16.21. Currently the ePR is accessible to all authorized clinicians throughout the enterprise. Images currently available include those from radiology, endoscopy, and surgery. These are produced by information systems from the different facilities and stored in a central data warehouse for life. Radiology images from different sources are transmitted to the central archive using dedicated WAN in DICOM format. Received images are stored after lossless compression in the central archive for one month. Because of the overwhelming amount of data and its associated cost, older images undergo lossy compression for long-term storage. When a request for an image is received from an ePR WS in the enterprise, the images are retrieved from the central archive and distributed using Web-based technology. Two actual clinical examples of the use of ePR illustrating its benefit are shown: For

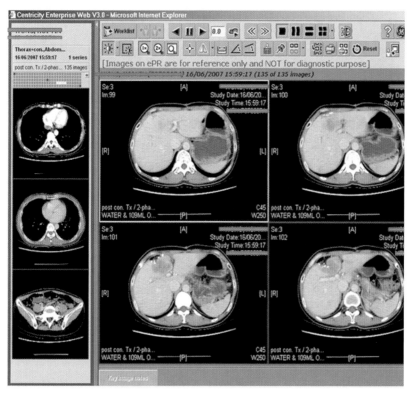

Figure 16.23 Patient A: Display of CT images archived in the ePR system. Images of an examination is requested by clicking on the image icon. The images are retrieved from ePR central image archive and displayed using the client image display software. The simple functions available include display format, zooming, windowing, and simple measurements like length and ROI measurements. Shown is a recurrent tumor after cholecystectomy for gallbladder cancer. (Courtesy of Dr. T. Chan)

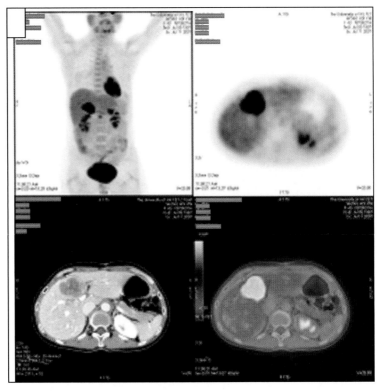

Figure 16.24 Patient A: A PET-CT performed at an outside institute that has access to the ePR. The intense FDG uptake (metabolically active) of the tumor (shown as the dark region of the liver on the PET image and the orange-colored region on the fused image) confirmed that the lesion in question shown in prior CT is a recurrent tumor rather than inactive postoperative scar tissue. (Courtesy of Dr. T. Chan)

patient A, Figure 16.22 to 16.24 show the ePR home page; CT and CT fused with PET, and for patient B, Figures 16.25 and 16.26 show CT and endoscopic images.

In 2006 a pilot project of the public–private interface–electronic patient record (PPI-ePR), which shares the clinical record in the HA repository with the private sector, was initiated. With consent of the patient, private practitioners enrolled in the scheme can access the information on line using a Web browser application, but data tramission is protected by encryption and a firewall. The information available from this project is the same as that available in ePR within the HA. This is a big step forward in realizing the eHR (electronic health record) system whereby individuals' health-related data may be shared among clinicians taking care of these individuals at different times and different locales. A basic schema of the project is shown in Figure 16.27 (see also Fig. 16.18).

16.12 SUMMARY OF FAULT-TOLERANT PACS AND ENTERPRISE PACS WITH IMAGE DISTRIBUTION

PACS is a large computer network and system integration of medical images and databases. The system is mission critical because it runs around the clock, 24/7.

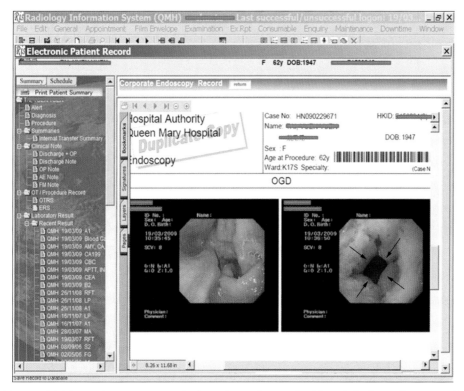

Figure 16.25   Patient B: Presurgical workup after an incidental finding of a tumor in the stomach by gastroscopy. Right: The subsequent reviewer can readily see the mucosal extent of the disease arrows and plan for treatment options. (Courtesy of Dr. T. Chan)

For this reason operation reliability is vital. The purpose of PACS fault-tolerant design is to maintain continuous operability of the system. To develop and operate an enterprise PACS continuously, system fault-tolerance is mandatory.

This chapter discusses two major components: fault-tolerant PACS and enterprise PACS. Without the fault-tolerant PACS design, it is very risky to develop an enterprise PACS. Enterprise PACS should be coupled with the teleradiology operation, and together they should be integrated to the ePR with image distribution.

Enterprise PACS with image distribution is the remaining frontier of PACS implementation. Enterprise PACS entails:

- Very large system integration
- Several years for implementation
- Expensive outlays
- Contributions by both the enterprise and the imaging manufacturer/system integrator
- Both PACS and Web-based technology in place
- Web-based ePR image distribution to referring and clinical sites

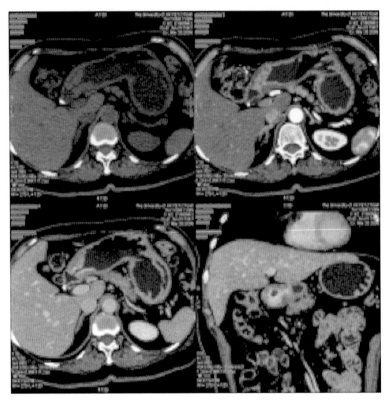

Figure 16.26   Patient B: Various views of contrast CT abdominal scan correlated with the endoscopy images. Notice that the enhancing mucosal thickening over the gastric pylorus indicates a malignant tumor. The CT shows deep mural involvement and regional lymphadenopathy. (Courtesy of Dr. T. Chan)

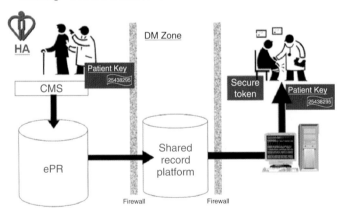

Figure 16.27   Public–private interface schematic showing the electronic patient record (PPI–ePR) sharing project of the Hospital Authority of Hong Kong (see also Fig. 16.18). (Courtesy of Dr. T. Chan)

Enterprise PACS with ePR-based image distribution would nevertheless be cost-effective and efficient for large-scale healthcare if implemented properly. The several large-scale enterprise-level PACS with image distribution around the world mentioned in this section and in Chapters 19 and 7.2 have proved their cost-effectiveness and improvement in healthcare delivery.

References

Avizienis A. Toward systematic design of fault-tolerant systems. *Computer* 30(4): 51–8; 1997.

Bajpai G, Chang BC, Kwatny HG. Design of fault-tolerant systems for actuator failures in nonlinear systems. *Proc Am Control Conf* 5: 3618–23; 2002.

Cao F, Huang HK, Liu BJ, Zhou MZ, Zhang J, Mogel GT. Fault-tolerant PACS server. *Radiology* 221(P): 737; 2001.

Cao F, Liu BJ, Huang HK, Zhou Z, Zhang J, Zhang X, Mogel G. Fault-tolerant PACS server. *SPIE Med Imag* 4685: 316–25; 2002.

Carrasco JA. Computationally efficient and numerically stable reliability bounds for repairable fault-tolerant systems. *IEEE Trans Comp* 51(3): 254–68; 2002.

Cheung NT, Lam A, Chan W, Kong HB. Integrating images into electronic patient record of the hospital authority of Hong Kong. *Computerized Medical Imaging and Graphics* 29: 137–142; 2005.

Compaq/Tandem. *Non Stop Himalaya*. http://www.tandem.comdel.

Gobbo D, Cukic B, Napolitano R, Easterbrook S. Fault detectability analysis for requirements validation of fault tolerant systems. *High-Assur Syst Eng*, Proc 4th IEEE Int Symp: 231–8; 1999.

Fabre JC, Perennou T. A meta object architecture for fault-tolerant distributed systems: the FRIENDS approach. *IEEE Trans Comp* 47(1): 78–95; 1998.

Huang HK. *PACS: Basic Principles and Applications*. New York: Wiley; 1999.

Huang HK, Cao F, Zhang JG, Liu BJ, Tsai ML. Fault tolerant picture archiving and communication system and teleradiology design. In: Reiner B, Siegel EL, Dwyer SJ, eds. *Security Issues in the Digital Medical Enterprise*. Great Falls, VA: SCAR, 57–64; 2000.

Huang HK, Cao F, Zhang J. Fault tolerant design and implementation of the PACS controller. RSNA InfoRAD Exhibit 9609; 2000.

Huang HK, Liu BJ. Coverage by diagnostic imaging. http://www.dimag.com/webcast00/archives.shtml; 27 Nov 2000.

Huang HK, Cao F, Zhang J, Liu B, Tsai ML. Fault tolerant picture archiving and communication system and teleradiology design. In: Bruce IR, et al., eds. *Security Issues in the Digital Medical Enterprise*. Great Falls, VA: SCAR; 2000a.

Huang HK, Cao F, Zhang JZ. Fault-tolerant design and implementation of the PACS controller. *Radiology* 217(P): 519, 709; 2000b.

Huang HK, Cao F, Liu BJ, Zhou MZ, Zhang J, Mogel GT. PACS simulator: a standalone educational tool. *Radiology* 221(P): 688; 2001a.

Huang HK, Cao F, Liu BJ, Zhang J, Zhou Z, Tsai A, Mogel G. Fault-tolerant PACS server design. *SPIE Med Imag* 4323: 83–92; 2001b.

Huang HK, Cao F, Liu BJ, Zhou MZ, Zhang J, Mogel G. A complete continuous-availability PACS archive server solution. 225(P): 692; 2002.

IBM S/390 Parallel Sysplex. http://ibm.com.

Institute of Electrical and Electronics Engineers. A compilation of IEEE standard computer glossaries. In: *IEEE Standard Computer Dictionary*. New York: IEEE; 1990.

Kanoun K, Ortalo-Borrel M. Fault-tolerant system dependability-explicit modeling of hardware and software component-interactions. *IEEE Trans Reliab* 49(4): 363–76; 2000.

Latif-Shabgahi G, Bass JM, Bennett S. History-based weighted average voter: a novel software voting algorithm for fault-tolerant computer systems. *Parallel and Distributed Processing. Proc 9th Euromicro Workshop*; 2001.

Liu BJ, Huang HK, Cao F, Documet L, Sarti DA. A fault-tolerant back-up archive using an ASP model for disaster recovery. *Radiology* 221(P): 741; 2001.

Liu BJ, Huang HK, Cao F, Documet L, Sarti DA. A fault-tolerant back-up archive using an ASP model for disaster recovery. *SPIE Med Imag* 4685: 89–95; 2002.

Liu BJ, Huang HK, Cao F, Documet L, Muldoon J. Clinical experiences with an ASP model backup archive for PACS images. *Radiology*, 225(P): 313; 2002.

Muller G, Banatre M, Peyrouze N, Rochat B. Lessons from FTM: an experiment in design and implementation of a low-cost fault tolerant system. *IEEE Trans Reliab* 45(2): 332–40; 1996.

Reiner BI, Siegel EL, Dwyer SJ, III. *Security Issues in the Digital Medical Enterprise*. Great Falls, VA: SCAR; 2000.

Resilience Corporation. Ultra2 Solaris servers. http://www.resilience.com.

Resilience Corporation. Technical Report. 2000. IMEX Research.com.

Smith DV, Smith S, Bender GN, et al. Evaluation of the medical diagnostic image support system based on 2 years of clinical experience. *J Digit Imag* 8(2): 75–87; 1995.

Some RR, Beahan J, Khanoyan G, Callum LN, Agrawal A. Fault-tolerant systems design— estimating cache contents and usage. *Proc IEEE Aerospace Conf* 5: 2149–58; 2002.

Sun Microsystem. http://www.sun.com.

Trivedi K, Dugan JB, Geist R, Smotherman M. Modeling imperfect coverage in fault-tolerant systems: fault-tolerant computing. *Highlights from Twenty-Five Years. 25th Int Symp*: 176; 1995.

Xu J, Randell B, Romanovsky A, Stroud RJ, Zorzo AF, Canver E, Von Henke F. Rigorous development of an embedded fault-tolerant system based on coordinated atomic actions. *IEEE Trans Comp* 51(2): 164–79, 402–9; 2002.

Bauman RA, Gell G, Dwyer SJ III. Large picture arching and communication systems of the world—Parts 1 and 2. *J Digit Imag* 9(3–4): 99–103, 172–7; 1996.

Dayhoff RE, Meldrum K, Kuzmak PM, Experience providing a complete online multimedia patient record. Session 38. *Healthcare Information and Management Systems Society*, 2001 An Conf and Exhib; 4–8 Feb 2001.

GE Medical Systems. Technical White Paper Cluster PACS. "Pilot project" proposal for Hong Kong Hospital Authority; Feb 2002.

Ha D-H, Moon M-S. Effectiveness of wireless communication using 100 Mbps infrared in PACS. Dept. of Diagnostic Radiology and PACS team, Pundang CHA General Hospital, Pochon CHA University, Sungnam, Korea. *Proc SPIE Med Imag*; 2002.

Huang HK. *PACS: Basic Principles and Applications*. New York: Wiley; 1999.

Huang HK. Consultancy study of image distribution and PACS in Hong Kong. Final report. HA 105/26 VII CL; 21 Mar 2002.

Huang HK. Development of a digital medical imaging archiving and communication system (MIACS) for services of Department of Health. HKSAR government. Final report; 15 Jul 2002.

Hur G, Cha SJ, et al. The impact of PACS in hospital management. Dept. of Radiology, Inje University Ilsan Paik Hospital, Korea. *Proc SPIE Med Imag* 4685, 64–71; 2002.

Inamura K, Kousaka S, Yamamoto Y, et al. PACS development in Asia *Comp Med Imaging Graphics* 27(2–3): 121–8; 2003.

Kim H-J. PACS industry in Korea. Dept. of Radiology, Yonsei University College of Medicine, Seoul, Korea. *Proc SPIE Med Imag* 4685, 50–57; 2002.

Kim JH. Technical aspects of PACS in Korea. Dept. of Radiology, Seoul National University Hospital, Seoul National University. *Proc SPIE Med Imag* 4685, 58–63; 2002.

Lemke HU, Niederlag W, Houser H. Specification and evaluation of a regional PACS in the SaxTeleMed project. Technical University Berlin, FR 3–3, CG & CAM. *Proc SPIE Med Imag* 4685, 1–15; 2002.

Lim JH. Cost-justification on filmless PACS and national policy. Dept. of Radiology, Samsung Medical Center, Sungkyunkwan University School of Medicine, Seoul, Korea. *Proc SPIE Med Imag*, 4685, 72–74; 2002.

Lim H, Kim DO, Ahn JY, et al. Full PACS installation in Seoul National University Hospital, Korea. *Proc SPIE Med Imag*, 4685, 75–82; 2002.

Philips Medical Systems. Image distribution and PACS system for Hong Kong Health Authority; Feb 2002.

Siemens Medical Solutions. *Future of Imaging and Beyond in Hong Kong*; Feb 2002.

Sim J, Kang K, Lim M-K., et al. Connecting and sharing medical images among three big full PACS hospitals in Korea. *Proc EuroPACS 20th Int Conf*, Oulu, Finland: 22–24; 5–7 Sep 2002.

CHAPTER 17

Image/Data Security

Medical image/data security is mandated by HIPAA (Health Insurance Portability and Accountability Act) to ensure that patients' records have protection of privacy. Although the DICOM standard provides a standard for the medical image industry to follow, this standard has not been enforced. This chapter discusses the concept of image/data security, some basic terminology, and methods used to secure data. Figure 17.1 (excerpted from Fig. 1.3) shows how this chapter corresponds to other chapters of Part III. Figure 17.2 shows the components (pink) involved image/data security in the PACS and teleradiology data flow.

17.1 INTRODUCTION AND BACKGROUND

17.1.1 Introduction

Data security becomes a critical issue not only when digital images and pertinent patient information are stored in an ASP off-site backup archive system but also during the transmission of these data through public networks in telemedicine and teleradiology applications. Generally, trust in digital data is characterized in terms of privacy, authenticity, and integrity of the data. Privacy refers to denial of access to information by unauthorized individuals. Authenticity means validating the source of a message, that is, that it was transmitted by a properly identified sender. Integrity refers to the assurance that the data had not been modified accidentally or deliberately in transit, by replacement, insertion, or deletion. Conventional Internet security methods are not sufficient to guarantee that image/data had not been compromised during data transmission through unsecured networks. Techniques including network fire walls, data encryption, and data embedding are used for additional data protection in other fields of applications like financial, banking, and reservation systems. However, these techniques were not systematically applied to medical imaging, partly because of the lack of urgency, until the recent HIPAA mandated requirements on patient data security.

In this chapter we present a digital envelope (DE) method used to ensure image/data security while the data reside in the archive and during data transmission through public communication networks. This method can also be used within an institution if image/data security is needed. In this chapter a medical image *digital signature* (DS) is defined as the encrypted message digest of the image using

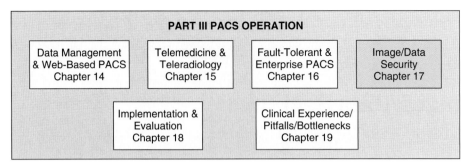

Figure 17.1 Position of Chapter 17 in the organization of this book. Color codes are used to highlight components and workflow in the chapters of Part III.

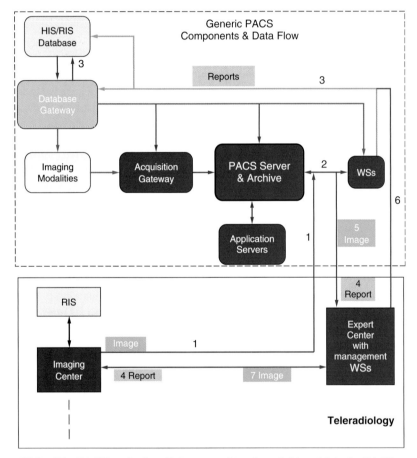

Figure 17.2 The PACS and teleradiology combined model in which the PACS supports imaging centers for teleradiology reading, or PACS and teleradiology support each other (excerpted from Fig. 7.7). The top rectangle is the PACS components and workflow (excerpted from Fig. 7.2), and the bottom rectangle is the teleradiology model modified from Fig. 7.6. Pink boxes and lines are components required image/data security. See Section 7.5.2 for explanation of workflow steps in numerals.

existing public domain hashing algorithms. A medical image *digital envelope* (DE) is defined as the DS plus the encrypted relevant patient information in the DICOM (Digital Imaging and Communication in Medicine) image header. The *residing site* is where the image is being stored, the *sending site* (SS) is where the image is originated, and the *receiving site* (RS) is where the image is received. *Image/data* means the image plus relevant patient information.

17.1.2 Background

Security is an extremely critical issue when image/data are residing in an archive, and transmitted across a public network (James et al., 1993; Berger and Cepelewicz, 1996; Berlin, 1998; Kamp, 1996). With current technology and know-how, it is not difficult to get access to the storage and network inserting artifacts within the image/data that defy detection. So image/data can be compromised without the knowledge of the owner. We give two examples in digital mammography (projection image) and chest CT (sectional image) to illustrate how easy it is to change medical digital images. Figure 17.3 shows a digital mammogram with 2-D artificial calcifications inserted (Zhou et al., 2001). Figure 17.3*A* is the original mammogram, 17.3*B* is the mammogram with artificial calcifications added, 17.3*C* is the magnification of a region containing some added artifacts, and 17.3*D* is the subtracted images between the original and modified mammograms. The calcifications are very small, subtle objects within a mammogram. If inserted, the artifacts will confuse the diagnostic process. Recall from Sections 15.5.2 and 15.5.3 the CT scan of the chest in Figure 15.8 (left) shows, and the 3-D artificial lesion inserted in Figure 15.8 (right).

Three major organizations in the United States are charged with ensuring medical image/data security. They have issued guidelines, mandates, and standards for image/data security. The ACR (American College of Radiology) Standard for Teleradiology, adopted in 1994, defines guidelines for "qualifications of both physician and nonphysician personnel, equipment specifications, quality improvement, licensure, staff credentialing, and liability." The Health Insurance Portability and Accountability Act (HIPAA) of 1996, Public Law 104-191, which amends the Internal Revenue Service Code of 1986 (HIPAA, 2000), requires certain patient privacy and data security. Part 15 of the DICOM Standard (PS 3.15-2000) specifies security profiles and technical means for application entities involved in exchanging information to implement security policies (DICOM, 1996). In addition SCAR (Society of Computer Applications in Radiology, the name of the society had been changed to the Society for Imaging Informatics in Medicine [SIIM] in 2006) has issued a primer on "Security issues in digital medical enterprise," which it presented before the 86th RSNA meeting in 2000, to emphasize the urgency and importance of this matter (Huang, 2000). Despite these initiatives the medical imaging community has yet initiate active systematic research and development efforts in tackling this issue. Data are still being protected by network fire walls, data encryption, and data embedding based on the different situations of data use. In telemedicine and teleradiology, because data cannot be limited within a private local area network protected by a fire wall, data encryption and data embedding are the most useful approaches.

Current cryptography can use either private key or public key methods (Garfinkel and Spafford, 1996; Schneier, 1995). Private key cryptography (symmetric cryptography) uses the same key for data encryption and decryption. It requires that

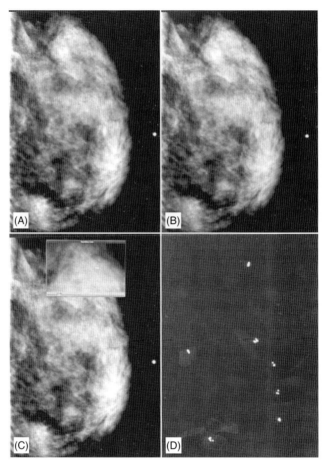

Figure 17.3 An example of a digital mammogram with inserted artificial calcifications. (A) Original mammogram, (B) with artifacts, (C) subtracted between (A) and (B) with a window confining the artifacts, (D) magnification of the artifacts within the window. The artifacts are highlighted with overexposure during display.

both the sender and receiver agree on a key before they can exchange a message securely. Although the computational speed of performing private key cryptograph is acceptable, it is difficult for key management. Public key cryptography (asymmetric cryptography) uses two different keys (a public key and a private key) for encryption and decryption. The keys in a key pair are mathematically related, but it is computationally infeasible to deduce the private key from the public key. Therefore, in public key cryptography, the public key can be made public.

Anyone can use the public key to encrypt a message, but only the owner of the corresponding private key can decrypt it. Public key methods are more convenient to use because they do not share the key management problem inherent in private key methods. However, public keep require longer times for encryption and decryption. In real-world implementation, public key encryption is rarely used to encrypt actual messages. Instead, it is used to distribute symmetric keys to encrypt and decrypt actual messages.

Digital signature (DS) is a major application of public key cryptography (Schneier, 1995). To generate a signature on an image, the owner of the private key first computes a condensed representation of the image known as an image hash value (or image digest), which is then encrypted by using mathematical techniques specified in public key cryptography to produce a DS. Any party with access to the owner's public key, image, and signature can verify the signature by the following procedure: First compute the image hash value with the same algorithm for the received image, decrypt the signature with the owner's public key to obtain the hash value computed by the owner, and compare the two image hash values.

The mechanism of obtaining the hash is designed in such a way that even a slight change in the input string would cause the hash value to change drastically. If the two hash values are the same, the receiver (or any other party) has the confidence that the image have been signed off by the owner of the private key and that the image had not been altered after it was signed off. Thus it ensures the image integrity.

In this chapter, an evolving image security system based on the digital envelope (DE) concept is introduced to ensure data integrity, authenticity, and privacy during image/data transmission through public networks. DE includes the DS of the image as well as selected patient information from the DICOM image header. Evolving means that any new and better encryption and security algorithms can replace those discussed in this chapter without affecting the DE principle. In telemedicine and teleradiology, data cannot be limited within a private local area network protected by a fire wall. Therefore DE offers the most useful security assurance. This method also provides additional image/data assurance to conventional data storage and network security protections.

17.2 IMAGE/DATA SECURITY METHODS

17.2.1 Four Steps in Digital Signature and Digital Envelope

The image/data security method presented in this chapter uses the DE concept. The DE method involves both the sender side and the receiver side. The sender side is data encryption and embedding, which consists of four steps:

1. Image preprocessing: To segment the image from its background and extract relevant patient information from DICOM image header.
2. Image hashing: To compute an image hash value of the segmented image using some existing hash algorithm.
3. Data encryption: To produce a DE containing the hash value of the encrypted image (DS of the image) and the relevant patient information.
4. Data embedding: To embed the DE into the image or the background of the image. The embedding should not affect the quality of the image. For digital radiography the embedding method is different than for the sectional image because the former may not have a background in the image for embedding the DE but the latter's background is very prominent. (In Section 17.7 we introduce the lossless DS embedding method by which the embedding can be done anywhere in the image without affecting the quality of the original image.)

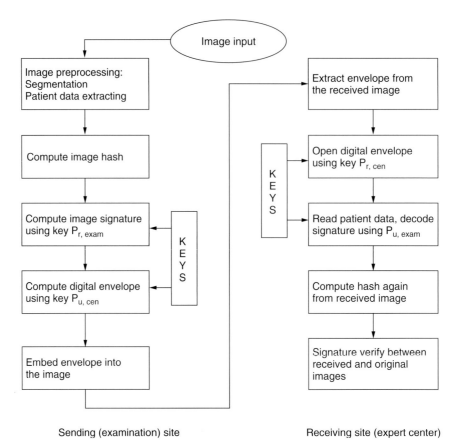

Figure 17.4   The block diagram of the encryption and embedding algorithm. (left) data encryption and embedding. $P_{r,exam}$, $P_{u,cen}$ are the private key of the examination site (sending site, SS) and the public key of the expert center (receiving site, RS), respectively. (right) data extraction and decryption. $P_{r,cen}$, $P_{u,exam}$ are the private key of the RS (expert center) and the public key of the SS (examination site), respectively.

The receiver side is data extraction and decryption, which reverses the process of these four steps.

17.2.2   General Methodology

The general methodology and description of the algorithm of the DS and DE are shown in Figure 17.4. In this description, sending site (SS) and receiving site (RS) are synonymous with examination site and expert center, respectively. Table 17.1 lists the symbols used in this section.

17.3   DIGITAL ENVELOPE

The digital envelope method involves data encryption and embedding in the sender side and data extraction and decryption in the receiver side.

TABLE 17.1   Symbols used in the digital envelope method

LSB	Least significant bit
ID	Image digest
IM	Segmented image
DS	Digital signature
DE	Digital envelope
SS	Sending site
RS	Receiving site
RSA_E	RSA public-key encryption algorithm
RSA_D	RSA public-key decryption algorithm
DES	Data encryption standard
DES_E	DES encryption algorithm
DES_D	DES decryption algorithm
$P_{r,\ exam}$	Private key of the examination site
$P_{u,\ exam}$	Public key of the examination site
$P_{r,\ cen}$	Private key of the expert center
$P_{u,\ cen}$	Public key of the expert center

17.3.1   Image Signature, Envelope, Encryption, and Embedding

17.3.1.1 Image Preprocessing   There are two parts to the preprocessing step. The first is segmentation with background removal or cropping of the image, which is done by finding the minimum rectangle covering the object (Huang, 1999; Zhou, 2000; see also Chapter 6). In digital radiography like the mammogram, the segmented image would be the breast region without the compression plate (Fig. 17.5*A* and *B*). In a sectional image like the MRI head, it would be the image inside the smallest rectangle enclosing the head. The first two columns in Figure 17.5*C* show the original and segmented sagittal, transverse, and coronal images, respectively. By cropping large amounts of background pixels from the image, the time necessary for performing image hashing within the image can be significantly reduced. Extracting the boundary of the image region can also guarantee that data embedding is performed outside of the image. If the minimum rectangle is the boundaries of the complete image, then embedding is performed in the least significant bit in the entire image. The second part of the embedding step is to extract patient information from the DICOM image header.

17.3.1.2 Hashing (Image Digest)   Begin by computing the hash value for all pixels in the image:

$$ID = H(IM) \tag{17.1}$$

where ID is the hash value of the image, H is the MD5 (message digest, see reference in this chapter) hashing algorithm, and IM represents the segmented image. MD5 has the characteristics of a one-way hash function (Rivest, 2000). It is easy to generate a hash given an image [H(IM) $\rightarrow$ ID] but virtually impossible to generate the image given a hash value (ID $\rightarrow$ IM). Also MD5 is "collision resistant." It is computationally difficult to find two images that have the same hash value. In other

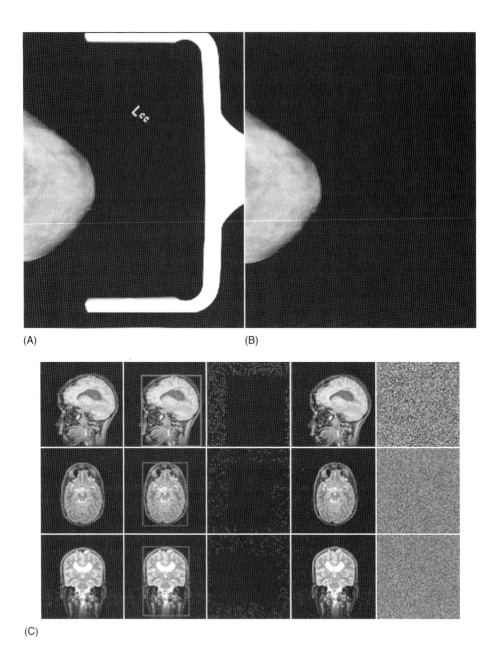

(A)   (B)

(C)

Figure 17.5 Example of background removal in a mammogram. (*A*) Original digital
mammogram with the compression plate; (B) mammogram with background removal.
(C) Rows 1, 2, and 3: sagittal, transverse, and coronal MRI, respectively. Columns 1, 2,
3, 4, and 5: the original, segmented, embedded, encrypted DS outside of the image (dots),
digital envelope = segmented + encrypted DS, and the encrypted digital envelope.

TABLE 17.2   Some core cryptography tools for generating digital envelope and managing digital certificate

Hash algorithm	MD5, SHA1, MDC, RIPEMD
Private-key encryption	DES, TripleDES, AES
Public-key encryption	RSA, ElGamal
Digital signature	RSA, DSS

Note: DES: data encryption standard; AES: advanced encryption standard; DSS: digital signature standard.

words, the chance of two images having the same hash value is small and dependent on the hash algorithm used (Kaliski, 1993). Currently there are better hash functions than MD5; some of these are shown in Table 17.2.

17.3.1.3 *Digital Signature*   Produce a digital signature based on the image hash value obtained in step 2:

$$DS = RSA_E \ (P_{r,exam}, ID) \qquad (17.2)$$

where DS is the digital signature of the segmented image, RSA_E represents the RSA public key encryption algorithm (Kaliski, 1993), and $P_{r,exam}$ is the private key of the examination site (sending site, SS). Figure 17.6A shows the MD5 hash value of the background-removed digital mammogram of Figure 17.5B, and Figure 17.6B is the corresponding DS.

17.3.1.4 *Digital Envelope*   Concatenate the DS and the patient data together as a data stream and encrypt them with the data encryption standard (DES) algorithm (Schneier, 1995).

$$data_{encrypted} = DES_E \ (key_{DES}, data_{concat}) \qquad (17.3)$$

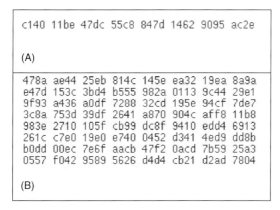

Figure 17.6   Hash value and the corresponding digital signature. (*A*) MD5 hash value of the background-removed mammogram shown in Figure 17.5*B*. (*B*) The corresponding digital signature.

where data$_{encrypted}$ represents data encrypted by DES, DESE is the DES encryption algorithm, key$_{DES}$ is a session key produced randomly by the cryptography library, and data$_{concat}$ is the concatenated data stream of the image DS and patient information.

The DES session key is further encrypted:

$$key_{encrypted} = RSA_E(P_{u,cen}, key_{DES})$$ (17.4)

where key$_{encrypted}$ is the encrypted session key and P$_{u,cen}$ is the public key of the expert center (receiving site, RS).

Finally, the DE is produced by concatenating the encrypted data stream and encrypted session key together:

$$DE = (data_{encrypted}) \text{ conc. } (key_{encrypted})$$ (17.5)

Figure 17.7*A* is the merged data file of DS and the patient information. Figure 17.7*B* is the corresponding DE to be embedded into the image.

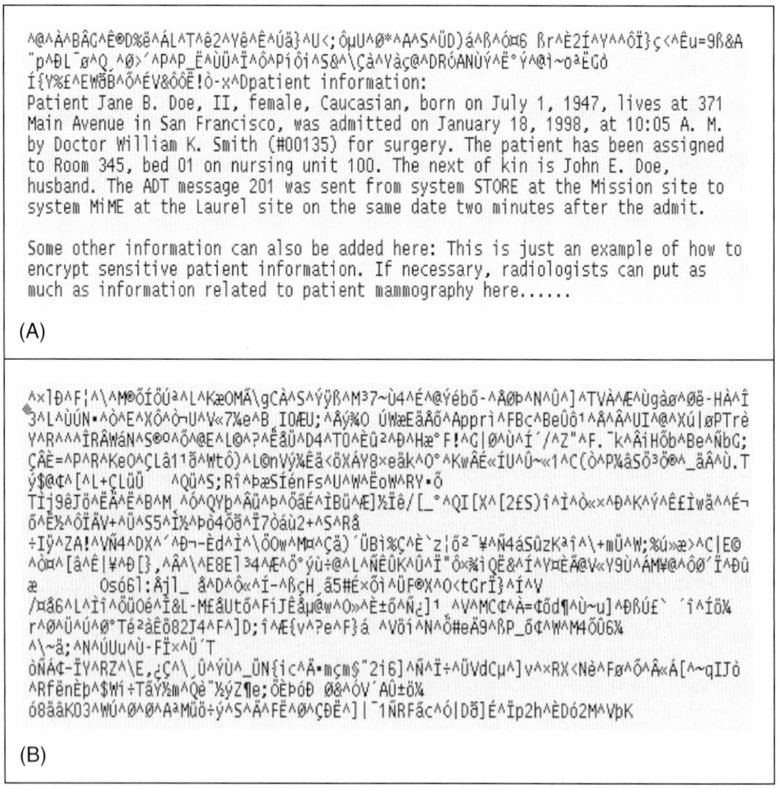

```
^@^À^BÂÇ^Ê©D%ë^ÁL^T^ê2^Yê^Ê^Úä}^U<;ÒµU^Ø*^A^S^ÚD}á^ß^Ó¤ß  ßr^È2Í^Y^^ÔÏ}ç<^Êu=9ß&A
"p^ÐL¯ø^Q¸^Ø>´^P^P_Ë^ÙÜ^Î^Ô^Pí Ôí^S&^\Çà^Yàç@^DRóANÙÝ^Ë°Ý^Øî~oªËÇô
í{Y%£^EWÖB^Õ^ÉV&ÒÒÊ!Ò-x^Dpatient information:
Patient Jane B. Doe, II, female, Caucasian, born on July 1, 1947, lives at 371
Main Avenue in San Francisco, was admitted on January 18, 1998, at 10:05 A. M.
by Doctor William K. Smith (#00135) for surgery. The patient has been assigned
to Room 345, bed 01 on nursing unit 100. The next of kin is John E. Doe,
husband. The ADT message 201 was sent from system STORE at the Mission site to
system MiME at the Laurel site on the same date two minutes after the admit.

Some other information can also be added here: This is just an example of how to
encrypt sensitive patient information. If necessary, radiologists can put as
much as information related to patient mammography here......
```
(A)

```
^×1Ð^F¦^\^AM®ÒÍÓÚª^L^Kæ0MÄ\gCÀ^S^Ýÿß^M37~Ù4^É^@Ýêbô-^A@Þ^N^Û^]^TVÀ^Æ^Ùgàø^Øë-HÀ^Î
¯3^L^ÙÜN•^Ô^É^X0^Ô^Ò¬U^V«7%ø^B¸I0ÆU;^AÝ%0 ÚW±ÉäÅô^Apprì^FBç^BeÜô¹^AÂ^Â^UI^@^Xú|øPTrè
Y^R^^^ÎRÂWáN^S®o^Ô^@E^L^Ø^?^ÉäÜ^D4^TO^Èü²^Ð^Hæ°F!^Ç|Ø^Ù^Î¯/^Z^^F.¯k^ÂîHÔb^Bе^ÑbÇ;
ÇÂÈ^=^P^R^Ke0^ÇLâ1¹Õ^Wtô}^L@nVÿ%Êä<ÒXÁÝ8xeäk^O°^Kw^AÉ«ÍU^Û~«1^C(Ò^P%äSÕ³Õ®^_äÂ^Ù.T
ÿ$@¢^[^L+ÇLÜÜ  ^QÛ^S;Rî^Þ�æSíénFs^U^W^ÆÊoW^RY•Õ
TÍj9êJÖ^ÊÂ^É^B^M ^Ô^QÝþ^Âü^Þ^ÕäÉ^ÎBÛ^Æ]%Îê/[_°^QI[X^[2£S)î^Î^Ô«×^Ð^K^Ý^É£Îwä^^É¬
Õ^Ê%^ÔÎÄV+^Û^S5^Î%^Þô4ÕÕ^Î7Òáú2+^S^Râ
+Iÿ^ZA!^VÑ4^DX^´^Ð¬-ÉdÎ^\ÕÕw^Mo^Çä) ´ÜBì%Ç^È`z¦ô²¯¥^Ñ4áSÙzK³î^\+mÛ^W;%ú»æ>^C|EÖ
^Ôo^[â^É|¥^Ð[},^ÂÂ^\^E8E1³4^AÈ^Ô°ÿü+@^L^ÑÉÜK^Û^Î"Õ×%ì QÊ&^Î^Y¤É^@V«Y9Ù^AM¥@^Ôø¯Î^Ðü
æ    Os06¦:Âj1_ ê^D^Ô«^Î-^Bçн_ä5HÉ×Õî^ÛF®X^A0<tÇrÎ}^Î^V
/¤â6^L^Îî^ÕÜ0ê^Î&L-MÊäUtÔ^FíJÊâµ@w^O»^È±Õ^Ñ¿]¹ ^V^MC¢^A=¢Õd¶^Ù~u]^Ð-ß-ÚÉ` ¯î^ÎÕ%
r^Ø^Ä^Ù^Ú^Ø°Té²âÊÕ82J4^F^]D;î^ÆÏ{v^?e^F}á ^VÕî^N^Ô#eÄ9^ßP_Õ¢^W^M^4^ÕÜ6%
^\~ä;^N^ÜUu^Ù-FÏ×^Ù´T
òÑÁ¢-ÎY^RZ^\E,¿Ç^\¸Û^YÙª_ÛN{íc^Â•mçm§"2í6]^Ñ^Î+^ÛVdCµ^]v^×RX<Nê^Fø^Ô^Â«Á[^~qIJò
^RFënÈþ^$Ŵí+TäÝ%m^Që¯%ÿZ¶e;ÒÈÞôÐ Ø&^ÕV¯AÛ±Õ%
ó8äâK03^WÚ^Ø^Ø^Aª^MÜö+ÿ^S^Â^FÊ^Ø^ÇÐË^]|¯1ÑRFáç^ÓÍ|Dõ]É^Îp2h^ÈÔ62M^VþK
```
(B)

Figure 17.7 (*A*) Combined data file of the digital signature and patient information. Two and a half lines (up to the word "patient ... ") of data is the digital signature displayed in ASC II format identical to Figure 17.6*B*, displayed in hexadecimal format. (*B*) Its encrypted format using the public key of the expert center.

17.3.1.5 *Data Embedding* Replace the least significant bit of a random pixel in the segmented image, outside of the image boundary or within the image (see Fig. 17.8*B*), depending on whether a minimum rectangle is found, by one bit of the digital envelope bit stream and repeat for all bits in the bit stream.

First, a set of pseudorandom numbers X_n is generated by using the standard random generator shown in Eq. (17.6):

$$X_{n+1} = (aX_n + C)\bmod m \qquad (17.6)$$

where a is a multiplier, C is an additive constant, and m is the mod denoting the modulus operation. Equation (17.6) represents the standard linear congruential generator; the three parameters are determined by the size of the image. In the example shown in Figure 17.8*B*, a, C, and m were set to be 2416; 37,444; and 1,771,875; respectively, based on the characteristics of the digital mammograms.

To start, both the SS and the RS decide a random number X_0, called the seed. The seed is then the single number through which a set of random numbers is generated by Eq. (17.6). Unlike other computer network security problems in key management, the numbers of SS and RS are limited in the teleradiology or telemedicine application; the seed management issue can be easily handled by a mutual agreement between the SS and RS.

Second, a random walk sequence in the whole segmented image is obtained:

$$\text{WalkAddress}_n = M\left(\frac{X_n}{m}\right) \qquad (17.7)$$

where WalkAddress$_n$ is the location of the nth randomly selected pixel in the segmented image, M is the total number of pixels in the segmented mammogram, and m is the mod defined in Eq. (17.6).

Finally, the bit stream in the envelope described in Eq. (17.5) is embedded into the least significant bit (LSB) of each of these randomly selected pixels along the walk sequence. Figure 17.8*A* is the digital mammogram shown in Figure 17.5*B*; Figure 17.8*B* is the mammogram with the DE embedded, and Figure 17.8*C* is the subtracted image between Figure 17.8*A* and 17.8*B*. Each dot in Figure 17.8*C* shows the location of the pixel in which DE data had been embedded in the LSB. Note that this embedding does not affect the quality of the image because the LSB is noise in a digital radiograph (mammogram in this case; see Zhou).

The four steps of image security: image segmentation, DE generation, data embedding, and encryption using the sagittal, transverse, and coronal MR images were shown in Figure 17.5*C*. We use the sagittal MRI in Figure 17.9 (upper) with mockup signature data as an example to demonstrate the complete process of data encryption and embedding at the sender side.

17.3.2 Data Extraction and Decryption

In the RS, the image and the DE are received. The image authenticity and integrity can be verified by using the DS in the envelope with a series of reverse procedures shown in the bottom of Figure 17.9 (Zhou et al., 2001). First, the same walk sequence

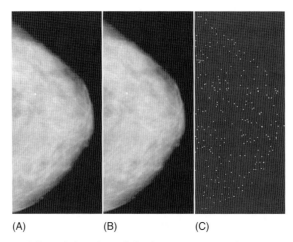

(A)   (B)   (C)

Figure 17.8   (From left to right): the original mammogram, the mammogram with digital envelope embedded, and the subtracted image between the original and the imbedded mammogram. Small white pixels in (*C*) are where DE is embedded in the LSB.

in the image is generated by the same seed known to the SS, so that the embedded digital envelope can be extracted correctly from the LSBs of these randomly selected pixels. Then the encrypted session key in the digital envelope is restored:

$$\text{key}_{\text{DES}} = \text{RSA}_{\text{D}}(\text{P}_{\text{r,cen}}, \text{key}_{\text{encrypted}}) \tag{17.8}$$

where RSA_{D} is the RSA public key decryption algorithm, $\text{P}_{\text{r,cen}}$ is the private key expert center (RS). After that, the digital envelope can be opened by the recovered session key, and the digital signature and the patient data can be recovered:

$$\text{data}_{\text{merged}} = \text{DES}_{\text{D}}(\text{key}_{\text{DES}}, \text{data}_{\text{encrypted}}) \tag{17.9}$$

where DES_{D} is the DES decryption algorithm. Finally, the image digest (ID, see Eq. 17.1) is recovered by decrypting the digital signature:

$$\text{ID} = \text{RSA}_{\text{D}}(\text{P}_{\text{u,exam}}, \text{DS}) \tag{17.10}$$

where $\text{P}_{\text{u,exam}}$ is the public key of the examination site (SS). At the same time a second image hash value is calculated from the received image with the same hash algorithm shown in Eq. (17.1) used by the sending site. If the recovered image hash value from Eq. (17.10) and the original image hash value match, then the receiving site can be assured that this image is really from the examination site and that none of the pixels in the image had been modified. Therefore the requirements of image authentication and integrity have been satisfied. The RSAREF toolkit (RSAref 2.0, released by RSA Data Security, Inc.) can be used to implement the data encryption part in this method.

   Although we use the terms sending site (SS) and receiving site (RS) in the case of teleradiology, in archive image/data assurance we consider the SS to be where the DS is generated, and the RS to be where the assurance is required.

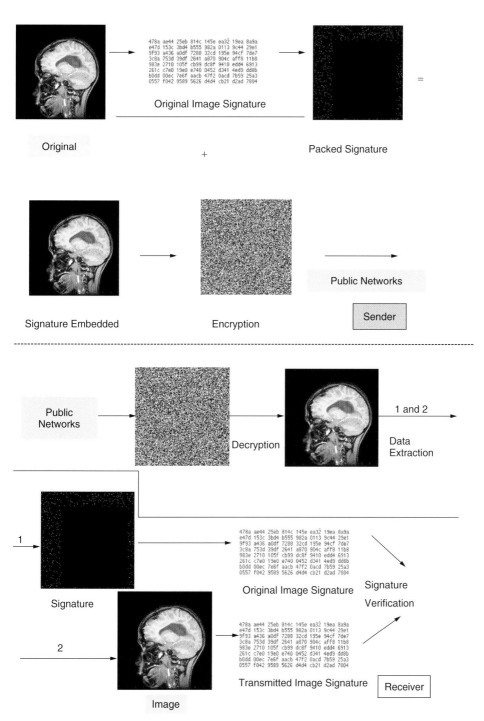

Figure 17.9 Principle of image integrity and steps of forming the digital envelope. (top) the sender; (bottom) the receiver. A mock-up of image signature data was used for demonstration purpose.

```
147a a78e a5c9 db08 d2fe dd6e 2447 1621

Different from the hash value in Fig. 17.6A
```

Figure 17.10 MD5 hash value of the data-embedded mammogram shown in Figure 17.8B after the value of one randomly selected pixel in the image was changed from a value of 14 to 12. It is totally different from the hash shown in Figure 17.6A.

17.3.3 Methods of Evaluation of the Digital Envelope

Three parameters—robustness of the method, percentage of the pixel changes, and time required to execute—can be used to evaluate the performance of the digital envelope method described in Section 17.3 (Zhou et al., 2001).

17.3.3.1 *Robustness of the Hash Function* The robustness of the hash function can be evaluated by changing one random pixel in the image with the digital signature and recalculating the hash value. In the example shown in Figure 17.8B, if one pixel in the embedded mammogram is changed from a value of 14 to 12, the hash value becomes completely different, as seen by comparing Figure 17.6A with Figure 17.10.

17.3.3.2 *Percentage of the Pixel Changed in Data Embedding* In the example shown in Figure 17.8B and C, the total pixels in which the LSBs were changed during data embedding are 3404, which accounts for 0.12% of the total pixels in the segmented mammogram. Since one character in the digital envelope has 8 bits, and there are 840 characters in the digital envelope that give a total of 6720 bits. During embedding, only 3404 bits were required to be changed and 3316 bits remain unchanged. The percentage of pixel change is a parameter for evaluating the performance of the algorithm, which is computed by

Total % pixel changed

$$= \left[\left(\text{Number of characters in envelope} \times 8\text{bits} - \frac{\text{Unaffected LSBs)}}{M} \right) \right] \times 100 \tag{17.11}$$

where M is the total number of pixels.

17.3.3.3 *Time Required to Run the Complete Image/Data Security Assurance* The time required to run the security assurance depends on the size of the segmented image, the algorithms used, and the efficiency of the software programming. Table 17.3 shows the time required with the AIDM to process the mammogram shown in Figure 17.5B. The results are based on one image, but that image provides a glimpse into the time required for such the assurance method. The procedures of embedding data, and extracting data refer to the time required for embedding the DE into the mammogram, and extracting back the DE from the embedded mammogram, respectively. For signing the document and verifying the signature, most of the computational time is taken by computing the image hash value. The purpose of this table is to show the relative time required for the encryption and decryption

TABLE 17.3   Time required for processing of mammogram shown in Figure 17.5*B* using the digital signature method of Section 17.3

Procedures in Examination Site	Time (s)	Procedures in Expert Center	Time (s)
Signing the signature	20	Extracting data	19
Sealing the envelope	<1	Opening the envelope	<1
Embedding data	17	Verifying the signature	17
Total	**<38**	**Total**	**<37**

processes, and method of evaluation. For this reason no special effort was made to optimize the algorithm or the software programming.

17.3.4   Limitations of the Digital Envelope Method

The method we described can only detect whether any pixel or any bit in the data stream had been altered, but it does not know exactly which pixel(s) or bit(s) had been compromised. It would be very expensive, in term of computation, to determine exactly where the change has occurred. Current data assurance practice is that once the RS determines that the image/data had been altered, it would discard the image, notify and alert the SS, and request the information to be retransmitted.

17.4   DICOM SECURITY PROFILES

This section has been excerpted from the DICOM Standard Part 15 (PS3.15-2001).

17.4.1   Current DICOM Security Profiles

DICOM Standard Part 15 (PS 3.15-2001) provides a standardized method for secure communication and digital signature (DICOM, 2001). It specifies technical means (selection of security standards, algorithms, and parameters) for application entities involved in exchanging information to implement security policies. In Part 15, four security profiles that have been added to the DICOM standard are secure use profiles, secure transport connection profiles, digital signature profiles, and media storage secure profiles. These address issues like use of attributes, security on associations, authentication of objects, and security on files.

17.4.1.1   Secure Use Profiles   The profiles outline how to use attributes and other security profiles in a specific fashion. The profiles include secure use of online electronic storage, basic, and bit-preserving digital signatures.

17.4.1.2   Secure Transport Connection Profiles   The profiles published in 2000 specify the technological means to allow DICOM applications to negotiate and establish the secure data exchange over a network. The secure transport connection is similar to the secure socket layer (SSL) commonly used in the secure Web on-line processing (see the SSL Web site) and VPN (virtual private network) encryption often used to extend an internal enterprise network to the remote branches. It is an application of public key cryptography, so the scrambled message by the sender can only be read by the receiver and no one else in the middle will be able to decode it. Currently the profiles specify two possible mechanisms for implementing secure transport connections over a network: TLS (transport layer security 1.0) and ISCL (integrated secure communication layer V1.00). It endows DICOM with a limited set of features that are required for implementation.

17.4.1.3 *Digital Signature Profiles*   Although the secure transport connection protects the data during transit, it does not provide any lifetime integrity checks for DICOM SOP (service-object pair) instances. The digital signature profiles published in 2001 provide mechanisms for lifetime integrity checks using DS. DS allow authentication of the identity entity that created, authorized, or modified a DICOM data set. This authentication is in addition to any authentication done when exchanging messages over a secure transport connection. Except for a few attributes, the profiles do not specify any particular data set to sign. The creator of a DS should first identify the DICOM data subset, then calculate its MAC and hash value, and last, sign the MAC into a DS. As with any DS, the receiver can verify the integrity of this DICOM data subset by recalculating the MAC and comparing it with the one recorded in the DS. Typically the creator of the DS would only include data elements that had been verified in the MAC calculation for the DS. The image digital envelope described in Section 17.3 has a very large data set that includes the segmented image and relevant patient information in the DICOM header. The profiles currently specify three possible ways of implementing DS, depending on what is to be included in the DICOM data set to be signed: base (methodology), creator (for modality and image creator), and authorization (approval by technician or physician) DS profiles.

17.4.1.4 *Media Security Profiles*   The DICOM media security profile that was also published in 2001 provides a secure mechanism to protect against unauthorized access to this information on the media with encryption. It defines a framework for the protection of DICOM files for media interchange by means of an encapsulation with a cryptographic "envelope." This concept can be called *protected DICOM file*. As an application of public key cryptography, it follows the steps similar to those of the DE method described in Section 17.3. The DICOM file to be protected is first digested, then signed with DS (optional in the profiles), and last, sealed (encrypted) in a cryptographic envelope, ready for media interchange.

17.4.2 Some New DICOM Security on the Horizon

The security needs in DICOM are under rapid development. Specifying a mechanism to secure parts of a DICOM image header by attribute-level encryption is probably a next step toward satisfying the patient privacy requirements of HIPAA. The principle is that any DICOM data elements that contain patient-identifying information should be replaced by the DICOM object with dummy values. Instead of simple removal, the dummy values of patient information, such as patient ID and names are required so that images can still be communicated and processed with existing DICOM implementations, security aware or not. The original values can be encrypted in an envelope and stored (embedded) as a new data element in the DICOM header. Using public key cryptography, the attribute-level encrypted envelope can be designed to allow only selected recipients to open it or different subsets can be held for different recipients. This way the implementation secures the confidential patient information and controls the recipients' access to the part of the patient data they are allowed to see. This selective protection of individual attributes within DICOM can be an effective tool to support HIPAA's emphasis that patient information is only provided to people who have a professional need.

17.5   HIPAA AND ITS IMPACTS ON PACS SECURITY

This section has been excerpted from materials available related to the HIPAA mandate. HIPAA was put in place by Congress in 1996, and this Act became a formal compliance document in April 14, 2003. HIPAA provides a conceptual framework for healthcare data security and integrity and sets out strict and significant federal penalties for noncompliance. However, the guidelines as they have been released (including the most technical assistance materials, July 6, 2001, modifying Parts 160 and 164) do not mandate specific technical solutions; rather, there is a repeated emphasis on the need for scalable compliance solutions appropriate to variety of clinical scenarios covered by HIPAA language.

The term "HIPAA compliant" can only refer to a company, institution, or hospital. Policies on patient privacy must be implemented institution-wide. Software or hardware implementation for image data security alone is not sufficient. Communication of DICOM images in a PACS environment is only a part of the information system in a hospital. One cannot just implement the image security using DICOM or the image-embedded DE method described in Section 17.3 and assume that the PACS is HIPAA compliant. All other security measures, such as user authorization with passwords, user training, physical access constraints, and auditing, are as important as the secure communication (Dwyer, 2000). However, image security as described in Section 17.3, which provides a means for protecting the image and corresponding patient information when exchanging this information among devices and healthcare providers, is definitely a critical and essential part of the provisions that can be used to support institution-wide compliance with HIPAA privacy and security regulations.

The Department of Health and Human Services (DHHS) publishes the HIPAA requirements in the so-called Notice of Proposed Rule Makings (NPRM). There are currently four key areas:

- Electronic transactions and code sets (Compliance date: October 16, 2002)
- Privacy (Compliance date: April 14, 2003)
- Unique identifiers
- Security

Transactions relate to such items as claims, enrollment, eligibility, payment, and referrals, whereas code sets relate to items such as diseases, procedures, equipment, drugs, transportation, and ethnicity. HIPAA mandates the use of unique identifiers for providers, health plans, employers, and individuals receiving healthcare services. The transactions, code sets and unique identifiers are mainly a concern for users and manufacturers of hospital information systems (HIS) and, to a much lesser extent, for radiology information system (RIS) users and manufacturers, whereas it has little or no consequence for users and manufacturers of PACS. Privacy and security regulations will have an impact on all HIS, RIS, and PACS users and manufacturers. Although

HIPAA compliance is an institution-wide implementation, PACS and its applications should have a great interest in making them helpful to become HIPAA supportive.

The image security discussed in this chapter and in Chapter 16 (Cao et al., 2002; Huang et al., 2000) includes methods for PACS continuous availability and disaster recovery and supports the HIPAA security regulations. In addition the basic requirement for a PACS that will help a hospital to comply with the HIPAA requirement is the ability to generate a list of information on demand related to the access of clinical information for a specific patient. From an application point of view, there should be a log mechanism to keep track of the access information such as the following:

- Identification of the person who accessed the data
- Date and time when data have been accessed
- Type of access (create, read, modify, delete)
- Status of access (success or failure)
- Identification of the data

Although each PACS component computer, especially UNIX machines, has its own system functions to collect all the user and access controls listed above as well as auditing information and event reporting if enabled, they are scattered around the system, and not in a readily available form. Also, because accessing of data is typically done from many WSs, tracking and managing each of them is a difficult task. With this in mind, a PACS should be designed in such a way that a single data security server can generate the HIPAA information without the need for "interrogating" other servers or WSs.

An automatic PACS monitoring system (AMS) jointly developed in SITP (Shanghai Institute of Technical Physics) and IPI laboratory, USC (Zhang, 2002), can be revamped as the PACS reporting hub for HIPAA-relevant user access information. The PACS AMS consists of two parts: a small monitoring agent running in each of the PACS component computers and a centralized monitor server that monitors the entire PACS operation in real time and keeps track of patient and image data flow continuously from image acquisition to the final WS. The PACS AMS is an ideal system to collect PACS security information and support HIPAA implementation.

The PACS alone cannot be claimed as HIPAA compliant. Secure communication of images using DE and DICOM security standards and continuous PACS monitoring have shown HIPAA support functionalities that are indispensable for hospital-wide HIPAA compliance.

In the next several sections, we introduce some novel concepts and methodology as a first attempt to tackle issues raised in the last two sections.

17.6 PACS SECURITY SERVER AND AUTHORITY FOR ASSURING IMAGE AUTHENTICITY AND INTEGRITY

17.6.1 Comparison of Image-Embedded DE Method and DICOM Security

The image-embedded DE method provides a strong assurance of image authenticity and integrity. The method has the advantage that the relevant patient information in the DICOM header is embedded in the image. It ensures image security for any individual image to be transmitted through public networks without using the DICOM image header. However, relevant patient information can be retrieved from the DE after being received. Meanwhile, because the actual data transfer will occur only after the DE has been successfully created and embedded, the most CPU-intensive cryptography does not have to be performed on the fly as in the SSL protocol used in Web transactions, or the TLS (transport layer secure) and ISCL (integrated secure communication layer) protocols specified in DICOM security standards. Both the sender and receiver do not have to be on-line at the same time to negotiate an on-line session. Therefore the image-embedded DE method is particularly suited well for store-forward type of systems like media interchange.

The DE method described has certain limitations of which we need to be aware:

1. Lack of standards It should be noted that this DE method does not cater for the automatic identification of the various algorithms and attributes used (e.g., hashing, encryption and embedding algorithms, DE data set to be sealed, communication protocols) while verifying the DE. Unlike the DICOM security profiles, which specify the means for the sender and recipient to negotiate the information, in the DE method they either must agree in advance or the sender must somehow transmit this information to the user by some out-of-band method.

2. Needs further evaluation The DE method is considered good for security communication of images only when it satisfies certain criteria such as robustness, percentage of the pixel changed in data embedding, and time required to run the complete image security assurance. The DE method with data embedded in the image is time-consuming to perform because of image processing and encryption algorithms that require heavy computation. It is necessary to optimize the DE method and fine-tune its performance for real-time applications. It is better to provide the user a choice of selecting less computationally intensive algorithms (see Table 17.2) or bypassing the integrity check altogether because the user's machine may not be powerful enough to handle the heavy DE processing.

3. Limited capability in image distribution The DE method is mostly suited for a controlled enterprise level and a small number of nodes in teleradiology application. It is not designed for large-scale network security. Because the DE is encrypted with the receiver's public key and then embedded in the image, this CPU-intensive process must be performed all over again for a different user or site because of the different public key.

The three shortcomings listed above would limit the image-embedded DE method in a well-controlled environment. Since the DICOM security profiles, described in Section 17.4, have been released and become the standard, the best image security strategy is to combine both the DE for image and the DCIOM security profiles. One method is to use DICOM-compliant communication to address the secure transmission of images between the sender (last step) and receiver (first step) as shown in Figure 17.9. Because the DICOM standard does not maintain the confidentiality and integrity of image data before or after the transmission, and the DS and DE in the DICOM header that is separated from the image data can be easily deleted and recreated by a hacker accessing the image, the image-embedded DE can be used to ensure image security. This way it can provide a permanent assurance of confidentiality and integrity of the image no matter when and how the image has been manipulated. In fact, even if one were to lose the key or, worse yet, be no longer in existence, the authentication and signature embedded in the image persist just as a written signature on paper does.

17.6.2 An Image Security System in a PACS Environment

As seen from the discussion above, one of the best designs for an image security system in a PACS environment is shown in Figure 17.11. The system is based on the combination of the image-embedded DE method for image and relevant patient information in the DICOM header and the DICOM security profile for communication. The DE method includes the modality gateway for image embedding and a dedicated *security server* to handle all PACS image- and patient-related security issues. The PACS security server has the following three major functions:

1. *A DICOM secure gateway to the outside connections* (Fig. 17.11, leftmost and rightmost). The gateway is in compliance with DICOM security profiles ensuring integrity, authenticity, and confidentiality of medical images in transit. The gateway plays a role in securing communication of DICOM images over public networks. It is important to build a separate DICOM secure gateway for handling CPU-intensive cryptography so as not to impact the performance of PACS in fulfillment of daily radiological services. The current DICOM security

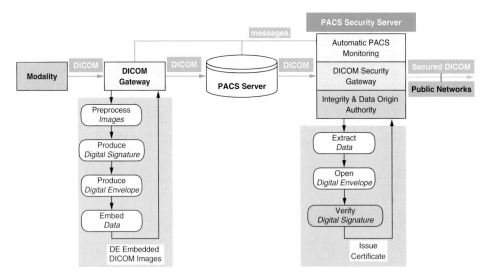

Figure 17.11 Combined DICOM secure transport connection profiles and Digital Signature image security system in a PACS environment. Blue box: data embedding performed, orange box: assurance of image authenticity and integrity performed; various green boxes: PACS security server; bright green: DICOM compliant network connection; pink line and box: public network.

standards are still evolving. It will take time for the standards to mature and to be fully implemented in PACS, so it is also important that the gateway can provide interoperability and evolve with the existing "non–security-aware" PACS.

2. *An image authority for image origin authentication and integrity* (Fig. 17.11, various green boxes at right). The authority server is designed to take away the limitations of the DE method discussed above and to integrate the method in a PACS environment. First, as a steganographic (hidden or digital signature) message, the DE embedded in the image should be permanent, associated only to the image itself and not intended to change every time with a new user. To solve the issue, a dedicated image authority server whose public key will be used to seal the DE of all images acquired locally. In this system, medical images from modalities will be first digitally signed at the modality gateway machine (Fig. 17.11, left, blue) by the image creator and/or through the physician's authorization or the PACS manufacturer. The signature plus relevant patient information can be sealed in a DE with the authority server's public key instead of the individual user's key.

   Whenever needed, a remote user can query the image authority to verify the origin authenticity and integrity of an image under review. The image authority (lower green box) is the only one who owns the private key that can be used to extract and decrypt the DE embedded permanently in the image. The image authority serves as the authority for checking the image originality and integrity, in the same way as a certificate authority (PKI Web) does for certifying the DS. The heavy computation jobs shown in Figure 17.9, of ensuring image authentication and integrity at the receiver side are now being taken over by the PACS security server, thereby reducing the workload at the client side. Meanwhile it is also relatively easy to keep the DE-embedding algorithms and attributes prearranged between the image security authority and the DE creators/senders in a local PACS environment without requiring the open standard to define them.

3. *A monitoring system for PACS operations.* This component can, at a minimum, keep a user access log and monitor security events, providing support for hospital-wide HIPAA compliance. The major monitoring functions and features (Zhang et al., 2002) include (1) real-time capture of all warnings and error messages in the PACS, (2) periodic checking of, PACS components' running status, (3) patient/image data flow tracking in PACS components and analyses of the image usages, (4) monitoring user log-on/off on remote display workstations and verification that images are securely read and used, (5) dynamic display of the image data flow, and (6) warnings to an administrator of serious errors via a pager.

In addition the PACS security server should be intelligent enough to deliver only the relevant information to a user. As the volume of clinical data, images, and reports has significantly increased with digital imaging technology, and government regulations continue to emphasize information privacy, they have imposed an implementation challenge for each individual user to access specific data from a specific location—where and how he/she can access the information in a timely fashion. Intelligent security management must find a secure way to match relevant information

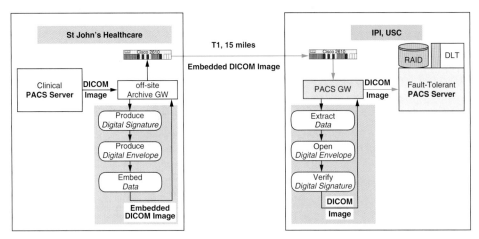

Figure 17.12 Interhospital connection between a clinical PACS and an off-line archive server with an ASL model. Compare with Figure 17.11. Blue box: data embedding performed; orange box: assurance of image authenticity and integrity performed; various green boxes: PACS security server.

with a particular user. The attribute-level DICOM security described in Section 17.4 and the image authority with an ability to check image attributes will definitely be a major step toward developing a smart and secured delivery system for medical images. Figure 17.12 shows a testbed of image security system for an off-site backup archive between St. John's Health Center and IPI Laboratory at USC.

17.7 LOSSLESS DIGITAL SIGNATURE EMBEDDING METHODS FOR ASSURING 2-D AND 3-D MEDICAL IMAGE INTEGRITY

17.7.1 Lossless Digital Signature Embedding

In Sections 17.1 through 17.6 we discussed some general methods to use in assuring image/data security. Two drawbacks of these methods are that (1) the DS (digital signature) and DE (digital envelope) are embedded in the original image and can permanently alter some pixels of the original image and (2) the examination entails hundreds or even thousands of two-dimensional images, so the time required to perform the DE assurance system can escalate quickly. Sections 17.7 through 17.10 present a three-dimensional (3-D) lossless digital signature embedding (LDSE) method for assuring the integrity of two-dimensional (2-D) and 3-D medical images in transit and in storage. The 3-D LDSE can overcome the two weaknesses of the conventional DS methods. First, while the LDSE also is based on the DS method, the DS is embedded losslessly in the original image. All of the original image can be recovered for viewing at a workstation (WS). Second, the 3-D LDSE generates only one DS for the 3-D volume. So LDSE method can be executed very efficiently.

We present the general LDSE in this section. In Section 17.8 we will focus first on 2-D and then on 3-D images. Examples in both 2-D sectional images and 3-D volume will be presented. Section 17.9 will be devoted to the interchange between 3-D DS and 2-D DS. This is important because in clinical practice, referring physicians may

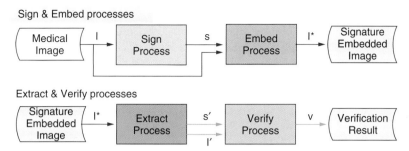

Figure 17.13 Data flow of sign and embed, and extract and verify processes in the LDSE method. I: original image; s: signature of the original image; I*: signature embedded image; s': recovered signature; I': recovered image; v: verification result.

only need several key images from the exam for their diagnosis and treatment of the patient.

17.7.2 Procedures and Methods

The goal of LDSE is to provide robust with their medical images integrity in fact to various application environments. In achieving this goal, it is important to permanently embed the digital signature (DS) in the image pixels without intruding on its quality. A permanently lossless embedded DS should provide image integrity assurance for the lifetime of the medical images.

17.7.3 General LDSE Method

The LDSE method consists of two processes as shown in Figure 17.13.

1. Sign and embed processes
   - Generate the DS of the image pixels with the image owner's private key

$$s = S_{k,\,priv}(I)$$ (17.12)

where s is the digital signature (DS) of the image, S denotes the signature signing process,[1] k,priv is the owner's private key, and I is the image.
   - Embed the bit stream of DS into the image pixels using lossless data embedding approaches:

$$I^* = I \oplus s$$ (17.13)

where I^* is the signature embedded image, $\oplus$ denotes the lossless data embedding process, and s is the DS.

---

[1]The signature signing begins with the computing of a hash value of all pixels of the image using cryptographic hash functions (e.g., SHA1), and this is followed by encrypting the hash value by the public key encryption method.

2. Extract and verify processes
   - Extract the DS from the signature embedded image and recover the image from the embedding process

$$(s, I') = \Theta I^* \tag{17.14}$$

where s is the DS, I' is the recovered image, Θ denotes the data extraction process, I^* is the signature embedded image.
   - Verify the extracted DS with the owner's public key

$$v = V_{k, \text{pub}}(I', s) \tag{17.15}$$

where v is the verification result, V denotes the signature verification process[2], k,pub is the owner's public key, I' is the recovered image, and s is the DS of I. If the verification result is true, which means the image has not been altered, image integrity is assured. If the verification is false, the image has been altered.

17.8 TWO-DIMENSIONAL AND THREE-DIMENSIONAL LOSSLESS DIGITAL SIGNATURE EMBEDDING METHOD

The goal is to obtain the digital signature of the image, and then embed it in the original image losslessly.

17.8.1 Two-dimensional LDSERS Algorithm

17.8.1.1 General 2-D Method Consider the original $N \times M$ medical image with pixel values in the set $P = \{0, \ldots, 4095, \text{or higher}\}$. The algorithm starts by preprocessing the original image to form an RS image. The digital signature is obtained from the preprocessed image along with the original image.

The RS image is obtained as follows: The algorithm divides the original image into disjoint groups of n adjacent horizontal pixels $(p_1, \ldots, p_n)$, for example, $(p_1, \ldots, p_4)$, where p stands for the value of pixel and n is an integer greater than 1. A discrimination function f, defined in Eq. (17.16), computes the correlation coefficients of each pixel group $G = (p_1, \ldots, p_n)$. The function f converts the vector G into a number f (G).

$$f(G) = \sum_{1}^{n-1} |p_{i+1} - p_i| \tag{17.16}$$

An invertible operation F on G called "flipping" is also defined. Flipping of a given bit in a pixel is defined as $0 \to 1$ or $1 \to 0$. The flipping would change the value of a pixel and the value change would depend on the bit locations in the pixel. Thus, for

---

[2]The signature verification process begins by decrypting the DS to get the original hash value and then comparing this hash value to a second hash value computed from the recovered image using the same hash function used in signing process.

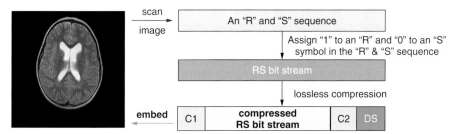

Figure 17.14 Embed the DS in an MR image using 2-D LDSERS. The U groups are not used. C1: counter 1 to record the length of the compressed RS bit stream; C2: counter 2 to record the length of the DS shown in bright green.

$f(F(G))$ compared with $f(G)$, there are three possibilities defined as three groups: R, S, and U:

$$\text{Regular (R) group: if } f(F(G)) > f(G)$$

$$\text{Singular (S) group: if } f(F(G)) < f(G)$$

$$\text{Unusable (U) group: if } f(F(G)) = f(G)$$

A new grouped image is formed with these three possible states in the selected bit plane.

17.8.1.2 Signing and Embedding
Refer to Figure 17.14. The embedding starts with the scanning of image pixels to find R and S groups. The U groups are skipped during scanning. For example, in most current medical images, we can select n = 4, then G = $(p_1, \ldots, p_4)$, field experimental results show that $f(F(G)) > f(G)$ after the flipping operation F. This is because F makes G less correlated, where the adjacent pixels are usually correlated. The relationship of the four pixels in every found group can be converted to an R (R group) or S (S group) symbol. As a result a new binary image consisting of R and S sequences is formed with 1 for R and 0 for S. The binary image with inter-mixed R and S (or 1s and 0s) sequences is converted to a bit stream of 1s and 0s, which is called an RS bit stream. The RS bit stream is then losslessly compressed using adaptive arithmetic coding [12]. The RS bit stream extraction and compression processes are complete until

$$l_{RS} - (l_{RScomp} + l_{DS}) \geq 0 \tag{17.17}$$

where l_{LSB} denotes the binary length of the RS bit stream, $l_{LSBcomp}$ denotes the binary length of the compressed RS bit stream, and l_{DS} denotes the binary length of the DS. It is noted that the lossless compression is not applied to the image, but to the digital signature of the image.

Afterward, the bit stream of DS is appended to the compressed RS bit stream to form a new bit stream. This new bit stream is then compared with the RS bit stream bit by bit. If there is no difference in the bit value, no change is made. If there is a difference, the corresponding group of pixels (R or S group) is flipped. After all the bits are compared, the embedding process is complete and the result is a signature embedded image.

Since the forming of R and S groups as well as the embedding is a reversible process, the original image can be completely recovered after the DS is extracted.

17.8.1.3 Extracting and Verifying The embedded bit stream is reconstructed from the R and S groups by the same scanning used to find R and S groups from the signature embedded image. The bit stream is first broken down into the compressed RS bit stream and the DS bit stream (see Fig. 17.14). The compressed RS bit stream is then decompressed to recover the original R and S groups. The original R and S groups are compared to the extracted groups, and the corresponding group of pixels is flipped if there is any difference. Since the flip operation is reversible, the original image pixels can be completely recovered. The recovered DS is verified with the restored image. If verification result is true, there is no alteration of the image and the image integrity is assured.

17.8.2 Three-dimensional LDSERS Algorithm

17.8.2.1 General 3-D LDSE Method Following the 2-D LDSERS concept, described in Section 17.8.1, the general 3-D LDSE method consists of two processes: (1) signing and embedding and (2) extracting and verifying. A 3-D volume of a single CT series with n images is used to illustrate the method in the following sections. If there are multiple series in an exam, the method can be applied to each series separately.

17.8.2.2 Signing and Embedding Refer to Figure 17.15, in order to make it more difficult to extract the embedded digital signature, randomization is utilized to re-arrange the image order in the CT volume before actual embedding. The random order is generated based on a set of pseudorandom numbers r_k computed by the random number generator. The new order of the CT volume, 2, n, ..., 1, is shown in Figure 17.15. After the re-arrangement, all pixels align into a pixel stream starting from the first pixel of the first image "1" to the last pixel of the last image "2." A hash value is computed for all pixels in the pixel stream using cryptography hash functions such as SHA1 (see Reference in this chapter). The hash value is then

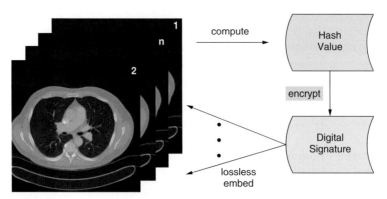

Figure 17.15 General 3-D lossless digital signature embedding (LDSE) method. A single digital signature is generated for a CT volume for assuring the integrity of the volume. The original 3-D volume set with 1, ..., n images has been randomized (2, n, ..., 1).

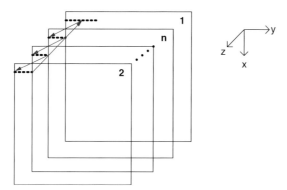

Figure 17.16 3-D LDSERS using Z-shape walking pattern (blue) to search the R and S groups for data embedding. Four voxels are used to form a group in order to increase the bit compression ratio to accommodate digital signature embedding.

encrypted to form a digital signature (DS) of the whole volume using a public key encryption method such as RSA (see Reference in this chapter). Finally, the DS is embedded in pixels of all images within the volume by using a lossless embedding algorithm similar to the one described in Section 17.8.1. Since the images are still in random order, the DS is embedded according to this order. The result of embedding is a signature embedded image volume. After embedding, the images within the volume are re-arranged back to the original order; therefore the LDSE method does not affect clinical data flow.

The embedding algorithm used in the 3-D LDSE method is different than the 2-D LDSE method in that it involves all images of the volume in the embedding. In comparison, the 2-D method embeds the 2-D image signature in each individual image within the volume. Figure 17.16 shows the 3-D LDSERS using a Z-shape walking pattern to search the R and S groups for data embedding. Four volexs are used to form a group to increase the compression ratio to accommodate the DS embedding. For more detail on the 3-D LDSERS algorithm, see the references at the end of this chapter.

17.8.2.3 Extracting and Verifying In extracting and verifying, the same random seed is used to reproduce the same random order as in the signature embedded volume. Images in the 3-D volume are then re-arranged according to this random order. Since embedding is an invertible process, the DS can be extracted and the original volume can be completely recovered. The extracted DS is then decrypted and verified with the hash value computed from the recovered volume. The verified volume is re-arranged back to the original order for clinical use.

17.9 FROM A THREE-DIMENSIONAL VOLUME TO TWO-DIMENSIONAL IMAGE(S)

17.9.1 Extract Sectional Images from 3-D Volume with LDSERS

In many clinical scenarios in which a referring physician retrieves images for clinical review, only several 2-D images from a 3-D volume may be needed, and not the entire volume. These images are usually critical images that the radiologists had selected for the referring physician's review. How to protect these several 2-D images in transit and in storage is a new data integrity issue.

For example, assume that only the third image in the CT volume is needed, and that the 3-D volume already has a signature embedded using the 3-D LDSERS algorithm described in Section 17.8.2. The procedure on how to protect the image integrity of this selected image is as follows:

1. The method starts by recovering the original 3-D CT volume using the extract and verify process of the 3-D LDSERS method.
2. Once the verification result assures the integrity of the CT volume, a copy of the required image is extracted.
3. A digital signature of this single CT image is generated and embedded in the image pixels using the 2-D LDSERS algorithm described in Section 17.8.1. The signature embedded image is sent to the physician for review.

If more than one single image is required, then steps 2 and 3 are repeated for each image.

By this method, the integrity of both the 3-D volume and the extracted 2-D images can be assured during the workflow where a physician is retrieving specific images from a 3-D volume. This method can be directly applied to the IHE (Integrating the Healthcare Enterprise) key image note profiles to be discussed in Section 17.10.

The 2-D LDSERS algorithms was tested with four major modality types of 2-D images used in current clinical practice, including CR, CT, grayscale US, and MR. Although color US images were not evaluated in the experiments, the LDSERS method can be used for color US images by embedding the digital signature in the three chrominance components of the color image. A total of 762 images, including 152 CR images, 204 CT images, 204 grayscale US images, and 202 MR images, have been collected. Most of the images collected have standard spatial and density resolution: MR ($256 \times 256 \times 12$), CT ($512 \times 512 \times 12$), and US ($640 \times 480 \times 8$), and CR images varying from $2010 \times 1670 \times 12$ to $2510 \times 2000 \times 12$.

Thirty image sets from three most common 3-D imaging modalities, CT, US, and MR, were collected for evaluating the performance of the 3-D LDSERS algorithm. The maximum number of images in these image sets was 176, while the minimum number was 10.

17.9.2 Two-dimensional LDSERS Results

17.9.2.1 Embedded LDSERS Pattern   In this section we give some examples of the LDSERS results shown in Figure 17.17. Figure 17.17*A* and *B* depict a signature embedded CT chest image using the 2-D LDSERS algorithm and the subtracted image between the signature embedded image and the original image, respectively; Figure 17.17*C* and *D* are the signature embedded US OBGYN image and the corresponding subtracted image, and Figure 17.17*E* and *F* are the signature embedded CR hand image and the corresponding subtracted image. The subtracted images were obtained by subtracting the original image from the corresponding signature embedded image. The subtracted image appears black in a regular window/level display. After window/level adjustments, the embedded data become visible. For example, a

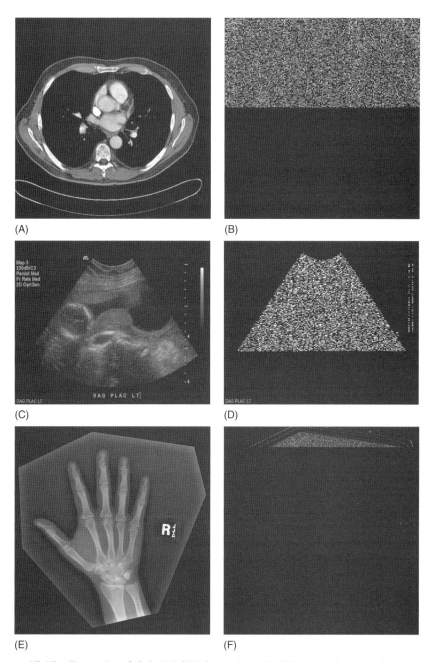

Figure 17.17 Example of 2-D LDSERS results. (*A*) CT chest image with signature embedded; (*B*) subtracted image between the original CT chest image and *A*, showing where the digital signature is embedded; (*C*) US OBGYN image with signature embedded; (*D*) subtracted image between the original US image and *C*; *E*. CR hand image with signature embedded; (*F*) subtracted image between the original CR image and *E*.

horizontal strip shape is the pattern observed in the subtracted images Fig. 17.17*B*. The strip shape shows that every bit embedding changes four adjacent pixels in the 2-D LDSERS image.

17.9.2.2 Time Performance of 2-D LDSERS   The time performances of the sign and embed processes as well as extract and verify processes of the 2-D LDSERS algorithm were recorded in hundredth seconds level for four types of images, MRI, CT, US, and CR (see Zhou, and the references to this chapter). This demonstrates that the 2-D LDSERS is efficient for assuring the integrity of a single 2-D image compared to the conventional methods presented in Sections 17.1 through 17.3. However, the image examination with hundreds of such images could still take a long processing time, though this can be shorten using 3-D LDSERS method.

17.9.3   Three-dimensional LDSERS Results

17.9.3.1 Embedded LDSERS Pattern   The 3-D LDSERS algorithm is evaluated in two steps. First, one digital signature is generated for the entire volume set and the signature is embedded in the volume set using the 3-D LDSERS algorithm. Second, the digital signature was extracted from the signature embedded volume set and verified. Figures 17.18, 17.19, and 17.20 show examples of an MRI breast, an US OBGYN, and a CT reformatted coronal chest volume set. Each figure depicts four consecutive images from each of the three volumes sets (each with a partial

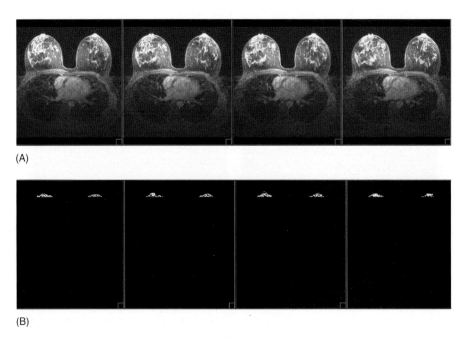

(A)

(B)

Figure 17.18   Example of the 3-D LDSERS results of MR breast volume. (*A*) Four consecutive images of the MRI volume, each image with a partial digital signature embedded; (*B*) subtracted images between the four original MR images and *A*, showing where the digital signature is embedded.

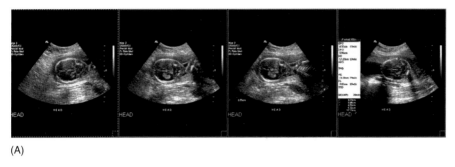

(A)

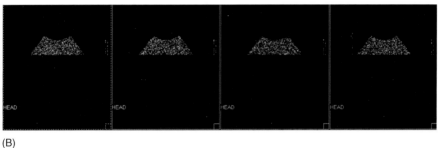

(B)

Figure 17.19   Example of the 3-D LDSERS results of US OBGYN volume. (*A*) Four consecutive images of the US volume, each image with a partial digital signature embedded; (*B*) subtracted images between the four original US images and *A*, showing where the digital signature is embedded.

signature embedded) and the subtracted images between the original and the corresponding signature embedded images. An intuitive view of the pixels changed after the data-embedding process can be observed from the subtracted images in Figures 17.18*B*, 17.19*B*, and 17.20*B*. A horizontal strip can be observed in every subtracted image of the volume set. The strip shows that every 1/0 bit embedding process changes four adjacent pixels in the 3-D LDSERS algorithm. As it can be seen, the portion of pixels being changed in every image is small, which means that plenty of space is still available for embedding more data. This is one of the advantages of the 3-D over the 2-D image-embedding methods, since the embedded data can then be distributed in the entire volume instead of just in a single image.

17.9.3.2   *Time Performance of 3-D LDSERS*   Use the three imaging modalities, MRI, US, and CT shown in Figs. 17.18, 17.19, and 17.20 as examples, the time performance of the 3-D LDSERS vs. the 2-D LDSERS method has been recorded and the results tabulated in Table 17.4. The results demonstrate:

Sign or Verify

- 3-D LDSERS performs much better than that of the 2-D LDSERS method, for example, see MR set3 vs. MR set14.
- The sign or verify process time increases steeply as the total size of the image sets increases. For instance, the time to sign is 0.12 seconds for the MR set3 with 3.16 Mbytes, whereas it is 2.52 seconds for the MR set14 with 94.4 Mbytes.

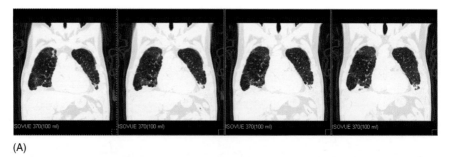

(A)

(B)

Figure 17.20 Example of the 3-D LDSERS results of a reformatted CT coronal chest volume. The images are reformatted and displayed from the anterior to posterior. (*A*) Four consecutive images of the CT volume, each image with a partial digital signature embedded; (*B*) subtracted images between the four original CT images and *A*, showing where the digital signature is embedded.

- The size of the image but not the number of images contained in an image set is the main factor in determining the process time of the digital signature.
- Different digital signature algorithms will affect the process time. Field experience has shown that SHA1with RSA has a faster process time for medical images than other digital signature algorithms, including SHA1with DSA and RIPEMD160 with RSA.

Embed or Extract   The embed or extract process time is mainly determined by the correlation of adjacent pixels of each image in an image set in accord with the concept of the LDSERS algorithm. For images with high correlation among adjacent pixels, the process time to embed or extract is short. For a comprehensive performance of the 3-D LDSERS, see Zhou et al. (2003).

17.10 APPLICATION OF TWO-DIMENSIONAL AND THREE-DIMENSIONAL LDSE IN CLINICAL IMAGE DATA FLOW

17.10.1 Application of the LDSE Method in a Large Medical Imaging System like PACS

The goal of the integration of the LDSE method with imaging systems is to assure the integrity of an image right after it is generated from an imaging modality. Thus,

TABLE 17.4   Time performance of the image volume sets using 3-D LDSERS vs 2-D LDSERS

3-D Volume sets (number of images)	3-D LDSERS		2-D LDSERS	
	Sign + Embed (seconds)	Extract + Verify (seconds)	Sign + Embed (seconds)	Extract + Verify (seconds)
MR set1 (20)	0.25 + 0.14	0.19 + 0.25	0.34 + 0.55	0.34 + 0.34
MR set2 (23)	0.11 + 0.05	0.05 + 0.11	0.42 + 0.51	0.40 + 0.38
MR set3 (23)*	0.12 + 0.06	0.06 + 0.11	0.38 + 0.38	0.53 + 0.38
MR set4 (23)	0.30 + 0.06	0.05 + 0.30	0.42 + 0.58	0.66 + 0.39
MR set5 (25)	0.12 + 0.06	0.06 + 0.12	0.38 + 0.53	0.62 + 0.43
MR set6 (36)	0.46 + 0.06	0.05 + 0.48	0.65 + 0.62	1.05 + 0.62
MR set7 (40)	0.59 + 0.05	0.05 + 0.58	0.78 + 0.65	0.67 + 0.66
MR set8 (40)	0.59 + 0.06	0.05 + 0.61	0.74 + 0.66	0.65 + 0.66
MR set9 (49)	0.22 + 0.06	0.06 + 0.20	0.70 + 0.94	0.88 + 0.77
MR set10 (57)	0.09 + 0.06	0.05 + 0.09	0.71 + 0.88	0.89 + 0.88
MR set11 (160)	1.69 + 0.37	0.51 + 1.67	2.51 + 4.30	3.03 + 2.65
MR set12 (160)	1.73 + 1.11	1.26 + 1.67	2.49 + 4.34	3.04 + 2.43
MR set13 (160)	1.69 + 0.52	0.64 + 1.67	2.59 + 4.09	2.51 + 2.55
MR set14 (176)*	2.52 + 0.34	0.19 + 2.42	3.21 + 3.27	2.89 + 2.97
US set1 (30)	0.28 + 1.10	0.53 + 0.28	0.42 + 0.99	1.26 + 0.39
US set2 (54)	0.48 + 0.86	0.39 + 0.76	0.82 + 1.48	1.89 + 0.85
US set3 (38)	0.34 + 0.05	0.03 + 0.34	0.53 + 1.25	1.60 + 0.49
US set4 (42)	0.39 + 0.05	0.05 + 0.37	0.59 + 1.38	1.76 + 0.55
CT set1 (10)	0.17 + 0.06	0.06 + 0.17	0.19 + 0.41	0.29 + 0.16
CT set2 (20)	0.33 + 0.06	0.08 + 0.31	0.38 + 0.82	0.58 + 0.32
CT set3 (29)	0.44 + 0.06	0.06 + 0.44	0.55 + 1.19	0.84 + 0.46
CT set4 (42)	0.62 + 0.06	0.06 + 0.61	0.80 + 1.72	1.22 + 0.67
CT set5 (51)	0.73 + 0.19	0.14 + 0.73	0.97 + 2.09	1.48 + 0.81
CT set6 (59)	0.84 + 0.08	0.06 + 0.83	1.12 + 2.42	1.71 + 0.94
CT set7 (72)	1.00 + 0.06	0.08 + 1.00	1.37 + 2.95	2.09 + 1.15
CT set8 (80)	1.12 + 0.06	0.08 + 1.11	1.52 + 3.28	2.32 + 1.28
CT set9 (90)	1.28 + 0.20	0.16 + 1.25	1.71 + 3.69	2.61 + 1.44
CT set10 (100)	1.42 + 0.19	0.11 + 1.39	1.84 + 3.42	2.17 + 1.63
CT set11 (69)	1.15 + 0.16	0.17 + 1.05	1.31 + 2.83	2.00 + 1.10
CT set12 (97)	1.37 + **0.06**	0.05 + 1.33	1.84 + **3.98**	2.81 + 1.55

*Set text.

the LDSE sign and embed process should be positioned near the imaging modality as close as possible. The PACS simulator discussed in Chapter 28 can be used as a testbed for evaluating the system integration of the LDSE method with a PACS.

Currently no network security, such as DICOM transport layer security (TLS), has been applied in current clinical PACS, so communication between any two PACS components may not be safe. As a matter of fact, not any of the PACS components has any image/data security assurance. The image integrity in every point after the image modality has therefore to be assured using the LDSE method. Figure 17.21 presents an ideal system integrating the LDSE method with the PACS simulator. The data flow is as follows:

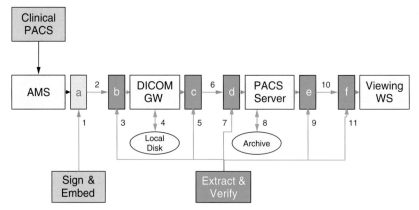

Figure 17.21 System integration of the LDSE methods with the PACS simulator without the DICOM transport layer security (TLS). The PACS simulator consists of an acquisition modality simulator (AMS), a DICOM gateway, a PACS server, and viewing workstations (WS). The connection between these components can be private or public networks. Boxes represent the LDSE processes. (*a*, orange) Signer (sign and embed processes); (*b*–*f*, green) verifier (extract and verify processes).

1. The modality simulator (AMS) passes the DICOM image to the signer (a) that calls the LDSE sign and embed process to embed the DS of the image in the pixels. Once the DS is embedded, it becomes a permanent part of the image. This is the only place where the digital signature is signed and embedded.
2. Signer (a) sends the signature embedded image to the verifier (b) using the DICOM communication protocol.
3. Verifier (b) calls the LDSE extract and verify process to verify digital signature. If the signature is valid, verifier (b) forwards the image to the DICOM gateway.
4. DICOM gateway receives the signature embedded image and stores it in its local disk. It then reads the image file back from the local disk and passes it to the verifier (c).
5–11. Steps 3 and 4 are repeated, verifying the digital signature in each imaging component and the communications between every two different components.

After the signature from (b) to (f) is verified, the image integrity is completely assured in transit and in storage within each component until the image reaches the viewing WS. If DICOM TLS is applied in the PACS simulator, then the protection of the image integrity in transit (e.g., verifiers b, d, and f) can be omitted. Besides these verifiers, other procedures are still necessary for assuring the image integrity in the archive of each component. By combining the LDSE method with DICOM TLS, the image integrity in PACS is completely assured.

If an image is found altered during the transmission, the verifiers (e.g., b) would reject the image and ask the sending component to re-send the image.

17.10.2 Integration of the Three-dimensional LDSE Method with Two IHE Profiles

The quality of a clinical diagnosis can be greatly improved by providing additional 3-D imaging modality features. For example, a series of reformatted CT coronal images generated from 3-D postprocessing provides more information for diagnosis when it is reviewed together with original axial CT images. However, novel clinical image data flow is required to integrate these features with clinical imaging systems like PACS seamlessly. Integrating the Healthcare Enterprise (IHE) has released two important profiles relevant to 3-D volume image data. One is the Key Image Note profile and the other is Post-Processing Workflow profile. In order to apply the 3-D LDSE method in PACS, the 3-D LDSE method must be able to integrate with these two profiles. The following two sections show the method of integration of these two IHE profiles in PACS with the 3-D LDSE method. In the integration of the 3-D LDSE method with these two IHE profiles, the focus is on how to protect the integrity of all images involved in the workflow profiles anytime and anywhere without interrupting the clinical data flow.

17.10.2.1 Integration of the Three-dimensional LDSE Method with Key Image Note
As Figure 17.22 shows, the image set of the exam stored in the archive already has a digital signature embedded when the exam is generated in the 3-D image modality. The lack of the protection occurs when several flagged 2-D images are sent to the WS for review. The 2-D LDSE method described previously in Section 17.9 can be used in this situation to embed the signature of every 2-D image in the flagged image correspondingly so that the physician at the WS can verify the integrity of the flagged images whenever they are viewed.

17.10.2.2 Integration of Three-dimensional LDSE with Three-dimensional Postprocessing Workflow
The integration of the 3-D LDSE method with the 3-D postprocessing workflow proceeds as shown in Figure 17.22:

1. The original exam is generated in a 3-D imaging modality. Before the exam is stored in the archive, a signature of each series of the exam is embedded in the image set of the series using the 3-D LDSE method. The signature embedded exam is then sent to the image server for archiving. Thus the integrity of the original image exam is assured when the exam is in transit and in archive.
2. The signature embedded exam is sent to a 3-D postprocessing WS.
3. When a series of reformatted images (e.g., a CT coronal reformatted series) is generated in the 3-D postprocessing WS, a signature of this coronal image set is also generated and embedded in the image set using the 3-D LDSE method that is installed in the WS.
4. The signature embedded series of reformatted images is sent to the image server for archiving. It is important to notice that no changes are made to the signature embedded original exam because the new signature is only embedded in the reformatted image series.

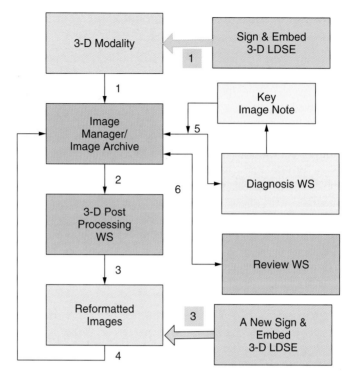

Figure 17.22 Integration of 3-D LDSE method with IHE 3-D postprocessing workflow (purple) and key image note (yellow) profiles in a clinical PACS.

5–6. Once the exam is retrieved to the diagnostic WS or the review WS, the integrity of the exam can be verified anytime on demand. If there is a key image note, then only several critical images are retrieved to the review WS. The integration method described previously in Section 17.9.1 can be used to protect the integrity of these critical images.

17.11 SUMMARY AND SIGNIFICANCE OF IMAGE SECURITY

The repercussions for information integrity in the fundamental shift of healthcare delivery toward telecommunications tools are not yet fully understood. The pressures generating concern about data security are both statutory—for example, the federally mandated Health Insurance Portability and Accountability Act of 1996 and Public Law 104-191, which amends the Internal Revenue Service Code of 1986 (HIPAA, 2000)—and social (a redefinition of patient-sensitive information). These pressures have the power to alter medical theory and practice at its core. Concommtent with the rapidly shifting technical and telecommunications tools at the disposal of healthcare providers and patients on this landscape is the need for research and development of robust, flexible, and easy-to-use methods of ensuring healthcare information security.

On October 1, 2000, the Electronic Signatures in Global and National Commerce Act went into effect. It was an extension of the standards of the Government Paperwork Elimination Act of 1997 that began to establish the definition of electronic signatures and their use in the federal government (21 CFR Part 11, Federal Register 62, 1997). The Electronic Signatures Act established the framework for using electronic signatures to sign contracts, agreements, or records involved in commerce. Although the bill does not specify any specific government technology standards, it allows parties to establish reasonable requirements regarding the use and types of electronic records and signatures.

In addition to the HIPAA and the Electronic Signatures Act in the domain of government regulation of electronic healthcare information, there are the industry standards, mainly DICOM within the medical community, that demonstrate concern for such research on image security.

Other medical federations will almost certainly follow the lead as practitioners and care delivery systems seek guidance on security issues. It is critical that objectively validated data be available as they set long-term policy in the coming years. The image and textual standards currently used in the medical community are DICOM and HL7. Although encryption technology has no similar standard at the present time, it is important for image security that the architecture be open with algorithms and systems that use a modular approach, in full concordance with all relevant HIPAA regulations and in compliance with DICOM security profiles. Technological development has traditionally been incremental by nature in any branch of science. In the aggregate, incremental advances in the scientific corpus often amount to qualitative changes in the level of understanding of a particular subject. It is common sense to develop image integrity and security in a modular fashion so that each component in the system can be replaced by newer technology when it becomes available. The system should be flexible and portable enough to respond to the multiplicity of demands that will unfold as standards, policy, and technology change.

As we mentioned in the beginning of this chapter that DICOM has certain image/data security assurance standard profiles, like those discussed in this chapter, for the medical image industry to follow; but none has yet been enforced. There are still no published records in the Publics on "how to implement," "when it will be," and "how robust and efficient is the assurance," among other issues. This chapter provides the background on image/data integrity assurance for the reader to be prepared for this challenge in dealing with telecommunications.

References

Graham IG. A (very) brief introduction to cryptography. http://www.onthenet.com.au/~grahamis/int2010/week10/crypto.html.

Acken JM. How watermarking adds value to digital content. *Commun ACM* 41(7): 75–7; 1998.

Berger SB, Cepelewicz BB. Medical-legal issues in teleradiology, *Am J Roentgenolo* 166: 505–10, 1996.

Berlin L. Malpractice issue in radiology-teleradiology. *Am J Roentgenolo* 170: 1417–22; 1998.

Cao F, Liu BJ, Huang HK, Zhou MZ, Zhang J, Zhang X, and Mogel G. Fault-tolerant PACS server. *SPIE Med Imag* 4685(44): 316–25; 2002. Complete e-Business Security for your Applications. http://www.rsa.com/products/bsafe/brochures/BSF_BR_1100.pdf.

Craver S, Yeo BL. Technical trials and legal tribution. *Commun ACM* 41(7): 45–54; 1998.

Digital Imaging and Communications in Medicine (DICOM). Part 15: Security and system management profiles;. 2004

Digital Imaging and Communications in Medicine (DICOM). National Electrical Manufacturers' Association. Rosslyn, VA: NEMA, 1996.

Dwyer SJ. Requirements for security of medical data. In Reiner B, Siegel EL, Dwyer SJ. *Security Issues in the Digital Medical Enterprise*. Great Falls, VA: SCAR, 9–14; 2000.

Garfinkel S, Spafford G. *Practical Unix and Internet Security*. O'Reilly & Associates, Inc., Chatsworth, CA, 139–90; 1996.

Fridrich J, Goljan M, Du R. Lossless data embedding for all image formats. in *Proc. SPIE Photonics West. Electr Imag* 4675: 572–83; 2002a.

Fridrich J, Goljan M, Du R. Lossless data embedding—new paradigm in digital watermarking. *EURASIP J Appl Sig Proc*, 2: 185–96; 2002b.

Hellemans A. Internet security code is cracked. *Science* 285: 1472–3; 1999.

HIPAA. U.S. Department of Health and Human Services. http://aspe.os.dhhs.gov/admnsimp.

HIPAA. http://www.rx2000.org/KnowledgeCenter/hipaa/hipfaq.htm.

Hodge JG Jr, Lawrence GO, Jacobson PD. Legal issues concerning electronic health information: privacy, quality, and liability. *J Am Med Assoc* 282(15): 1466–1471; 1999.

Huang HK. Teleradiology technologies and some service models. *J Comp Med Imag Graphics* 20(2): 59–68; 1996.

Huang HK, Wong AWK, Lou SL, Bazzill TM, et al. Clincial experience with a second generation PACS. *J Digit Imag* 9(4): 151–66; 1996.

Huang HK, Wong AWK, Zhu X. Performance of asynchronous transfer mode (ATM) local area andd wide area networks for medical image transmission in clinical environment. *J Comp Med Imag Graphics* 21(3): 165–73; 1997.

Huang HK. *Picture Archiving and Communication Systems: Principles and Applications*. New York: Wiley, 521; 1999.

Huang HK, Lou SL. Telemammography: a technical overview. *RSNA Categorical Course in Breast Imaging*: 273–81; 1999.

Huang HK, Zhang J. Automatic background removal in projection digital radiography images. U.S. Patent 5,903,660; 11 May 1999.

Huang HK, Cao F, Zhang JG, Liu BJ, Tsai ML. Fault tolerant picture archiving and communication system and teleradiology design. In: Reiner B, Siegel EL, Dwyer SJ. *Security Issues in the Digital Medical Enterprise*. Great Falls, VA: SCAR, 57–64; 2000.

Huang HK, Cao F, Liu BJ, Zhou M, Zhang J, Mogel GT. PACS simulator: a standalone education tool. 87th *Radiological Society of North America, Presentations. Chicago: RSNA; 25–30 Nov* 2001.

Information processing systems, Open systems Interconnection. Basic reference model—Part 2: Security architecture *ISO* 7498-2; 1989.

Introduction to SSL. http://developer.netscape.com/docs/manuals/security/sslin/ index.htm.

Integrating the Healthcare Enterprise (IHE). www.ihe.net *Technical Framework*. Vol. I: *Integration Profiles*; 2005.

James AE Jr, James E III, Johnson B, James J. Legal considerations of medical imaging. *Leg Med* 14: 87–113; 1993.

Kaliski BS Jr. An overview of the PKCS standards. RSA Laboratories Technical Note; 1993.

Kamp GH. Medical-legal issues in teleradiology: a commentary. *Am J Roentgenolo* 166: 511–2; 1996.

Law MYY, Zhou Z. New direction in PACS education and training. *Comput Med Imag Graph* 27: 147–56; 2003.

Lehmer DH Mathematical methods in large-scale computing units. in *Proc 2nd Symp Large-Scale Digital Calculating Machinery*, Cambridge, MA, MIT Press, 141–6; 1949.

Lou SL, Sickles EA, Huang HK, et al. Full-field direct digital mammograms: technical components, study protocols, and preliminary results. *IEEE Trans Info Technol Biomed* 1(4): 270–8; 1997.

Liu BJ, Huang HK, Cao F, Documet L, Sarti DA. A fault-tolerant back-up archive using an ASP model for disaster recovery. Presentation 87th *Radiol Soc N Am*. Chicago: RSNA; 25–30, Nov 2001.

Machin D, Campbell M, Fayers P, Pinol A. *Sample Size Tables for Clinical Studies*, 2nd ed. Malden, MA: Blackwell Science; 1997.

McHugh RB, Lee CT. Confidence interval estimation and the size of a clinical trail, *Contr Clin Trails* 5: 157–63; 1984.

Memon N, Wong PW. Protecting digital media content. *Comm ACM* 41(7): 35–43; 1998.

Menezes AJ, Oorschot PC, Vanstone SA. *Handbook of Applied Cryptography*. CRC Press; 1997.

Mogel GT, Huang HK, Cao F, Liu BJ, Zhou M, Zhang J. PACS simulator: a standalone education tool. Presentation, Scientific Papers. 87th *Radiological Society of North America*. Chicago: RSNA; 25–30 Nov 2001.

Nelson M. Arithmetic coding + statistical modeling = data compression. http://dogma.net/markn/articles/arith/part1.htm; 1991.

Park SK, Miller KW. Random number generators: good ones are hard to find. *Comm ACM* 31: 1192–201; 1988.

PGP SDK User's Guide. ftp://ftp.pgpi.org/pub/pgp/sdk/PGPsdkUsersGuide.pdf.

Pietka E. Image standardization in PACS. In: Rangayyan RM, Woods RP, Robb RA, Huang HK, eds. *Handbook of Medical Imaging*. San Diego: Academic Press, 783–801; 2000.

PKCS #1 v2.1: RSA Cryptography Standard, RSA laboratories. http://www.rsasecurity.com/rsalabs.

Public Key Infrastructure (PKI). http://home.xcert.com/~marcnarc/PKI/thesis/characteristics.html.

Quade D. Rank analysis of covariance. *JASA* 62: 1187–1200; 1967.

RIPEMD-160 page. http://www.esat.kuleuven.ac.be/~bosselae/ripemd160.html.

Rivest R. The MD5 message-digest algorithm. Document. MIT Laboratory for Computer Science and RSA Data Security; 1992.
ftp://ftp.funet.fi/pub/crypt/hash/papers/md5.txt.

Rivest R, Shamir A, Adleman L. A method for obtaining digital signatures and public-key cryptosystems. *Comm ACM* 21(2): 120–6; 1978.

RSA Crypto FAQ. http://www.rsasecurity.com/rsalabs/faq.

Schneier B. *Applied Cryptography: Protocols, Algorithms, and Source Code in C*. New York: Wiley, 250–9; 1995.

Secure Hash Standard. Federal Information Processing Standards Publication 180-1; 1995.

Secure Socket Layer (SSL). http://wp.netscape.com/eng/ssl3/draft302.txt.

SHA1 secure hash algorithm—Version 1.0. www.w3.org/PICS/DSig/SHA1_1_0.html.

Stahl JN, Zhang J, Chou TM, Zellner C, Pomerantsev EV, Huang HK. A new approach to tele-conferencing with intravascular ultrasound and cardiac angiography in a low-bandwidth environment. *RadioGraphics* 20: 1495–1503; 2000.

Stahl JN, Zhang J, Zeller C, Pomerantsev EV, Lou SL, Chou TM, Huang HK. Tele-conferencing with dynamic medical images. *IEEE Trans Info Technol Biomed* 4(2): 88–96; 2000.

Telemedicine and Advanced Technology Research Center (TATRC). Integrated research team radiology imaging. Program review. TATRC, U.S. Army Medical Research and Materiel Command, Fort Detrick, MD; 20 Sep. 2000.

Telemedicine and Telecommunications: Option for the New Century. HPCC program review and summary. Program book. National Library of Medicine, NIH, Bethesda, MD; 13–14 Mar 2001.

Veracity Tutorial Manual. Appendix A: Glossary. http://www.veracity.com.

Verisign Onsite. http://www.verisign.com/products/onsite/onsite.pdf.

Walton S. Image authentication for a slippery new age. *Dr. Dobb's Journal*; April 1995.

Wong STC, Abundo M, Huang HK. Authenticity techniques for PACS images and records. *SPIE Med Imag* 2435: 68–79; 1995.

Yeung MM. Digital watermarking. *Comm ACM* 41(7): 31–3; 1998.

Yu F, Hwang K, Gill M, Huang HK. Some connectivity and security Issues of NGI in medical imaging applications. *J High Speed Net* 9: 3–13; 2000.

Zhang J, Huang HK. Automatic background recognition and removal (ABRR) of computed radiography images. *IEEE Trans Med Imag* 16(6): 762–71; 1997.

Zhang J, Stahl JN, Huang HK, Zhou X, Lou SL, Song KS. Real-time teleconsultation with high resolution and large volume medical images for collaborative health care. *IEEE Trans Info Technol Biomed* 4(2): 178–85; 2000.

Zhang J, Han R, Wu D, Zhang X, Zhuang J, Huang HK. Automatic monitoring system for PACS management and operation. *SPIE Med Imag* 4685(49): 348–55; 2002.

Zhao J, Koch E, Luo C. In business today and tomorrow. *Comm ACM* 41(7): 67–72; 1998.

Zhou X, Huang HK, Lou SL. Authenticity and integrity of digital mammogrpahy image. *IEEE Trans Med Imag* 20(8): 784–91; 2001.

Zhou XQ, Lou SL, Huang HK. Authenticity and integrity of digital mammographic images. *Proc SPIE Med Imag* 3662: 138–44; 1999.

Zhou XQ, Huang HK, Lou SL. A study of secure method for sectional image archiving and transmission. *SPIE Med Imag* 3980: 390–9; 2000.

Zhou Z. Lossless digital signature embedding for medical image integrity assurance. PhD dissertation Chapter 2, University of Southern California, Los Angeles, Aug 2005.

Zhou Z, Huang HK, Cao F, Liu BJ, Zhang J, Mogal GT. Educational RIS/PACS simulator. *SPIE Med Imag* 4: 139–47; SPIE Annual Conference 2003.

Zimmerman PR. *PGP User Guide*; MIT Press, Fifth Print, 2000.

CHAPTER 18

PACS Clinical Implementation, Acceptance, and Evaluation

The preceding chapters of this book are prerequisite knowledge for implementing PACS in the clinical environment. This chapter is on the implementation and deployment methodology, and the next chapter (Chapter 19) on clinical experience and lessons learned. Figure 18.1 (excerpted from Fig. 1.3) shows how this chapter relates to other chapters of Part III.

18.1 PLANNING TO INSTALL A PACS

Our philosophy of PACS design and implementation is that regardless of the scale of the PACS being planned, we should always leave room for future expansion, including integration with the enterprise PACS and ePR with image distribution. Thus, if the planning objective is to have a large-scale PACS now, the PACS architecture should allow for its future growth to an enterprise PACS with ePR image distribution features. On the other hand, if only a PACS module is being planned, consideration of the connectivity and compatibility of this module with future modules or a larger scale PACS is essential. The terms we discussed in previous chapters, namely open architecture, connectivity, standardization, portability, modularity, and IHE workflow profiles, should be included in the PACS design.

18.1.1 Cost Analysis

A frequent question asked is, When is a good time to change the film operation to a digital operation by implementing PACS as a clinical necessity and/or a business investment? Many radiology consulting firms nationwide provide models tailored to individual services after analyzing operation and cost benefits. In these models the participating radiology department or health organization inputs information on its workflow and operating environment, including resources used and expenses; the model will compare predicted costs of the current film-based operation with the digital-based operation. In this section we present a spreadsheet model developed by the Department of Diagnostic Radiology, Mayo Clinic and Foundation, Rochester, Minnesota. The assumptions of this model are that the institution modeled only considers the change from a totally film-based to a totally digital-based operation, and

PACS and Imaging Informatics, Second Edition, by H. K. Huang
Copyright © 2010 John Wiley & Sons, Inc.

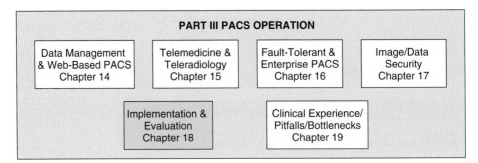

Figure 18.1 Position of Chapter 18 in the organization of this book. Color codes are used to highlight components and workflow in the chapters of Part III.

that only differential costs, including equipment and staff, are included. The model tracks operations from patient admission to resulting events across departmental boundaries. Through this workflow, staff and equipment requirements are determined, leading to the total costs of the two systems. Using this model, spreadsheets for three fictitious institutions with 25,000, 50,000, and 105,000 procedures per year were simulated. Cost comparisons were drawn between the film-based and the digital-based operations. Results are given in Figure18.2 A, B, and C. Figure 18.2A shows the annual operating expenses, with the film-based operation costs rising as the number of procedures increases. Figure 18.2B indicates that capital investment in a digital-based operation costs more when the number of procedures is lower and that the gap between the two operations narrows as the number of procedures increases. The total costs for the film-based and digital-based operations, including capital investment and the annual operating budget, are given in Figure 18.2C. Note that the costs intersect when the institution performs over 50,000 procedures a year but favor the digital-based operation.

This model allows a first approximation of the cost issue in comparing the film-based and digital-based operations. Results from simulation with a mathematical model can be biased by the assumptions of the model as well as the method of data collection. Care should be exercised in interpreting the results. The spreadsheet file used by the authors can be found at the anonymous ftp site:

ri-exp.beaumont.edu/pub/diag/Dos/pac-cost.xls

or

ri-exp,beaumont.edu/pub/diag/Mac/pac-cost.xls

It must be noted that the model was developed in the mid-1990s; many parameters used then may not fit with today's equipment and operation situation and costs. For example, the costs of PC-based workstations and the Web-based image distribution method have changed dramatically and facilitate PACS operation environments. In addition the large numbers of CT and MRI images produced have tilted the lever more toward clinical necessity than just business investment. In Chapter 1 we gave an example of the South Korean models that were obtained from actual field data.

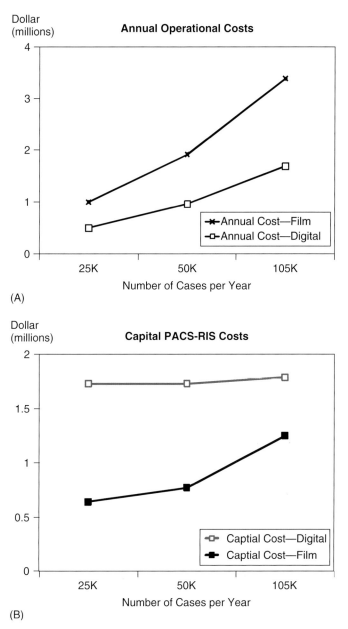

Figure 18.2 Cost comparison between a film-based and a digital-based operations based on a mathematical simulation of three institutions with 25,000, 50,000, and 105,000 procedures a year (Langer, 1996). (*A*) Annual operating budget; (*B*) annual capital budget; (*C*) capital plus annual operating budget. The crossover is at 50,000 procedures.

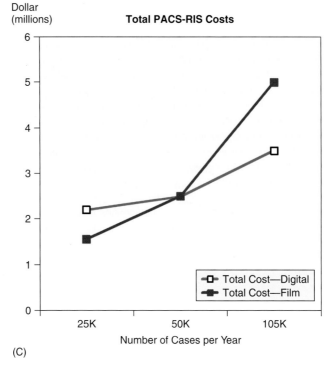

Figure 18.2 (*Continued*).

18.1.2 Film-Based Operation

The first step in planning a PACS is to understand the existing film-based operation. In most radiology departments, the film-based operation procedure is as follows: Conventional diagnostic images obtained from X-ray or other energy sources are recorded on films, which are viewed from alternators (light boxes) and archived in the film library. Images obtained from digital acquisition systems—for example, nuclear medicine, ultrasound, transmission and emission computed tomography, computed and digital radiography, and magnetic resonance imaging—are displayed on the acquisition device's monitor for immediate viewing and then recorded on disks for digital archiving. In addition the images are recorded on films for viewing as well as for long-term archival purposes. Because films are convenient to use in a clinical setting, clinicians prefer to view digital images on film, even though the film method may reduce the digital image quality. As a result many departments still use film as a means for diagnosis and as a storage medium regardless of the image origin. In general, films obtained within six months are stored in the departmental film library and older films are stored at remote hospital sites. The time it takes to retrieve older films is from 0.5 to 2 hours.

Most radiology departments arrange their operations on an organ and body region basis, with exceptions in nuclear medicine, ultrasound, and sometimes MRI and CT type images. Some hospitals group MRI and CT into neuroradiology and body imaging sections. It is advantageous during planning to understand the costs of each film-based operation. The following sample tables are useful for collecting statistics in the planning stage. Table 18.1 shows an example of the procedures, film uses, and film costs, providing an overall view of the number of procedures and film uses for each specialty. This information, readily available at the radiology administrative office, can be used to design the PACS server routing mechanisms, to determine the required number of WSs, and to assess the local storage capacity needed for each WS (the PACS thin client model does not need this parameter). The estimate of the cost of the film-based operation is derived from the total film used and compared with the cost of the digital-based or PACS operation.

The film-based operation cost estimate from Table 18.1 is applied in Table 18.2. Direct and indirect film library expenses included under item 1 in Table 18.2 are X-ray film jackets, mailing envelopes, insert envelopes, negative preservers, rental on film storage both internal and external to the department, fleet services for film delivery, direct (equipment) and indirect (operational) film processor expenses (item 2), developing solutions, replacement parts, facilities repairs and installations, and other miscellaneous supplies. In a typical film-based operation in a large teaching hospital, 70% of the film-based operation budget is allocated to the film library (item 3).The film cost (item 5) should be derived from the number of procedures performed and films used each year, given in Table 18.1. The film operation (not including film viewing) requires a large amount of premium space within the radiology department, which should be translated to overhead cost in the same estimate.

Use of Table 18.2 and the PACS checklist (Section 18.1.3.3) will allow a comparison of the PACS installation and operation costs with those of the film-based operation. Tables 18.1 and 18.2 give an overview of the film-based operation

TABLE 18.1 Record of number of procedures, film used, and film cost

Section (Specialty)	Number of Procedures Year 1 ... Year N	Film Used (sheets) Year 1 ... Year N	Film Cost[a] (dollars) Year 1 ... Year N
Nuclear medicine			
Ultrasound			
CT/MRI			
Pediatrics			
Gentitourinary, gastrointestinal (abdominal)			
Neuroradiology			
Cardiovascular			
Interventional radiology			
General outpatient[b]			
General inpatient[b]			
Mammography			
Emergency radiology			
ICUs[c]			
TOTAL			

[a]Film cost is for X-ray film purchased only; film-related cost is not included.
[b]Include chest and musculoskeletal examinations.
[c]Include all portable examinations.

TABLE 18.2   Multiple-year estimation of film and film-related costs

	Year 1	. . .	Year N
1. Film library	$		$
Indirect expenses	$		$
2. Film Processor	$		$
Indirect expenses	$		$
3. Personnel:	$ (FTE)[a]		$ (FTE)[a]
Darkroom	$ (FTE)[a]		$ (FTE)[a]
Film library			
4. Film-related costs Total $(1 + 2 + 3)$	$		$
5. Film Cost (from Table 17.1)	$		$
Total Costs	$		$

[a]Full-time equivalent (FTE)

and its cost, whereas Table 18.3 provides comparative statistics among radiology sections. Table 18.3 gives an estimated breakdown of the percentage distribution of procedures performed and efforts required in conventional projection X-ray examinations according to body region in a large urban hospital in northeastern United States. A similar table can be generated for digital sectional images including CT, MR, and US. The effort required is a measure of time and labor required to perform the procedure. The hospital or the department contemplating installation of a PACS should generate similar tables to facilitate proper planning.

Several two-phase cost analysis models are available in the market to help a hospital analyze the cost impact of PACS. The first phase is to assess the current film-based operation costs. In this phase, the user completes data forms similar to Tables 18.1 and 18.2, and the model predicts in detail the associated costs of the film-based operation. In the second phase, the user evaluates how these costs might differ from the implementation of PACS. A model like this allows a hospital to have

TABLE 18.3   Percentage of conventional projection X-ray procedures performed and effort required according to body region in a radiology department

Procedure	Percentage in Department	Effort Required[a]
Chest	40	18%
Musculoskeletal	39	25%
Gastrointestinal	9	22%
Genitourinary	1	8%
Neuroradiology	1	9%
Others	7	15%

[a]Effort required means that in the first row, it takes 18% effort to perform all chest X-ray examination, which amounts to 40% of all departmental examination, and so forth. Breast imaging was not included in this estimation. Generally, it is about 8% in the department. 3-D imaging has changed the percentages shown in this table drastically.

a clearview of the financial differences between its current film-based operation and a future PACS operation.

18.1.3   Digital-Based Operation

18.1.3.1   Planning a Digital-Based Operation

Interfacing to Imaging Modalities and Utilization of Display Workstation   In a digital-based operation, two components (see Fig. 1.2) are not under the control of the PACS developer/engineer, namely interfacing to imaging modalities and the use of PACS WS. In the former, the PACS installation team must coordinate with imaging modality manufacturers to work out the interface details. When a new piece of equipment is purchased, it is important to negotiate with the manufacturer on the method of interfacing the imaging modality to the PACS server through a DICOM

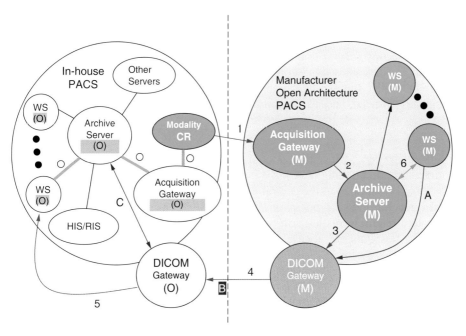

O: original PACS and dataflow path
M: manufacturer's new PACS to be implemented

1-5 and 6: transitional path
1-2-6: new path
A-B-C: first route of retrieving old images from the original
         archive server
6-3-4-C: a better route

Figure 18.3   Integration of an existing in-house PACS through a partnership with a manufacturer that is in the process of implementing a larger scale PACS for the institution. Two DICOM gateways, one in the in-house PACS and the second in the new PACS with open architecture, are used for the integration. Numerals and alphabets indicate paths of the integration.

gateway. Communication with the manufacturer should include the DICOM standard compliance statement in the equipment specifications.

For the WS, radiologists and clinicians are the ultimate users approving the system. For these reasons human interface and image workflow have an important role in planning the installation. It is necessary to consider IHE workflow profiles in the planning; and to detail specifications of the WSs and design proper environments to house them. Input from radiologists and technologists is essential, and several revisions may be necessary to ensure user satisfaction.

Cabling   We described the cabling and the hub room concept in Section 8.2. This section discusses the overall cable plan. Proper cabling for the transmission of images and patient text information within the department and within the hospital is crucial for the success of a digital-based operation. The traditional method of cabling for computer terminals is not recommended because, as the magnitude of the digital-based operation grows, the web of connecting wires very quickly becomes unmanageable.

Cabling is much simpler if the entire department is on the same floor. Greater complications ensue when the communication cable must traverse the whole hospital, which can occupy several floors or even several building complexes.

Layout of the cables that support the digital-based operation should be thought through carefully. Intranet and high-speed Ethernet switches and routers should be strategically situated, and a conventional Ethernet backup system should be considered

Air-Conditioning   Most digital equipment in a digital-based operation requires additional air-conditioning (A/C). If a new radiology department is planned, adequate A/C should be supplied to the central computing, server, and image-processing facilities. In general, WSs do not require special A/C considerations, but certain room temperature requirements are still necessary.

Because hospitals are always limited in space, it may be difficult to find additional central A/Cs for the large area housing the PACS central facility. Sometimes individual, smaller local A/C units can be installed. The individual A/C can be a stand-alone floor unit or a ceiling-mounted unit.

Each time another A/C unit is installed, an additional cool water source from the hospital is required. Thus the hospital's capacity for cooling water should be considered. Also, as noted earlier, additional A/C units can create a lot of noise in a room. To ensure that the room housing the WSs is suitable for viewing images, adequate sound proofing should be used to insulate these areas from the extra noise created by the A/C and cooling system.

Staffing   The hospital or department should allocate special technical staff with proper training to support the digital-based operation. In particular, system programming, digital engineering, and quality assurance personnel are necessary to make a digital-based operation run smoothly and efficiently. These new full-time equivalents (FTEs) can be re-allocated by terminating the existing FTEs in the film-based operation. Even if the manufacturer installs a department's digital-based operation and provides support and maintenance, the department is left with the responsibility of supplying trained personnel to oversee the operation. In general, the staff requirements consist of one hardware engineer, one system/software engineer, and a quality assurance technologist, all under the supervision of a PACS manager/coordinator.

18.1.3.2 Training Training of the department or hospital staff should include four categories:

Continuing Education for Radiologists/Clinicians Adequate training by the department/manufacturer should be provided to staff radiologists/clinicians on the concept of a digital-based operation as well as on the use of WSs. This training should be continued with periodic training as new equipment or upgraded WSs are implemented.

Resident Training The training for radiology and other specialty residents should be more basic. The radiology residency program should include training in digital-based operations. A one-month elective in PACS would be advantageous to radiology residents, for example. During this period, one or two residents would rotate through the PACS unit and obtain basic training in computer hardware architecture, software overview, architecture of the image processor, communication protocols, and the concept of WS.

Residents also can learn all basic image-processing functions that are useful for image manipulation as described in Section 12.5. The training schedule should be in the first or second year of residency so that residents can learn the concept and the complete procedure involved in a digital-based operation early in their training. This will facilitate future digital-based operations for the department and the healthcare center. In addition a quick refresher course once a year in July, when new house staff members start in radiology and other specialties, will minimize WS downtime and potential chaos in the reading area

Training of Technologists Retraining of technologists in the radiology department must precede the changeover to a digital-based operation. Digitization of X-ray films with the laser scanner, use of computed and digital radiography with imaging plates, and the digital radiography system are quite different from the screen/film procedure familiar to technologists. Also the use of PACS WS for image viewing, RIS WS for patient information retrieval and image transmission from image acquisition devices to the PACS gateway are new concepts that require additional training. The department should provide regular training classes, emphasizing hands-on experience with existing digital equipment.

Training of Clerical Staff Past experience in training secretarial staff to use word processors rather than typewriters has proved that the switch to digital operations at the clerical level is not difficult. The training should emphasize efficiency and accuracy. Ultimately the move to a digital-based operation will reduce the number of FTEs in the department.

18.1.3.3 Checklist for Implementation of a PACS This section provides a checklist for implementation of a hospital-integrated PACS. The implementation cost and operational cost can be estimated by multiplying the component price by the number of units and adding the subtotals. The component prices can be obtained from various vendors.

A. Acquisition gateway computers
    (one computer for every two acquisition devices) No._____
    Local disk
    ATM or fast Ethernet connection
    Interface connections

B. PACS server
    Database machine No. __2__
    File server No._____
    Permanent storage library No._____
    Temporary storage No._____
    Backup archive No._____
    Intranet and/or high-speed Ethernet connection No._____

C. Communication networks cabling (contracting)
    Intranet and high-speed Ethernet switches No._____
    Ethernet switches No._____
    Router No._____
    Bridge No._____
    Video monitoring system No._____

D. Display workstation (LCD WS)
    Four-monitor 2K WS No._____
    Two-monitor 2K WS No._____
    Four-monitor 1K WS No._____
    Two-monitor 1K WS No._____
    One-monitor 1K WS No._____
    Web-based WS No._____

E. Teleradiology component
    Yes_____ No_____

F. Interface with other databases
    HIS Yes_____ No_____
    RIS Yes_____ No_____
    Other database(s) Yes_____ No_____

G. Software development
    The software development cost is normally about 1 to 2 times the hardware cost.

H. Equipment maintenance
    10% of hardware + software cost.

I. Consumable
    Optical disks, tapes/year No._____

J. Supporting personnel

FTE (full-time equivalent) No._____

18.2 MANUFACTURER'S PACS IMPLEMENTATION STRATEGY

18.2.1 System Architecture

There are many PACS manufacturers that can install PACS of various scales. For larger manufacturers, the strategy is to install a full PACS for the institution either at one time or incrementally attached with a service and maintenance contract with upgradable features. Smaller vendors tend to carve a niche in the PACS market (e.g., in teleradiology or special imaging center mini-PACS) that larger manufacturers do not consider financially promising. Regardless of the approach, with the advances and lower cost in the PC-based WSs, high-speed networks, and RAID, and the practically free Internet technology, the manufacturer's WS architecture design is more generic and allows full or incremental implementation.

18.2.2 Implementation Strategy

A manufacturer's generic PACS business unit consists of R&D, service, training, design, implementation, consulting, marketing, and sale components. The market and sales components handle the presale, contributing to the design and site planning consultation. Information is fed back to R&D for product development. The post-sale is responsible for system design and implementation. Normally the manufacturer assigns a PACS manager to work closely with the hospital team in overseeing the implementation process. Operations after the implementation is the responsibility of service and training subunits. It is interesting to observe the difference in the manufacturer's point-of-view of selling a PACS with that of selling an imaging modality to a hospital, as shown in Table 18.4. In PACS, the implementation cost to the manufacturer is 60%, compared with only 20% for the imaging device. Table 18.5 shows the view of the manufacturer in the allocation of workers to a PACS negotiation and implementation. Over the past several years most institutions have felt that the postimplementation personnel support is not adequate at the institution level because of the high demand by clinical staff in the use of the PACS WSs throughout the hospitals, at least one to two IT personnel have been added to the PACS daily operation team.

TABLE 18.4   Comparing the manufacturer's perception of effort in selling an imaging devices versus a PACS

	Imaging Device % Effort	PACS % Effort
Marketing	40	20
Sale	40	20
Implementation	20	60

TABLE 18.5   Manufacturer's estimation of allocation of human resources required for PACS implementation (33- to 500-bed hospital)

	Pre-sale as needed	Design 4–6 weeks	Implementation 6 weeks	Application 4 weeks	Post Implementation
Institution		2 RT 1 manager	1 manager	2 RT	1 manager, 2RT +institution's staff
Manufacturer	1	2	2	2	1

Note: The estimation is based on the institution installing the first PACS module with an expandable permanent image archive. The human resources refer to persons assigned to the task but not necessary full time.

18.2.3 Integration of an Existing In-house PACS with a New Manufacturer's PACS

Larger manufacturers provide strategies for upgrading or integrating an existing in-house PACS through partnership. Figure 18.3 shows an example of using two DICOM Gateways for integration, one at the in-house PACS and the second at the manufacturer's open architecture PACS.

In Figure 18.3, the existing in-house PACS (left, yellow) is in daily operation and a much larger scale PACS (right, blue) supplied by the manufacturer with open architecture is being designed and implemented. The goal is to continue utilizing the in-house PACS for daily operation until the full implementation of the manufacturer's PACS is ready for operation. In the process the new design takes full advantage of the open architecture of the manufacturer's PACS during the transitional phase. Let us use an example to illustrate the steps involved. Consider the intensive care unit (ICU) original PACS operation in which CRs are used for image acquisition, and WSs for display.

Step I. Original dataflow: (O, orange): CR (green)–acquisition gateway (O, orange)–archive server (O, orange)–WS (O, orange).

During the transitional phase:

Step II. (1–5 and 6): CR (green, 1) sends a second copy of images to the new acquisition gateway (M, green, 2)–archive server (M, green, 3)–DICOM gateway (M, dark blue, 4)–DICOM gateway (O, yellow, 5)–WS (O, orange).

A second copy of the Images are also sent from the archive server (green, M, 6) to WS (M, green). When the workflow in the step II path is completed, the ICU directory has two identical copies in both archive servers O (orange) and M (green). This phase can be completed in about two weeks, since the average stay of ICU patients is normally less than one week. Then the original path (O) can be disconnected. All CR images will be routed through "1" to the archive server (M) only; and WSs (M, green) replace WSs (O, orange).

Step III. To retrieve historical images from the original archive server (O, orange) from the new WS (M, green) through bright blue route (A–B–C): WS (M green, path A)–DICOM gateway (M, dark blue, path B)–DICOM gateway (O, yellow, path C)–archive server (O, orange).

The disadvantage of this path is that the older images of the same patient stored in the original archive server (O, orange) would appear in separate files when they are retrieved from WS (M, green). A better routing path is WS (M, green, 6)–archive server (M, green, 3)–DICOM gateway (M, dark blue, 4)–DICOM gateway (O, yellow, path C)–archive server (O, orange). The latter path will require the archive server (M, green) to add the older images to the patient's folder in the archive server (M, green) once they have been retrieved, before sending them to the WS (M, green). That is, the manufacturer's archive server has two additional tasks: retrieving images from the old archive, and integrating them with the recent images in patient's folder. This discussion presents a first glimpse of data migration. The integration of old and new image data in the new archive server (M) is not a trivial task as we will discuss further in the topic of data migration in this chapter.

18.3 TEMPLATES FOR PACS RFP

There are several templates for PACS RFPs (requests for proposals) in the public domain. One, A PACS RFP Toolkit (http://www.xray.hmc.psu.edu/dicom/rfp /RFP.html), is by John Perry, who was with the Siemens Gammasonic Unit and developed the Medical Diagnostic Imaging Support (MDIS) system. Two others were developed by the military: One was for the original MDIS, and the second was the DIN/PACS II (www.tatrc.org) by Commander Jerry Thomas of the U.S. Navy. Another RFP was developed by D. G. Spigos of the American Society of Emergency Radiology's Committee on New Techniques and Teleradiology. These RFPs contain much useful information for those who plan to start the PACS acquisition process. Web sites can be terminated from time to time by the sponsors, readers are suggested to check the original sources for connection.

18.4 PACS IMPLEMENTATION STRATEGY

When implementing a PACS within a clinical environment, it is important to recognize two key concepts for a successful implementation. First, PACS is an enterprise-wide system or product. It is not just for the radiology or imaging department. It is crucial for a successful implementation that key constituents within the healthcare institution adopt implementation of PACS. These include administration, radiology department, IT department, and high-profile customers of radiology (e.g., orthopedics, surgery). Furthermore a champion should be identified to claim the ownership of the PACS implementation process. Usually this person is the medical director of radiology. Second, because PACS is a system with multiple complex components interacting with each other, all these components must be assessed carefully. The following subsections describe some critical steps to PACS implementation.

18.4.1 Risk Assessment Analysis

A risk assessment analysis performed before implementation can map out problem areas and challenges and accordingly timeline schedules to accommodate potential roadblocks. Some areas to focus on are the network infrastructure that supports the

PACS operation, the integration of acquisition modalities with PACS, and physical space for housing PACS equipment. Resource availability is crucial because a successful PACS implementation hinges on the support provided by the in-house radiology department. In making risk assessments, it is helpful to determine clinical specialties like critical care, orthopedics, and surgery that require many imaging examinations, but the return rate of films to the radiology department after the use is low. These clinical service areas should be the first areas for PACS implementation.

18.4.2 Phases Implementation

Implementation of PACS should be done in phases based on results from risk assessment. Usually the first phase is the implementation of main components such as network infrastructure, PACS server, archive server, and HIS–RIS–PACS interfaces with several imaging modalities, as well as some WSs targeting for special clinical services. The next phases would be strategically deploying modalities connection, and a Web server for enterprise-wide and off-site distribution of PACS image data. The phased approach allows for a gradual introduction of PACS to the clinical environment, with the ultimate goal being a filmless department/hospital operation.

18.4.3 Development of Work Groups

Because PACS serves many clinical areas in the hospital, it is important to develop work groups to handle some of the larger tasks and share responsibilities. In addition a PACS implementation team should be in place to oversee the timely progress of the implementation. The following are some key work groups and their responsibilities:

1. PACS network infrastructure: Responsible for all design and implementation of the network infrastructure to support PACS.
2. RIS–PACS interface and testing: Responsible for integration/testing of RIS–PACS interfaces including the modality worklist in the imaging acquisition devices.
3. Imaging modalities and PACS system integration: Responsible for the technical integration of modalities with PACS, installation of all PACS components, and space renovation.
4. Image acquisition workflow and training: Responsible for developing image input workflow and training for clerical and technical staff.
5. PACS system workflow and training: Responsible for developing PACS system workflow; and training for radiologists and clinicians to use WSs; and the design and monitoring the construction of PACS reading rooms.

It is crucial for these work groups to identify particular in-house resources to facilitate the implementation process. These should include the technical supervisor of each modality, the clerical supervisor, an experience film librarian or film clerk, a seasoned RIS support person, and an IT network support person. These staff members are excellent sources of information for issues related to PACS such as technologist workflow, clerical workflow, film distribution workflow, designing and performing RIS interface testing with PACS, and the overall hospital IT infrastructure of the hospital.

TABLE 18.6   Sample heading for an implementation checklist

Done	When	Who	WG	Event
X	5/14/07	John	2	Review modality integration list

Note: The first column indicates whether the task is complete; the second column shows the date the task was assigned; the third column indicates who the task responsibility is assigned to; the fourth column (WG) is the workgroup that the task belongs to; and the last column shows the task description.

In addition to the aforementioned work groups, a PACS implementation team should be formed to oversee the implementation process. Members should include at least one point person from each work group, and additional members should include the PACS implementation manager, the medical director of imaging, the administrative director of imaging, a IT representative, and an engineering/facilities representative. This team should meet at least every two weeks and more often as the on-line live date is approaching. The goals of this team are to update implementation progress, highlight potential stumbling blocks and potential solutions. In addition this team meeting provides a forum for higher level administrators of the hospital to observe the progress of the implementation.

18.4.4 Implementation Management

Developing a schedule and implementation a spreadsheet checklist can assist management of the implementation process. This template includes topics such as the task description, date scheduled for the task, owner of the task, and a checkmark box to indicate completion of the task. Table 18.6 shows a sample heading of an implementation checklist and a sample task. This template allows for finer granularity of the implementation process to protect against overlooked implementation tasks. Input for the checklist can come from the PACS implementation team meetings. Furthermore the checklist can be broken down into smaller subtask checklists for tracking of issues within each of the work groups.

18.5 IMPLEMENTATION

18.5.1 Site Preparation

The first step in PACS implementation is to plan and carry out space design and construction. One challenge in many healthcare institutions is to utilize existing space to renovate and build around it to accommodate a new project. This process involves coordination and communication with a wide spectrum of personnel because there may be many areas in the hospital that may need renovation to accommodate special PACS hardware and communication equipment. Among these is the design and construction of ergonomically conforming reading rooms for radiologists to read and referring physicians to visit and consult. Careful attention should be paid in designing a work space environment so that a radiologist can read softcopy cases for a long period of time comfortably. Figure 18.4 shows four transition stages of converting a clinical area into an ergonomic reading room. In addition, during the transition from a film to a filmless environment, the reading area should include the

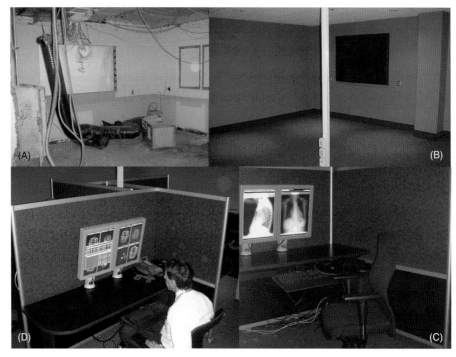

Figure 18.4   Conversion of clinical space into an ergonomic reading room with features like glare proof, ambient luminance, acoustic noise, privacy for individual radiologist and for group discussion and consultation. Different stages of the construction are shown, clockwise: (*A*) demolition; (*B*) space ready; (*C*) WS installation; and (*D*) WS being used.

ability of viewing hard copy films and soft copy images in the same work space conveniently.

During the construction an equally important task is the planning and installing the network infrastructure for the PACS connectivity. One of the first decisions to make is whether to utilize existing hospital networks or implement a new network specifically dedicated to PACS with connection to the hospital network. It will be more costly to implement a separate network for PACS; however, it would be necessary if the hospital does not have enough bandwidth to support images distribution of the PACS. The network infrastructure should be in place before the deployment of any PACS components. Baseline performance tests should be made before PACS goes live and afterward to confirm if the network performance is clinically acceptable.

18.5.2 Define Required PACS Equipment

Another step in the implementation process is to define the PACS equipment needed for the hospital operation. This task is most challenging because the determining factors include financial budget and workflow-related issues. The end results will undoubtedly vary from institution to institution. Some areas to be considered are workstation requirements, storage capacity, and storage types and image data migration.

18.5.2.1 Workstation Requirements   The PACS team needs to know the number of diagnostic WSs for radiologists, review WSs in the critical care areas, and the number of clients WS for the Web server. In addition, because sectional image acquisitions are complex, especially for CT and MR, several quality control (QC) WSs may be needed. These QC WSs will help the technologist to arrange the large number of images in particular orders and presentation format for the radiologist, as well as remove any unnecessary images before archiving. In clinical practice a technologist reviews CT and MR images at the QC WS before they are sent to the PACS archive. In case of CR and DR, he/she reviews it at the CR/DR own image processing WS for QC before they are sent for storage. However, in most practice, radiologist does not want the technologist to adjust the window and level of the image before they are sent to their WSs.

18.5.2.2 Storage Capacity   The storage capacity for all image data is crucial for a clinical PACS and should be estimated based on three parameters: capacity for the total archive, the backup archive, and the WS local storage (for the client and server PACS model, no local storage is required). These parameters can be estimated based on the number of exams acquired daily that would be sent to the local WS, the exam type, the average number of images per exam, and the image data size, as well as the length of time desired for the exams to remain on line. This task is sometimes known as a procedural volume analysis.

18.5.2.3 Storage Types and Image Data Migration   A decision to be made is what kind of long-term storage should be utilized; for example, digital linear tape, DVD, MOD, large-scale RAID, SAN, and the off-site ASP model. During the initial planning stage, some future advanced storage technology may not yet be available. A plan for future upgrade should be included, which leads to the topic of image data migration discussed more fully in Chapter 16.

18.5.3 Develop the Workflow

The next two steps of the PACS implementation process are the development and implementation of new radiology workflow and the starting of the training program. These two tasks are vital because they involve the users of PACS, who ultimately become the yardstick to measure the true success of PACS. In the past the focus was more related to whether the technology could support the needs of the users. However, with the maturing of PACS technology, it is more apparent now that the focus has shifted to how well the users can embrace the technology. To develop and design a new workflow, the workflow work group should include the clerical supervisor, the technologist supervisor, a radiologist, the PACS system administrator, and a training and modalities representative. The work group initially defines the current baseline work flow which can address a lot of unnecessary functions steps that were currently performed. The new workflow for PACS is developed in an iterative process during biweekly meetings. PACS manufacturer's engineers should install new WSs on site, and trainers to train the PACS users to use the WSs at least three months before the go-live date.

18.5.4 Develop the Training Program

Development of the training program for PACS is another key step toward a successful implementation. A PACS training team should be formed before the implementation consisting of the PACS system administrator and two key point persons identified from the clinical and technical area together they will attend intensive training class provided by the manufacturer. The training team has four major responsibilities:

1. As the team members become the experts, they will train other users in the hospital. This is commonly known as the "train the trainer" model.
2. The training team provides feedbacks from the PACS users to the manufacturer, and any user input is documented.
3. The team will develop training documents for the PACS users. These include easy instructions for the use of the more complex WS functions. These instructions can be posted at high-visibility areas next to the WS, and
4. The team will develop an in-house user manual completed with a troubleshooting guide and contact personnel numbers for support.

Once the training team becomes competent, they will train other PACS users in the hospitals. PACS users and user groups must first be identified because each user group performs different PACS functions. Some such group users would include radiologists, technologists, clerks, physicians, nursing staff, and system administrators. It is important that all users be trained not just on the specific PACS devices but on any other functions related to the device's workflow. Eventually the training team may evolve into the PACS management and support team.

18.5.5 On Line: Go Live

Before the PACS is on line in the clinical environment, there are some steps that can facilitate the transitional period. First, a "countdown to go-live" checklist and script should be developed to ensure against any overlooked tasks on the "go-live" date. Second, the go-live date should not be the beginning (Monday) or the end of the weekday (Friday).The training team should identify the PACS local user support (PLUS) representatives who will provide the initial frontline support for specific wards that utilize the PACS review WS, and radiology diagnostic WSs. These PLUS representatives can also notify the PACS management team of any outstanding issues that can be discussed on a weekly basis during the initial "go-live" phase of the implementation.

The training program schedule should begin three months before the go-live date and should focus on training the users and PLUS users on demonstration WSs. About two weeks before go live, a refresher WS training session should be offered. During the "go-live" week there will be many areas where on-the-spot training is necessary. For example, radiologists usually would not appreciate the full extent of application training until they must read cases on PACS WS as part of their real clinical workflow. An advanced WS training session can be offered as a follow-up for those users interested in learning more about advanced WS functions. During the "go-live" phase, at each review WS in the ward areas, radiology staff and PLUS representatives can be stationed there to provide immediate support and confidence to the ward physicians and users. Analog films would be gradually phased out as patients are discharged from the wards and the department, and those films needed for comparison studies would be digitized immediately by PLUS representatives for physicians to view them. Finally, exams acquired from the modalities would not be printed on film any more, to promote rapid PACS utilization. During the initiation of the "go-live" week, an issues list should be developed. This list will help track any outstanding issues that evolved from the "go-live" week and the list should be managed, resolved, and updated on a regular basis.

18.5.6 Burn-in Period and System Management

The PACS management and support team is a key component in the successful implementation and management of the system during the burn-in or stabilization period. The team members could be the same group as in the training team, they are responsible for any issues related to the daily operation and maintenance of the PACS system.

The PACS system administrator should have a medical imaging background. This member is responsible for the integration and implementation of PACS devices, maintenance and support of PACS, and coordination of any issues related to PACS (i.e., upgrades, service, troubleshooting). The PACS technical assistant can be an in-house FTE with a technical background in computer science. This member is responsible for troubleshooting PACS workflow issues, assists in the training of PACS devices, and performs backup maintenance and support for PACS. The PACS training and modalities support representative can be an in-house technologist FTE with training and support skills. This member is responsible for coordinating and training of PACS devices and modalities, troubleshooting technologist PACS-related workflow issues, and maintenance and support of the modalities.

During the burn-in period some of the issues carried over during the "go-live" phase need to be addressed and resolved as soon as possible. During this time period it would be advantageous to tune the workflow accordingly because the initial workflow developed by the work group may not be exactly as predicted. This is where workflow development will play an important role in the full utilization of the PACS for a filmless environment.

18.6 SYSTEM ACCEPTANCE

The key milestone in PACS implementation is the completion of the acceptance testing (AT) of PACS for the following reasons. AT provides:

1. vendor accountability for delivering the final product that was initially scoped and promised,
2. accountability for the in-house administration that there is documentation that the system was tested and accepted,
3. a glimpse into determining the characteristics of PACS uptime and whether it will function as promised, and
4. a proof of both PACS performance and functionality as originally promised by the vendor.

Most vendors provide their own AT plan, but usually the plan is not thorough enough; it is a template that is not customized to the specific healthcare institution's needs. The following sections describe some of the steps in designing and developing a robust AT that can be used for the final turnover of PACS in the clinical environment.

18.6.1 Resources and Tools

One of the first steps is to identify resources that will be involved in both AT design and implementation. Usually the PACS manufacturer will supply one resource person to be involved in the AT, and it is typically the vendor's PACS project manager. However, it is necessary for some in-house personnel to be involved in the AT. For example, the PACS system administrator can gain knowledge or even provide knowledge about the new PACS during AT development and implementation. A technologist representative can assist in the acquisition portion of end-to-end testing of PACS. Finally, a RIS support person can assist in the RIS portion of the end-to-end testing of PACS. As for the AT tools, the vendor usually provides a system acceptance document/checklist. However, it is usually a boiler plate document and not customized to the client's needs. Therefore it is important to ensure that all acceptance criteria and test development are client-driven. The checklist should include the following:

1. Test description
2. Pass/fail criteria and comments
3. Who performed the test
4. Any performance times

In addition, a consistent data set of PACS exams containing various modality types and a large image file size should be used for all tests.

18.6.2 Acceptance Criteria

Acceptance test criteria are divided into two categories. The first category is quality assurance. This includes PACS image quality, functionality, and performance. The second category is technical testing, which focuses on the concept of "no single point of failure" throughout the complete PACS workflow. The test should include simulation of downtime scenarios (see Chapter 16).

Acceptance criteria should include identifying which PACS components are to be tested. Figure 18.5*A* and *B* provides an example of a PACS component setup prepared for the technical acceptance testing. Figure 18.5*A* shows the hot swap main network switch. Figure 18.5*B* shows the components included in this PACS technical testing:

1. RIS–PACS interface
2. PACS broker
3. Modality scanner(s)
4. PACS server/storage

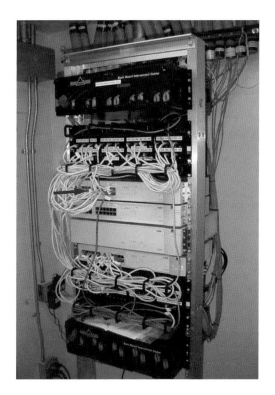

(A)

Components used in PACS Acceptance Testing

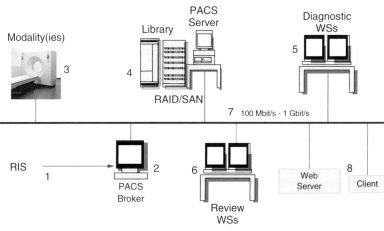

(B)

Figure 18.5   PACS acceptance testing (AT) design. (*A*) PACS network AT showing hot swap main network switch (red arrow); (*B*) an example of the components setup for the PACS acceptance testing (AT). Numerals described in text are the components needed to be included in the AT. Red: 100 Mbit/s; blue: 1 Gbit/s.

5. Diagnostic WS
6. Review WS
7. Network devices
8. Web server and client

Table 18.7*A*, *B*, *C*, and *D* provides a PACS acceptance testing outline, including AT components (see Fig. 18.5), what should be tested, technical testing design, and when the technical testing should be performed. The following subsections describe acceptance test parameters. Section 18.8 presents a system evaluation methodology.

18.6.2.1 Quality Assurance   The quality assurance portion of the acceptance testing plan can be grouped into three categories: (1) PACS image quality, (2) PACS functionality, and (3) PACS performance (see Table 18.7*A*).

PACS image quality is the evaluation of the display monitor and whether a particular display monitor is suitable for the radiologists. Because the radiologists will be reading directly from the display monitors it is important that they are satisfied with the quality of the image display. Currently there are two options, 5MP (mega pixels) and 3MP LCD (see Chapter 12). Radiologists from each specialty should be involved in the evaluation because each specialty may have specific needs. The five characteristics to be evaluated are as follows:

1. Sharpness: Identification of structures within the PACS image (e.g., interstitial lung markings, renal filling defects, bony trabecular markings).
2. Brightness: Ability to display high brightness while maintaining the best gray scale dynamic range.
3. Uniformity: Perception of uniformity in different brightness while viewing an image.
4. Angle of view: Ability to view images at extreme side angles.
5. Glare or reflection: Amount of glare emanating from an ambient light source on the display monitor.

In general, the 3MP LCD WS is acceptable for general sectional and 3-D radiology reading. The 5MP LCD WS is acceptable for CR and DR, and for digital mammogram with the enlargement feature.

The second category of quality assurance is PACS functionality. Usually vendors focus mostly on WS functionality such as displaying the worklist, images, and image tool sets. Some WSs may feature 3D postprocessing tools as well (see Chapter 12). The acceptance of WS functionality mostly occurs during applications training for the radiologists. However, back-end functionality (e.g., RIS–PACS interface, archiving and distributing functions, and QC WSs) tends to be overlooked during acceptance testing even though it is a vital part of the entire PACS workflow. The end-to-end testing is one of the few methods that can truly track the functionality of PACS as a whole. This includes ordering a radiology exam in the RIS, acquiring the PACS exam on a modality scanner, archiving, distributing, and displaying on all corresponding PACS components. In addition verification that all necessary RIS and PACS data are captured and stored in PACS (e.g., patient demographics, image characteristics) DICOM header.

TABLE 18.7   PACS acceptance testing outline

A. Acceptance testing components

1. Quality assurance
   - PACS image quality
   - PACS functionality
   - PACS performance
2. Technical testing
3. Tools

B. What should be tested —focus on no-single-point-of-failure concept in PACS

1. PACS server: stand-alone verses client-server
2. Short-term storage
3. Archive storage: SAN, RAID, tape, others
4. DICOM gateway
5. RIS/PACS interface
6. Network devices
7. Web server: client-server
8. Diagnostic WSs
9. Review WSs
10. Contingency plans

C. Technical testing design

1. Simulate real-world downtime clinical scenarios
2. Observe downtime effects on PACS with technical testing
3. Provide a level of comfort for the PACS system administrator with tangible simulated downtime experiences
4. Confirm any redundancy features as functional during downtime scenarios (e.g., redundant servers, redundant network switch)

D. When should the technical testing be performed?

1. Each implementation phase should have acceptance testing
2. The approach should be two-phased:
   - Phase 1 (1 week before live date): technical components testing points of failure, end to end, contingency solutions, and baseline performance measurements
   - Phase 2 (about 2 weeks after live date): workstation functions, PACS dynamic and performance testing on loaded clinical network

The last category is PACS performance. It is extremely important to separate as much as possible the performance of the network from the performance of the PACS. If possible, a network baseline performance should be performed before the PACS is on line. This can be accomplished by querying and retrieving a test set of PACS exams. When the PACS is on line, a second network performance test should be performed to measure the network bandwidth capability of a live network.

In addition to the network performance tests the PACS vendor normally suggests performance numbers that are expected from the PACS application. These performance numbers should be agreed on by both the client and the vendor to ensure the acceptance. For PACS performance numbers the time measured should always be from the time the first image of the PACS exam arrives at the WS until the last image of the entire exam can be displayed on the WS. This measurement will yield realistic performance that reflects real clinical scenarios. Most vendors only present the performance time of the first arrival image, which is not a realistic measurement. Table 18.8 shows measurements made during an acceptance test of a clinical PACS. These measurements were performed several years back, and general PACS performance numbers have improved considerably since then. Nevertheless, the method used in generating this table can be used as a general guideline for recording the performance test.

18.6.2.2 Technical Testing

The technical testing component of AT focuses on identifying single points of failure (SPOF, Chapter 16) in the PACS, and then acts to circumvent them through a backup mechanism so that the PACS can continue to operate clinically, if not at full performance level (see Table 18.7C). While doing this testing, it should be under a downtime scenarios. The following technical acceptance testing items are often ignored during the acceptance test.

Storage Systems As an example let us test the reliability of the storage systems in the PACS server shown in Figure 18.5*B*. The archive component (4) includes a RAID, a SAN, and a library. One of these storage systems is shut down to simulate a downtime scenario of the storage system. If the purchased PACS system has a backup storage mechanism, the other storage systems will backup the shutdown system, and no images will be lost during the storage downtime. We repeat the testing by shutting down the second storage system, and so on. After testing the downtime scenario, it is important to bring the storage system back to verify that normal operation is intact, as both backup and return to normal are vital to technical testing acceptance.

PACS Broker The PACS broker (see Fig. 18.5*B*, 2) should be shut down to observe the contingency workflow provided by the PACS server and to verify whether the PACS can continue to operate even if it is limited.

TABLE 18.8 Performance numbers gathered from a PACS Acceptance Testing

	CR Exam 2 Images	MR Exam 80 Images	CT Exam 90 Images
RAID (short-term storage)	12	45	73
MOD (long-term storage)	45	107	140

Note: Times measured in seconds were when the entire exam was loaded onto the local WS and the test was performed on a loaded clinical network.

Network Infrastructure Another component that is often overlooked is the network infrastructure (see Fig. 18.5*B*, 7). If a hot spare network switch is available on site as the redundant switch, it is necessary to perform the scenario of shutting down the live network switch, and of replace it with the hot spare as part of the acceptance test (see Fig. 18.5*A*). Once the spare is turn on, the network should function properly.

In summary, each PACS component that has the potential for hardware failure should undergo a downtime scenario and be brought back up to ensure that the clinical PACS operation is continuous. This technical testing provides several assurances (see Table 18.7*C*):

1. It simulates real-world potential downtime clinical scenarios.
2. Observations can be made of the effect of downtime on the clinical PACS when certain components are shut down.
3. It provides a level of comfort for the PACS support personnel, as they will be encountering tangible downtime experience.
4. It can confirm any redundancy features as functional (e.g., a redundant network switch, redundant servers).

18.6.3 Implement the Acceptance Testing

Each of the implementation phases of the PACS process should have an acceptance testing performed. Acceptance at each of the phases is also crucial for the vendor because it is only after the acceptance that the vendor can collect the remainder of the fee balance, which is negotiated beforehand. Carrying out the AT is a two-phase approach (see Table 18.7*D*). The first phase should be performed approximately one week before the go-live date. The content of phase one includes the technical component testing focusing on single points of failure, end-to-end testing, contingency solutions for downtime scenarios, and any baseline performance measurements. The second phase should be performed approximately two weeks after the go-live date, after the PACS has been stabilized in the clinical environment. The contents of phase two include PACS functionality and performance testing as well as any additional network performance testing, all carried out with a full loaded clinical network.

18.7 CLINICAL PACS IMPLEMENTATION CASE STUDIES

The following section will describe experiences encountered during the implementation of PACS at four clinical facilities. Each of the facilities, from a small community hospital, to two large enterprise level healthcare facilities in the United States, to an International hospital cluster, which is similar in the PACS implementation approach but contains challenges and issues that make them unique. The terminology and methodology introduced in this chapter are used to present these case studies.

18.7.1 Saint John's Healthcare Center, Santa Monica, California

Background   Saint John's Healthcare Center (SJHC) is a high-profile community-size hospital of approximately 200 beds located in an extremely competitive area in southern California. Damage sustained from the Northridge–Los Angeles Earthquake in 1994 led SJHC to decide on building an entirely new state-of-the-art hospital with a filmless imaging department. The PACS installation commenced in April 1999 so that a completely digital environment would be in place once the new inpatient wing opened in 2004. The PACS process was implemented in two phases.

Phase One   Phase one marked the implementation of the core PACS with CR imaging for all critical care areas. Phase two included the implementation of all the digital modalities and Web distribution to off-site physician's offices. Phase two occurred approximately 8 months after the go-live date of phase one. Since the hospital decided on transitioning from a film environment to a filmless environment, special emphasis was placed on workflow development and training. Some of the highlights for phase one include:

1. A go-live checklist (see Section 18.6) was used extensively to plan the immediate 12 hours before the go-live date and time, which was determined to be 7:00 AM on a Monday and coincided with the start time of radiologist's daily reading.
2. All chest films of patient within the critical care areas were digitized 12 hours ahead of time prior to the go-live time.
3. Since the CR system was a vital part of the going live, CR applications training and support were initiated at the go-live date.
4. IT support and training was provided to the ER Staff and their PACS workstations.
5. Additional IT supports were stationed at each of the PACS WSs within the critical care areas to promote user acceptance and utilization.
6. As patients were discharged from the critical care areas, the corresponding films were phased out and not utilized in the daily workflow.
7. In order to promote rapid PACS acceptance and utilization, studies acquired from the CR were not printed to film, even though there was a laser film printer available.

The final result was that the critical care areas, including ER, were filmless within 48 hours of the go-live date and since then have never reverted to film. Any issues that arose during and immediately following the go-live date were tracked and managed with an extensive and detailed issues list as part of the PACS support mechanism.

Phase Two   A similar go-live strategy was implemented for phase two. Two additional issues needed to be addressed: (1) referring physicians needing training and support in navigating the more complex volumetric imaging studies such as CT, MR, and US and (2) extra training for the clerks performing the film print protocols, which are more complex for the digital modalities. The reprints were previously performed by the technologists, but since the studies were archived to PACS, the film librarians and clerks needed to print them for off-site referring physicians.

Epilogue   The SJHC PACS operation was accepted by radiologists and the clinical staff immediately after its deployment, and it has been running very smoothly without any major pitfalls even after several major upgrades. In 2007 SJHC merged its healthcare information operation with the Sisters of Charity Leavenworth Health System Headquarter in Kansas. The RIS and PACS technical operations had since been under the management of the National Enterprise.

18.7.2 University of California, Los Angeles

Background   The University of California, Los Angeles (UCLA) Healthcare enterprise is a large-scale academic healthcare institution with multiple campuses. UCLA had developed its own homegrown PACS since the early 1990s and so had a long history and experience in PACS utilization. In 2003 UCLA decided to partner with a PACS manufacturer to implement an enterprise-wide commercial off-the-shelf PACS integrated with the previously implemented commercial RIS (see Fig. 13.4*B*).

From a Legacy PACS to Off-the-shelf PACS   Given the background of such a facility, the fact that the medical staff had utilized a homegrown PACS for a number of years was both a blessing and a curse. The blessing was the expectations and experience gained through workflow, training, and support of an existing PACS. The curse was the expectations of what a new, off-the-shelf commercial PACS should be able to do. The challenge was to balance the high expectations of the new PACS while sacrificing some of the customization that occurred with the legacy homegrown PACS. Because the new enterprise PACS was based on a client–server architecture (see Chapter 11) replacing a legacy homegrown PACS, some of the following features were built-in for PACS implementation:

1. Data migration of the legacy PACS data to the new PACS to begin eight months prior to the go-live date.
2. No phased approach during the PACS implementation—all modalities were to be integrated to the new PACS altogether prior to the go-live date.
3. A contingency plan with a backup PACS server to be implemented, and tested prior to the go-live data.
4. Redundancy built in to the PACS server, including a mirrored cluster server architecture, redundant fiber channel path to the SAN storage (see Fig. 11.4*B*).
5. PACS network infrastructure upgrades to provide adequate PACS performance including network switches with redundant supervisors and power supplies and new fiber cabling.
6. Multiple DICOM gateways to group the digital modalities together and provide redundancy.
7. A triple clustered Web server architecture for the hospital floors.
8. Local SAN storage designed to store 1.5 years of PACS studies as short-term storage.
9. An ASP archive off site with an ATM OC-3 connection and a DS-1 connection for backup as long-term storage.

Current Status   The implementation planning took one year from the kickoff meeting in 2004 to the go-live date. During that year the implementation tasks were broken down into the five work groups discussed in Section 18.4.3. This arrangement for such a large-scale PACS implementation ensured a successful installation. Because the medical staff was already familiar with PACS, the most challenging aspect of going live was the training and support related to the new application features. The careful planning and prior training made the implementation of the new PACS installed at UCLA extremely smooth. Chapter 19 will cover the UCLA data migration strategy.

18.7.3 University of Southern California, Los Angeles

Background   In the 2003 the Department of Radiology at the University of Southern California (USC) was offered a unique opportunity to install a total digital solution within an outpatient imaging center called Healthcare Consultation Center 2 (HCC2), operated under the total management, both business and technical, of the radiology department (see Chapter 16). The project included the integration of HIS, RIS, PACS, and voice recognition (VR), by which speech is converted to text during the radiologist dictation for diagnostic reporting. An IT team with six people was formed for the service and maintenance of the enterprise PACS operation.

Challenges   Among the number of challenges, the biggest was that the go-live date for CR studies only was scheduled for six months after the kickoff implementation meeting, and this provided a unique set of implementation parameters:

1. Total digital solution included the introduction of RIS-driven workflow.
2. The USC orthopedics group was the first referring customer, so a special effort was made to support the PACS WSs installed in every patient room within the orthopedic department.
3. As part of the total digital solution, an integrated RIS/PACS/VR WS was implemented for the radiologists—three separate system (RIS, PACS, and VR) applications in simultaneous operation.
4. Although the initial building plans did not include a data center, space dedicated to a future second MRI chiller unit was utilized because the cooling parameters were of similar specifications. Eventually the clinical IT systems and hardware were moved to its primary data center location.

Go Live   After going live, PACS user acceptance was higher at the orthopedic clinic than in the radiology department. This is a unique outcome as, generally, radiologists are more accepting of PACS than referring physicians. The main explanation appears to be that the integration of three separate clinical systems of RIS/PACS/VR in one reading WS within the concept of RIS-driven workflow had not been fully worked out at the go-live time.

RIS-Driven Workflow   RIS-driven workflow is basically having the RIS provide a reading worklist for the radiologist instead of PACS. Once the radiologist selects the study from the RIS reading worklist, the studies are automatically loaded into the

PACS application. Traditionally VR systems integrated with PACS applications were developed by PACS manufacturers familiar with the Radiologist's reading workflow. The integration of VR with RIS, while conceptually appearing to be the best approach in a RIS-driven workflow, in reality proved to be a barrier for the radiologist. The RIS turned out to not be tailored for diagnostic reading especially in an academic teaching environment.

The Divorce   The inadequacy of the integrated reading WS provided by the PACS manufacturer was eventually resolved by replacing this PACS manufacturer by a different manufacturer. Then the VR system was integrated with a new PACS instead of with the existing RIS. More detail on the PACS replacement is provided in Chapter 19.

18.7.4 Hong Kong New Territories West Cluster (NTWC): Tuen Mun (TMH) and Pok Oi (POH) Hospitals

Background   The Hong Kong NTWC is under the auspices of the Hong Kong Hospital Authority (see Chapter 16). Four separate hospitals and several clinics form a cluster of facilities dedicated to the care of the patients in the West New Territories, northwest of Kowloon, Hong Kong. Two of the facilities, Tuen Mun (TMH, 1500 beds) and Pok Oi (POH, 1000 beds), are considered the main hospitals, and PACS servers were to be installed there first. One of the objectives of the NTWC was to integrate the separate hospital RIS and PACS so as to provide an infrastructure to support the HA enterprise ePR system with image data distribution. An implementation team with five members was commissioned to IPILab, USC for two-week advanced PACS and imaging informatics training in September 2008 (see Chapter 28). Figure 18.6 shows the NTWC current workflow with emphases in PACS operation and ePR with image distribution to all clinicians.

The Challenges   POH recently undertook major renovations to expand the number of hospital beds from 200 to 1000. During the expansion a new PACS was purchased and installed. This meant meeting new challenges with regard to the NTWC PACS implementation strategy:

1. POH's integration with TMH required a PACS operation redesign. TMH operation consists of four separate PACS modules from four separate manufacturers. Each PACS module contains specific imaging modality data and was generally tied to the purchase of the modalities.
2. Before integration with POH, the imaging studies from these disparate PACS modules needed to be migrated into a single PACS.
3. Both TMH and POH had to be redesigned to serve as each other's redundant backup of PACS studies.
4. A single PACS user interface was desired across the entire NTWC so a single PACS vendor had to be selected.
5. The RIS under the HA enterprise CMS (clinical management system) was combined to serve the two hospitals.

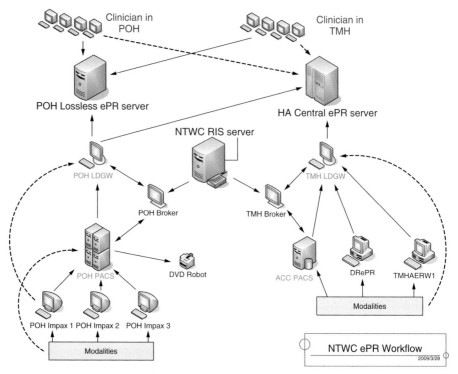

Figure 18.6   NTWC current workflow with emphases in PACS operation and ePR with image distribution to all clinicians. The NTWC is connected to the HA (Hospital Authority) enterprise ePR server (upper left) through the POH LDGW and TMH LDGW gateways. The gateways receive patient data and PACS images from both TMH and POH hospitals. The NTWC has its own RIS server (center) under the HA CMS (clinical management system). The figure also depicts the new POI PACS connection, and the four PACS modules at TMH connections.

6. The radiology service in NTWC had to be designed to support all clinicians' queries and retrieve patient information including image data from the HA enterprise ePR system.

Data Migration   Among the challenges the first one priority was the data migration by which the disparate PACS would be integrated into one central archive at TMH. This began in fall of 2008. Once the data were completely migrated, the hospital began the implementation process of a new single vendor PACS to replace the current four disparate systems. This implementation process is currently ongoing.

Current Status   The NTWC purchased a single vendor PACS for the cluster operation. The PCAS implementation is proceeding in four phases. The first phase was to install the PACS in POH; this was completed in late 2008 and is in clinical operation. The second phase is in data migration, which is still in progress. The POH PACS archive system is being used as the staging tool for TMH data migration, and the manufacturer is working with both TMH and POH on the project. The third phase is to stage the PACS implementation in TMH, and this is also in progress. The final phase will be total system integration.

18.7.5 Summary of Case Studies

Each facility of the aforementioned four case studies is different in its configuration and needs. Nevertheless, common to all four, as well as to other PACS implementations, is the fact that regardless of vendor choice, successful PACS implementation depends on the expertise and skill level of the in-house PACS support staff. As PACS go live, well trained support staff will enable a smooth transition to PACS utilization. Additionally one of the staff elects to champion the drive to implement PACS and works to remove barriers to PACS implementation.

18.8 PACS SYSTEM EVALUATION

In Section 18.6 we presented a PACS acceptance testing that is performed before the system is put into daily clinical operation. After the PACS has been in operation for several months, the impact of the PACS on the clinical environment has to be evaluated too. In this section we discuss three methods of PACS system evaluation. The first is to valuate PACS subsystem throughputs. The second is a direct comparison between the film-based and digital-based operations. The third is a standard ROC (receiver operating characteristic) analysis, comparing image quality of hard copy versus soft copy display. Sections 18.8.1 through 18.8.3 give examples of each method.

18.8.1 Subsystem Throughput Analysis

The overall throughput rate of the PACS is the sum of the throughput time of all individual PACS subsystems, including acquisition, archive, display, and communication network. Table 18.9 shows how to account for acquisition, archival, retrieval, distribution, display, and network residence times.

The throughput of a PACS subsystem can be measured in terms of the average residence time of individual images in the subsystem. The residence time of an image in a PACS subsystem is defined as the total time required to process the image in order to accomplish all tasks within the subsystem. The overall throughput of the PACS is the sum of total residence time of an image in all subsystems.

Each of the PACS subsystems may perform several tasks, and each task may be accomplished by several processes. An archive subsystem, for example, performs three major tasks: image archiving, image retrieval, and image routing. To perform the image retrieval task, a server process accepts retrieve requests from the WS, a retrieve process retrieves an image file from the permanent archive, and a process sends the image file to the destination WS. These three processes communicate through a queuing mechanism and run cooperatively to accomplish the same task. The retrieval residence time of an image file in the archive subsystem can be measured by the elapsed time from the moment an archive server receives the retrieve request, and retrieves the image file from the archive, to the time the server sends the image file to the WS.

TABLE 18.9   Definitions: Acquisition, archival, retrieval, distribution, display, and network residence times used for PACS system evaluation

Image Residence Time	Measurement Performed at	Definition
Acquisition	Acquisition	Total time of receiving an image file from an imaging device, reformatting images, and sending the image file to the PACS controller.
Archival	Archive	Total time of receiving an image file from an acquisition gateway, updating the PACS database, and archiving the image to the permanent storage.
Retrieval	Archive	Total time of retrieving an image file from the archive library and sending the image file to a WS.
Distribution	Archive	Total time receiving an image file from an acquisition gateway, updating the PACS database, and sending the image file to a WS.
Display (2 K)	Display	Total time of receiving an image file from the PACS Server, transferring the image file to the disk or RAID and displaying it on a 2 K monitor.
Display (1 K)	Display	Total time of receiving an image file from a PACS Server and displaying it on a 1 K monitor.
Network	Network manager	Total traveling time of an image from one PACS component to another via a network.

Once these residence times are broken down into computer processes, a time stamp program can be implemented within each process to automatically log the start and the completion of each process. The sum of all processes defined in each task is the measured residence time. The following subsections define various residence times.

18.8.1.1 Residence Time

Image Acquisition Residence Time   An acquisition subsystem performs three major tasks:

1. Acquires image data and patient demographic information from devices.
2. Converts image data and patient demographic information to DICOM format.
3. Sends reformatted image files to the PACS server.

Archive Residence Time   Images in the PACS server are archived to permanent storage. However, the archival residence time of an image may be significantly affected by the job prioritizing mechanism (Section 18.8.1.2) utilized in the PACS server. Because of its low priority compared with the retrieve and distribute processes running on the archive subsystem, an archive process is always compromised—that is, it must wait—if a retrieve or distribute job is executing or pending.

Image Retrieval Residence Time   Images are retrieved from the permanent storage to the PACS controllers. Among three major processes carried out by the PACS server, retrieve requests always have the highest priority. Thus images intended for study comparison are always retrieved and sent to the requested WS immediately before archive and distribute processes.

Distribution Residence Time   All arriving images in the PACS server are distributed immediately to their destination WSs before being archived in the permanent storage. Images can also be sent directly from the acquisition gateway to the WS.

Display Residence Time   A WS configured with a local disk storage or RAID may need to first receive images from the PACS server's RAID or SAN and thus delay the image display time on the monitor.

Communication Subsystem: Network Residence Time   The residence time of an image in the multiple communication networks can be measured as an overlapped residence time of the image in the acquisition, archive, and display subsystems (see preceding subsections). The Intranet or high-speed Ethernet throughput is limited by the magnetic disk input/output rate.

PACS Overall Throughput: Total Image Residence Time   The overall throughput of the PACS can be determined by the total residence time of an image from its original source (a imaging device) to its ultimate destination (a WS or the permanent archive).

18.8.1.2 Prioritizing   The use of job prioritizing control allows urgent requests to be processed immediately. For example, a request from a WS to retrieve an image from the permanent archive has priority over any other processes running on the archive subsystem and is processed immediately. On completion of the retrieval, the image is queued for transmission with a priority higher than that assigned to the rest of the images that have just arrived from the acquisition nodes and are waiting for transmission. During the retrieval, the archive process must be compromised until the retrieval is complete. Suppose, for example, that the retrieval of a 20-Mbyte image file from the permanent archive takes 54 seconds if this image file is retrieved while another large image file is being transmitted to the same archive, reducing the retrieval time for the former image file to 96 seconds, the time delay of the retrieval without job prioritizing is 42 seconds.

18.8.2 System Efficiency Analysis

We can use image delivery performance, system availability, and user acceptance as a means of measuring system efficiency. This section presents the comparison between a film-based versus a digital-based system operation.

18.8.2.1 Image Delivery Performance   One method of evaluating PACS system efficiency is to compare image delivery performance from the film management system and from the PACS. For example, consider the neuroradiology PACS component—in particular, for CT and MR images. We can decompose both the film-based and the digital-based operation into four comparable stages. In the film-based system, the four stages are as follows:

1. At each CT and MR scanner, a technologist creates films by windowing images, printing images, and developing films.
2. The film librarian delivers the developed films to the neuroradiology administration office.
3. The neuroradiology clerk retrieves the patient's historical films and combines them with the current examination films.
4. Radiology residents or film library personnel pick up the prepared films and deliver them to a readout area (or neuroradiology reading room).

The four stages in the PACS are similar:

1. The period during which the acquisition gateway receives images from the imaging device and formats the images into DICOM standard.
2. The elapsed time of transferring image files from the gateway to the PACS server.
3. The processing time for managing and retrieving image files at the PACS server.
4. The time needed to distribute image files from the server to the WS.

The time spent in each film management stage can be estimated and recorded by experienced personnel. Certain circumstances should be excluded from the calculation because their performance variances are too large to be valid, such as retrieval of a patient's historical films from a remote film library and the lag time between pickup and delivery of films through various stages in the film management system described above. These exclusions could make the film-based operation more competitive with the PACS.

The performance of the PACS can be automatically recorded in the database and log files by software modules. The data included in these files are (1) date, time, and duration of each modularized process and (2) size of the image file acquired.

18.8.2.2 System Availability

PACS system availability can be examined in terms of the probability that each component will be functional during the period of evaluation. In the neuroradiology example, several components are considered to affect the availability of the neuroradiology PACS:

1. the image acquisition subsystem, including all CT and MR scanners and interface devices between the scanners and the acquisition gateway.
2. the PACS server and the archive library.
3. the display subsystem with its WS and display monitors.
4. the communication network.

Calculations of the probability that each component will be functional can be based on the 24-hour daily operating time. The probability P that the total system will be functional is the product of each component's uptime probability in the subsystem, defined as follows:

$$P = \prod_{i=1}^{n} P_i \tag{18.1}$$

where P_i is the uptime probability of each component i, n is the total number of components in the subsystem, and π is the product of all terms.

18.8.2.3 User Acceptance   The acceptability of the WS can be evaluated by surveying users' responses and analyzing data from a subjective image quality questionnaire. Table 18.10 shows a sample item in a user acceptance survey, and Table 18.11 is a typical subjective image quality survey.

18.8.3 Image Quality Evaluation — ROC Method

A major criterion in determining the acceptance of PACS by users is the image quality in soft copy display compared with that for the hardcopy. In Table 18.10 we briefly noted a subjective image quality survey method. In this section we discuss a more rigorous method based on the receiver operating characteristic (ROC; see Section 6.5.4). Although the method is tedious, time-consuming, and expensive to perform, ROC has been accepted by the radiology community as the de facto method for objective image quality evaluation. The ROC analysis consists of the following steps: image collection, observer testing, truth determination, and statistical evaluation. Consider a sample comparison of observer performance in detecting various pediatric chest abnormalities—say, pneumothorax, linear atelectasis, air bronchogram, and interstitial disease—on softcopy (a 2K monitor) versus digital laser-printed film from computed radiography. Sections 18.8.3.1 through 18.8.3.5 describe basic steps of carrying out an ROC analysis.

18.8.3.1 Image Collection   All routine clinical pediatric CR images are sent to the primary 2K WS and the film printer for initial screening by an independent project coordinator with extensive experience in pediatric radiology. The project coordinator selects images of accepted diagnostic quality, subtle findings, disease categories, and

TABLE 18.10   Display workstation user survey form

Attribute	Poor	Fair	Good	Excellent	Ave.
	(1)	(2)	(3)	(4)	Score
Image quality					
Speed of image display					
Convenience of image layout					
Performance of manipulation functions					
Sufficiency of patient information					
Sufficiency of image parameters					
Ease of use					
Overall impression					
Overall average					

TABLE 18.11   Subjective image quality survey form for comparing the film viewing versus the display workstation

Display System	Ranking Scales (Perception of Confidence)					
	Least					Most
	1	2	3	4	5	6
Film-and-light box						
Display workstation						

also selects a set of matched normal images to set of abnormal images. To ensure an unbiased test, half of the selected images should be read from the soft copy and the other half from the hard copy. A reasonably large-scale study should consist of about 350 images to achieve good statistical power.

The two selected image sets should be screened one more time by a truth committee of at least two experts who have access to all information related to those patients whose images had been selected, including clinical history and images. During this second screening some images will be eliminated for various reasons (e.g., poor image technique, pathology too obvious, overlying monitoring or vascular lines clouding the image, and/or overabundance of a particular disease type). The remaining images are then entered into the ROC analysis database in both hardcopy and soft copy forms.

18.8.3.2 Truth Determination   Truth determination is always the most difficult step in any ROC study. The truth committee determines the truth of an image by using clinical history of each case, hard copy digital film image, softcopy on LCD with all available image processing tools, and biopsy results if available.

18.8.3.3 Observer Testing and Viewing Environment   The WS should be set up in an environment similar to a viewing room, with ambient room light dimmed and no other extraneous disruption. Film images should be viewed in a standard clinical environment. Observers are selected for their expertise in interpreting pediatric chest radiographs. Each observer is given a set of sample training images from which they are trained in four steps: (1) learn how to interpret an image with softcopy display, (2) read the assigned softcopy set from LCD, (3) complete the ROC form for the softcopy reading results (e.g., see Fig. 18.7), (4) read the assigned hardcopy film using a light box, and (4) complete a second ROC form for the hardcopy reading results.

18.8.3.4 Observer Viewing Sequences   An experimental design is needed to cancel the effects due to the orders in which images are interpreted. The images selected can be randomized and divided into four subsets (A, B, C, and D), containing approximately equal numbers of images per subset. Identical subsets are included in both hardcopy and softcopy viewing. But softcopy and hardcopy can not be mixed in the same subset. Each observer participates in two rounds of interpretation. Round 1 consists of four sessions as shown in Table 18.12 (but it depends on the total number of images in the ROC study). During each session either the softcopy subset or the hardcopy subset is read. To minimize fatigue, each observer interprets about 30 images of the same kind (i.e., either hard or softcopy) during a session. In round 1, the assigned observers interpret all four subsets, half from hard copy and the other

Case Number _____   Board Number _____

Patient Name _____   Procedure Date _____ Time _____

Patient I.D. _____   Reading Date _____ Size _____

Instructions: If abnormality is present, please indicate your level of confidence.

Confidence Scale:

0 . . . . 1 . . . . 2 . . . . 3 4

Sure Not Present   50% sure   100% sure
   (default)   It is present   It is present

Radiographic Condition	Enter Confidence Ratings					
	Absent	Diffuse	R.U.	R.L.	L.U.	L.L.
1. Pneumothorax						
2. Interstitial Disease						
3. Linear Atelectasis						
4. Air Bronchograms						

Comments:

Figure 18.7 Structured form of the receiver operating characteristic used in a typical ROC study of chest images. For each disease category, a level of confidence response is required. Chest quadrants assessed were right upper (RU), right lower (RL), left upper (LU), and left lower (LL).

half from soft copy. During the round 2, which should be three to five months later to minimize the learning effect, the observers again interpret all images, but for each subset with the viewing technique not used in round 1. After round 2, each observer has read eight sessions covering all images twice, one with hardcopy and the other with softcopy. The viewing sequence is shown in Table 18.12.

18.8.3.5 Statistical Analysis The two ROC forms for each image (softcopy and hardcopy reading) filled in by each observer for all eight sessions are entered in the ROC program for statistical analysis. Nowadays, graphical user interface (GUI) is

TABLE 18.12   Order of interpreting image sets used in the ROC study

Observer Number	Order of Interpreting Technique Subsets	
	Round 1	Round 2
I	A1, B1, C2, D2	A2, B2, C1, D1
II	A2, B2, C1, D1	A1, B1, C2, D2
III	C1, D1, A2, B2	C2, D2, A1, B1
IV	C2, D2, A1, B1	C1, D1, A2, B2
V	C1, D1, A2, B2	C2, D2, A1, B1

Note: A, B, C and D are the four image sets, each with equal number of images. The number 1 and 2 refer to the viewing technique (soft or hardcopy). For example, observer I views image sets A1, B1, C2, D2 during round 1 and later (>3 months) in round 2 reviews the image sets A2, B2, C1, and D1.

used to alleviate the burden to the observers, the form shown in Figure 18.7 has been computerized for easier to input reading results to the ROC program.

A standard ROC analysis program—for example, CORROC2 developed by Dr. Charles Metz of the University of Chicago—can be used to calculate the area under the ROC curve (see Fig. 6.10) along with its standard deviation for a given observer's results for both the hardcopy and softcopy viewing method. The ROC area can be compared by the disease category with the paired t-test. The results provide a statistical comparison of the effectiveness of using softcopy and hardcopy reading on these two sets of images in diagnosis of the four diseases. This statistical analysis forms the basis of an objective evaluation of image quality of the hardcopy versus softcopy reading based on these two image sets.

18.9 SUMMARY OF PACS IMPLEMENTATION, ACCEPTANCE, AND EVALUATION

In this chapter we present terminology, methodology, and road maps for PACS implementation, acceptance testing, and evaluation. In implementation and acceptance testing, we stress in-house staff training prior to, during, and post installation. An in-house champion should claim the PACS ownership from the beginning to daily operation. Our philosophy of PACS design and implementation is that regardless of the scale of the PACS being planned, room should always be left for future expansion, including integration with the enterprise PACS and ePR with image distribution. We give step-by-step guidelines in all phases for the PACS implementation. Four PACS implementation case studies from a small community hospital, to two large-scale enterprise PAC systems, to an International hospital cluster are presented. Reasons for their success and failure are highlighted and discussed.

References

Huang HK, Andriole K, Bazzill T, Lou ASL, Wong AWK. Design and implementation of PACS—the second time. *J Digit Imag* 9(2): 47–59; 1996.

Huang HK, Wong AWK, Lou SL, Bazzill TM, et al. Clinical experience with a second generation PACS. *J Digit Imag* 9(4): 151–66; 1996.

Huang HK. Introduction to Paper by H. K. Huang, D.Sc., et al. Digital radiology at the University of California, Los Angeles: a feasibility study. *J Digit Imag* 16(1): 69; 2003.

Huang HK, Barbaric Z, Mankovich NJ, Molar C. Digital radiology at the University of California, Los Angeles: a feasibility study. *J Digit Imag* 16(1): 70–6; 2003.

Liu BJ, Huang HK, Cao F, Zhou MZ, Zhang JZ, Mogel G. A complete continuous-availability PACS archive server. *Radiographics* 24: 1203–9; 2004.

Liu BJ, Cao F, Zhou MZ, Mogel G, Documet L. Trends in PACS image storage and archive. *Comput Med Imaging Graph* 27: 165–74; 2003.

Osman R, Swiernik M, McCoy JM. From PACS to integrated EMR. *Comp Med Imag Graph* 27(2–3): 207–15; 2003.

Siegel EL, Huang HK. PACS and integrated medical information systems: design and evaluation. *Proc SPIE*. 4323: 426; 2001.

CHAPTER 19

PACS Clinical Experience, Pitfalls, and Bottlenecks

This chapter's presentation of clinical experience and lessons learned is excerpted from the last edition of this book and based on the clinical experiences of two medical centers: the Baltimore VA Medical Center and the St. John's Healthcare Center in Santa Monica, California. The Baltimore VA case is a study of a successful filmless PACS operation. The St. John's Health Center case is a study of two PACS operation issues and solutions that resulted in an upgrade of the archive server and off-site backup archive. We predicted in our 2004 edition that many existing and future PAC systems would face similar issues; we provide two new case studies at UCLA and at the University of Southern California, that substantiate our prediction. The remaining topics in this chapter explore PACS pitfalls, PACS bottlenecks, and pitfalls in DICOM conformance. Figure 19.1 (excerpted from Fig. 1.3) shows how this chapter corresponds to other chapters of Part III.

19.1 CLINICAL EXPERIENCE AT THE BALTIMORE VA MEDICAL CENTER

This section is based on a retrospective of the filmless radiology department at the Baltimore VA Medical Center by Drs. Eliot Siegel and Bruce Reiner that appeared in *Computerized Medical Imaging and Graphics* (Siegel and Reiner, 2003).

The Baltimore VA Medical Center (VAMC) started its PACS implementation in the late 1980s and early 1990s. The VAMC purchased a PACS in late 1991 for approximately $7.8 million, which included $7.0 million for PACS and $800,000 for CR. It should be pointed out that the cost was based on the estimated value of the 2003 U.S. dollar extrapolate to the then-current PACS technology; both the dollar value and the technology have changed considerably since those years. The manufacturers involved were Siemens Medical Systems (Erlangen, Germany) and then took over by Loral Western Developed Labs (San Jose, California); the product line was later acquired by Loral/Lockheed Martin and then General Electric Medical Systems. The objective of the VAMC project was to integrate with the VA homegrown clinical patient record system (CPRS) with a VistA imaging system (see Section 22.2). The project was headed by Dr. Eliot Siegel, chair of the radiology department. The system was in operation by the middle of 1993 in the new Baltimore VAMC, but has

PACS and Imaging Informatics, Second Edition, by H. K. Huang
Copyright © 2010 John Wiley & Sons, Inc.

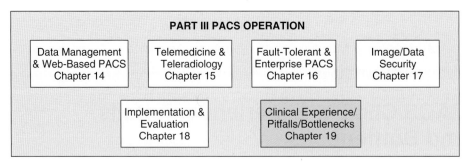

Figure 19.1   Position of Chapter 19 in the organization of this book. Color codes are used to highlight components and workflow in chapters of Part III.

since evolved and been integrated with other VA hospitals in Maryland into a single imaging network. The following subsections summarize the benefits, costs, savings, and cost-benefit analyses.

19.1.1   Benefits

The clear benefits for Baltimore VAMC in changing its radiology operation to filmless were reductions in unread cases and in retake rates, and consequently a drastica improvement in the clinical workflow. In the early 1990s healthcare establishments were still debating the wisdom of why PACS should be installed at all. Demonstration of these benefits was crucial in convincing VAMC to consider PACS. Figure 19.2 shows the drop from the 8% unread imaging study rate before PACS to approximately 0.3% in 1996.The remaining number of unread studies was identified in a weekly audit with the HIS/RIS system and subsequently made available for interpretation or reinterpretation with PACS. The transition to filmless was the direct benefit of using a CR system.

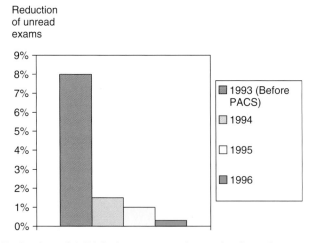

Figure 19.2   Reduction of 96% in lost or unread examinations, but not complete elimination, within three years of the transition to filmless operation.

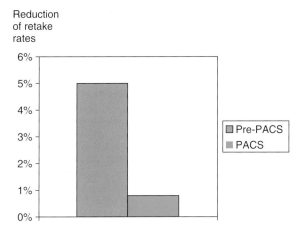

Figure 19.3   Wide dynamic range of computed radiography, and the ability to manipulate images at the WS, resulting in a reduction of retake rate by 84% from 5% (orange) when film was used for general radiographic examinations. There was also a shift in the most common reason for the retakes, from error in technique (images too light or too dark) to problems with patient positioning.

CR also contributed to reducing the rate of retake due to unsatisfactory examinations. This retake rate was reduced by 84% from 5% when film was used to approximately 0.8% after the transition to the CR and filmless operation shown in Figure 19.3.

The transition to filmless operation resulted in the elimination of a number of steps in the process in which imaging studies were made available for interpretation by radiologists. Figure 19.4 shows the 59 steps required in a film-based operation in 1989, and the sharp drop to 9 steps after the transition to PACS operation. Figure 19.5 The time interval from the point where a study is begun to where it is reported was reduced from several hours (often running into the following days) to less than 30 minutes (during a normal workday). A further reduction in reporting (from when a study was performed until it was dictated) time, which was reduced from 24 hours to 2 hours as shown in Figure 19.6, facilitated "real-time" reporting and had a positive impact on the quality of patient care and on the referring clinicians. The time savings in radiology services are associated with the strong (92%) preference for PACS over film (3%, with 5% undecided) by the clinicians at the Baltimore VAMC when an initial survey was conducted about two years after the implementation of PACS. According to the survey, in the clinicians' view, the biggest benefit of PACS to their practice was that it saved them time and allowed them to be more productive. In response to a formal survey in the mid-1990s, 98% of the respondents indicated that the PACS resulted in more effective utilization of their time.

19.1.2   Costs

Initially the two major cost considerations of PACS were depreciation and the service contract. The VA depreciates its medical equipment over a period of 8.8 years, whereas computer equipment was typically depreciated over a 5-year time period

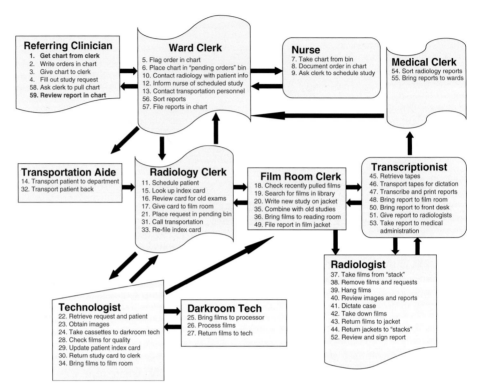

Figure 19.4   In 1989 a workflow study conducted at the Baltimore VA Medical Center determined that 59 steps (blue) were involved in a film-based environment from the point of request to the report on an inpatient's chest radiograph. (Courtesy of Dr. E. Siegel)

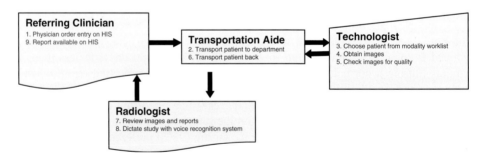

Figure 19.5   After introduction of PACS and integration of the system and imaging modalities with the hospital and radiology information systems, the number of steps required for an inpatient chest radiograph decreased substantially to 9 (blue). (Courtesy of Dr. E. Siegel)

(that was depreciation in 2003; today the market puts it in the neighborhood of three years). Other significant contributors to the cost of the PACS was the service, which includes the following:

1. Personnel required to operate and maintain the system.
2. Service contracts to the manufacturers.

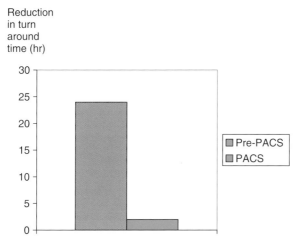

Reduction
in turn
around
time (hr)

Pre-PACS
PACS

Figure 19.6   Combination of workflow reduction and rapid availability of images. After images were obtained, the time was reduced from approximately 24 to 2 hours, starting from when an image was acquired until it was transcribed.

3. Software upgrades and replacement of all hardware components that fail or demonstrate suboptimal performance.
4. Replacement of any monitors that do not pass periodical quality control tests.

In the Baltimore VAMC, the radiology administrator, chief technologist, and chief of radiology shared the administrative duties of a PACS departmental system administrator.

19.1.3   Savings

19.1.3.1   Film Operation Costs   Films were still used in certain circumstances. Mammography exams still depend on films, but they were digitized and integrated to PACS. Films were also printed for patients who need to have them for hospital or outpatient visits outside the VA Healthcare network. Despite these two services, film costs had been cut by 95% compared with the figure that would have been required in a conventional film-based department. Additional savings include reductions in film-related supplies such as film folders and film chemistry and processors.

19.1.3.2   Space Costs   The ability to recover space in the radiology department because of PACS contributed to a substantial savings in terms of space indirect costs.

19.1.3.3   Personnel Costs   The personnel cost savings included radiologists, technicians, and film library clerks. An estimate was made that at least two more radiologists would have been needed to handle the current workload at the VAMC had the PACS not been installed. The efficiency of technologists had improved by about 60% in sectional imaging exams, which translated to three to four additional technologists had the PACS not been used. Only one clerk was required to maintain the film library and to transport film throughout the medical center.

19.1.4   Cost-Benefit Analysis

In Section 18.1.1 we describe a cost analysis model that compares film-based operation and PACS operation. There is a crossover point at which PACS becomes
more cost-effective to use than the conventional film-based operation (see Fig.
18.2*C*).

The Baltimore VAMC PACS underwent a similar study by a group of investigators
from the Johns Hopkins University; the results are shown in Figure 19.7. The study
found that in a conventional film-based environment the cost per unit examination
was relatively flat as the volume of studies performed in the radiology department
increased from 20,000 to 100,000 studies a year. As the number of studies increases,
additional space, personnel, and supplies were necessary. With a PACS, there was a
rapid decrease in unit cost per study because equipment costs for the system were
fixed and did not increase substantially with added volume. At a volume of 90,000
studies per year, there was an approximately 25% savings in cost per unit study with
a PACS compared with film. The breakeven point between film-based and filmless
operation occurred at approximately 39,000 studies a year. At volumes greater than
that, the study found filmless operation to be more cost-effective than a conventional
department operation.

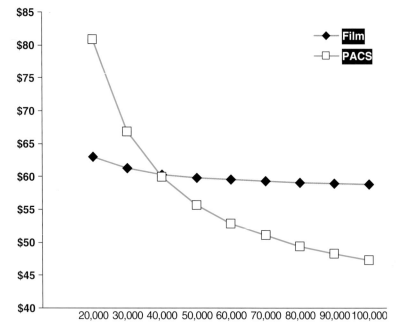

Figure 19.7 Relatively flat cost per unit examination in the film operation (orange)
as volume of studies performed in the radiology department increased from 20,000 to
100,000 studies a year. There was nevertheless a rapid decrease in unit cost per study with
a PACS (green). At 90,000 studies per year there was an approximately 25% decrease
in cost per unit study with a PACS in comparison to film. The breakeven point occurred
at approximately 39,000 studies each year. (Courtesy of Dr. E. Siegel)

19.2 CLINICAL EXPERIENCE AT ST. JOHN'S HEALTHCARE CENTER

19.2.1 St. John's Healthcare Center's PACS

In Section 18.7.1 we described the PACS implementation experience at Saint John's Healthcare Center (SJHC) in Santa Monica, California. This section recaps that PACS operation and presents the two archival issues that SJHC faced after the implementation. Saint John's had a filmless PACS that acquired roughly 130,000 radiological exams annually. As the first phase St. John's implemented the PACS with CR for all critical care areas in April 1999. The second phase, completed in April 2000, comprised the integration of MR, CT, US, digital fluorography, and digital angiography within the PACS. Since then, St. John's PACS volumes have increased steadily. The original storage capacity of the PACS archive was a 3.0 TB MOD Jukebox, which meant that older PACS exams had to remain off line before a year was over. Also the archive had only a single copy of the PACS data. Therefore in a natural disaster St. John's stood to lose all the PACS data because there was no backup (see Chapter 16). Based on this consideration, St. John's determined to overhaul its PACS archive system with the following goals:

1. Upgrade the archive server to a much larger capacity
2. Develop an off-site image/data backup system
3. Conduct an image/data migration during the archive system upgrade.

These goals were accomplished in late 2001 using the concepts discussed in Chapter 16 (fault-tolerant server) and Chapter 18 (acceptance test).

With the archive upgrade, all new PACS exams are archived through a Sun Enterprise 450 platform server with a 270 GB RAID. The exams are then archived to a network-attached digital tape storage system comprising an additional Sun Enterprise 450 with a 43 GB RAID and a 7.9 TB storage capacity digital tape library.

19.2.2 Backup Archive

19.2.2.1 The Second Copy The recovery solutions for image/data following a natural disaster are as follows.

1. Keep a second copy within the PACS. This is usually not recommended because of the high likelihood of it being destroyed along with the primary copy.
2. Create the secondary copy to be stored somewhere on site in a fireproof safe or storage compartment. While this decreases the possibility of data loss, in a widespread disaster throughout an entire local area, the PACS data would still susceptible to destruction.
3. Store the data media off site in a storage vault. This strategy is adopted by most data centers and is considered the best solution among the others.

19.2.2.2 The Third Copy To satisfy the fault-tolerant definition of PACS, a third copy of the data is needed. This strategy provides for a disaster that occurs right as the most recent tape is being filled to capacity and has not been sent off site, since then the hospital could lose up to a few weeks' worth of PACS exams.

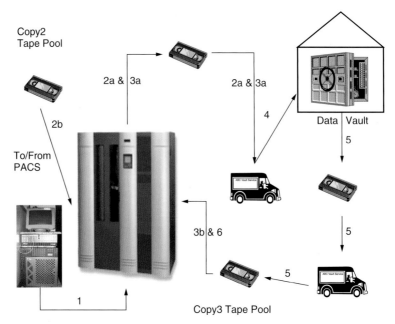

Figure 19.8   Third copy tape used as a disaster recovery procedure for PACS data at Saint John's Healthcare Center. The purple color library in the center is the digital linear tape archive system. Numerals are the workflow steps.

Creating a third copy would cover the turnover period between secondary copy tapes. A disaster recovery strategy that includes a daily third copy of the PACS data is necessary to cover the turnover period.

PACS digital linear tape usually has large capacity media. Each tape can hold several weeks' worth of PACS data (depending on the size of the PACS). These tapes can be used to hold a third copy that can be stored either on or off site in a data storage vault. It is estimated that one digital tape medium can currently hold 5 days' worth of PACS data at St. John's. The following steps, along with Figure 19.8, provides a procedure that an operator can performs manually. External to the tape library, there are three tape pools, copy1, copy2, and copy3; in the library there are always copy1, copy2, and copy3 tapes. Copy1 tape stays permanently in the library; copy2 tape resides in library until it is 95% full, and then is sent off to the data vault; copy3 tape is recycled daily in the data vault, first in–first out.

1. When a PACS exam arrived, it is archived in three copies to three separate tapes. Copy1 is the primary copy and always resides in the tape library.
2. Copy2 tape also resides in the tape library and is the backup; at 10 AM daily it is checked manually by the operator for its available capacity.
   a. As the copy2 tape becomes 95% full, it is ejected (approximately every 5 days) and sent off site to the data vault as the backup copy.
   b. A new copy2 tape is loaded into the library from the copy2 tape pool.
3. Copy3 tape is replaced daily, as coverage for the period when the copy2 tape reaches 95% full.

    a. Copy3 tape is ejected at 10 AM every day and sent off site. If copy2 tape is 95% full, copy3 tape of that specific day is returned to the copy3 tape pool for reuse.

    b. Two new Copy3 tapes are loaded into the library from the copy3 tape pool to fill the gap vacated by the 10 AM copy3 tape. Two tapes are loaded in case the first tape has been filled to capacity during the previous day and overflowed onto the second tape.

4. Data vault storage service picks up tapes daily for transfer to a secure location. Copy2 tapes are stored permanently there for disaster recovery. Copy3 tapes are stored temporarily.

5. The copy3 tape pool is replenished from the data vault if needed, covering for the period when the copy2 tape reaches 95% full. More than one tape might be necessary if the daily data rate is higher than one tape. When a copy2 tape arrives at the data vault storage facility, all used copy3 tapes stored are returned to St. John's copy3 tape pool.

6. When a copy3 tape is 95% full, the copy3 tape contents are erased and readied for reuse.

Some disadvantages to this approach are that there must be enough recyclable data media for each day of the coverage period and that the procedures are tedious and prone to human errors because they were labor intensive. Although this solution can provide the necessary redundancy of all acquired PACS data, the hospital must logistically still wait for new hardware to replace the damaged components in order to import the data media after a disaster. This can take days or even a week, depending on availability of the hardware. In the meantime radiologists are dependent on the previous exams for a diagnosis until the replacement hardware arrives and is installed. The concept of the Data Grid, which will be presented in Chapter 21, is an elegant and error-free solution for backup archive.

19.2.2.3 Off-site Third Copy Archive Server   With the option of storing the third copy of data in a backup archive server off site, the copy can be stored automatically; there is no need for an operator to perform the daily backup chore. In addition the backup storage capacity is easily configurable based on the needs of the hospital. A downside to this option includes the logistics of purchasing, maintaining, and supporting a backup archive server off site by the hospital. During a disaster there is a high probability that the network connection will be down and therefore the backup copies of the PACS exams will not be accessible. The existence of the third copy archive server may eliminate the need for the second copy.

    With these issues as a backdrop, there have been new attempts at developing not only a fault-tolerant main archive server but also data redundancy and recovery during either scheduled downtime events or unscheduled disasters like the off-site ASP fault-tolerant backup archive described in Chapter 21.

19.2.3 ASP Backup Archive and Disaster Recovery

Among these options St. John's chose the ASP fault-tolerant off-site backup archive method in preparing for its archive upgrade as well as for its disaster recovery scheme for the following reasons:

1. A copy of PACS exam is created and stored automatically.
2. Backup archive server is CA (continuously available) and fault tolerant with 99.999% availability.
3. There is no need for operator intervention.
4. Backup storage capacity is easily configurable and expanded based on requirements and needs.
5. Data are recovered and imported back into hospital PACS within one day with a portable data migrator.
6. System is DICOM compliant and ASP model based.
7. System does not impact normal clinical workflow.
8. Radiologists can read with previous exams until hospital PACS archive is recovered.

The detail of this ASP model has been presented in Section 11.6, and Figures 11.11 and Figure 11.12.

19.3   UNIVERSITY OF CALIFORNIA, LOS ANGELES

As we previously discussed in Chapter 18, in 2002 UCLA partnered with a large PACS manufacturer to replace their legacy homegrown PACS with an off-the-shelf system. During the implementation and subsequent go-live two major challenges arose. The first was the challenge of migrating data from the legacy DICOM archive to the new PACS archive. The second was the implementation, testing, and evaluation of a long-term ASP archive. Both topics will be discussed more fully in the following sections.

19.3.1   Legacy PACS Archive Data Migration

Figure 19.9*A* shows the timeline strategy of data migration. There are four terms we use: legacy PACS, legacy PACS archive, new PACS, and new PACS archive. As the figure shows:

1. The timeline endpoint is anchored by the go-live date (right green line).
2. Once the go-live date is fixed, the next step is to determine the next anchor point, which is when the new PACS server ad archive pass the acceptance testing and become operational (center red line). Pass the acceptance testing includes the Installation of the new PACS server and archive system with its integration to the RIS and imaging modalities. The two integrations mean that the RIS and imaging modalities have to be interfaced with the legacy PACS as well as the new PACS.
3. At this point (center red line) the dual archive process starts, that is, while the legacy PACS is running the daily clinical operation, the new PACS archive as well as the legacy PACS archive are archiving the same studies. The image volume is approximately 25 GB daily on weekdays and 10 GB daily on weekends. The dual archival step has certain advantage because there is no need for data migration for all studies acquired on and after the date when the new

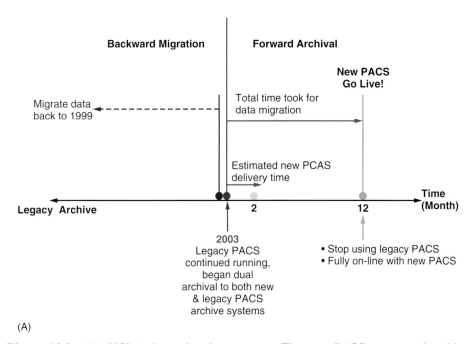

(A)

Figure 19.9 (*A*) UCLA data migration strategy. The new PACS server and archive system along with integrations with RIS and modalities were installed in 2003 (red dot) and the new PACS was anticipated in operation in two additional months (purple dot and line). Data migration from the legacy archive system dated back to 1999 (blue dot and line). Data migration took more than a year (green dot and lines), and the new PACS took that long before it was ready for daily operation. (*B*) Workflow of data migration results: (1) Historical PACS data retrieved from second copy tapes of the backup archive system, and exams are transmitted to the Data migration gateway server in DICOM format. (2) The legacy data migration system (LDMS) handled by a SUN E420 computer with RAID and a data migration gateway server with a quality assurance (QA) Workstation (WS). (3) Successfully exams with correct patient ID and DICOM format transmitted automatically to the new PACS archive; exams with discrepancies are held in the LDMS queue for routine manual intervention, correction, and then transmission. (*C*) Current UCLA enterprise PACS using the client-server model: (I) Input; (II) PACS server and archive; (III) Web client and server; (IV) SP backup archive; (V) contingency archive server. Black: Normal operation workflow. The PACS server is using a mirrored server system; and dual archive, with one copy on site with SAN technology, and the second copy is off-site using the ASP model. Yellow: Major PACS components during normal workflow. Green: Off-site ASP backup archive workflow. Orange: PCAS and RIS interface. Purple: Web server, review WSs and PC desktop. Blue background: Various types of WS. Red: Contingency workflow when the PCAS server and archive system are down. The contingency operation is much slower than the normal workflow. (Courtesy of the UCLA PACS team)

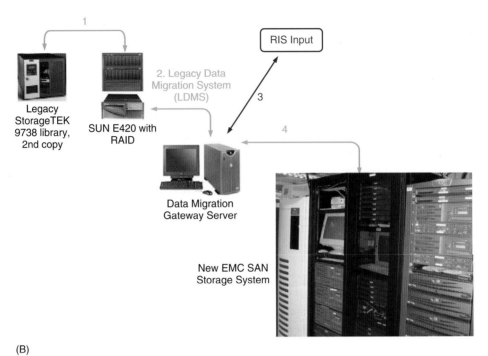

(B)

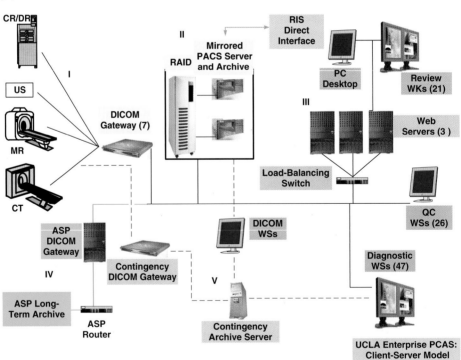

(C)

Figure 19.9 *(Continued)*

PACS archive was put on line, even though the new PACS was not ready for clinical use. The dual archival at this time is important because even though the new PACS archive is operational, the estimate is that at least two months before all other PACS hardware and software would be ready for daily operation. During this time the users continue utilizing the legacy PACS until the go-live date. Had all PACS studies archived in the legacy PACS storage only, they would have to be migrated to the new PACS archive after the new PACS becomes operational.

4. A concurrent step in the migration strategy during the dual archival is to migrate all the data from the legacy storage, going back to a predefined date (left, blue dotted line). For UCLA the decision was to archive studies dating back to 1999. This meant about 20 TB from approximately 750,000 procedures would be transferred, to the new PACS archive—quite a substantial amount of data to be migrated to the new PACS archive.

5. For the data migration process a challenge was to migrate the data during the time period when the legacy PACS was still in daily clinical operation. Figure 19.9B shows a schematic of this data migration procedure. To accomplish this, UCLA took advantage of the fact that the legacy PACS archive stored two copies of any procedure on two separate digital linear tape systems. This allowed UCLA to migrate the data from the second copy tape system and left the first tape system for daily operation (see Fig.19.9*B*, 1.) Therefore the data migration had no effect on daily clinical operation of the legacy PACS. The migration procedure was as follows: First, UCLA installed a legacy data migration system (LDMS), which consisted of a SUN E420 computer with a RAID, and a data migration gateway server with a WS to be used for staging the migration (see Fig. 19.9*B*, 2). Images from the second tape system were copied into the RAID. A stand-alone DICOM QC WS connected to the RAID in the LDMS was used to reconcile any missing DICOM header demographics with the RIS input (Fig. 19.9*B*, 3) prior to sending images from the RAID to the new PACS archive (see Fig. 19.9*B*, 4). Successive exams with correct patient ID and DICOM format received from the LDMS were transmitted automatically to the new PACS archive. Exams with discrepancies were held in a queue of the LDMS for routine manual intervention, correction, and then transmission.

The total data migration took more than one year, 10 more months than estimated. This turned out to be a blessing in disguise in that UCLA had all the legacy PACS exams migrated to the new PACS archive before the new PACS went live (see item 4 above).

19.3.2 ASP Backup Archive

Figure 19.9*C* shows UCLA new PACS (current) configuration and various workflow. There are five major components shown in Figure 19.9*C*:

1. Input devices (I, upper left)
2. Normal PACS operation (II, upper middle, yellow) and diagnostic WSs (lower right, blue) including all black lines in III.

3. Web server and clients (III, upper right) for clinical use (black lines). A system of three Web servers (purple) is used to ensure a fault-tolerant design (see Chapter 16).
4. ASP (application service provider) backup archive (IV, lower left, green) (see Chapter 16).
5. Contingency archive server and workflow as a backup in case the enterprise PACS fails (V, middle and lower right, red dotted lines).

For the new PACS archive, the local short-term storage SAN was configured to store 1.5 years of PACS studies. For long-term storage, an ASP (application service provider) PACS archive located in a data center in Chicago (see green lines in Fig. 19.9C) was commissioned. The main network connectivity was an ATM OC-3 line (see Chapter 8) with a backup DS-1 line. (Recall that similar functional components in the Saint John's Health Center ASP backup archive had an ASP router and a DICOM gateway, which are key components for an ASP backup archive solution; see Fig. 11.11). During the initial evaluation and acceptance testing, the network's performance was acceptable, but the ASP archive located in Chicago needed to be reconfigured. Currently UCLA is utilizing the ASP archive for long-term storage, but the ASP off-site data center is planning on moving to Burbank, California, closer to UCLA. Long-term storage will be supported by a T-3 line instead of an OC-3 line to keep costs at an acceptable level.

19.4 UNIVERSITY OF SOUTHERN CALIFORNIA

19.4.1 The Ugly Side of PACS: Living through a PACS Divorce

Inevitably there are times when a clinical site encounters a situation that leads to the institution filing for a divorce from the current PACS manufacturer. In general, the following combinations of circumstances can bring on a PACS divorce:

1. Dissatisfaction with support or service.
2. Lack of functionality.
3. Lack of integration with other systems and applications.
4. Inability for the PACS to scale to facility's needs.
5. Blank or unfulfilled vendor promises.
6. Unintuitive workflow and GUI designs.
7. High maintenance–PACS IT team requires too much time to support even after the go-live period.

Initially USC implemented a total digital solution with an integrated HIS/RIS/PACS/VR clinical system. In addition to the above-mentioned issues encountered by USC during implementation and go-live period, two critical issues accelerated the need to reevaluate the current PACS relationship and consider a PACS divorce:

1. Delayed delivery on a promise of an improved, upgraded PACS from the manufacturer that would address some of the issues USC was experiencing with the current PACS.

2. USC was simultaneously undergoing a campus-wide initiative for a single PACS vendor across the enterprise.

Because of these compounding issues, USC began the process for evaluating the need for a PACS divorce.

19.4.2   Is Divorce Really Necessary? The Evaluation Process

USC conducted a PACS Replacement (by a new vendor) Readiness Assessment to determine whether USC would be ready for a change should it occur. USC considered five important issues:

1. Have the issues at USC been escalated to the appropriate levels via the right channels and the vendor is aware of the gravity of the situation?
2. Has the vendor been given adequate opportunities to respond?
3. Has the customer implemented all reasonable solutions suggested by the vendor?
4. Has the customer determined that the long term strategy of the vendor is unlikely to resolve the issues at hand?
5. Have the major issues been well documented and presented to the vendor?

Only after this final analysis, did USC make the difficult decision to begin the PACS divorce process.

19.4.3   Coping with a PACS Divorce

19.4.3.1 Preparing for the Divorce   Once the decision was made to enter into the divorce proceedings and change the PACS vendor, two major steps had to be planned: data migration and the implementation of a new PACS. To enable the decision to change PACS vendors, certain steps had to already be in place to minimize the difficulties and challenges of a divorce, should it become a reality:

1. Documentation: Always require full documentation from the current PACS vendor on storage and database schemas as well as potential proprietary information such as annotations, customizations, and teaching files or key images.
2. Tools: Ensure that the current PACS vendor provides tools for managing and extracting data from the database as well as time and materials needed for conversion of proprietary data into the industry standards of DICOM and HL7.
3. Data Standardization: Ensure that the current PACS vendors has the ability to provide the imaging and informatics data utilizing the DICOM and HL7 standards, especially the DICOM image files. This is crucial for a smooth data migration.
4. Costs: Determine what costs go forward should a divorce occur, specifically, data migration costs and hardware and equipment costs. Negotiate beforehand that should a contract be terminated, who owns the existing PACS equipment and whether the agreement is cost-effective for the institution.

During the divorce process, USC had performed "due diligence" in preparing for such an event and what to look for in a new PACS manufacturer. These included negotiations with other PACS vendors.

19.4.3.2 Business Negotiation   As USC began negotiations with potential new PACS vendors, this part of the negotiation was very similar to the PACS process for selecting a new vendor from the beginning described in Chapter 18. The difference was in the knowledge and experience gained from the previous PACS manufacturer and understanding the shortcomings of the PACS predecessor. These considerations factored in this first step of the decision-making process of the selecting a new PACS vendor.

19.4.3.3 Data Migration   The next step was the data migration. Usually PACS manufacturers are unlikely to go above and beyond what is expected from them by the institution during this transition period. However, because a manufacturer's reputation as a reliable PACS vendor is important, the manufacturer will agree to do what is necessary to facilitate the data migration. In most cases the burden of the data migration costs will fall on the new PACS vendor, and it is important that the institution include migration costs as part of the agreement when entering into a contract with the new manufacturer. For USC the new PACS manufacturer saw the data migration problem as a benefit because the experience gained in performing a data migration at an academic institution was a significant ROI (return of investment) for the new PACS vendor and would bolster their portfolio as a reputable PACS manufacturer.

The data migration plan was executed in a fashion similar to that described in the previous section regarding UCLA; that is, all data migration occurred off line and the new PACS did not go live until all historical data were migrated. In the USC case there was only a total of 1.5 TB data that was migrated from the old PACS to the new PACS. The migration process was manual, performed by the new PACS manufacturer, and was accomplished in a six-month time frame. The following were workflow steps:

1. An initial data survey was performed to determine an estimate of the length of data migration. The 1.5 TB data represented approximately 80,000 procedures of various modalities and image sizes.
2. A DICOM gateway WS was installed to query and retrieve PACS studies from the old PACS archive.
3. Studies with duplicate exam numbers were evaluated on a case by case basis by verification with the RIS. One of the studies was retrieved while the second copy was left behind.
4. Studies with erroneous exam numbers or irregular format were not migrated.
5. Upon successful retrieval, the DICOM gateway WS forwarded the PACS studies to the new PACS archive.

19.4.3.4 Clinical Workflow Modification and New Training   During the implementation of the new PACS, the clinical workflow was modified slightly to accommodate the new functionalities and additional training was provided on the new PACS applications. The clinical workflow modifications as well as new training were minimal, since USC was careful in choosing a new PACS vendor based on the initial analysis performed in previous subsections.

19.4.4 Summary of USC and Remaining Issues

USC began the process of divorce and retained a new PACS manufacturer to install an enterprise PACS in the spring of 2007. Since then the new PACS has been widely accepted by the users and fewer problems have occurred than previously. In addition, as expected, the replacement PACS paved the way for a single PACS vendor across the entire USC Healthcare Campus, which is the case as of 2008.

Three major issues remain: (1) certain integration issues like uniform patient ID, accession number, and data consistency still occur periodically; (2) the single database for the entire enterprise and the fault-tolerant backup archive are still in the progress of resolving; and (3) the design and implementation of an ePR system with image distribution has not yet begun. Figure 19.10*A*, *B*, and *C* shows the current single vendor enterprise PACS in operation at USC Health Science Campus. Figure 19.10*A* gives the USC campus map with buildings circled in red being the hubs in the enterprise PACS. There are also two off-campus outpatient imaging centers, and one student health center at the main campus). Figure 19.10*B* gives a schematic of the PACS related components' locations and distribution. Figure 19.10*C* shows some of the main buildings housing PACS-related equipment.

19.5 PACS PITFALLS

PACS glitches are mostly due to human error, whereas bottlenecks are due to an imperfect design and/or image acquisition devices, and to network contentions. These drawbacks can only be understood through accumulated clinical experience. We discuss bottlenecks in Section 19.6.

Glitches due to human error can occur at imaging acquisition devices and at WSs. The three common errors that can cause acquisition devices to malfunction are entering the wrong input parameters, stopping an image transmission process improperly, and incorrect patient positioning. Human errors occur most often at the WSs, where a user may enter too many key strokes at once or click the mouse too frequently before the WS can respond. Other errors at the WS that are not of human origin are missing location markers in a CT or MR scout view, images displayed with unsuitable lookup tables, and white borders in CR images from X-ray collimation. Errors created by human intervention can be minimized by a better quality assurance program, periodic in-service training, and interfacing image acquisition devices directly to the HIS–RIS through a DICOM broker to minimize typing mistakes.

19.5.1 During Image Acquisition

19.5.1.1 Human Errors at Imaging Acquisition Devices
At the older generation computed radiography (CR) units, two common errors are using the wrong imaging plate ID card at the reader and entering the wrong patient's ID, name, accession number, or birth date and invalid characters at the scanner's operator console. These errors can result in a loss of images, images being assigned to the wrong patient, a patients image folder containing another patient's images, orphaned images, and acquisition device crashes because of illegal characters. Routine quality assurance (QA) procedures at the CR WS (see Chapter 12) that check the CR operator log book or the RIS examination records against the PACS patient's folder normally can

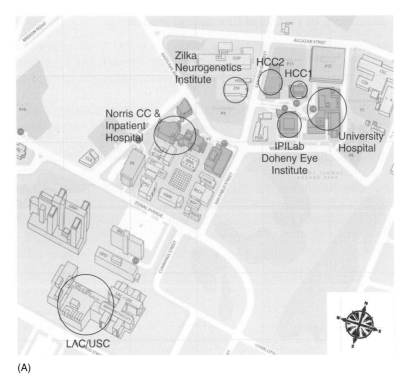

(A)

Figure 19.10   USC enterprise PACS. (*A*) USC Health Science Campus map; (*B*) schematic of USC enterprise PACS (Courtesy of K. Huang); (*C*) USC Health Science Campus building photos. The current single vendor enterprise PACS in operation at USC Health Science Campus consists of *B*, lower left: (1) Norris CC (Cancer Center) and (3) Norris CC Inpatient Hospital. *B*, lower left middle: (2) UH (University Hospital), including (6) Zilka Neurogenetics Institute and (7) IPILab, Doheny Eye Institute. *B*, upper right: (4–5) New and old LAC/USC (Los Angeles County) Hospital. *B*, upper left corner: (8) HCC1 (Health Consultation Center 1). *B*, upper middle left: (9) HCC2 (Health Consultation Center 2). *B*, lower right: OP IC1, and OP IC2 (Outpatient Imaging Center 1 and 2) not inside USC campuses. *B*, lower middle: SHC (Student Health Center at USC main campus). (Courtesy of the IT team of the Department of Radiology, USC, for compiling set of information, and M. Fleshman for the campus map)

discover these errors. If a discrepancy is detected early enough, before images are sent to the PACS server, WS, or the long-term archive, the technologist/PACS coordinator can perform the damage control by manually editing the PACS database to:

1. correct for patient's name, ID, and other typographical errors;
2. delete images not belonging to the patient; and
3. append orphaned images to the proper patient's image folder

Lost images from a patient's folder can usually be found in the orphaned image directory. If images have already been sent to the WS before the PACS manager has a chance to do the damage control described above, the PACS coordinator should

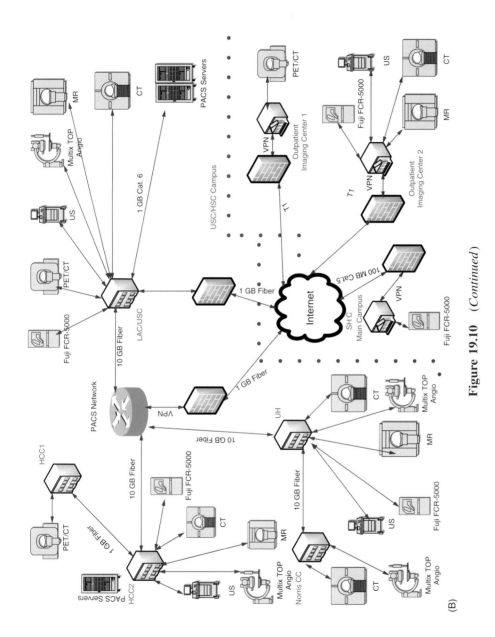

Figure 19.10 (*Continued*)

617

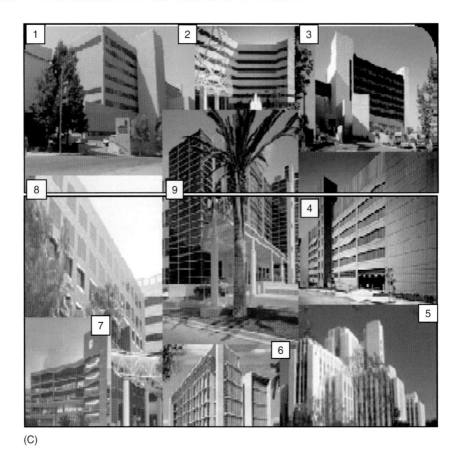

(C)

Figure 19.10 (*Continued*)

alert the users immediately. If, however, these images have already been archived to the long-term storage before the damage control is performed, recovery of the errors can be more complicated. To anticipate this case, the PACS server should have a mechanism allowing the PACS manager to correct such errors at the PACS database. More current CR units can accept the patient worklist from the RIS to minimize possible human errors.

19.5.1.2 Procedure Errors at Imaging Acquisition Devices
Procedure errors can be categorized according to CT, MR, and CR.

CT and MR in General Three common errors are as follows:

1. Terminating a study while images are being transmitted.
2. Manually interrupting an image transmission process.
3. Realigning the patient during scanning.

These errors can result in missing images in CT/MR image files, images out of sequence, and scanner crashes because of the interruption of image transmission.

Wrong Orientation in CT Coronal Scan   A nonhuman error during CT acquisition is in the coronal head scan protocol. In this scan protocol the image appearing on the CT display may have the left and right directions reversed. If film output is used, the technologist can manually annotate the orientation of the patient on the screen, which is then printed on the film with the correct orientation. However, such an interactive step in the PACS is not possible because the graphical user interface on the CT display console does not Include the DICOM image header. A way around this difficulty is for the technologist to go through the scanning protocol from the DICOM image header and annotate the orientation in the image during its display on the PACS WS as shown in Figure 19.11. The solution is implemented in the PACS WS automatically in the later generation CT scanners.

Wrong Direction of the Image Plate during the Scan   In CR, the technologist placing the imaging plate under the patient in the wrong direction during a portable examination and manual interruption of the transmission procedure can result in the loss of images. Incorrect CR orientation during display can be checked by an algorithm with automatic rotation (see Fig. 19.12, and Section 10.6) as shown in Figure 19.12, or by an interactive rotation during the QA procedure. Errors due to manual interruption of the transmission procedure can be remedied by using the DICOM communication protocol for automatic image verification and recovery during the transmission. Images archived out of sequence order can be manually edited during the CR QA procedure.

Scheduling regular in-service training and continuing education for technologists can minimize malfunctions caused by human error. However, the most effective method is to use a direct HIS–RIS DICOM broker interface between the image acquisition device and the PACS acquisition gateway, which can minimize the human interaction for inputting improper patient-related data. Currently a commercial product for interfacing CR, CT, and MR to the RIS through a DICOM broker is available for direct patient data input.

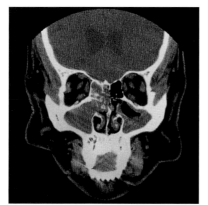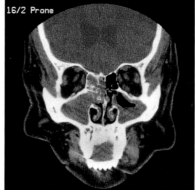

Figure 19.11 Left: Coronal view of a CT scan without a "left" or "right" indicator. Right: Label "16/2 prone" can be generated using the DICOM header information to identify the left and the right of the patient scan.

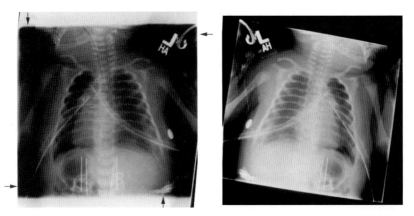

Figure 19.12 CR image. Left: White boarders (red arrows) and wrong orientation. Right: Background removal providing better display quality, and automatic rotation to correct for the orientation with the heart in the left side of the patient.

19.5.2 At the Workstation

19.5.2.1 Human Error Human error can occur when the WS response is slow. An impatient user may then enter the next few commands while the WS is still executing the very first request. As a result one of several things may happen:

1. The display program may crash or hang the display software.
2. The WS may not respond to the next command,
3. The user may forget to close the window of a previous operation,
4. The user may forget what commands he/she had entered when an unexpected display appears on the screen.
5. If the user panics and enters other commands, errors similar to those described in the first scenario may occur.

A possible remedy is to provide a large visible timer on the WS screen for the user to know that the last command or request is still being processed; this will minimize errors due to the user's impatience. A better solution is to have an improved WS design to tolerate this type of human error.

19.5.2.2 Display System Deficiency We consider here four system deficiencies at the WS:

1. Omission of localization markers in the CT/MR scout view (Fig. 19.13*A*, *B*).
2. Incorrect lookup table for CT/MR display (Fig. 19.14*A*, *B*, *C*, *D*).
3. Wrong orientation of the CT head image in the coronal scan protocol discussed earlier (Fig. 19.11).
4. White borders in CR due to X-ray collimation (Fig. 19.12).

Omission of localization markers in a CT/MR scout view can be remedied by creating the localization lines with the information from the DICOM image header (see

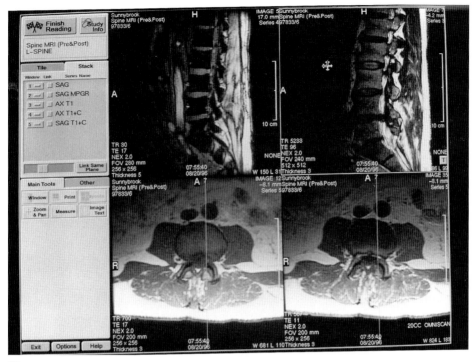

(A)

Figure 19.13 (*A*) Scan lines (bottom) can be generated from the DICOM header information to correlate scans between various planes (examples show the Sagittal: top, the transverse: bottom). (*B*) A better correlation between the sagittal view (left) and the transverse view (right) where multiple black lines showing the correlation between the two planes with the two red lines designating the two views depicted in the figures.

Fig. 19.13, bottom two images). The use of an incorrect lookup table for a CT/MR display is case dependent. Using the histogram technique can generate correct lookup tables for CT. There are still some difficulties in obtaining a uniformly correct lookup table for all images in an MR sequence because of the possibility of nonuniformity of the body or surface coils used. Sometimes it is necessary to process every image individually by using the histogram method (see Fig. 19.14). The correction for the CT head coronal scan was discussed above (Fig. 19.11). White boards in CR due to X-ray collimation can be corrected by an automatic background removal technique (see Fig. 12.10*C* and Fig. 19.12).

19.6 PACS BOTTLENECKS

Bottlenecks affecting the PACS operation include network contention; CR, CT, and MR images stacked up at acquisition devices; slow responses from WSs; and long delays for image retrieval from the long-term archive. Improving the system architecture, reconfiguring the networks, and streamlining operational procedures through a gradual understanding of the PACS clinical environment can alleviate bottlenecks.

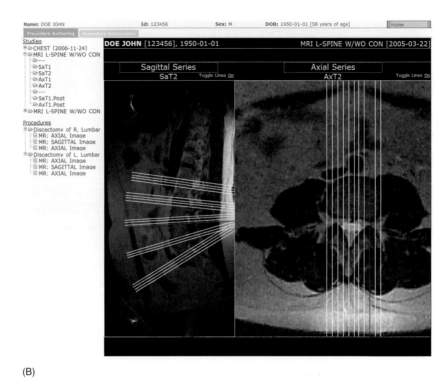

(B)

Figure 19.13   (*Continued*)

Utilization of the IHE workflow profiles discussed in Chapter 9 could help circumvent some bottleneck problems.

19.6.1 Network Contention

Network contention can cause many bottlenecks. First, CR/CT/MR images could stack up at the image acquisition gateway. The result is an overflow in the computer disks and eventually loss of some images. Other effects are that it will take longer for the PACS server to collect a complete sequence of images from one MR or CT examination, which can consequently delay the transmission of the complete sequence file to the WS for review. Network contention can also cause a long delay for image retrieval from the long-term archive, especially when the retrieved image file is large.

19.6.1.1 Redesigning the Network Architecture   Methods of correction can be divided into general and specific. The general category includes redesigning the network architecture, using a faster network, and modifying the communication protocols. An example of redesigning the network architecture is to separate the network into segments and subnets and to redistribute the heavy traffic routes to different subnets. For example, CT/MR acquisition and CR acquisition can be divided into two subnets. Assigning priorities to different subnets based on the amount network traffic and time of day is one way to address the user's immediate needs.

Using a faster network can speed up the image transfer rate. If the current network is the conventional Ethernet, consider changing it to fast Ethernet switches and

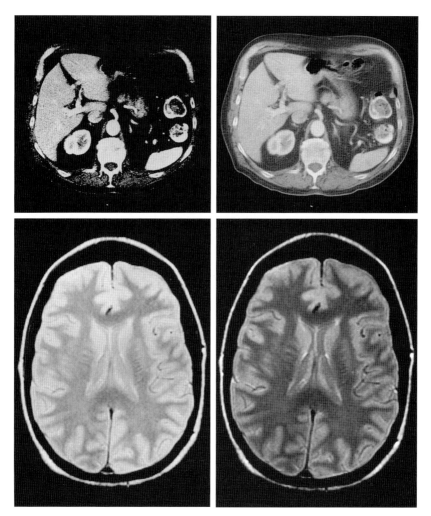

Figure 19.14 Body CT (top) and MR (bottom) head scan. Left: Incorrect LUT. Right: Correct LUT.

WSs with Ethernet connection. Conventional network protocols often use default parameters that are only suitable for small file transfer. Changing some parameters in the protocol may speed up the transfer rates, for example, enlarging the TCP window size and the image buffer size.

19.6.1.2 Operational Environment Methods in the specific category are based on the operational environment. Methods of correction may involve changing the operational procedure in the radiology department. Consider two examples: CR images stacked up at the CR readers and CT/MR images stacked up at the scanners. Most CR applications are for portable examinations and are mostly performed in early morning. An obvious method of correction is to rearrange the portable examination schedule at the wards.

CT/MR images stacked up at the scanners can be caused by a design fault in the communication protocol at the scanners. There are two methods of correction. First,

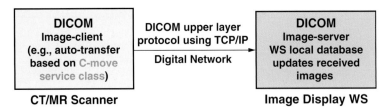

Figure 19.15 Push operation at the scanner to transmit an image out of the scanner as soon as it is generated.

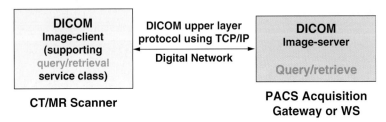

Figure 19.16 Pull operation at the acquisition gateway or the WS to receive an image from the scanner as soon as it is generated.

use the DICOM auto-transfer mode to "push" images out from the scanner as soon they are ready to be sent to the acquisition gateway or the WSs (see Section 9.4.5, and Fig. 19.15). Second, from the acquisition gateway or the WS, use DICOM to "pull" images from the scanner periodically (see Section 9.4.5 and Fig. 19.16).

19.6.2 Slow Response at Workstations

A slow response at the WS is mostly due to bad WS local database design with insufficient image memory in the WS. An example of a bad WS database design is when the database uses a large file in the local disk for image storage. During the initial configuration of the WS software, this storage space is contiguous. As the WS starts to accumulate and delete images while it is being used, this space becomes fragmented. Fragmented space causes an inefficient I/O transfer rate, rendering a slow response in bringing images from the disk to the display. Periodic cleanup is necessary to retain contiguous space in the disk. Insufficient image memory in the WS requires continuous disk memory swaps, slowing down the image display speed. This is especially problematic when the image file is large.

Several methods for correcting a slow response at the WS are possible. First, increasing the image memory size to accommodate a complete image file will minimize the requirement for memory-disk swapping. The use of RAID technology is another way to speed up the disk I/O for faster image display. A better local database design and image search algorithm along with RAID at the WS can speed up the image seeking and transfer time (Fig. 19.17). PACS uses a client server model that does not require local storage in the WS, and does not have this problem. But a similar situation may occur at the archive server, as will be described in the next section.

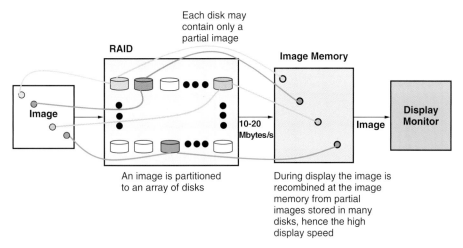

Figure 19.17 A preloaded image from the RAID to the image memory to speed up the required display time.

19.6.3 Slow Response from the Archive Server

A slow response from the long-term archive can be caused by:

1. slow optical disk or digital linear tape library search,
2. slow disk or tape read/write operations, and
3. the same patient images scattering in different storage media when many simultaneous requests are taking place.

For example, the optical disk read/write data rate normally is about 400 to 500 Kbytes/s, but when many large image files have images scattered in many platters or disks, the seek time and disk I/O will be slow. This will cause a slow retrieval response of these files from the long-term archive.

There are three possible methods of improvement:

1. An image platter or tape manager software can be used to rewrite scattered images of the same patient to contiguous optical disk platters or tapes periodically (Fig. 19.18). This mechanism will facilitate the future retrieval time for images.
2. To use an image prefetch mechanism (Fig. 19.19), which anticipates what images will be needed by the clinician for a particular patient. A combination of the prefetch mechanism and mechanism 1 will speed up the response time from the long-term archive.
3. To upgrade the disk/tape library with multiple read/write drives, which can improve the overall throughput of the retrieval operations.

Pitfalls and bottlenecks are the two main obstacles to smooth PACS operation after installation. Sections 19.5 and 19.6 identify most of these problems based on clinical experience. Methods are also suggested to circumvent these pitfalls and to minimize the occurrence of bottlenecks.

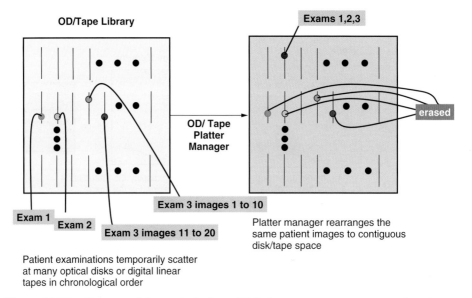

Figure 19.18   Concept of the optical platter/digital tape manager to save patient images from exams 1, 2, and 3 in a contiguous space (red dot).

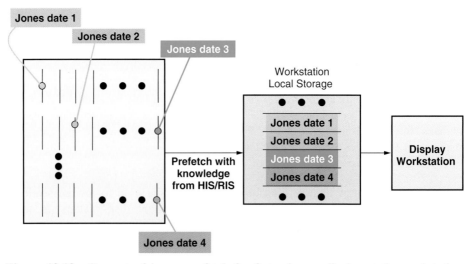

Figure 19.19   Concept of image prefetch for faster image display at the workstation. Patient Jones date 1, date 2, date 3, and date 4 images had all been prefetched in the workstation local storage.

19.7 DICOM CONFORMANCE

19.7.1 Incompatibility in DICOM Conformance Statement

During the integration of multivendor PACS components, even though each vendor's component may come with a DICOM conformance statement, they still may not be compatible. We have identified some deficiencies caused by such incompatibility as follows:

1. Missing image(s) from a sequence during an acquisition process: When a CT or MR scanner (storage SCU) transmits individual images from a sequence to an image acquisition gateway (storage SCP), the scanner initiates the transfer with a push operation (see Chapter 7). The reliability of the transmission is dependent on the transfer mechanism implemented by the scanner. An abnormal manual abortion of the scanning process can sometimes terminate the transmission, resulting in missing the image being transferred.

2. Incorrect data encoding in image header: Examples of incorrect data encoding include missing type 1 data elements that are mandatory attributes in the DICOM standard, incorrect value representation (VR) of data elements, and encoded data in data elements exceeding their maximum length.

3. SOP service class not fully supported by the SCP vendor: This happens when a SCU vendor and a SCP vendor implement an SOP service class with different operation supports. For example, a C-GET request initiated from a display WS is rejected by an archive server because the latter only accepts C-MOVE requests, even though both C-GET and C-MOVE are DICOM standard DIMSE-C operations that support the Q/R service class.

4. DICOM conformance mismatching between individual vendors: When an SCU vendor and an SCP vendor implement the Q/R service class in different information models or with different support levels, a C-FIND request in Patient Level initiated from a WS is rejected by a CT scanner because the latter only supports the Q/R study root model, which does not accept any query requests in Patient Level.

5. Shadow group conflict between the individual vendors: When vendor A and vendor B store their proprietary data in the same shadow group, data previously stored in the shadow group by vendor A are overwritten by vendor B's data.

19.7.2 Methods of Remedy

These pitfalls can be minimized through the implementation of two DICOM-based mechanisms, one in the image acquisition gateway and the second in the PACS server, to provide better connectivity solutions for multivendor imaging equipment in a large-scale PACS environment, the details of which have been discussed in Sections 9.4 and 9.5.

19.8 SUMMARY OF PACS CLINICAL EXPERIENCE, PITFALLS, AND BOTTLENECKS

This chapter presents PACS clinical experience from four hospitals: the Baltimore VA Medical Center; St. John's Healthcare Center, Santa Monica, CA; University of California, Los Angeles; and University of Southern California. Lessons learned from these four sites include PACS malfunctions, bottlenecks, and deficiencies in manufacturers' implementation of DCIOM compliance.

References

Dayhoff R, Siegel EL. Digital imaging within and among medical facilities. In: Kolodner R, ed. *Computerized Large Integrated Health Networks: The VA Success*. New York: Springer, 473–490; 1997.

Liu BJ, Cao F, Zhou MZ, Mogel G, Docemet L. Trends in PACS image stroage and archive, *Comput Med Imag Graph* 27(2–3): 165–74; 2003.

Reiner BI, Siegel EL, Pomerantz SM, Protopapas Z. The impact of filmless radiology on the frequency of clinician consultations with radiologists. Presentation. American Roentgen Ray Society Annual Meeting, San Diego, 5–10 May 1996.

Reiner BI, Siegel EL, Hooper FJ, Glasser D. Effect of film-based versus filmless operation on the productivity of CT technologists. *Radiology* 207(2): 481–5; 1998.

Reiner BI, Siegel EL, Flagle C, Hooper FJ, Cox RE, Scanlon M. Effect of filmless imaging on the utilization of Radiologic services. *Radiology* 215(1): 163–7; 2000.

Siegel EL, Diaconis JN, Pomerantz S, Allman RM, Briscoe B. Making filmless radiology work. *J Digit Imag* 8: 151–5; 1995.

Siegel EL, Protopapas Z, Pickar E, Reiner BI, Pomerantz SM, Cameron E. Analysis of retake rates using computed radiography in a filmless imaging department. Abstract. Radiological Society of North America Annual Meeting, Chicago, 3 Dec 1996.

Siegel EL. We're off to see the wizard: consultations in the 21st century. *Diagn Imag* (5): 31, 33, 79; 2000.

Siegel E, Reiner B, Abiri M, Chacko A, Morin R, Ro DW, Spicer K, Strickland N, Young J. The filmless radiology reading room: a survey of established picture archiving and communication system sites. J Digit Imag 13 (2 suppl 1): 22–3; 2000.

Siegel EL, Reiner B. Work flow redesign: the key to success when using PACS. *Am J Roentgenol* 178(3): 563–6; 2002.

Siegel EL, Reiner BI. Filmless radiology at the Baltimore VA Medical Center: a nine year retrospective. *Comput Med Imag Graph* 27(2–3): 101–9; 2003.

PART IV

PACS- AND DICOM-BASED IMAGING INFORMATICS

CHAPTER 20

DICOM-Based Medical Imaging Informatics

Biomedical Informatics (BMI) is loosely categorized into four levels of study: bioinformatics (molecular level), imaging informatics (cellular, tissue, and organ system level), clinical informatics (individual healthcare system), and public health informatics (population level). The concepts of and methodologies used in these four levels overlap each other. In this chapter we focus on imaging informatics.

Medical informatics has gradually evolved and established itself as a rigorous scientific discipline during the past fifteen years. There are now at least 10 to 15 major training programs supported by the National Library of Medicine (NLM), and more from other U.S. federal government agencies and institutions around the world, training students the concepts and methods of health information gathering, data structure, information extraction, retrieval and distribution, and knowledge representation.

Medical Imaging Informatics is a subset of medical informatics that studies image/data information acquisition; processing; manipulation; storage; transmission; security; management; distribution; visualization; image-aided detection, diagnosis, surgery, and therapy; as well as knowledge discovery from large-scale biomedical image/data sets. Although imaging informatics is based on many existing concepts, theories, terminology, and methodology derived from medical informatics, different types of data are involved, including multidimensional medical images, graphics, waveforms, and text. Accordingly imaging informatics requires new concepts and new tool sets to handle these types of data. Although there are training programs in medical imaging and telemedicine, focused training dedicated to imaging informatics is limited because of its novelty.

Recent advances in medical imaging technology, such as PACS (picture archive and communication system), image-guided surgery and therapy, CAD (computer-aided diagnosis), ePR (electronic patient record) with image distribution have propelled imaging informatics as a discipline to manage and synthesize knowledge from medical images for effective and efficient patient care as well as outcome analysis. "DICOM-based" is used as a keyword in the chapter title to signify the data communication and formatting aspect of medical imaging informatics and the emphasis on images, waveform, and text. The concept of DICOM-based medical imaging informatics presented in this chapter forms the foundation of and serves as an introduction to the following eight chapters (see Fig. 20.1).

PACS and Imaging Informatics, Second Edition, by H. K. Huang
Copyright © 2010 John Wiley & Sons, Inc.

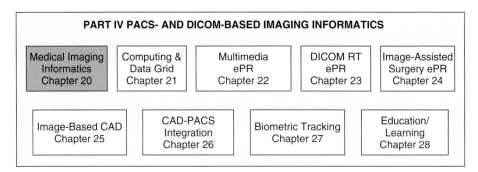

Figure 20.1 Concept of medical imaging informatics in relation to the topics in later chapters discussing various technologies, tools, and applications; the last chapter is devoted to medical imaging informatics training.

20.1 THE MEDICAL IMAGING INFORMATICS INFRASTRUCTURE (MIII) PLATFORM

Medical imaging informatics infrastructure (MIII) is a platform designed to take advantage of PACS and ePR resources and related images, waveforms, and related textual data for large-scale horizontal and longitudinal clinical service, research, and education applications that could not have been performed before because of insufficient data and connectivity. MIII is the vehicle to facilitate the utilization of PACS, ePR, and other medical images for applications in addition to their daily clinical service. The DICOM standard is emphasized in the platform.

Medical image informatics infrastructure (MIII) platform can be loosely divided into five logical layers: (1) data sources, (2) tools, (3) database and knowledge base, (4) application middleware, and (5) customized software, shown in Figure 20.2. Major components in these layers are as follows:

1. Medical images and associated data (including PACS and ePR databases)
2. Tools for image processing, visualization, graphical user interface, communication networking, and data security
3. Database and knowledge base management, simulation and modeling, Data Grid and data mining
4. Application oriented software
5. Customized system integration software

Figure 20.3 depicts the connection of the medical imaging informatics platform to PACS and other imaging resources.

20.2 HIS/RIS/PACS, MEDICAL IMAGES, ePR, AND RELATED DATA

20.2.1 HIS/RIS/PACS and Related Data

HIS/RISPACS data and related health information system data constitute the major data sources in MIII. These data consist of patient demographic data, case

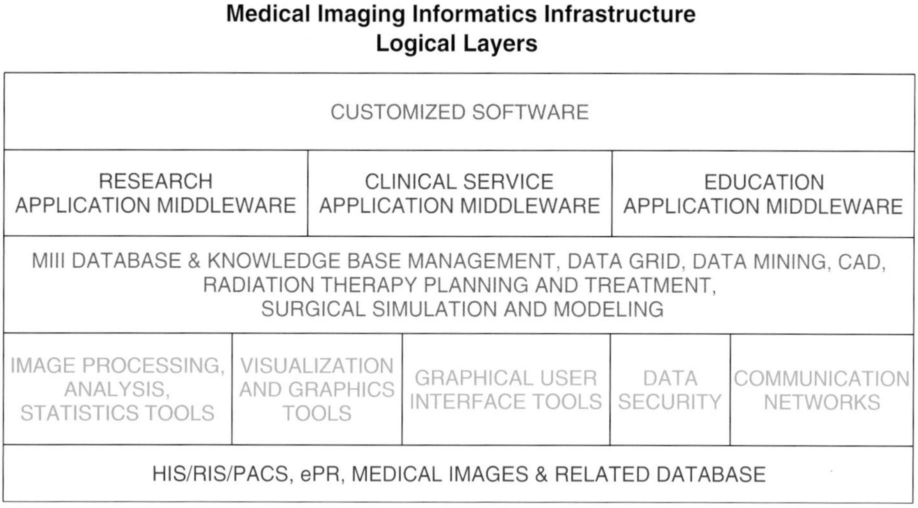

Medical Imaging Informatics Infrastructure
Logical Layers

CUSTOMIZED SOFTWARE				
RESEARCH APPLICATION MIDDLEWARE	CLINICAL SERVICE APPLICATION MIDDLEWARE		EDUCATION APPLICATION MIDDLEWARE	
MIII DATABASE & KNOWLEDGE BASE MANAGEMENT, DATA GRID, DATA MINING, CAD, RADIATION THERAPY PLANNING AND TREATMENT, SURGICAL SIMULATION AND MODELING				
IMAGE PROCESSING, ANALYSIS, STATISTICS TOOLS	VISUALIZATION AND GRAPHICS TOOLS	GRAPHICAL USER INTERFACE TOOLS	DATA SECURITY	COMMUNICATION NETWORKS
HIS/RIS/PACS, ePR, MEDICAL IMAGES & RELATED DATABASE				

Figure 20.2   Five logical layers of Imaging Informatics infrastructure platform: data sources including data from HIS/RIS/PACS, ePR, other medical images and related data; various tools commonly used in medical images; databases and knowledge base management, Data Grid and data mining, surgical simulation and modeling, and image-based radiation therapy treatment planning; application middleware for research, clinical service, and education; customized software and system integration. Color codes are used for reference with the informatics data sources, concepts, technologies, and applications shown in Figure 20.9.

histories, diagnostic radiological images and corresponding diagnostic reports, and laboratory test results and are organized and archived with standard data formats and protocols, such as DICOM for image and HL7 for text (see Chapter 9). A controlled health vocabulary is the standard used for medical identifiers, codes, and messages, as is recommended by the American Medical Informatics Association.

20.2.2   Other Types of Medical Images

Some types of medical images are not included in diagnostic radiological domain but are used for patient care required for diagnosis or treatments of the patient. Some such images are the real-time images used in surgery and radiation therapy related images and graphics, as described in Chapters 3, 4, 5, 22, 23, 24, 25, and 26.

20.2.3   ePR and Related Data/Images

The electronic patient record (ePR, or EMR [electronic medical record]) and related data/images are object-oriented information. While ePR contains textual information, it normally is linked to images, graphic overlays, and waveforms to form a more complete description of the object under consideration (see Chapters 13, 22, 23, 24, 25, and 26).

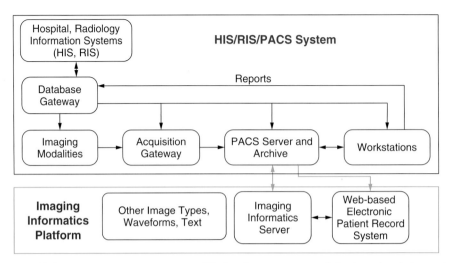

Figure 20.3 Relationship between PACS dataflow (upper) and the imaging informatics platform (lower). DICOM images and related data are transmitted from the PACS server to the imaging informatics server as well as the web-based ePR system. Data from the imaging informatics server can be linked but not necessary directly transmitted back to the PACS archive server, from the medical imaging informatics platform processed data can be retrieved by and displayed on PACS workstations.

20.3 IMAGING INFORMATICS TOOLS

20.3.1 Image Processing, Analysis, and Statistical Methods

Image processing and analysis software can be very broad to allow for extracting relevant parameters from images for quantitative measurements. Measurement functions can include segmentation, region of interest determination, texture analysis, content analysis, morphological operations, image registration, and image matching. The output from image processing and analysis can be an entirely new image or a detail extracted from an image. Image processing functions can be performed automatically or interactively on image data by an input gateway or analysis server. Data extracted from the image processing functions can be appended to the image data file in the DICOM Structured Report format.

Measurements are basic ingredients for the development of imaging informatics tools described in Section 20.3. Measurements can be used for deriving databases and knowledge base management for data mining, and for image content indexing and retrieval mechanism. Statistical methods applied to collective measurements from a large database can be further used to draw meaningful clinical results.

20.3.2 Visualization and Graphical User Interface

Visualization and graphical user interface (GUI) are used for output summarization and proper display. Both components are related to workstation (WS) design (see Chapter 12). Visualization includes 3-D rendering, image data fusion, static and dynamic imaging display. These tools utilize extracted data from image processing (i.e., segmentation, enhancement, and shading) for output rendering. Visualization can be performed on a standard WS or with high-performance graphic WS or engine. The latter is sometime referred to as postprocessing WS (see Chapter 12). For lower performance WS, the final visualization can be pre-computed and packaged at the WS, whereas with a high-performance graphic WS or engine, the rendering can be performed in real-time at the WS.

Graphical user interface optimizes the workstation design for information retrieval and data visualization with a minimal effort from the user. A well-designed GUI is essential for effective real-time visualization and image content retrieval. GUI can also be used for extraction of additional parameters for nonstandard interactive image analysis.

20.3.3   Three-dimensional Rendering and Image Fusion

Three-dimensional and surface rendering and image fusion use computer graphic methods to display 3-D or 4-D and multimedia data on a 2-D screen (see Chapters 4 and 5). Computer graphics can also be used to retrieve multidimensional data through visual interaction.

20.3.3.1   3-D Rendering   PACS is designed as a data management system; it lacks the computational power for image content analysis at the PACS workstation or at the PACS controller/server. For this reason it is necessary to allocate a computational and 3-D rendering resources or WS in the MIII infrastructure for high-performance computational tasks should such tasks be requested by MIII workstations. On the completion of a given 3-D computation, the results can be displayed on a 3-D WS with visualization capability or be distributed to other image workstations through high-speed networks. A computational and 3-D rendering with visualization resource shown in Figure 20.4 is needed in the PACS environment: the PACS database is at the left; the computational 3-D rendering visualization resource is on the top, connected to the PACS or/and MIII networks with high-speed networks (100 Mbits/s or higher). The Web server in the MIII provides a connection to the PACS for image query/retrieve. Both Web clients and PACS workstations can access 3-D rendered images from the Web server. To view 3-D images after rendering, 3-D visualization tools are needed, for example, on a postprocessing WS monitor (see Chapter 12).

Steps in 3-D Visualization   A volumetric visualization within the 3-D rendering, postprocessing (PP) WS and visualization component are MIII resources. The user at a satellite site wishing to view 3-D or fusion volumetric images from different imaging modalities (e.g., MRI CT, PET) in the PACS database from a workstation can use the rendering and visualization tools. Figure 20.5 shows the steps to accomplish this task through the visualization engine or PP WS. The workflow is as follows:

1. The PACS workstation (WS, center) sends the volume data file already in the WS, or the PACS WS requests the PACS database (right) to retrieve the volumetric image set.
2. The image set is sent to the visualization engine or PPWS (left).

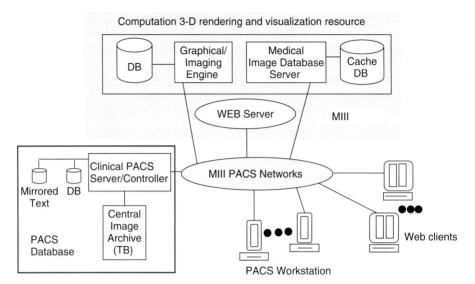

Figure 20.4 Connectivity of a PACS with the MIII server containing computational 3-D rendering and visualization resources, and a Web server. Both PACS workstations and Web clients through the MIII can request 3-D rendering and visualization services. In recent display technology, postprocessing (PP) WS is available to replace some functions of the graphics/imaging engine. 3-D rendered images can be displayed on the PP WS dedicated monitors. DB: database. TB: Terabytes.

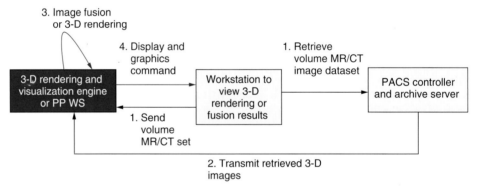

Figure 20.5 Workflow of using the client-server to download 3-D volumetric images to a rendering and visualization engine or postprocessing (PP) WS, and to receive the results. The rendering and visualization engine is a major resource of the MIII.

3. The visualization engine/PPWS (blue fonts) performs the necessary 3-D computational and rendering functions.
4. Results are sent back (blue arrow) to the PACS WS for viewing after the task is completed.

Step 4 allows the user also to communicate with the rendering and visualization resource directly and to provide any further instructions or manipulations. Let us consider two application scenarios.

Scenario 1: Volumetric Visualization of Clinical Images   A user wishes to view fusion volumetric images from different imaging modalities (e.g., CT with PET, or MR with CT) in the PACS database, either from the PACS workstation or from a Web client through the Web server. Suppose that the existing PACS and workstations at the site do not support such capability. Figures 20.4 and 20.5 illustrate the steps that the user would need to accomplish this task through the computational resource. In this scenario the workstation, like a PP WS, has the hardware and software capability to view 2-D and 3-D images with graphics. Figures 5.8–5.11 show examples of whole body CT and PET fusion images.

Scenario 2: Video/Image Conferencing with Image Database Query Support   The referring physician at a PACS workstation viewing a patient's image case requests a video conference with a radiologist located at separate location. Figure 20.6 shows the workflow and demonstrates how to utilize the medical image database server and the computational resource to accomplish the task. The workflow proceeds as follows:

1. The referring physician requests and establishes a video conference session between two PACS or image workstations.
2. The physician requests the case from the PACS database and sends necessary queries to the MIII server (black, then black and blue lines).
3. The MIII server queries images from PACS database (blue then black line), which transmits data through high-speed networks (black then blue line) to the MIII computational resource.

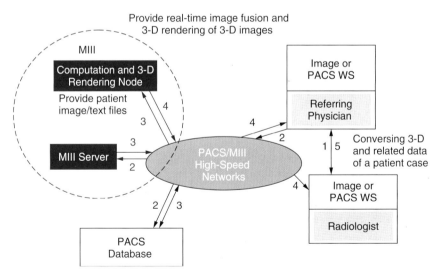

Figure 20.6   Three-dimensional rendering and fusion image tools in MIII and its connection with PACS in teleconference application. Application in scenario 2: teleconference with high-resolution 3-D image set. Light yellow: PACS domain; blue: MIII computational engine and postprocessing WS; light blue: high-speed networks connecting PACS and MIII. Numerals representing the teleconference workflow steps described in the text.

4. The computational resource performs necessary 3-D rendering and sends the results back almost in real time to the PACS WSs at both sites (blue line followed by two black lines).

5. The real-time video conference with the 3-D high-resolution image file available in both WSs proceeds.

Note that to accomplish this video/image conferencing, in addition to the PACS database, three components are necessary: the MIII server (blue), the computational node (blue), and the high-speed network (light blue). However, the conferencing does not allow the manipulation of images by either site. Synchronization and instantaneous image manipulation of require the teleconsultation resources described in Section 15.6.

20.3.3.2 Image Fusion   Image fusion is used to combine multimodality images into one single display. To optimize the display result, proper manipulation and contrast matching of the lookup table of each modality image are critical. In addition, using pseudocolor on one modality image and gray scale on the second is important (see Section 5.1.5).

20.3.4 Data Security

Data security encompasses data authenticity, access, and integrity. Data authenticity relates to the originality of the data, access relates to who can view what data and when, and integrity relates to data remaining unaltered during transmission. After images and data have been processed, some validation mechanisms are needed to ensure their security, accuracy, and completeness. See Chapter 17 for details.

20.3.5 Communication Networks

Communication networks include network hardware and communication protocols that are required to connect MIII components together as well as with HIS/RIS/PACS, other image types, and ePR data. The MIII communication networks can have two architectures: individual MIII networks with a connection to the HIS/RIS/PACS networks, or shared communication networks with HIS/RIS/PACS. In the former, the connection between the MIII networks and HIS/RIS/PACS networks should be transparent to the imaging informatics users, providing necessary high-speed throughput for the MIII to request HIS/RIS/PACS images and ePR related data and to distribute results to user's workstations. In the latter, the shared of MIII networks with that of PACS, the MIII networks should have a logical segment isolated from the PACS networks that does not interfere with the HIS/RIS/PACS daily clinical functions. High-speed networks with fast Inter- and Intra-Ethernet switches or connections to the Internet 2 routers can facilitate the data transfer rates when large volume of images is required for the study.

20.4 DATABASE AND KNOWLEDGE BASE MANAGEMENT

The database and knowledge base management component software has several functions. First, it integrates and organizes pertinent HIS/RISPACS images and related data, extracts image features and keywords from image processing, and arranges medical heuristics rules and guidelines into a coherent multimedia data model. Second, it supports on-line database management, content-based indexing and retrieval, and formatting and distribution for visualization and manipulation. This component software can be run on a commercial database engine with add-on application software. Third, data-mining tools with knowledge bases as guides can be used to obtain relevant information from the databases.

20.4.1 Grid Computing and Data Grid

Grid computing is the integrated use of geographically distributed computers, networks, and storage systems to create a virtual computing system environment for solving large-scale, data-intensive problems in science, engineering, commerce, and healthcare. A grid is a high-performance hardware and software infrastructure providing scalable, dependable, and secure access to the distributed resources. Unlike distributed computing and cluster computing, the individual resources in grid computing maintain administrative autonomy and are allowed system heterogeneity; this aspect of grid computing guarantees scalability and vigor. Therefore the grid's resources must adhere to agreed-upon standards to remain open and scalable. A Computational Grid with the primary function for resilient data storage is called Data Grid. Both the Computational Grid and the Data Grid are important in medical imaging informatics, with the latter for PACS data storage and large-scale clinical applications. A formal taxonomy composed of five layers, defined by the open source software Globus Toolkit 4.0 of Grid Computing, will be described in more detail in Chapter 21.

20.4.2 Content-Based Image Indexing

HIS/RIS/PACS and ePR databases are designed to retrieve information by artificial keys, such as patient name and hospital ID. This mode of operation is sufficient for traditional radiology operations but not adequate for image data storage of large-scale research and clinical applications. Therefore various enhanced databases in MIII are needed that contain not only keywords in diagnostic reports, patient history, and imaging sequences but also certain features of images for content-based indexing of underlying PET/MR/CT/US/CR images in the HIS/RIS/PACS databases.

Using artificial indexing like the patient's name, ID, age group, disease category, and so on, through one-dimensional keyword searches is a fairly simple procedure. On the other hand, indexing through image content is complicated because the query first has to understand the image content, which can include abstract terms (e.g., objects of interest), derived quantitative data (e.g., area and volume of the object of interest), and texture information (e.g., interstitial disease).

There are two basic methods using the image contents as a means for image retrieval: concept-based and content-based Rasmussen. In the concept-based method, the image is associated with metadata, that is, data about the image data. The metadata can include the image type (e.g., CT, MRI, and radiography), the brain and its substructures, their functions and blood supply, and so forth. Metadata describing the actual content and relationship can be free text or keywords chosen from a structured vocabulary. In PACS, the most important metadata are contained in the DICOM header file. Indexing and retrieval methods similar to those in text-based

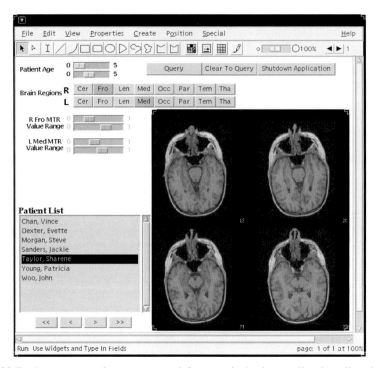

Figure 20.7 Image query by content and features in brain myelination disorders. Easy to use graphical user interface allows image query by image content through visualization. The sliding bars on the left can be used to control retrieved images shown in the right. R (L) FRO MTR: right (left) front magnetization transfer ratio. (Courtesy of Drs. K. Soohoo and S. Wong)

retrieval can then be used to organize and access the images. Since in the study of any organ, almost all images depict some sort of anatomical entity, an important component of a structured vocabulary should be an anatomical terminology that is also arranged to show relationships among the anatomical structures and their functions. Therefore the concept-based method is more anatomically oriented.

In content-based methods, image processing and mathematical techniques are used to analyze the actual content of the images. For example, the gray level distribution, or the different shapes and relationships, then match these features against a query image. Ideally one would like to be able to ask for images that "look like this one." Content-based image retrieval requires extensive image processing and sophisticated mathematical techniques.

Figure 20.7 shows the concept of image content indexing developed for brain myelination disorder research. Indexing via image content is a frontier research topic in image processing, and the HIS/RIS/PACS-rich databases will allow the validation of new theories and algorithms.

20.4.3 Data Mining

20.4.3.1 The Concept of Data Mining Data mining (DM) is a way to discover knowledge based on data in the data warehouse or data mart. A data warehouse is a collection of integrated, subject-oriented databases designed to support the decision-making functions, where each unit of data is relevant to some moment in time and locality. Large data warehouse may own several specialized warehouses, often called data marts. However, neither data warehouses nor data marts makes decisions, they are only for the repository of data. The process of DM, on the other hand, studies models, summaries, and derived values within a given collection of data in the data warehouse and data marts. So DM is not simply a collection of isolated tools; it uses the tools to make a decision. In practice, it is an iterative process, although a single and simple application of a method may not suffice to achieve the mining goal. DM focuses on the entire process of knowledge discovery, including data cleansing, learning, and integration and visualization of results. There are two categories of data mining: predictive DM and descriptive DM. The former is to produce the model of the system described by the given data set, and the latter is to develop new, nontrivial information based on the available data.

The data mining process consists of the following steps:

1. State the problem and formulate the hypothesis.
2. Collect the data.
3. Preprocessing the data including segmentation; detection and removal, scaling, encoding and selecting features.
4. Estimate the model.
5. Interpret and validate the model and draw conclusion.

Some data mining tools are machine learning, statistics, and visualization; they are applied to data in the data warehouses and data marts for knowledge discovery. In particular, some statistical methods are cluster analysis, decision trees and decision rules, association rules, artificial neural network, genetic algorithms, fuzzy Inference systems, and N-dimensional visualization methods. These methods are standard techniques taught and used in computer science and statistical methods curricula.

20.4.3.2 An Example of Discovering the Average Hand Image

In Chapter 25, we will discuss a CAD method is used to assess the bone age of a child from a hand radiographic image. In the process we need to find the average hand image of a child of a subgroup of given race, age, and gender from a large normal database comprising of children hand image data of different races from age 1 to 18 years old, both female and male. Let us use this example to illustrate the concept of using data mining to find the average hand image from a children radiographic hand image database following the DM five-step process described in the aforementioned paragraph:

1. *State the problem*: To find the average hand image.
2. *Collect the data*: The normal children hand radiographic image database.
3. *Preprocessing the data*: Each hand has over 20 quantitative parameters extracted from the image by image processing methods. These parameters are used as the gauge to determine the average hand image in a subgroup in the hand database (see Chapter 25 for methods).

4. *Estimate the model*: Criteria are set up to discover the average hand in a subgroup of children based on these parameters from the database.

5. *Interpret and validate*: Comparing the discovered average image with all available hand images based on visualization (see Fig. 20.8).

Figure 20.8 depicts the discovered average hand images per year old in a subgroup of African-American females from age 1 to 12 years old in the hand database using the data-mining method.

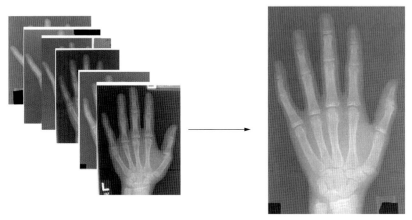

(A). Average image (right) selected from a group of images (left)

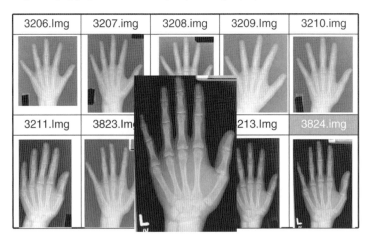

(B). Example of average image of a AAF11 group

Figure 20.8 An example of the data mining process used to locate an average hand image of African-American female (AAF) from 1 to 12 years old. (*A*) The objective is to find the average image (right) from a group of images (left). (*B*) Example of the average image overlaid on a group of 11-year-old AAF11 hand images from the database. (*C*) The average hand images of a group of African-American girls from 1 to 12 years old from a child hand database. One average image is provided per year group; see the example in (*B*) for the 11-year-old group.

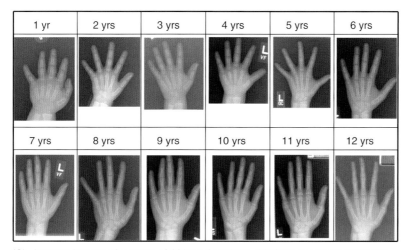

1 yr	2 yrs	3 yrs	4 yrs	5 yrs	6 yrs

7 yrs	8 yrs	9 yrs	10 yrs	11 yrs	12 yrs

(C). Average images of a group of African-American girls from one to 12 years old

Figure 20.8 *(Continued)*

20.4.4 Computer-Aided Diagnosis (CAD)

Computer-aided diagnosis (CAD) research started in the early 1980s and has gradually evolved as a clinically supported tool. In mammography, CAD has in fact become a part of the routine clinical operation for detection of breast cancers in many medical centers and screening sites in the United States. Various CAD schemes are being developed for detection and classification of many different kinds of lesions obtained with the use of various imaging modalities. The concept of CAD is broad and general as a tool in assisting radiologists by providing the computer output as a "second opinion." The usefulness and practicality of CAD, however, depend on many factors, including the availability of digital image data to train the CAD algorithm, computer power, and high-quality display and image-archiving systems. Therefore CAD needs to be integrated into a part of HIS/RIS/PACS in order to obtain sufficient data for CAD knowledge base development. Image-based knowledge discovery and decision support by use of CAD are a new trend in research that translates CAD diagnostic results to assist in short- and long-term treatments. Integration of CAD with HIS/RIS/PACS would take advantage of the image resources in PACS and enhance the value of CAD. Because of this, CAD applications have emerged into mainstream image-aided clinical practice in imaging informatics. The concept and methods of CAD will be discussed in detail in Chapter 25, its clinical applications and integration to PACS in Chapter 26.

20.4.5 Image-Intensive Radiation Therapy Planning and Treatment

Comprehensive clinical image data and relevant information is crucial in the image-intensive radiation therapy (RT) for the planning and treatment of cancer. Multiple stand-alone systems utilizing technological advancements in imaging, therapeutic radiation, and computer treatment planning systems acquire key data during the RT treatment course of a patient. Currently the data are scattered in various RT systems throughout the RT department. These scattered data compromise an efficient clinical workflow since the data crucial for a clinical decision may be time-consuming to retrieve, temporarily missing, or even lost. The DICOM standard has been extended from radiology to RT by ratifying seven DICOM RT objects, which helps set standard for data integration and interoperability between RT equipment from different vendors (see Chapter 9). An integrated image-based radiation therapy planning and treatment ePR system is a fundamental knowledge base in the medical imaging informatics infrastructure for cancer treatment. The concept and application of RT ePR will be discussed in Chapter 23.

20.4.6 Surgical Simulation and Modeling

Image-guided minimally invasive spinal surgery is a relatively new branch of surgery that relies on multimodality images for guiding the surgical procedure. The surgical procedure is relatively simple and safe if performed by the expert, and with a rapid patient recovery time. Despite the overall advantageous and benefits of this type of surgery compared to conventional open surgery, there are still challenges with respect to informatics remained to be addressed:

1. Scattered data acquisition systems within the operating room (OR) during surgery, including multiple sources of images, video, and waveforms.
2. Enhanced the surgical workflow with data acquisition, management, and distribution all in a single imaging information system.
3. The need of a one-stop integrated data repository during pre-, intra-, and post-surgical workflow.
4. Outcomes analysis for the patient undergoing the surgical procedure.
5. Training of new surgeons to perform this type of surgical procedure.

The solution to these challenges is an image-guided minimally invasive surgery ePR system. In Chapter 24, a comprehensive discussion will be given in minimally invasive spinal surgery as an example.

20.5 APPLICATION MIDDLEWARE

Sections 20.2, 20.3, and 20.4 discuss various aspects and components of the first, second, and third layer of MIII shown in Figure 20.2. Each application will require specific subsets of data, tools, and knowledge bases to form the nucleus of the application. Once it is accomplished, target-oriented middleware can be designed and developed to integrate and streamline these components for the application, whether it be for the purpose of clinical service, research, or education. This will provide rapid prototyping and reduce costs required for the development of every application. It is in this application middleware layer that the user will encounter the advantage and the power of the MIII. In Chapter 26 the topic of bone age assessment for children used to illustrate the middleware designed for research will be followed by its extension to the design of middleware for clinical service. Chapter 28 will provide a middleware example of an interactive digital breast teaching file designed for education.

20.6 CUSTOMIZED SOFTWARE AND SYSTEM INTEGRATION

20.6.1 Customized Software and Data

Customized software is high-level software tailored for a specific application site using the MIII infrastructure. The five logical levels shown in Figure 20.2 form a general infrastructure, and when implemented in a specific environment, certain components may need to be modified. Using the bone age assessment for children as an example, the normal children hand data used for the bone age assessment was collected in Los Angeles. When the CAD method was implemented in another site, namely in Hong Kong, the children these have a slight difference in the hand data's normal representation. In order to use the CAD method effectively in Hong Kong, the data collected in Los Angeles may have to be replaced by new data recollected in Hong Kong. This may result in a customized data collection software and database with data collected in Hong Kong. Thus, even though the bone age assessment methodology may be identical in both Los Angeles and Hong Kong sites, the database need to be customized to be applicable for children in Hong Kong. Chapter 25 will discuss certain aspects of the customized software and data.

20.6.2 System Integration

System integration includes components integration, subsystems interface, and shared data and workspace software. Subsystem interface software utilizes existing communication networks and protocols to connect all infrastructure components into an integrated information system. Shared data and workspace software allows the allocation and distribution of resources that include data, storage space, and workstation to the on-line users. System integration is the last step in the implementation and deployment of a MIII infrastructure platform to a specific site.

20.7 SUMMARY OF MEDICAL IMAGE INFORMATICS INFRASTRUCTURE (MIII)

Medical image informatics infrastructure (MIII) platform is an organized method to perform large-scale longitudinal and horizontal studies to advance research, enhance education, and better clinical service. It takes advantage of the richness of the HIS/RIS/PACS data, other medical image types, and related data from ePR. It may also share some of the HIS/RIS/PACS and ePR resources. There are certain resources that HIS/RIS/PACS do not have because the primary mission of HI/RIS/PACS was designed for clinical services. Therefore MIII needs to embed additional resources that are necessary for performing large-scale knowledge base management development. These include image content indexing, 3-D rendering and visualization engine, grid computing and data grid, CAD methods, surgical and radiation therapy

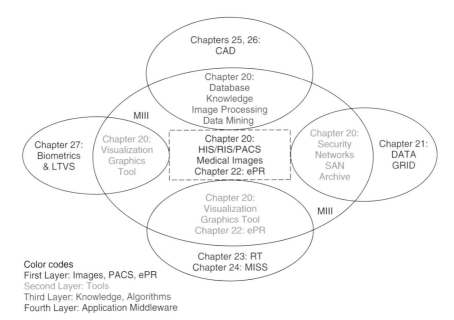

Figure 20.9 Relationships among imaging informatics data sources (rectangle), concepts, technologies, and applications (large and small ellipses) discussed in Part IV. MIII: Medical imaging informatics infrastructure (within the largest ellipse) that consists of the data sources and fundamental tools used by applications); Data Grid: used for fault-tolerance medical image archive, SAN (storage area network); CAD: computer-aided detection and diagnosis; LTVS: location tracking and verification system using biometric technologies; MISS: minimally invasive spinal surgery, RT: radiation therapy treatment and planning; HIS/RIS/PACS, medical images; ePR, are data components of MIII used by all other applications. Color codes are used for references to the five-layer informatics infrastructure shown in Figure 20.2.

technologies discussed in this chapter. Additional innovative resources may be needed in time as we advance our understanding from the current level of medical imaging informatics to a higher level. The relationships among data, tools, and applications to be discussed in Part IV are shown in Fig. 20.9.

References

Brinkley JF, Wong BA, Hinshaw KP, Rosse C. Design of an anatomy information system. *Comp Graph Appl* 19: 38–48; 1999.

Fuller A, Kalet I, Tarczy-Hornoch P. Biomedical and health informatics research and education at the University of Washington. *Yearbook Med Inform 2000, Res Educ* 11: 107–13; 2000.

Gell G, Errath M, Simonic KM. Research at the Department of Medical Informatics, Statistics and Documentation of the University of Graz. *Yearbook Med Inform 2000, Res Educ* 11: 1114–9; 2000.

Graves JR, Amos LK, Huether S, Lange LL, Thompson CB. Description of a graduate program in clinical nursing informatics. *Comp Nurs* 13(2): 60–70; 1995.

Greenes RA, Shortliffe EH. Medical informatics: an emerging academic discipline and institutional priority. *JAMA* 263(8): 1114–20; 1990.

Greenes RA. Ed. *Clinical Decision Support: The Road Ahead*. Burlington, MA, Elsevier; 2007.

Hasman A, Talmon JL. Education and research at the Department of Medical Informatics Masstricht. *Yearbook Med Inform 2000, Res Educ* 11: 100–6; 2000.

Heathfield HA, Wyatt J. Medical informatics: hiding our light under a bushel, or the Emperor's new clothes? *Meth Inform Med* 32(2): 181–2; 1993.

Huang HK, Wong STC, Pietka E. Medical image informatics infrastructure design and applications. *Med Inform* 22(4): 279–89; 1997.

Huang HK. *PACS: Basic Principles and Applications*. New York: Wiley, 521; 1999.

Huang HK. *PACS and Imaging Informatics: Principles and Applications*. Hoboken, NJ: Wiley; 2004.

Johns ML. The development of a graduate program in health information management. *Meth Inform Med* 33: 278–81; 1994.

Kangarloo H, Huang HK. Training program for imaging based medical informatics. NIH/NLM, IT15LM07356; 2002.

Kantardzic M. *Data Mining: Concepts, Models, Methods, and Algorithms*. Hoboken, NJ: Wiley; 2003.

Leven FJ, Haux R. Twenty-five years of medical informatics education at Heildelberg/Heilbronn: discussion of a specialized curriculum for medical informatics. *Yearbook Med Inform 2000, Res Educ* 11: 120–7; 2000.

McCray AT. Medical informatics research and training at the Lister Hill National Center for Biomedical Communications. *Yearbook Med Inform 2000, Res Educ* 11: 95–9; 2000.

Musen MA. Stanford medical informatics: uncommon research, common goals. *MD Comput* 16(1): 47–8; 1999.

Patton GA, Gardner RM. Medical informatics education: the University of Utah experience. *J Am Med Inform* 6(6): 457–65; 1999.

Pietka E, Pospiech-Kurkowska S, Gertych A, Fao F. Integration of computer assisted bone age assessment with clinical PACS. *Comput Med Imag Graph* 27(2–3), 217–22; 2003.

Rasmussen EM. Indexing multimedia: images. *Ann Rev Info Sci Technol* 32: 169–196; 1997.

Shortliffe EH. Medical informatics training at Stanford University School of Medicine. *Yearbook Med Inform:* p. 6; 1995.

Shortliffe EH, Patel VL, Cimino JJ, Barnett GO, Greenes RA. A study of collaboration among medical informatics research laboratories. *Artif Intell Med* 12: 97–123; 1998.

Shortliffe, E.H. (ed) and Cimino, J.J. (assoc. ed. 3rd). *Biomedical Informatics: Computer Applications in Health Care and Biomedicine*. New York: Spriger-Verlag, 2006.

Staggers N, Gassert CA, Skiba DJ. Health professionals' views of informatics education: findings from the AMIA 1999 Spring Conference. *J Am Med Inform* 7(6): 550 8; 2000.

Tagare HD, Vos FM, Jaffe CC, Duncan JS. Arrangement: a spatial relation between parts for evaluating similarity of tomographic sections. *IEEE Trans Pattern Anal Mach Intell* 17: 880–93; 1995.

Tagare HD, Jaffe CC, Duncan JS. Medical image databases: a content-based retrieval approach. *J Am Med Inform Assoc* 4: 184–98; 1997.

Van der Maas A, Johannes Ten Hoopen A, Ter Hofstede A. Progress with formalization in medical informatics? *J Am Med Inform*, 8(2): 126–30; 2001.

Warner HR. Medical informatics: a real discipline? *J Am Med Inform Assoc* 2(4): 207–14; 1995.

CHAPTER 21

Data Grid for PACS and Medical Imaging Informatics

In Chapter 20, we presented the framework of DICOM-based medical imaging informatics Figure 21.1 shows the topics and concepts covered in Part IV with regard to the five logical layers of the medical imaging informatics infrastructure (see Fig. 21.2). This chapter discusses the Data Grid and its applications in PACS and medical imaging informatics.

21.1 DISTRIBUTED COMPUTING

21.1.1 The Concept of Distributed Computing

Data Grid, which is a component of grid computing, a concept that has evolved from distributed computing. The basic idea behind distributed computing is that if several computers are networked together, the workload can be divided into smaller pieces for each computer to work on. In principle, when n computers are networked together, the total processing time can be reduced down to $1/n$ of the single-computer processing time. It should be noted that this theoretical limit is unlikely to be achieved because of various unavoidable overheads, for example, data communication latency.

Two important factors affect the design of a distributed computing schema. Processor speed variations in different computers make it important to implement the mechanism to balance the workload in distributed computing in a way that allows faster computers to be given more work to do. Otherwise, the speed of the processing will be slowed down by the slower computers in the distributed computing network. Data communication speed is another factor to consider. If workstations are connected by conventional Ethernet, with a maximum data transfer rate of 10 Mbits/s, the slower data transfer rate will limit the application of the distributed computing. Increased implementation of the asynchronous transfer mode (ATM) and gigabit Ethernet technologies will widen the parameter regime in which distributed computing is applicable.

The minimum requirement for distributed computing is a networked computer system with software that can coordinate the computers in the system to work coherently to solve a problem. There are several software implementations available for distributed computing; an example is the Parallel Virtual Machine (PVM) system

PACS and Imaging Informatics, Second Edition, by H. K. Huang
Copyright © 2010 John Wiley & Sons, Inc.

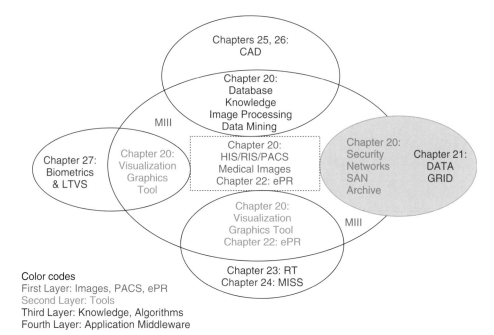

Figure 21.1   Imaging informatics data sources (rectangle), concepts, technologies, and applications (large and small ellipses) as discussed in Part IV. MIII (within the largest ellipse) consists of the data sources and fundamental tools used by applications; Data Grid is for fault-tolerance medical image archive SAN for storage area network, CAD for computer-aided detection and diagnosis, LTVS for location tracking and verification using biometric technologies, Surgery for minimally invasive spinal surgery, RT for radiation therapy treatment and planning, HIS/RIS/PACS for medical images, and ePR for electronic patient record. All are data components of MIII used by other applications. Color codes refer to the five-layer informatics infrastructure shown in Fig. 20.2. Orange color for the Data Grid.

developed jointly by Oak Ridge National Laboratory, the University of Tennessee, and Emory University. PVM supports a variety of computer systems, including workstations by Sun Microsystems, Silicon Graphics, Hewlett-Packard, DEC/Microvax, and IBM-compatible personal computers running the Linux operating system.

After the PVM system is installed in all computer systems, one can start the PVM task from any computer. Other computers can be added to or deleted from the PVM task interactively or by a software call to reconfigure the virtual machine. For computers under the same PVM task, any computer can start new PVM processes in other computers. Intercomputer communication is realized by passing messages back and forth, thus allowing the exchange of data among the computers in the virtual machine.

The parameter regimes for applicability of distributed computing are both problem and computer dependent. For distributed computing to be profitable, t_1, the time interval required to send a given amount of data between two computers across the network, should be much shorter than t_2, the time needed to process them in a host computer. In other words, the network data communication rate (proportional to $1/t_1$) should be much higher than the data processing rate (proportional to $1/t_2$). The smaller the ratio of t_1 to t_2 or the higher the ratio of the two rates, the more advantages for distributed computing. If the ratio of the two rates is equal to or less than 1, there is no reason to use distributed computing, since too much time would be spent waiting for the results to be sent across the network back to the host computer. Thus, for $t_1 \leq t_2$, it is faster to use a single computer to do the calculation.

Although the data communication rate can be estimated based on the network type and the communication protocol, the data processing rate depends both on the computer and on the nature of the problem. For a given workstation, more complex calculations lower the data processing rate. Since the computer system and the network are usually fixed within a given environment, the data processing rate depends more on the nature of the problem. Therefore, whenever a problem is given, one can estimate the ratio of the two rates and determine whether distributed computing is worthwhile. Figure 21.2*A* depicts the concept of distributed computing based on the data communication rate and processing rate. The data were obtained using the Sun SPARC LX computers and the Ethernet (1.0 Mbits/s) communication protocol. Although the data in this example were obtained several years ago when both the Internet and the computing speed in WSs were slow, the results are useful for demonstrating the concept of distributing computing. However, even with the advances of gigabit Ethernet technologies and the fast CPU cycle time in desktop computers, the concept of when distributing computing should be used remains valid; that is, distributive computing is applicable only when the communication rate is above the computation rate. Immediate applications using distributed computing are image compression, unsharp masking, enhancement, 3-D rendering, image fusion, and computer-aided diagnosis. Some of these topics will be discussed in later chapters.

21.1.2   Distributed Computing in PACS Environment

Each image workstation in a PACS, when it is not in active use, consumes only a minimum of its capacity for running background processes. As the number of image workstations grows, this excessive computational power can be exploited to perform value-added image processing functions for PACS. Image processing is used extensively in the preprocessing stage, which does not require as much computational power as in unsharp masking and background removal in CR, but it has not been used extensively in image postprocessing. One reason is that preprocessing can be done quickly through manufacturer's imaging modality hardware and software, which is application specific and the execution time is fast. On the other hand, postprocessing depends on the image workstation (WS) which, in general, does not provide hardware image processing functions beyond such simple functions as lookup table, zoom, and scroll. For this reason, at the image workstation, the user very seldom uses time-consuming image processing functions even though some, like unsharp masking and image fusion are necessary and effective. The multi-image workstation PACS environment and MIII infrastructure connected with many servers and workstations suggest the configuration of distributed computing and, for image processing, the advantage to be gained if the extensive computational power were available at workstations and servers. Conceptually, distributed computing should raise interest in image processing applications to the extent that there will be demand for image

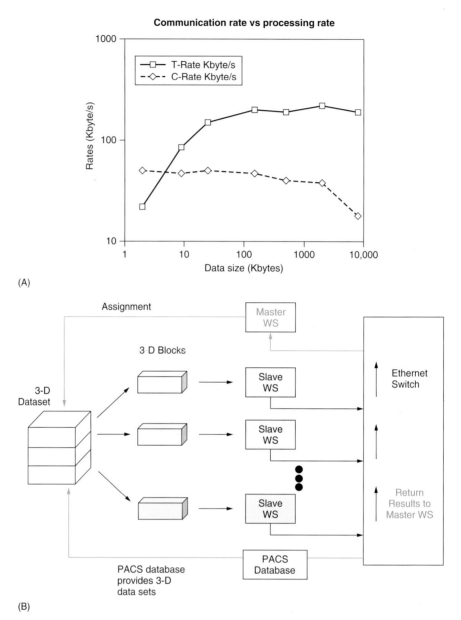

(A)

(B)

Figure 21.2 (*A*) Distributed computing in a PACS environment. The solid curve represents the computer-to-computer transmission rate (T-rate) under PVM (parallel virtual machine) and TCP/IP Ethernet (1.0 Mbits/s) connection, as a function of data size (horizontal axis). The dotted curve represents data processing rate (C-rate) required to perform a 2-D FFT in a Sun SPARC-LX computer. The squares and diamonds represent the measured data points. Distributed computing is applicable only when the solid curve is above the dotted curve. (Courtesy of Dr. X. Zhu) (*B*) Procedure in distributed computing. Master workstation requests 3-D volume image data from the PACS database and assigns 3-D blocks to each slave workstation (WS) for the computation task. Each slave WS returns results to the master WS, which compiles all results for the task. (Courtesy of Dr. J. Wang)

postprocessing tools that can improve medical service by providing near real-time performance at the image workstations. Currently heavier image processing functions like 3-D rendering and CAD, on specially designed postprocessing WS, are used in the clinical environment.

As in distributed computing, several networked PACS WS could be used for computationally intensive image processing functions by distributing the work load to these workstations. Thus the image processing time could be reduced at a rate inversely proportional to the number of workstations used. Distributed computing requires that several workstations be linked to a high-speed network; these conditions are within the realm of PACS and MIII in the number of available WSs workstations and gigabit intra Ethernet technologies. Figure 21.2*B* shows how distributed computing in a PACS and MIII network environment would process a three-dimensional data set.

Notice in the figure that if for a data security purpose the computation is for the encode/decode digital signature of the 3-D image volume, and if some slave WSs do not have the encryption software, grid computing can be used to send the encryption software (middleware) with the individual 3-D block data sets to the slave WSs.

21.2 GRID COMPUTING

21.2.1 The Concept of Grid Computing

Grid computing represents the latest and most exciting computing technology to evolve from the familiar realm of parallel, peer-to-peer and client-server models, and then distributed computing. Grid computing includes many of the concepts of distributed computing and networked computing. In distributed computing, a given task is performed by distributing it to several or more networked computers (see Figure 21.2*B*). Grid computing has one more major ingredient—the middleware—that goes with the data while it is being distributed. Middleware can be computational resources, a software package, a security check, some display functions, or even data to facilitate the designated computer if it does not have the necessary resources for the task. For example, if image content indexing task is being requested that depends on high-power computational algorithms, the middleware that goes with the image data will contain the necessary computational algorithms. Grid computing also has more organization than distributed computing, and each grid within the grid framework may have different resources and even data. When needed, the administrative federation of the grid networked computers can poll resources from different grids for a specific task. Grid computing in medical imaging informatics applications is still in its infancy, but MIII should include grid computing as a resource in its infrastructure plan.

21.2.2 Current Grid Computing Technology

Grid computing is the integrated use of geographically distributed computers, networks, and storage systems to create a virtual computing system for solving large-scale, data-intensive problems in science, engineering, and commerce. A grid is a high-performance hardware and software infrastructure providing scalable, dependable, and secure access to the distributed resources. Unlike distributed computing and

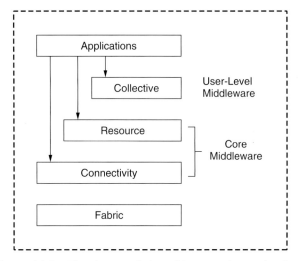

Figure 21.3   Five layers of the grid computing technology.

cluster computing, the individual resources in grid computing maintain administrative autonomy and are allowed system heterogeneity; this aspect of grid computing guarantees scalability and vitality. Therefore the grid's agreed-upon standards must remain open and scalable. A formal taxonomy, composed of five layers (as shown in Figure 21.3) has been created to enssure its standardization:

1. *Fabric layer:* The lowest layer includes the physical devices or resources, such as computers, storage systems, networks, sensors, and instruments.
2. *Connectivity layer:* The layer above the fabric layer includes the communication and authentication protocols required for grid network transactions, such as the exchange of data between resources, and the verification of the identity of users and resources.
3. *Resource layer:* This layer contains connectivity protocols to enable the secure initiation, resource monitoring, and control of resource-sharing operations.
4. *Collective layer:* The layer above the resource layer contains protocols, services, and APIs (application programming interfaces) to implement transactions among resources, such as resource discovery, and job scheduling.
5. *User application layer:* This highest layer calls on all other layers for applications.

At its core, grid computing is based on an open set of standards and protocols—such as the Open Grid Services Architecture (OGSA). The grid computing provides the user with the following types of service:

1. *Computational services* support specific applications on distributed computational resources, such as supercomputers. A grid for this purpose is often called a Computational Grid.
2. *Data services* allow the sharing and management of distributed datasets. A grid for this purpose is often called a Data Grid.

3. *Application services* allow access to remote software and digital libraries, and provide overall management of all applications running.

4. *Knowledge services* provide for the acquisition, retrieval, publication, and overall management of digital knowledge tools.

There are several large-scale grid projects underway worldwide: the Ninf from the Tokyo Institute of Technology; Globus from ANL (Argonne National Laboratory) and Information Science Institute (ISI), USC; Gridbus from the University of Melbourne; European Datagrid, and others. However, there is only limited investigation of the impact of this emerging technology in biomedical imaging, with an exception being a project called e-Diamond, which is a Grid-enabled federated database of annotated mammograms.

21.2.3 Grid Technology and the Globus Toolkit

Grid computing is based on an open set of standards and protocols in its core infrastructure. In this chapter we use the Open Grid Services Architecture (OGSA) as an example to discuss the computational services and the data services (see Section 21.2.2) of the Globus Toolkit 4.0 co-developed by ANL (Argon National Laboratory), University of Chicago and ISI (Information Sciences Institute), University of Southern California for PACS and Medical Imaging Informatics applications.

Figure 21.4 shows the five layers of the grid computing technology defined by the Globus toolkit 4.0 and the layers correspondence with the OSI (Open System Interconnection) architecture.

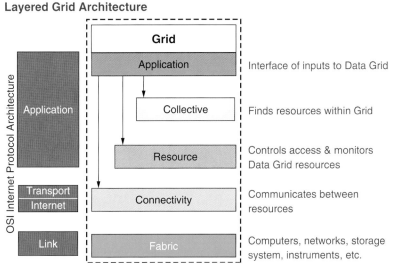

Figure 21.4 Five layer grid architecture defined by the Globus Toolkit 4.0: Fabric, connectivity, resource, collective, and application. The left-hand side depicts its correspondence to the OSI (open system interconnection) seven-layer Internet protocol. The right-hand side describes its functions.

21.2.4 Integrating DICOM Technology with the Globus Toolkit

The Globus Toolkit can be used for specific PACS operations by integrating it with a selected customized subset of DICOM resources. For examples, Globus can be customized as a fault-tolerant archive system and a Computational Grid for enterprise PACS operations (see Chapter 16). Sections 21.3 to 21.5 present PACS fault-tolerant archive and some related clinical applications. PACS fault-tolerant archive includes topics on PACS image storage, backup archive and disaster recovery operations using the DICOM image store's query and retrieve (Q/R) services through the Data Grid.

Figure 21.5 describes the resources and tools available in each of the five layers after the integration. The majority of these tools are directly from the Globus, and others are through customization using DCIOM services. Figure 21.5 also depicts the positions of these DICOM services and the Metadata in the Globus Grid's five-layer infrastructure. The customized components are shaded, and the color boxes indicate components developed at the IPILab, USC.

21.3 DATA GRID

Three topics will be presented in this section: use of the Data Grid in a large-scale enterprise PACS operation, methods of integrating multiple PAC systems with the Data Grid, and three Data Grid tasks during a PACS disaster recovery.

21.3.1 Data Grid Infrastructure in the Image Processing and Informatics Laboratory (IPILab)

Figure 21.5 illustrates the integration of DICOM image store and DICOM image Q/R in the application layer of the Globus Toolkit to form the Data Grid for fault-tolerant storage backup of multiple PAC systems. Figure 21.6 depicts the existing Data Grid with the integrated Globus Toolkit and DICOM services (green) presented in Figure 21.5 in the Image Processing and Informatics Laboratory (IPILab). The existing Data Grid is ready to be used for PACS and medical imaging informatics applications with customized software. Some of the key customized software, including PACS and DICOM GAP (Grid Access Point; see Fig. 21.7, white box), SAN (storage area network), Medadata DB, Replica DB, Grid Services, and Data Grid Simulator, are illustrated in Figure 21.7.

21.3.2 Data Grid for the Enterprise PACS

The first application of the Data Grid is in a large-scale enterprise PACS operation. The example enterprise to be discussed consists of three PACS sites, as shown in Figure 21.8 (three yellow boxes) plus a research site at IPILab (green box) used for monitoring the operation. The three operations used for demonstration are the image/data archive, query/retrieve, and server and archive disaster recovery fault-tolerance features of the Data Grid.

The operation environment is as follows: Three PACS sites operate independently as three separate PAC systems, each supporting its own clinical site. Each site has a stand-alone PACS with its own server, workstations (WSs), SAN (storage area network; see Chapter 11) archive and storage backup. Without the Data

IPI Data Grid Layered Infrastructure Integrating Globus and DICOM

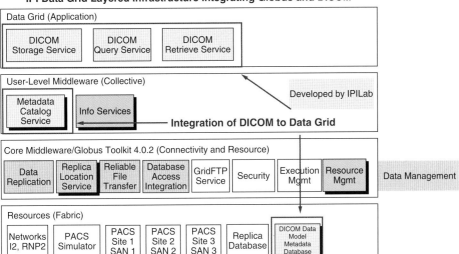

Figure 21.5   The five-layer Data Grid architecture integrating DICOM services and the Globus Toolkit for PACS and MIII applications. *Resources (fabric) layer*: The five leftmost clear boxes are existing resources from PAC systems; I2 (Internet 2); RNP2 (Rede Nacional de Ensino e Pesquisa); SAN (storage area network) is for PACS archive (see Chapter 11). The Replica Database is a Globus tool; the rightmost metadata database is for fault-tolerant Data Grid and Computing Grid (shadow) application. *Core Middleware (connectivity layer and resource layer)*: The four leftmost boxes are Globus tools used for data management in PACS Data Grid; the rest are other Globus tools. Replica (shadow) and Resource Management (green shadow) are also used for the Computing Grid. *User-level middleware (collective layer)*: Metadata catalog service and the Globus info services tool are included for fault tolerance. Both resources are also used for Computing Grid applications (shadow boxes). *Data Grid application layer*: This consists of the DICOM storage, query, and retrieve services. Light shaded boxes with bold red external rectangles are DICOM resources, and the metadata database for fault tolerance. Services in these boxes were developed at the Image Processing and Informatics Laboratory (IPILab), USC.

Grid (green in Fig. 21.8), any WS at a PACS site can Q/R images from its own SAN to display image data. In addition any WS of any of the three PAC systems can Q/R images from other sites using a Web client imaging routing mechanism (IRM, dotted lines in Fig. 21.6) if the PACS manufacturers supports such function.

There are several disadvantages to using this method of integrating multiple PACS operations:

1. The two single points of failures (SPOFs) in each PACS are the server and the SAN archive, assuming that the networks have backup.
2. If the server of a PACS goes down, its WS is not able to retrieve images from the SAN of its own PACS or review images of other PAC systems because

Existing Data Grid at IPILab, USC

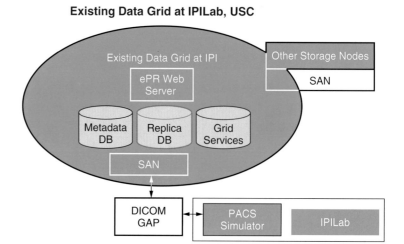

Current Applications

• Second-tier PACS backup
• Imaging Center's resource for clinical trial
• Molecular Imaging Center's archive

Figure 21.6   Existing Data Grid and its three current applications developed at IPILab, USC.

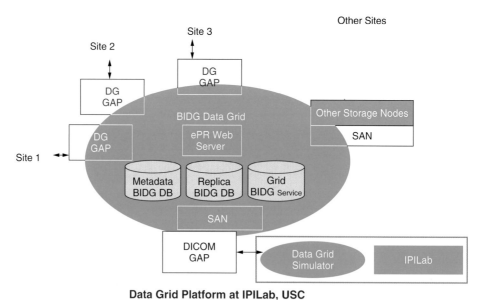

Data Grid Platform at IPILab, USC

Figure 21.7   Data Grid platform at IPILab used to customize for PACS and MIII applications. The major components are the DG GAPs (Grid access point) and the DICOM GAP for connection to PACS sites, other MIII servers, and the Data Grid simulator. The Data Grid simulator can be used for prototyping other Data Grid applications.

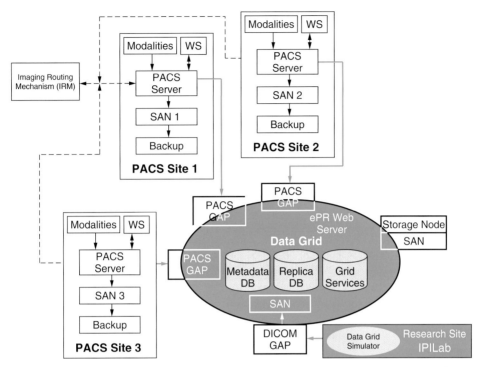

Figure 21.8 Enterprise PACS with three PACS sites (light yellow boxes). Each site has a stand-alone PACS with its own server, workstations (WSs), SAN (storage area network) archive and storage backup, and each site operates independently. An enterprise PACS is when these three PAC systems (or more) are connected together to share images. In an enterprise PACS, a WS at each site can Q/R images from its own SAN for image display. A WS of any three PAC systems can also Q/R images from other sites using an imaging routing mechanism (IRM, yellow box) shown in the left. The weakness of this method of connecting the three PAC systems is that two single points of failure can occur. When a PACS server or the SAN fails, the interconnectivity of the three PAC systems breaks down. On the other hand, the fault-tolerant Data Grid architecture shown in green can restore each site's backup and their connections to the IRM. It maintains interconnectivity of these three systems in real-time without human intervention. There are two types of PACS GAPs in this architecture, DICOM GAP (bottom) and PACS GAP (middle left). The former is for the PACS WS that uses the DICOM standard for image Q/R, the latter is for none DICOM file transfer used by some PAC systems.

the workflow (see dotted lines workflow arrows in Fig. 21.8) relies on the availability of the PACS server.

3. It the SAN of a PACS goes down, two things can happen. First, its WS will not be able to view its own images from the SAN. Even though the PACS may have a backup archive, it will take time for the IT (information technology) team to bring the backup on line and supply images to its own WS. This is because most of the backup storage nowadays is low cost, and the

priority is to preserve a second copy of the archived data instead of immediately failover to support a continuing operation. The backup is usually without an automatic switch function to take over the primary operation. Second, a WS from other PAC systems will not be able to Q/R images from this PACS.

Therefore two major goals for of the Data Grid are to minimize the impact due to the failure of the server or the SAN of each PACS.

21.3.3 Roles of the Data Grid in the Enterprise PACS Daily Clinical Operation

The PACS Data Grid can be designed to link the three sites together (1) to support the archive and the backup, and disaster recovery for all three sites, and (2) to allow a WS of any site to retrieve and review image/data from any other sites. The more critical responsibility of the fault-tolerant Data Grid is taking care of PACS own archive, backup, and disaster recovery, though its role in image distribution to and receiving from other PAC systems is useful.

Figure 21.8 illustrates the architecture of the DICOM-imbedded Data Grid located at the IPI, USC (or at any site with sufficient capability); SANs are located at the three clinical PAC systems as shared storage resources. The three primary components in the Data Grid are as follows:

1. *Storage node:* Resources from the three PAC systems, including the SAN 1, SAN 2, and SAN 3, (see Fig. 21.5, resources layer; and Fig. 21.8, three yellow boxes), provide storage resources for the Data Grid. Each SAN will have one copy of every image for a given PACS.
2. *Database:* A Grid Service that keeps track of metadata as well as file locations of different storage nodes within the Data Grid. Dynamic and robust access to data is provided by the Data Access Interface (DAI, see item 3 below) in the Globus Toolkit integrated with the database (Fig. 21.8, three light blue cylinders inside the Data Grid [green])
3. *Metadata Database:* Metadata contain all DICOM image header and data model information extracted from an image when it is acquired from the imaging modality. This information is organized and stored in the metadata database (Fig. 21.5), which provides all necessary information about the image, including a pointer to where the image is located in the Data Grid SANs. Upon a proper query, any image data in the metadata database can be retrieved by the WS through the GAP. The metadata database without backup databases can be a single point of failure in the Data Grid. For this reason a middle layer called the DAI (data access interface) in the Global Toolkit servers is added in-between GAPs and metadata storage nodes. Therefore there are two layers in the metadata database, the multiple DAI servers and multiple metadata storage nodes (or SANs), as shown in Figure 21.9, that allow multiple GAPs to access multiple DAI servers and multiple metadata storage nodes. The three main functions of the DAI server are centralization of metadata access, replication of metadata into multiple storage nodes, and handling metadata for different PACS archives.

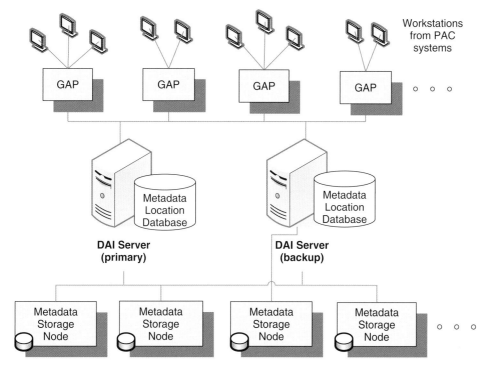

Figure 21.9 General Architecture of the fault-tolerance metadata system for the Data Grid. There are three levels of fault tolerance: (Top) Multiple GAPs, (middle) DAI (Data Access Interface) servers, and (bottom) multiple metadata storage nodes (SANs). (Courtesy of J. Lee)

4. *PACS or DICOM Grid Access Point (GAP):* A service provides access data within the Data Grid with DICOM compliant storage and query/retrieve capabilities for the WS of any PAC system. There are multiple PACS GAPs in the Data Grid (see Fig. 21.8, connected to WSs of each PACS and embedded in the Data Grid) that can be used as the backup for each other.

21.4 FAULT-TOLERANT DATA GRID FOR PACS ARCHIVE AND BACKUP, QUERY/RETRIEVAL, AND DISASTER RECOVERY

In Figure 21.8 ignore the IRM and the dotted line connections, and consider the three PACS sites that are now fully connected (green lines) to the Data Grid (green). In each PACS, the SAN has been partioned into P1 and P2, with P1 for its own PACS images/data storage and P2 for contribution to the other two PAC systems for their backup copies (see Chapter 11). As the enterprise fault-tolerant PACS Data Grid, it has three major responsibilities: (1) archives its own image/data and backup it up with two extra copies at P2 of two other PACS SANs, (2) queries/retrieves image/data from other PAC systems, and (3) performs disaster recovery when either its server or SAN goes down.

21.4.1 Archive and Backup

Under normal conditions of operation (Fig. 21.10, left, solid lines), the first copy of the image acquired at site 1 is sent to partition 1 of its own SAN, the second and third backup copies are sent utilizing the GAP 1 to P2 of SAN 2 and P2 of SAN 3 contributed by other PACS sites to the Data Grid. The fault-tolerance (FT) of the GAP can be demonstrated by the dotted lines in the figure. During the backup procedure, suppose that GAP 1 fails (red cross-lines), then the Data Grid would automatically assign GAP 2 to replace GAP 1. GAP 2 would then complete the task original assigned to GAP 1 by storing copy 2 to P2 of SAN 2, and P2 of SAN 3.

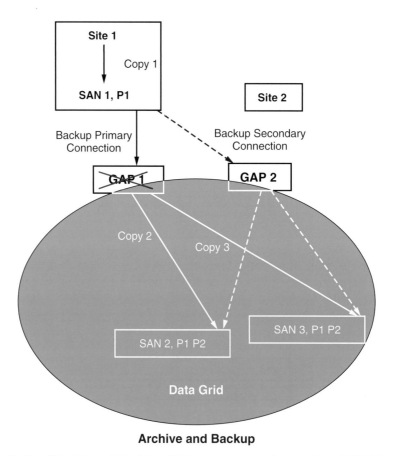

Archive and Backup

Figure 21.10 Workflow of the Data Grid during image data archive. Solid black lines (left), show the normal archive and backup operations, the first copy of the image file is sent from the acquisition to its SAN1 P1, and two backup copies to the Data Grid SAN2 P2, and SAN3 P2 for backup storage through its designated GAP1. Dotted blue line shows when GAP 1 fails (red cross-lines), and GAP 2 takes over GAP 1 functions automatically.

21.4.2 Query/Retrieve (Q/R)

There are two scenarios:

1. *Q/R its own PACS image file:* Refer to Figure 21.11*A* where the solid lines (left) show the normal operation of DICOM Q/R from WS at site 1. If the image file is in its own SAN 1 P1, then it is normal PACS operations. But if SAN 1 P1 fails, Q/R will go to its PACS backup through GAP 1 to either SAN 2 P2, or SAN 3 P2. Then Q/R will initiate GAP 1 to the Data Grid to query and then retrieve the image file from the storage nodes, in this example, SAN 2, P2. On the other hand, if during the process SAN 2 fails (red cross-lines), Data Grid identifies SAN 3, P2, from which the file is then retrieved (blue dotted lines). If during the off site Q/R, GAP 1 fails, GAP 2 will replace the function of GAP 1, as described in Figure 21.10.

2. *Q/R other PACS image file:* The Q/R goes to GAP 1 to query, then retrieve the image file from SAN 2 P1, as shown in Figure 21.11*B*. If SAN 2 fails (red lines), then Data Grid will automatically switch to SAN 3 P1, from which the file is then retrieved (blue dotted lines). If GAP 1 fails, GAP 2 will replace the function of GAP 1, as described in Figure 21.10.

21.4.3 Disaster Recovery — Three Tasks of the Data Grid When the PACS Server or Archive Fails

In the Data Grid architecture shown in Figure 21.8, there are two single points of failures (SPOFs) at each site, the server/archive and the SAN storage device. When any of these two SPOF, or both, fails, the Data Grid has to overcome three major tasks (disaster recovery) in order to be fault tolerant.

First, it has to maintain continuous clinical operation allowing WSs at this PACS site to Q/R images from its backup in the Data Grid. Second, after the server and the SAN have been repaired, the Data Grid has to rebuild the SAN P1 at this site for its own primary archive. Third, it has to rebuild the backup archive SAN P2 that contributes to other PAC systems in the enterprise for their backup. Figure 21.12 describes, using site 3 as an example, these three tasks when the server and/or SAN fail (red cross-lines). SAN 3 is partitioned into P1 and P2. P1 is the archive for its own site and P2, in green fonts, is site 3's SAN storage resource committed to the Data Grid for other sites' backup archive. Task 1 has the highest priority among three tasks shown in heavy green lines. All three tasks are performed automatically without human intervention. The archive's backup Q/R functions described earlier can be used to compete all three tasks.

21.5 DATA GRID AS THE IMAGE FAULT-TOLERANT ARCHIVE IN IMAGE-BASED CLINICAL TRIALS

21.5.1 Image-Based Clinical Trial and Data Grid

Clinical trials play a crucial role in testing new drugs or devices in modern clinical practice. Medical imaging has become an important tool in clinical trials because images provide a unique and fast diagnosis with visual observance and quantitative

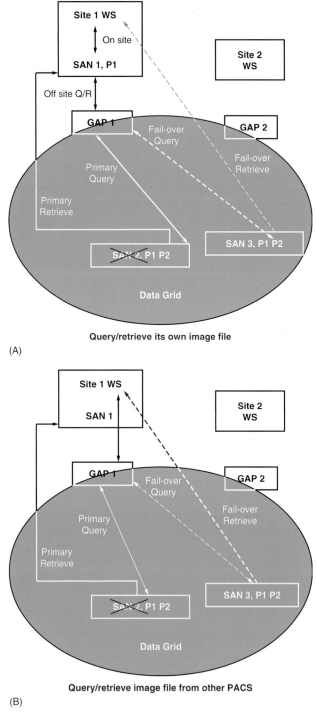

Figure 21.11   Workflows of Data Grid during query/retrieve of an image file. (*A*) The PACS WS Q/R its own PACS image file or from the Data Grid; (*B*) the PACS WS Q/R other PACS image file from the Data Grid.

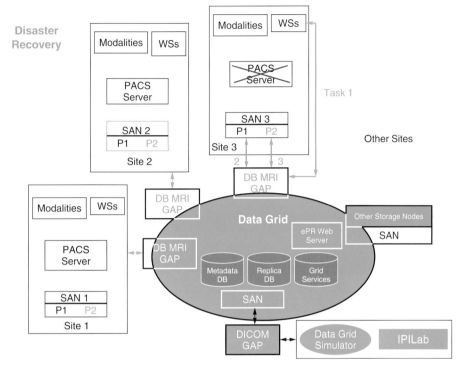

Figure 21.12 Three tasks (upper right, heavy green lines) of the Data Grid during disaster recovery when either a PACS server or the SAN fails. Site 3 is used as an example. Task 1: Allow site 3 PACS WS to Q/R its own images from the Data Grid for continuing clinical operation. Task 2: After its server and SAN have been restored, the Data Grid rebuilds P1 of SAN 3 installing its own images. Task 3: After its server and SAN have been restored, the Data Grid rebuilds P2 of SAN 3, which has the backup images of other PAC systems connected to the Data Grid. All three tasks are performed without human intervention. Workflows and operations of Figures 21.10, and 21.11A and B allow the Data Grid to automatically complete the three tasks.

assessment. A typical imaging-based clinical trial consists of (1) a well-defined rigorous clinical trial protocol; (2) a radiology core that has a quality control mechanism, a biostatistics component, and a server for storing and distributing data and analysis results, and (3) many field sites that generate and send clinical trial image studies to the radiology core. With ever-increasing number of clinical trials, it becomes a great challenge for a radiology core that handles multiple clinical trials to have a robust server to administrate multiple trials as well as satisfy the requirements to quickly distribute information to participating radiologists/clinicians worldwide to assess the trials' results. Data Grid as a grid computing technology can satisfy the aforementioned requirements of imaging-based clinical trials.

21.5.2 The Role of a Radiology Core in Imaging-Based Clinical Trials

Medical imaging is taking on a prominent role in early detection and quantization of new diseases or change in diseases. Multiple imaging-based clinical trials provide the required number of cases examined by using images from unbiased populations required to test new diagnostic, therapeutic techniques, or agents. Through the years the methodology and protocols of clinical trails have changed gradually, and Figure 21.13 remains a good representation of a general organization chart of a medical imaging-based clinical trial. The radiology core in this figure has the responsibilities of collecting imaging data from multiple field sites with quality control, and a server for storing and distributing trial results to field sites. The field sites recruit patients and generate images and send to the radiology core. The general workflow of an imaging-based clinical trial (Fig. 21.13) is shown in Figure 21.14:

1. Field sites $(1-n)$ generate DICOM format image data related to the patients enrolled in a specific clinical trial and transmit the image data to the radiology

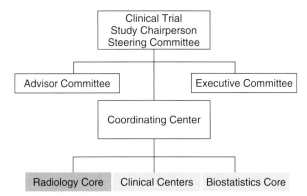

Figure 21.13 Organizational chart of an imaging-based clinical trial. Radiology core (blue) is responsible for all image-related operations.

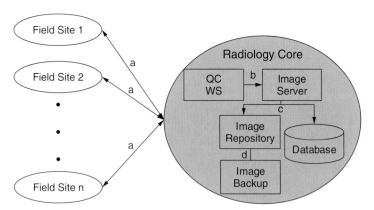

Figure 21.14 Typical workflow of imaging-based clinical trial. (*A*) The images are sent from field sites (1, 2, . . . , n) to a radiology core (blue), where the images are checked by a QC (quality control) WS (workstation). (*B*) Images are stored in the image server. (*C*) The server archives images in an image repository and stores the metadata of the image in the database. (*D*) The images in the Repository are backed up.

core through various digital networks or storage media (e.g., a CD). The image data are de-identified before they are sent out.

2. The images received by the radiology core go through a QC (quality control) WS (workstation) to assure image quality, for example, regarding patient positioning, equipment calibration, space localization, acquisition parameters, and patient demographic information. Once the quality of the images is approved, the images are sent to a centralized image server.

3. The image server extracts the metadata from the DICOM header of the image and stores the metadata and related patient information in the database of a data repository, such as RAID (redundant array of independent disks). The images are distributed to assigned radiologists of field sites worldwide to make diagnosis. The diagnosis results, usually quantity numbers, are returned and stored in the metadata database.

4. The images stored in the repository are also backed up in an off-line manual storage device.

This workflow and setup at the radiology core can satisfy a small number of clinical trials. With the ever-increasing number of clinical trials, it becomes a great challenge for a radiology core that handles multiple clinical trials to have a robust server to administrate multiple trials as well as satisfy the requirements to quickly distribute information to participating radiologists/clinicians worldwide to assess trials' results. In addition different clinical trials can vary in the parameters of results. A dynamic database model is necessary for the image server in the radiology core to accommodate new clinical trials. All these issues underline the need for a new infrastructure that can satisfy the requirements of imaging-based clinical trials. Data Grid, an emerging image storage and distribution computing technology, is an ideal solution to this new demand.

21.5.3 Data Grid for Clinical Trials — Image Storage and Backup

In order to form the Data Grid, participated radiology cores have to join a Data Grid confederation, something very similar to the enterprise PACS discussed in Sections 21.3 and 21.4. Three radiology cores are modeled to illustrate the Data Grid concept using DICOM store for data and backup, query/retrieve, and recovery. The premises are that during the implementation phase, the Data Grid cannot affect the current radiology core data storage backup operation, and that once the Data Grid is in operation, the existing radiology core storage backup can be dismantled and the radiology core workflow replaced by the Data Grid. The Data Grid concept can be extended to support more than three radiology cores.

Figure 21.15 shows the system design of the three-core Data Grid for clinical trials image backup. Each core has the same setup (Figure 21.14) described previously. The image backup storage (e.g., storage area network [SAN]) in every radiology core is separated into partition P1 and P2; P1 is for local radiology core backup, while P2 is contributed to the Data Grid to form a virtual large backup storage for other radiology cores participated in the Data Grid. The image server in each core sends a second copy of the image to the Data Grid, which automatically replicates it into two additional copies stored in the other two cores. In this case, images from core A will be stored in P2 at cores B and C. This will ensure fault tolerance (FT) within the Data

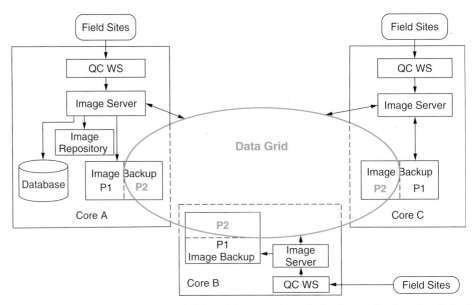

Figure 21.15 Three-core Data Grid architecture (green) for image backup in clinical trials. Cores A, B, and C have the same setup. The image backup storage (e.g., SAN) in every radiology core is separated into two partitions, P1 and P2. P1 is used for local backup, while P2 is contributed to the Data Grid for backup of images from other cores. Notice that the Data Grid has not intruded on the core's backup operation in the image repository. Figure 21.17 describes the data migration process from the current local hard disk backup to P1 of the SAN.

Grid in case a storage resource is unavailable. Remember, in the current operating radiology core, the backup uses standard hard disks as shown in Figure 21.14. The archive and backup, query/retrieve, and disaster recovery procedures follow the Data Grid workflow described in Figures 21.10, 21.11A and B, and 21.12.

21.5.4 Data Migration from the Backup Archive to the Data Grid

The major reason for using the Data Grid for clinical trials is to replace existing storage backup while the Data Grid is deploying. This section discusses the data migration steps to (1) start to archive all new images to its own SAN and (2) replace the existing local backup at the radiology core by the Data Grid. Following the Data Grid configuration described in Figure 21.15, Figure 21.16 and Figure 21.17 show how to migrate images from the local backup to the Data Grid.

The clinical trial radiology core test bed with three international sites is used as an example. They are the Image Processing and Informatics Laboratory (IPI), University of Southern California; the PACS Lab, Hong Kong Polytechnic University (PolyU); and the Heart Institute (InCor) at University of Sao Paulo, Brazil. All three sites have the same version of the Globus Toolkit integrated with DICOM services and are connected with the International Internet 2. The IPI SAN in core A (Fig. 21.16) is used as a Data Grid confederation for illustration purpose.

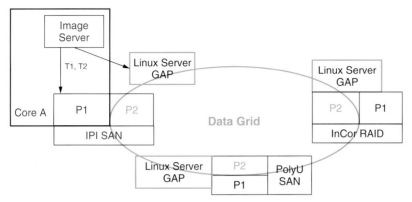

Figure 21.16 Data Grid test bed (green) with three International sites at the Image Processing and Informatics Laboratory (IPI), University of Southern California; the Hong Kong Polytechnic University (PolyU); and the Heart Institute (InCor) at University of Sao Paulo, Brazil. The test bed used two real clinical trials images (T1 and T2) for the validation of the Data Grid. IPI (blue) is used as the site for testing data migration.

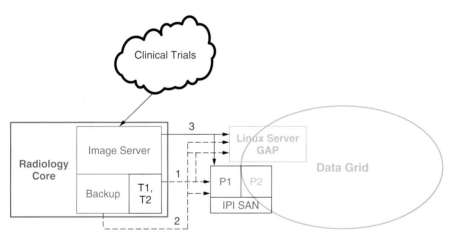

Figure 21.17 Data migration from existing backup storage to the Data Grid (green) during Data Grid deployment. Image migration from the local backup of the radiology core (blue) to P1 of the IPI SAN and the Data Grid is through a three-step procedure. In this scenario, after completion of the Data Grid deployment, SAN becomes the local backup archive for the clinical trials' images of the IPI. P1 is the core's own backup, and P2 is used to backup for other cores.

1. Following the workflow shown in Figure 21.17, two clinical trials (T1 and T2) start with a small number of enrolled patients. For any *new* image received by the image server sent by a clinical trial site (see Fig. 21.14), one copy of the image is stored within the radiology core existing local backup storage. The local backup sends a copy to P1 of the IPI SAN as the archive in the core, which designates as the migrated new image from the existing local backup to its SAN (IPI SAN), one image at a time. Meanwhile the local backup also

sends a copy to the Linux server (GAP) at the Data Grid for backup. The Data Grid will maintain two copies of the image in two remote storages (see Fig. 21.16, two P2s at PolyU and InCor).

2. Once all testing and evaluation of step 1 are satisfactory, one copy is sent of all *historical backup images* of the same patient enrolled in T1 and T2 in the local backup to P1 of the IPI SAN, and another copy is sent to the Linux server at the Data Grid, which replicates it to two more copies stored at P2s of two remote cores. Step 1 continues if more *new* images are coming in during step 2.

3. When step 2 is completed, IPI SAN P1 has all backup images of trials T1 and T2, both *new and historical*. The image server then stops sending images to the local backup. But the image server will begin to send any *new* images of trials T1 and T2 to P1 of the SAN as the local archive, and also send a copy to the Data Grid for backup, which replicates two copies in two P2s of other cores. The data migration procedure for trials T1 and T2 is completed, and traditional local backup at the core can be dismounted.

21.5.5 Data Grid for Multiple Clinical Trials

With the use of more digital mammography, multislice CT, MRI, and US imaging in clinical trials and the ever-increasing number of clinical trials, the current information system infrastructure of the radiology core that handles multiple trials can no longer satisfy the requirements of fault tolerance of image data and analysis results and accomplish quick distribution of images and results to worldwide experts involved in the trials. In this section we present the use of Data Grid for the radiology core in clinical trial. A Data Grid test bed with three international sites for backup of clinical trial images from multiple imaging cores is also presented with a data migration scheme. The Data Grid concept can be extended to multiple trial databases. Such a Data Grid can provide three benefits to the trials databases: (1) fault tolerance, (2) data and result sharing, and (3) dynamic creation and modification of data model to support any new trial or change of trials.

A further advancement in using the Data Grid in clinical trials is that radiology/imaging cores inside the Data Grid can be embedded so that the computer process or analysis software from multiple cores can be shared and be fault tolerant. The ultimate goal of the Data Grid in clinical trials is to provide a large virtual distributed fault-tolerant data system for a variety of clinical trials to store, back up, and share images and results. Such a Data Grid infrastructure would allow trials images and results to be pooled and mined for hidden knowledge, which could eventually improve clinical trials outcomes. Since the use of Data Grid in clinical trials is a new concept, extensive current research results are given in references provided in this chapter.

21.6 A SPECIFIC CLINICAL APPLICATION – DEDICATED BREAST MRI ENTERPRISE DATA GRID

This section presents an application which is the dedicated breast MRI enterprise Data Grid.

21.6.1   Data Grid for Dedicated Breast MRI

During the past decade health centers have emerged that specialize in women's health needs, particularly breast imaging. The Breast imaging centers perform all types of breast imaging examinations: digital mammography (DM), ultrasound imaging (US), 3-D US, US biopsy, and MRI as discussed in Chapters 4 and 5. Each of these imaging modalities is dedicated to specialized breast imaging except MRI. The reason is that the MRI calls for very expensive imaging equipment, so it is not cost-effective to have a general MRI system to take care of only breast imaging. This situation has created a niche in the development of dedicated breast (DB) MRI, a much lower cost MRI modality yet providing the required quality in breast imaging. However, because DB MRI is lower cost compared to a generalized MRI system, it may not have the common DICOM connectivity, file format and structure, backup archive to be readily integrated in the daily PACS operation. In last several years DB MRI has found a market in breast imaging centers, due to either the cost of a DB MRI becoming financial affordable by a breast imaging center or the MRI manufacturer making a profit-sharing arrangement with the center. In certain favorable situations the manufacturer may even finance several DB MRI systems in a given geographic region forming an enterprise DB MRI. In all these situations Data Grid has become an ideal add-on component in helping the center integrate the purchased DB MRI with other breast imaging modality and to the daily PACS operation. In the case of enterprise DB MRI, the manufacturer may manage the many DB MRI systems in a region and even in multiple regions. The next section presents the Data Grid for the DB MRI enterprise.

21.6.2   Functions of a Dedicated Breast MRI Enterprise Data Grid

The DICOM-based enterprise dedicated MRI breast imaging Data Grid (BIDG) is an infrastructure that supports the management of a large-scale breast imaging archive and distribution. The AURORA dedicated breast MRI enterprise is used as an example. The BIDG has the following functions:

1. It archives AURORA 3-D dedicated breast MRI images, and patient records related to the MRI study, including other modality type breast images in DICOM format and diagnostic reports.
2. The Data Grid provides fault tolerance to all archived data.
3. The BIDG also utilizes DICOM structured report (SR) standard and IHE (integrating healthcare enterprise) workflow profiles linking special quantitative DICOM metadata, reports, and breast images for patient record distribution through the Data Grid.
4. Within the AURORA enterprise BIDG, any site can access patient record including images and reports from other sites, provided that permission has been granted by the enterprise. In addition access rights to patient records from different sites can be controlled through security protocols within the BIDG.
5. Following item 4, any Aurora workstation (WS) can display AURORA 3-D dedicated breast MRI images from other sites, including the quantitative metadata through DICOM-SR.

21.6.3 Components in the Enterprise Breast Imaging Data Grid (BIDG)

Three dedicated breast MRI systems in the enterprise BIDG are used as an example. Figure 21.18 shows the BIDG and its connection to the three MRI sites. Compare the similarity in architecture between Figure 21.12 and Figure 21.18. Four main components in the BIDG are as follows:

1. SAN with P1 and P2 partitions: The SAN storage device at each site is divided into two partitions, P1 and P2. P1 is used for its own patients' records, and P2 is contributed to other sites for their backup archive within the BIDG. Each image in each site has three copies, one in its own SAN P1 and two in SANs P2 of two other sites that are stored within the BIDG. However, while P2 in each SAN is physically located in the SAN of the site, logically, once P2 is committed to the BIDG for other sited backup, it serves only the BIDG. (See Fig. 21.18, where all P2s designate storage nodes dedicated to the BIDG.)

2. DCIOM Conversion Unit (DCU): The DCU converts AURORA 3-D MRI images or any other related breast images (DM, US, etc.) of the patient to the DICOM standard if necessary. It also converts a specialized MRI report to DICOM structured report (SR) format allowing the linkage between the report, images, and quantitative metadata. This feature allows (a) tracking the patient progress from multiple studies, (b) performing data mining for patient outcome analysis, and (c) developing breast imaging teaching files. The converter also coverts AURORA 3-D MRI DICOM images to AUROR WS display format.

3. Dedicated Breast (DB) MRI and DICOM Grid Access Point (GAP): The DB MRI GAP (black box with green fonts) provides storage and query/retrieve services for any DICOM-compliant WS of any MRI system to access data within the Data Grid. There are multiple GAPs in the Data Grid (see Fig. 21.18, green fonts) and can be used as the backup for each other. The DICOM GAP provides the transfer of DICOM files from other DICOM-compliant breast imaging modality. If the AURORA enterprise conforms to the DICOM standard in the foreseeable future, the DICOM Gap may not be necessary.

4. Database Services: A service that keeps track of DICOM metadata as well as file locations of different storage nodes within the Data Grid (see components within the green ellipse in Fig. 21.18). Dynamic and robust access to data is provided by the Data Access Interface (DAI) in the Globus Toolkit integrated with the database (see Fig. 21.19).

21.6.4 Breast Imaging Data Grid (BIDG) Workflows in Archive and Backup, Query/Retrieve, and Disaster Recovery

Figure 21.18 depicts the general connection to the three sites and workflow of the BIDG (compare with Fig. 21.8). The three major functions in BIDG, archive ad backup, query/retrieve, and automatic disaster recovery are similar to those shown in Figures 21.10, 21.11*A* and *B*, and 21.12, respectively. Site 3 is used to demonstrate the disaster recovery. An ePR Web server is added in the Data Grid to demonstrate the use of ePR as a means to manage the BIDG in an enterprise level.

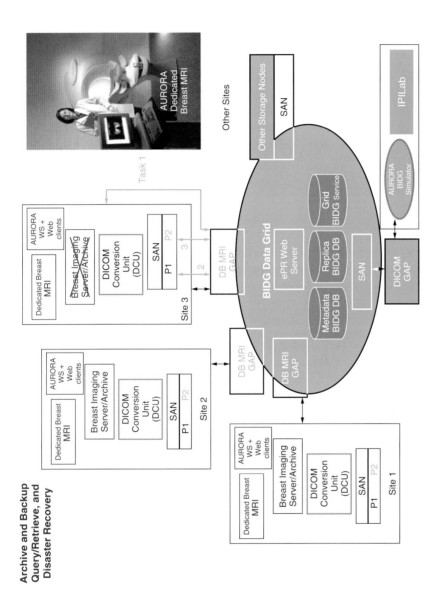

Figure 21.18 DICOM-based enterprise dedicated MRI breast imaging Data Grid (BIDG) is an infrastructure that supports large-scale breast imaging archive and distribution management. The AURORA dedicated breast MRI enterprise is used as an example. Compare the similarity between this figure and the general Data Grid architecture shown in Figure 21.12. Two additional components in this figure are the ePR Web server and the DIOCM conversion unit (DCU) explained in text. (Courtesy of AURORA Imaging Technology, Inc.)

21.7 TWO CONSIDERATIONS IN ADMINISTRATING THE DATA GRID

In this section we discuss two issues that should be considered when a Data Grid is being planned. The first is the data security in the Data Grid, and the second is the sociotechnical considerations in administrating the Data Grid.

21.7.1 Image/Data Security in Data Grid

We discussed data security in PACS in Chapter 17, the same methodology can be extended to the Data Grid. Although backup policies and grid certificates guarantee privacy and authenticity of grid access points (GAP), there still lacks a method to guarantee that the sensitive DICOM images have not been altered or corrupted while at a trial site and during transmission across a public domain. This section provides a general framework toward achieving full image storage and transfer security within the Data Grid by utilizing DICOM image authentication and a HIPAA-compliant auditing system discussed in Chapter 17.

The 3-D lossless digital signature embedding (LDSE) procedure involves a private 64-byte signature that is embedded into each original DICOM image volume, whereby on the receiving end the signature can be extracted and verified following the DICOM transmission. The HIPAA-compliant auditing system (H-CAS) is required to monitor embedding and verification events, and allows monitoring of other grid activity as well. The H-CAS system federates the logs of transmission and authentication events at each grid access point and stores it into a HIPAA-compliant database. The auditing toolkit is installed at the local grid-access-point and utilizes Syslog, a client-server standard for log messaging over an IP network, to send messages to the H-CAS centralized database. By integrating digital image signatures and centralized logging capabilities, DICOM image integrity within the Medical Imaging and Informatics Data Grid can be monitored and guaranteed without loss to any image quality. Figure 21.19 shows the locations of LDSE and H-CAS when an image source sends images to and the user queries image/data from the Data Grid.

Figure 21.20*A* describes the workflow involved for a clinical trial (Section 21.5) utilizing the IPILab Data Storage Grid with LDSE embedding and verification. The red (darker) dots represent the embedding procedure of the digital signature into DICOM images. The green (lighter) dots represent the physical workflow locations where the digital signature is extracted and verified for image integrity. The H-CAS system receives LDSE logs from all GAP's and storage nodes using Syslog messaging and SSL (secure socket layer) encryption. A Web-based monitoring application can also be developed to communicate with the H-CAS database and function as the audit layer's monitoring tool and user interface for the system administrator. Figure 21.20*B* uses a 3-D CT image set as an example to illustrate the LDSE to assure data integrity.

21.7.2 Sociotechnical Considerations in Administrating the Data Grid

21.7.2.1 Sociotechnical Considerations   Data Grid, when used properly, is a cost-effective backup and disaster recovery solution for large-scale enterprise PACS and medical imaging informatics applications. Geographic separation provides fault-tolerance against localized disasters. Pooling of storage resources across organizations

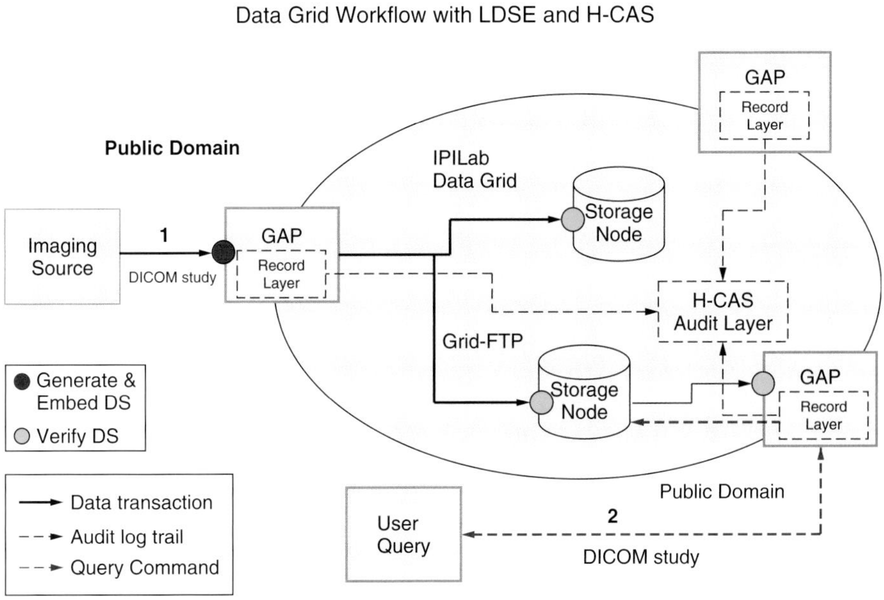

Data Grid Workflow with LDSE and H-CAS

Figure 21.19 Data Grid workflow with LDSE (Lossless Digital Signature Embedding) and H-CAS (HIPAA-Compliant Auditing System) implemented. Red circle: Generate and embed digital signature (DS). Green circle: Verify DS. There are two data lines, (1) Left middle: Imaging source sends image/data to the Data Grid. (2) Lower middle: User queries image/data.

is facilitated by the low marginal costs of storage area network (SAN) technology. However, the control and administration of the Data Grid is now spread across multiple organizations, which increases the complexity of a Data Grid deployment. There are now multiple stakeholders networked together in a series of relationships that must agree on every operational detail.

The introduction of a DG means stakeholders in various organizations are now linked together over issues such as security, service level agreements, and liability in the event of a security breach. Many other issues should be considered such as human issues on allocating responsibility for managing and operating the hardware and software of the grid, policy issues on to how much storage will be shared and how much bandwidth can be used, and the administrative issues on the allocation of costs and protection against liability.

King (2006) has studied the intertwined personnel relationships within a Data Grid linking three clinical sites. Each site is composed of two groups of shareholders, the administrators and the operators shown in Figure 21.21. Before there was a Data Grid, the personnel relationships at the sites were straightforward, as indicated in the figure by the double line and the hexagons labeled $1-1$, $2-2$, and $3-3$ for administrators and operations personnel working side by side. After the Data Grid was added $3^2 = 9$ new primary relationships resulted, as shown in the original three double lines plus six solid lines. In addition there is potential for $3 \times 2 = 6$ optional relationships, as marked by the dotted lines. The personnel relationship grows as the number of sites n grows, so there will be n^2 new primary relationships, and $n \times 2 = 2n$ optional relationships. Clearly, Data Grid administration has become a complex issue.

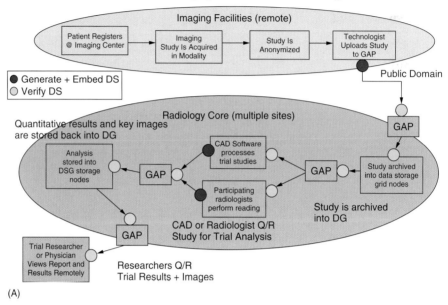

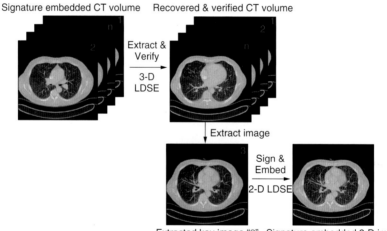

Figure 21.20 (*A*) Simulated LDSE workflow in a clinical trials setting using the Data Grid (see Fig. 21.16). This simultaneously tests the LDSE (lossless digital signature embedding) verification system and HIPAA-compliant (HIPAA-compliant auditing system) user authentication. (*B*) LDSE process to assure data integrity. A CT image set is used in this example (see also Chapter 17).

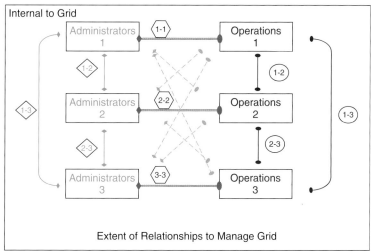

Figure 21.21 Interwined nature of personal relationships within a Data Grid consisting of three clinical sites. Each site is composed of two groups of shareholders, the administrators and the operators. Double (blue) and solid (green and blue) lines are for primary relationships, dotted lines (purple) are for optional relationships. The personal relationships become complex as the number of sites in the Data Grid grows. (Courtesy of Dr. N. King.)

21.7.2.2 *For Whom the Data Grid Tolls?*

Data Grid indeed may not be suitable for every clinic, especially for those clinics that have a culturally independent operation philosophy and aversion to external risk. However, Data Grid is very suitable for large-scale enterprise level PAC systems and medical imaging informatics applications. Examples are enterprise PACS, enterprise imaging center, HMO (healthcare maintenance) PACS operation, dedicated breast imaging enterprise operation, radiology core in a large-scale image-based clinical trials, as have been discussed in previous sections.

A site that prefers to operate independently may join a suitable Data Grid organization to take advantage of fault-tolerant backup and disaster recovery of its image/data without contributing their own storage and personnel to the Data Grid. This arrangement can avoid Data Grid's administrative complexity and necessary security relationships. The security protection is similar to that of the ASP (application service provider) model discussed in Chapter 16.

21.8 CURRENT RESEARCH AND DEVELOPMENT ACTIVITIES IN DATA GRID

In this section we present four current medical imaging and informatics research and development activities in Data Grid: IHE Cross-Enterprise Document Sharing (XDS), IBM Grid Medical Archive Solution (GMAS), Cancer **B**iomedical **I**nformatics **G**rid (caBIG), and Medical Imaging and Computing for Unified Information Sharing

(MEDICUS). Readers with thorough appreciation of materials discussed in Sections 21.1 through 21.7 should be able to follow the concepts behind these projects, the grid infrastructure and data workflow, as well as to browse their Web sites.

21.8.1   IHE Cross-Enterprise Document Sharing (XDS)

Some of the information in this section is excerpted from the Web site http://wiki.ihe.net/index.php?title=Cross_Enterprise_Document_Sharing. The Cross-Enterprise Document Sharing (XDS) Integration Profile is a workflow profile of IHE (integrating the healthcare enterprise; see Chapter 9). It "facilitates the registration, distribution, and access across health enterprises of patient electronic health records." An enterprise level healthcare system adopting this profile can use the Data Grid concept to implement its operation.

Cross-Enterprise Document Sharing (XDS) aims to provide a standards-based specification for managing document sharing with any healthcare enterprise, ranging from a private physician office to a clinic to an acute care inpatient facility and personal health record systems. XDS is managed through a federation of document repositories. A document registry maintains patients' medical histories and can create a record of information about a patient for a given clinical need. The responsibilities of these four distinct entities are: the *Document Repository* for storing documents is provided by *Document Sources*; the *Document Registry* information about the documents is accessed by *Document Consumers*. The file transfer mechanism can be HTTP, HL7, or DICOM. Since XDS is a profile or a document transfer model, the responsibilities of data management and fault tolerance are left to the healthcare organization. Potential users are national EHR (Electronic Health Record) healthcare centers supported by regional health information organizations and others. As of November 2008, the following organizations have joined the XDS: UK CfH (Radiology WF), France DMP, Demark (Funen), Italy (Veneto), Spain (Aragon), Austria (Q4–2006), Italy 2005 (Conto, Corrente Salute), Canada (Quebec, Toronto, Alberta, British Columbia, Canada Infoway 2007–8), China (Shanghai Imaging Info Sharing), China-MoH (Lab Results Sharing), Japan–Nogaya Imaging Info Sharing), THINC–New York, NCHICA–North Carolina, Philadelphia HIE 2005, State Project–NY, and MA Share–MA 2006–7. Figure 21.22 shows the IHE Cross-Enterprise frameworks.

21.8.2   IBM Grid Medical Archive Solution (GMAS)

Some of the information in this section was excerpted from the IBM Web site http://www-03.ibm.com/grid/pdf/fsgmas.pdf. The IBM Grid Medical Archive Solution is a commercial data storage product based on the BycastGRID© gird infrastructure. It was built as a set of services leveraging a service-oriented architecture with real-time fail over protection against data loss. The data transfer services are deployed across the organization as a set of interrelated software nodes that reside as part of IBM's System Storage Multilevel Grid Access Manager Software. Data are encrypted and compressed for security and speed. If data transfer to a remote site is required, the data is replicated first to the local storage node cache and then sent from the local cache to the remote site storage node.

IHE Cross-enterprise Frameworks

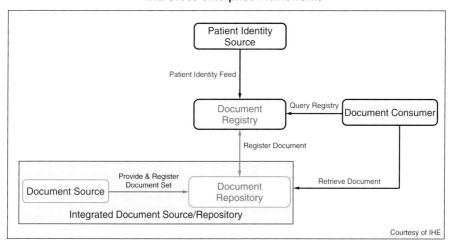

Figure 21.22 Enterprise-wide information systems that manage a patient's electronic health record, such as a hospital information system, may benefit by following the IHE XDS profile for document exchange, which includes images. Actors and transactions are shown in the drawing. (See also Chapter 13, Source: IHE XDS Workflow)

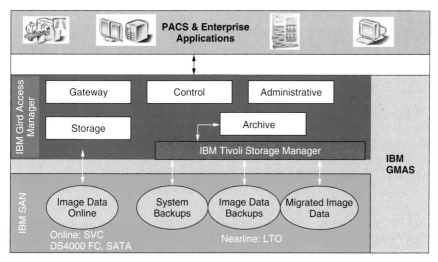

Figure 21.23 IBM Grid Medical Archive Solution (GMAS) using the medical archive grid storage architecture. There are three layers in the architecture, the first two are the IBMSAN and Grid Access Manager, and the third layer is the user's PACS and Enterprise Application interface layer. (Courtesy of Frost and Sullivan, IBM GMAS)

The GMAS targets mid- to large-scale hospitals' PACS archives. Some major components in the GMAS are IBM servers, total storage, multilevel grid access manager software, IBMSAN, and ByCAST storage grid running on the Linux operating system software. Current limitations are not using the DICOM standard and IHE profiles for data transfer. The robustness of the ByCast StorageGrid layers remains to be validated. Figure 21.23 shows the GMAS Grid layer architecture.

21.8.3 Cancer Biomedical Informatics Grid (caBIG)

Some of the information contained in this section is excerpted from the caBIG Web site https://cabig.nci.nih.gov/overview. The cancer Biomedical Informatics Grid™ (caBIG™) is an information network enabling all constituencies in the cancer community to share data and knowledge; the network is also open to experts in other fields. Its organization is funded by the National Institute of Cancer (NCI) and the National Institutes of Health (NIH). The mission of caBIG™, is as stated on its Web site, "to develop a truly collaborative information network that accelerates the discovery of new approaches for the detection, diagnosis, treatment, and prevention of cancer, ultimately improving patient outcomes."

caBIG uses an open source Globus Toolkit as the infrastructure and Web service but is currently not directly connected to sites using the DICOM standard for image transmission and format. Each institution connected to caBIG maintains local control over its own resources and data. caBIG has strict compliance requirements in data information model, vocabularies, data elements, and message interfaces. These requirements may ultimately lead to a steep learning curve and difficulty for a site to join or implement. Current limitations are that image transfer speed and performance have not been measured to satisfaction, and that no data are available in the system nor data fault tolerance. Figure 21.24 depicts caBIG implementation scenarios.

21.8.4 Medical Imaging and Computing for Unified Information Sharing (MEDICUS)

Some of the information contained in this section is excerpted from the MEDICUS Web site http://dev.globus.org/wiki/Incubator/MEDICUS. MEDICUS (Medical Imaging and Computing for Unified Information Sharing) is an incubator project to federate Medical Imaging and Computing Resources for clinical service and research of children diseases.

The open source Globus Toolkit is used as the platform providing infrastructure and resources for this diverse research field. Two major research projects using this grid infrastructure are: The Children's Oncology Group (COG), grid (www.curesearch.org), funded by NCI/NIH and the New Approaches to Neuroblastoma Therapy (NANT), grid (www.nant.org), funded by the Neuroblastoma Cancer Foundation. Many children hospitals and cancer centers in the United States are affiliated with this project. Figure 21.25 depicts the DICOM image workflow within a Globus grid and implementation. Compare the logical similarity in the Globus components between the architecture and the dataflow of this diagram with those shown in previous sections of this chapter. In the current development, MEDICUS seems limited by no life-cycle management, by use of static backup policies, and by lack of Web-based management tools and system fault-tolerance design.

21.9 SUMMARY OF DATA GRID

In the previous eight sections we showed that Data Grid's powerful infrastructure can advance PACS clinical service and imaging informatics research. The R&D of the Data Grid has advanced remarkably over the past five years.

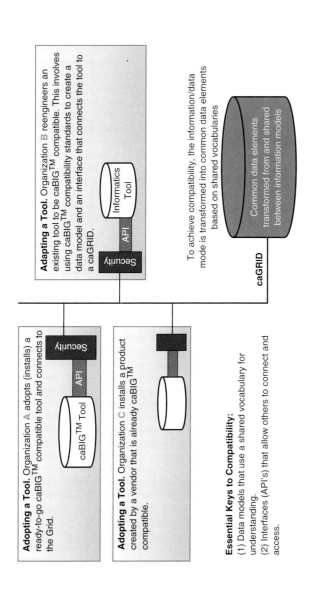

Adapting a Tool. Organization B reengineers an existing tool to be caBIG™ compatible. This involves using caBIG™ compatibility standards to create a data model and an interface that connects the tool to a caGRID.

Informatics Tool

API

Security

Adapting a Tool. Organization A adopts (installs) a ready-to-go caBIG™ compatible tool and connects to the Grid.

caBIG™ Tool

API

Security

Adapting a Tool. Organization C installs a product created by a vendor that is already caBIG™ compatible.

Essential Keys to Compatibility:
(1) Data models that use a shared vocabulary for understanding.
(2) Interfaces (API's) that allow others to connect and access.

To achieve compatibility, the information/data mode is transformed into common data elements based on shared vocabularies

caGRID

Common data elements transformed from and shared between information models

Courtesy of caGrid

Figure 21.24 cancer Biomedical Informatics Grid™ (caBIG™) is an information network using the open source Globus Toolkit. The figure depicts three different scenarios of connecting three sites to the caBIG infrastructure. Top left: Organization A adopts a tool, organization C installs a caBIG compatible product created by a vendor; Top right: Organization B reengineers an existing "tool." All data go to the caBIG Information/data model for compatibility check, store, then ready for distribution. (Courtesy of caBIG)

681

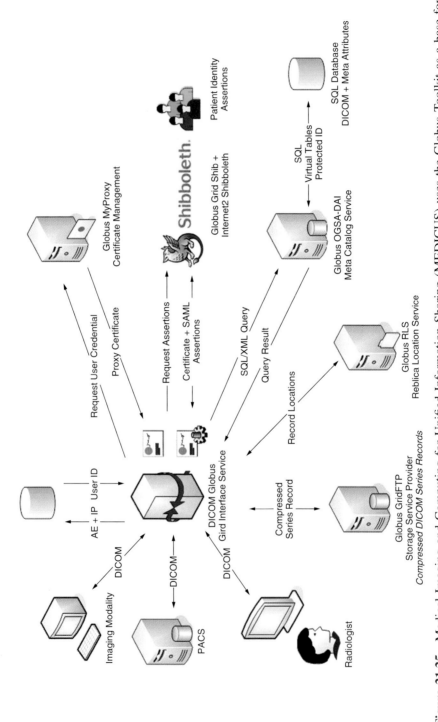

Figure 21.25 Medical Imaging and Computing for Unified Information Sharing (MEDICUS) uses the Globus Toolkit as a base for image communication. Its workflow is shown in this figure. Compare the logical similarity in the Globus components between the architecture and the dataflow of this diagram with those of Figures 21.6, 21.8, 21.12, and 21.18. (Courtesy of MEDICUS)

We reviewed the distributed computing that led to grid computing and presented the grid computing open source Globus Toolkit. Although the topic is complex and requires certain understanding, it forms the foundation of the Data Grid whose concept has applications in PACS. The fault-tolerant concept with three tasks of data archive/backup, query/retrieval, and disaster recovery using Data Grid is discussed along with two Data Grid applications in image-based clinical trials and dedicated breast MRI enterprise.

References

Allcock W, Bresnahan J, Kettimuthu R, Link M, Dumitrescu C, Raicu I, Foster I. The Globus striped GridFTP framework and server. *Proc Super Comput*; Nov. 12–18 ACM, Seattle, Washington, 1–11; 2005.

alRen, http://www.cenic.org/calren/index.htm, accessed on March 14, 2006.

Brown MS, Shah SK, Pais RC, Lee Y, McNitt-Gray MF, Goldin JG, Cardenas AF, Aberle DR. Database design and implementation for quantitative image analysis research. *IEEE Trans. Info Techno Biomed* 9: 99–108; 2005.

Chan LW, Zhou MZ, Hau SK, Law MY, Tang FH, Documet J. International Internet-2 performance and automatic tuning protocol for medical imaging applications. *Comput Med Imag Graph* 29: 103–14; 2005.

Chervenak A, Foster I, Kesselman C, Salisbury C, Tuecke S. The Data Grid: towards an architecture for the distributed management and analysis of large scientific datasets. *J Net Comput Appl* 23: 187–200; 2001.

Chow SC, Liu JP. *Design and Analysis of Clinical Trials: Concepts and Methodologies*. Hoboken, NJ: Wiley; 2004.

Conducting a HIPAA security audit. Digital Imaging and Communications in Medicine (DICOM) 2004. http://medical. nema.org/dicom/2004.html, accessed 14 Mar 2006.

Foster I. *Globus Toolkit Version 4: Software for Service-Oriented Systems*. New York: Springer, 2005, 2–13; 2005.

Foster I. The grid: a new infrastructure for 21st century science. *Phys Today* 55: 42–7; 2002.

Fridrich J, Goljan M, Du R. Lossless data embedding—new paradigm in digital watermarking. *EURASIP J Appl Sig Proc* (2): 185–96; 2002

HARNET. http://www.jucc.edu.hk/jucc/content_harnet.html, accessed 14 Mar 2006.

HIPAA Security Standard. http://www.hipaadvisory.com/regs/finalsecurity/

http://searchdomino.techtarget.com/news/article/0,289142,sid4_gci912158,00.html.

https://cabig.nci.nih.gov/overview.

http://wiki.ihe.net/index.php?title=Cross_Enterprise_ Document_Sharing.

http://www-03.ibm.com/grid/pdf/fsgmas.pdf.

http://dev.globus.org/ wiki/Incubator/MEDICUS.

Huang HK, Zhang A, Liu B, Zhou Z, et al. Data Grid for large-scale medical image archive and analysis. *Proc. 13th ACM Int Conf Multimedia*: 1005–13; 2005.

Huang HK. *PACS and Imaging Informatics: Basic Principles and Applications*. Hoboken, NJ: Wiley; 2004.

Internet2, http://www.internet2.edu/, accessed 14 Mar 2006.

King NE. Information systems and healthcare XVII: operational stakeholder relationships in the deployment of a data storage grid for clinical image backup and recovery. *Comm*

Assoc Info Sys 23(1). http://www.globus.org/solutions/data_replication/, accessed 14 Mar 2006.

Law MYY, Zhou Z. New direction in PACS education and training, Comput Med Imag Graph 27: 147–56; 2003.

Liu B, Zhou Z, Huang HK. A HIPAA-compliant architecture for securing clinical images. *SPIE Med Imag Conf Proc PACS and Imaging Informatics*; 2005.

Liu B, Zhou Z, Documet J. Utilizing Data Grid architecture for the backup and recovery of clinical image data. *Comput Med Imag Graph* 29: 95–102; 2005.

Liu BJ, Cao F, Zhou MZ, Mogel G, Documet L. Trends in PACS image storage and archive. *Comput Med Imag Graph* 27: 165–74; 2003.

Liu BJ, Zhou Z, Gutierrez MA, Documet J, Chan L, Huang HK. International Internet2 connectivity and performance in medical imaging applications: bridging Americas to Asia, *J High Speed Networks*, 16.1, 5–20; 2007.

McNitt-Gray MF, Aramato SG, Clarke LP, McLennan G, Meyer CR, Yankelevitz DF. The lung imaging database consortium: creating a resource for the image processing research community. *Radiology* 225: 739–48; 2002.

Meinert CL. *Clinical Trials: Design, Conduct, and Analysis*. Oxford: Oxford University Press; 1986.

Moge Gl, Huang HK, Cao F, Zhou Z, Dev P, Gill M, Liu BJ. NGI performance in teleradiology applications. *Proc. SPIE Med Imag* 3: 25–30; 2002.

Ouchi NK. System for recovering data stored in failed memory unit. US Patent 714/5, 714/6, 714/807; 1977.

Piantadosi S. *Clinical Trials: A Methodologic Perspective*. New York: Wiley, 1997.

Redundant Array of Independent Disks (RAID). http://en.wikipedia.org/wiki/ Redundant_ array_of_independent_disks, accessed 14 Mar 2006.

RNP2. http://www.rnp.br/en/, accessed 14 Mar 2006.

Schopf JM, Nitzberg B. Grids: top ten questions. *Sci Progr* 10: 103–11; 2002.

Syslog. http://www.loriotpro.com/Products/SyslogCollector/SyslogDataSheet_ENv3. php, accessed Dec 2007.

TeraGrid. http://www.teragrid.org/, accessed 14 Mar 2006.

Zhou XQ, Huang HK, Lou SL. Authenticity and integrity of digital mammography images. *IEEE Trans. Med Imag* 20(8): 784–91; 2001.

Zhou Z, Liu B, Huang HK et al. A RIS/PACS simulator integrated with the HIPAA-compliant auditing toolkit. *SPIE Med Imag Conf Proc*; 2005.

Zhou Z, Huang HK, Liu B. Digital signature embedding for medical image integrity in a Data Grid off-site backup archive. *SPIE Med Imag Conf Proc PACS and Imaging Informatics*; SPIE Publication, 2005.

Zhou Z, Dodumet J, Chan L, et al. *The Role of a Data Grid in Worldwide Imaging-Based Clinical Trials*. USC UPU: Marina del Rey; 2006.

Zhou Z, Liu BJ, Huang HK, Zhang J. Educational RIS/PACS simulator integrated with the HIPAA compliant auditing (HCA) toolkit. *Proc SPIE Med Imag* 6: 491–500; 2005.

CHAPTER 22

MULTIMEDIA ELECTRONIC PATIENT RECORD (ePR) SYSTEM

The concept of an electronic patient record (ePR) was introduced in Chapter 13 when the integration of HIS/RIS/PACS was presented. The traditional ePR contains mainly textual information. This chapter discusses the multimedia ePR system that includes with the textual data also images, videos, waveforms, and other data from acquisition devices within and outside of the radiology profession. First we review the traditional ePR system; then we present the ePR with images and follow this by a discussion of the multimedia ePR system. Two case studies of ePR with images in the US Veterans Affairs Healthcare Enterprise (VAHE) and the Hospital Authority (HA) of Hong Kong are used as examples. The concept of multimedia ePR is presented with examples in radiation therapy treatment and minimally invasive spinal surgery. These two topics will be detailed in Chapters 23 and 24, respectively.

Figure 22.1 illustrates the topics and concepts to be covered and their interrelationship with the five logical layers of the medical imaging informatics infrastructure (see Fig. 20.2).

22.1 THE ELECTRONIC PATIENT RECORD (ePR) SYSTEM

22.1.1 Purpose of the ePR System

The electronic patient record (ePR) system is an emerging concept that offers a way to supplement or extract relevant data of the patient from small-, medium-, or large-scale clinical-based hospital information system (HIS) or clinic management system (CMS). The basic concept of ePR is described in Chapters 7 and 13. The major functions of ePR are as follows:

- Accept direct digital input of patient data.
- Analyze across patients and providers.
- Provide clinical decision support and suggest courses of treatment.
- Perform outcome analysis and patient and physician profiling.
- Distribute information across different platforms and health information systems.

PACS and Imaging Informatics, Second Edition, by H. K. Huang
Copyright © 2010 John Wiley & Sons, Inc.

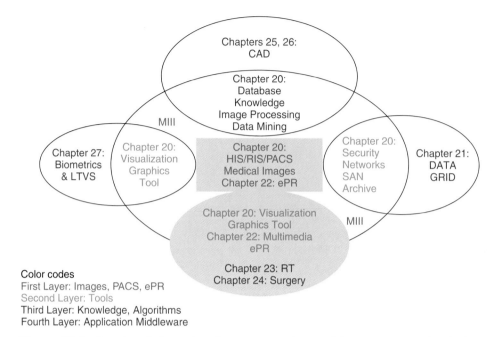

Color codes
First Layer: Images, PACS, ePR
Second Layer: Tools
Third Layer: Knowledge, Algorithms
Fourth Layer: Application Middleware

Figure 22.1   Imaging informatics data sources (rectangle), concepts, technologies, and applications (large and small ellipses) as discussed in the chapters of Part IV. Color codes refer to the five-layer informatics infrastructure shown in Figure 20.2. This chapter presents multimedia ePR which requires visualization tools discussed in Chapter 20.

The importance of ePR is that data travels with the patient and contains all pertinent medical information about the patient. The traditional ePR system very seldomly contains images or multimedia data. The multimedia ePR systems presented in this chapter, and in Chapters 23 and 24, include all forms of media data in the ePR database. So the multimedia ePR constitutes a complete information system.

22.1.2   Integrating the ePR with Images

In traditional ePR the textual base requires using pointers to locate and retrieve relevant patient data from many connected information systems, be these systems very small and low end or very large and sophisticated. The data extracted are usually small files without images. Nevertheless, the characteristic textual ePR requires very complex software even though the system interfacing devices, storage, data communication, and hardware requirements are minimal compared to those of PACS and imaging informatics data. When ePR is integrated with imaging data, that, of course, raises the complexity of the ePR in that software requirements of the system's interfacing devices; storage, data communication, and imaging hardware become more demanding. For this reason, after the development of textual-based ePR, many years passed before technologies could catch up to integrate ePR with images. Among these technologies are the Web-based client-server, high-speed networks, large and reliable storage devices, text and imaging standards, and the specialized search engine. The ePR software thus becomes extremely complex when images are added to the system. Currently there is yet to be developed a fully integrated ePR with images for a large hospital or an enterprise, the two systems to be described come close. Sections 22.3 and 22.4 present these two large-scale ePRs integrated with images systems that are the best going in the daily clinical environment. The main attributes of these two systems are (1) large scale, (2) government or quasi-government operation, and (3) under management by a single authority and team. However, in general, because large-scale system integration still has not overcome the constraints of the pre-operational environment, large-scale ePR with image distribution will take years of preparation and planning, as was the case of the two examples to be described. So today ePR with images are mostly available for small-scale special clinical applications with well-defined goals and endpoints.

22.1.3   The Multimedia ePR System

The database in the ePR system with images can point to the location of the waveform data or other relevant nontextual data in other information systems and retrieve them in image format, for example, as an EKG waveform converted to a display screen in a JPEG format or a digital scanned waveform. Multimedia ePR can have besides images, other multimedia medical data that have not been converted to image format. The integration has to be done in static or dynamic mode. Integration in the static mode for multimedia data that has been acquired and stored somewhere in its raw original form is off line; the multimedia ePR integrates these raw textual and image data into the ePR database using a certain data model, and archives them in the storage media to be retrieved and displayed for later clinical use. A full description of the static multimedia ePR system relating to radiation therapy planning and treatment is provided in Section 22.5 and in Chapter 23.

The dynamic multimedia ePR model is a system whereby some multimedia data has be live, that is, used and displayed in real time as acquired by the ePR. The ePR has to handle both static and live data integration in real time for clinical use. An example is its use in minimally invasive spinal surgery, as discussed in Section 22.6 and in Chapter 24.

22.2   THE VETERANS AFFAIRS HEALTHCARE ENTERPRISE (VAHE) ePR WITH IMAGES

22.2.1   Background

The U.S. Department of Veterans Affairs Healthcare Enterprise (VAHE) information system, called VistA, is the earliest developed enterprise level ePR to be integrated with images. VAHE consists of a nationwide network of 172 VA medical centers (VAMCs) and numerous outpatient clinics serving a patient population of 25 million veterans. VAHE is organized according to locations as VISNs (VA Capitol Health Care Network, VISN 5, 1995), which is an area level VA entity consisting of VA hospitals, clinics, outpatient centers, and so forth. There are 22 VISNs. In this section we describe its basic system architecture, data flow, and operation.

22.2.2 The VistA Information System Architecture

The VAHE Information System Technology Architecture (VistA) consists of four major Veterans Health components:

- VistA, the hospital information system (HIS)
- VistA, the radiology information system (tightly coupled with HIS)
- VistARad for diagnostic radiology
- VistA Imaging

The VistA Hospital and Radiology Information Systems (HIS/RIS) is used in all VAHE sites. In these systems DICOM and HL7 standards are used for images and text information, respectively. The HIS is internally developed and comprehensive enough to support all clinical services, and it uses a client-server architecture that allows clinical workstation clients to communicate with HIS servers. The database is the vintage Mumps beetree. The database files are all in Mumps, some stored on the hospital side to enable access from anywhere in the facility, and others kept locally. VistARAD is the radiology PACS used for primary image diagnosis. Some VAMCs purchase PACS from vendors; other, smaller centers rely on the VAHE IT department to supporting a homegrown PACS. VistA Imaging is an ePR integrated with images within a multimedia imaging distribution system for clinicians and healthcare providers, which we describe below in Section 22.2.3. Note that the term "multimedia" is used in VistA when images or data are converted to an image format. The VAHE IT department supports all centers in the integration of the four Vista A components listed above. The connectivity of these four components is shown in Figure 22.2.

22.2.3 The VistA Imaging

22.2.3.1 Current Status The **VistA Imaging System** is an extension of the Veterans Health VistA hospital information system that captures images and makes them part of the patient's electronic patient record (ePR). VistA Imaging is the multimedia access and display component of the VistA. There are about 60 VistA imaging centers, of which about 50 are fully implemented. The number of VistARad implementations is about 40. The size of Jukebox in the VistA Imaging, archiving 1,000,000 images plus, is about 10 terabytes. All images come through the DICOM gateways, are placed on the server's RAID, and archived via the background processor to the Jukebox (Fig. 22.2). Figure 22.3*A* and *B*, shows a typical workstation and its connectivity as used in the VistA HIS and VistA Imaging, respectively. Figure 22.4 shows the diagnostic and clinical disciplines supported by VistA Imaging. Figure 22.5*A* shows a VistA Imaging WS displaying images with a patient record, and Figure 22.5*B* the thumbnail images, microscopic images, MRIs, and EKGs.

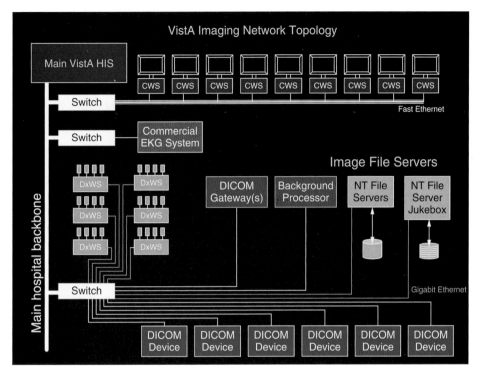

Figure 22.2 Connectivity of the four components in the VistA Information System: VistA HIS, VistA RIS, VistA RAD, and VistA Imaging. (Courtesy of Drs. H. Rutherford and R. Dayhoff).

22.2.3.2 VistA Imaging Work Flow The window used to input patient information in the VistA Imaging is the CPRS (Computerized Patient Record System), which is the main workstation used by the medical support personnel for logging, scheduling procedures, and viewing data, reports, and images in the patient's folder. VistA Imaging is launched from a menu item in CPRS, and all patient images, reports, and notes are available through the VistA Imaging Clinical Display Workstation. When the medical provider has completed a review of the data, VistA Imaging may be closed and the control reverts back to CPRS to access another patient. Each VistA Imaging clinical workstation can be used to address patient information with images, reports, and notes. Furthermore CPRS can be launched from a clinical workstation and linked to the medical data about the patient in images and reports.

The imaging system is operable from a workstation through access to patient information in the HIS and RIS, or it is accessible through the general CPRS hospital capabilities where orders, chart records, lab results, documents, and other items connected with the patient are stored. Text information utility (TIU) is the primary method of connecting a patient with a medical order and the results from that order. Figure 22.6 shows the multimedia object database schema with an example showing multiple access to three database files.

Prefetch and routing are facilities that note that a patient has checked in for a procedure. The RIS automatically sends an HL7 message to be processed by the

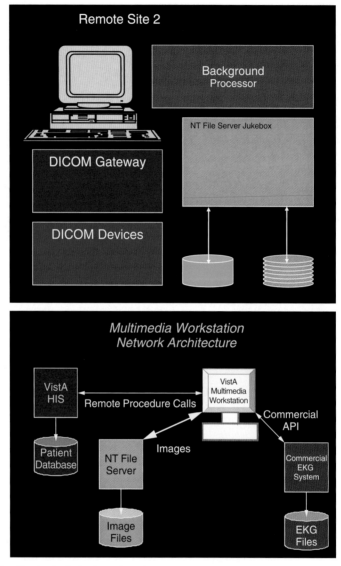

Figure 22.3 Typical clinical workstation and its connectivity in the VistA HIS and Vista Imaging. (Courtesy of Drs. H. Rutherford and R. Dayhoff).

DICOM gateways. As a result the prior cases are prefetched and made available on the appropriate workstation for the user. Also the appropriate cases are routed to a predetermined remote site to be read as required. Both of these operations are accomplished by placing an entry in the background processor queue.

Additionally the background processor runs a purge process to detect images on hard disk that have a time stamp older than a user-determined date. The personnel maintaining the system must start this process. As a result a schedule has to be established whereby in the morning certain parameters are examined and potential problems isolated regarding space and image availability for the user.

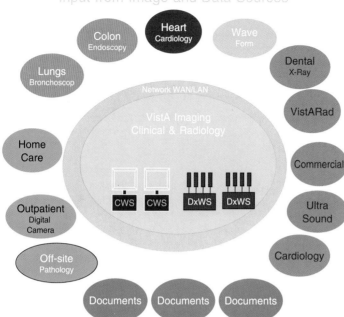

Figure 22.4 Clinical disciplines supported by VistA Imaging. (Courtesy of Drs. H. Rutherford and R. Dayhoff).

22.2.3.3 *VistA Imaging Operation*

VistA Imaging is a mechanism that enables physicians and other care providers to have complete and immediate access to all patient data, including images. Documents can also be scanned in under document imaging. This is in fact an ePR data model architecture.

The patient record includes notes that schedule a procedure, reports on findings in images, and attached images that result from the procedure. The HIS has CPRS as the GUI (graphical user interface) front end and the VistA database (with the RIS database for radiology) to provide the lookup of patient information. The access is via a few letters of the patient's last name or the patient's social security (SS) number. There is the usual problem with duplication of names when the patient communicates verbally rather than with a SS card, driver's license, or birth certificate. Even with one of these forms of identification, the clerk may click on an adjacent patient from the list. One way of confirmation is to verify that the patient with the presented identification has coverage in the system.

Radiology images are pulled or pushed from the radiology modalities through the DICOM text and image gateways. HL7 messaging is used to "listen" on the gateway end, and the HIS initiates the TCP/IP channel communication to send the images from the modalities. Like all other PAC systems, one of the ongoing problems is to determine when a study is complete. Confusion arises when the technologist wants to send "just one more" image, for whatever reason. Timing out can be used, but there are occasions when even a commonsensible time-out is exceeded (see Chapter 10). Modality dictionary file entries and modality worklist entries are set up for each

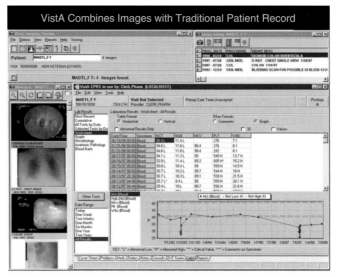

(A)

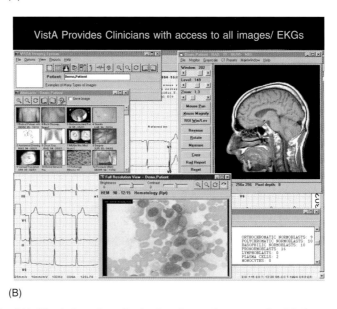

(B)

Figure 22.5 (*A*) VistA Imaging displaying the patient record with images. (*B*) VistA Imaging displaying thumb-nail medical images, and microscopic images, MRI, and EKG. (Courtesy of Drs. H. Rutherford and R. Dayhoff)

DICOM modality. This also includes the "-oscopies" (endo-, etc.), ophthalmology, dental, and others as the DICOM communications are put into place.

Once images are acquired in the DICOM gateway, a task called "image process-ing" assigns an image identifier in the master image file that is maintained on the HIS to make it available from anywhere in the enterprise. A queue entry is generated to the background processor queue to (1) archive the image to the Jukebox, (2) generate

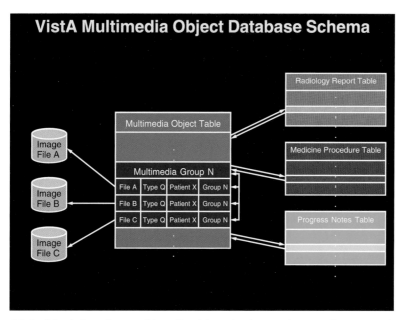

Figure 22.6   VistA Imaging multimedia object database schema. (Courtesy of Drs. H. Rutherford and R. Dayhoff)

a thumbnail image as a preview (abstract) image, and (3) place the images and the created abstract on a server for viewing access. When images are part of a group, an entry is made to indicate with an icon the group associated with the images. Because the system was designed when DICOM was not a common capability, the images are separated into a text file (the DICOM header) and an image with a limited header attached. The image is subsampled to support viewing on standard 1280×1024 monitors (1024×768 monitors are used at physician desktops).

22.3   INTEGRATING IMAGES INTO THE ePR OF THE HOSPITAL AUTHORITY (HA) OF HONG KONG

22.3.1   Background

In chapter 16, we presented enterprise PACS, which is the system used by the Hospital Authority of Hong Kong (HA HK), along with its integrated clinical information system (Clinical Management System [CMS]). To recap briefly, administratively, HA HK was established in 1990 to manage all the public hospitals in Hong Kong, namely 43 hospitals and institutions and numerous specialist and general outpatient clinics. The HA manages 29,000 beds and employs 49,000 staff taking care of over one million inpatients, over two million accident and emergency visits, and six million specialty outpatients. This section extends the discussion to HAHK's territorywide longitudinal electronic patient record (ePR), as the second example of the use of ePR with images.

The HA HK CMS and ePR systems mostly deal with textual data and have used by over 4000 doctors and 20,000 other clinicians to document and review care. The ePR has nearly 3 TB of data covering 44 million episodes for 6.4 million patients.

Because PACS technology is increasingly being adopted in the HA, the administration started a strategic plan to integrate images into the existing ePR, and deployed the ePR with images for clinical use hospital by hospital, beginning in late 2006. The objective is to make ePR with images available throughout the HA as part of the patient's longitudinal record, leveraging the ePR to distribute radiological and other images in an integrated, affordable, and sustainable manner.

22.3.2 Clinical Information Systems in the HA

To summarize the four major clinical information systems in the HA described in Chapter 16 are knowledge systems, clinical management systems (CMS), informational systems, and the textual-based ePR (see Fig. 22.7B). In addition there are many mini and full PAC systems distributed among the many HA hospitals; these systems are connected by a an HA systemwide network infrastructure (see Fig. 22.7A).

22.3.3 Rationales for Image Distribution

As with any site that has digital imaging in place, it makes sense to make the best use of these images by delivering them electronically wherever they are required. In the HA there are two rationales behind the ePR-image integration project: (1) patient mobility and (2) remote access to images.

22.3.3.1 *Patient Mobility*   In Hong Kong, patient mobility is routine practice due to the small geographic size of the territory. Hospitals are organized into seven clusters. Patients are moved between hospitals within a cluster because the services are rationalized and different aspects of care are often provided at different hospitals in the cluster. The movement of patients has been a major reason for the adoption of ePR, as the ePR makes key clinical data available no matter where the data were collected. Increasingly clinicians are asking for images to made available wherever the patients are moved. Thus the ePR is the method of choice for delivering the images.

22.3.3.2 *Remote Access to Images*   One big advantage of electronic images is that they can be used it for teleradiology whereby images are read by off-site radiologists. Many hospitals with mini-PACS images to have been wanting to utilize teleradiology's capability of sending the radiologists' homes for afterhours reviews. Because the HA has very strict security controls on network traffic beyond the corporate firewall, these requests have become nontrivial endeavors. An ePR-image integration project that includes a common image gateway for accessing images from outside the HA corporate firewall would be an ideal solution.

22.3.4 Design Criteria

To design and build a system with the most reliable and best image quality, but yet to avoid a costly system, the HA ePR with images system design emphasized the following criteria:

1. Existing resources be leveraged, including PACS, networks, storage, WS and ePR in HA,
2. The system be deployed to nearly 10,000 existing WSs throughout the HA to access the CMS and ePR with images,

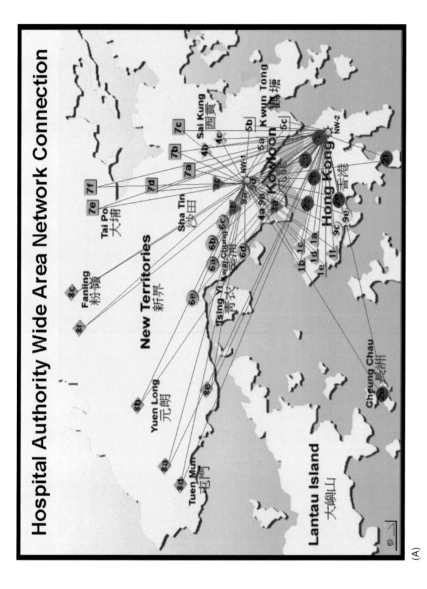

(A)

Figure 22.7 (A) Hong Kong Hospital Authority wide area network connection. (Courtesy of the Hong Kong Hospital Authority) (B) Hong Kong Hospital Authority Clinical Information Systems and the planned ePR with image distribution architecture. Before the planning, these clinical information systems and the textual ePR were already in place for daily clinical operation. The planned ePR with image had to follow the existing architecture, which the designed criteria are based on. (Courtesy of the Hong Kong Hospital Authority)

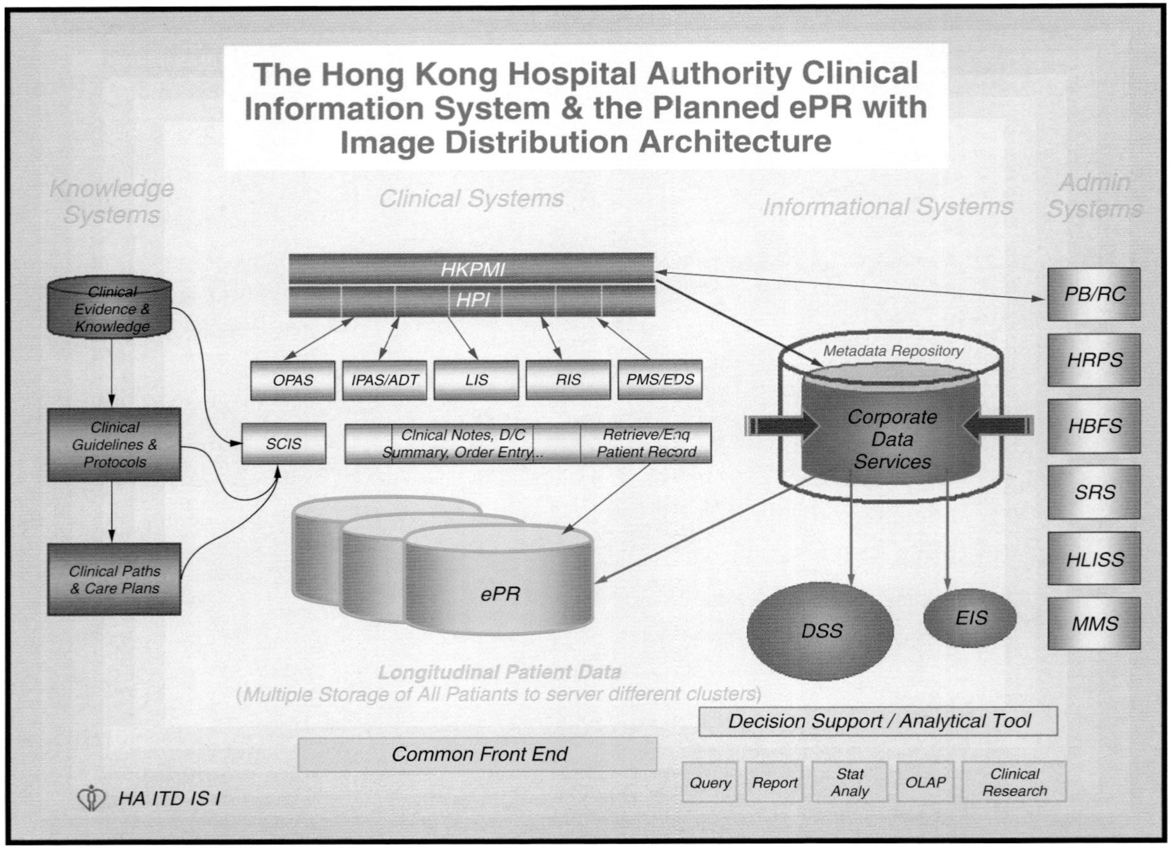

The Hong Kong Hospital Authority Clinical Information System & the Planned ePR with Image Distribution Architecture

Figure 22.7 (*Continued*)

3. The system be easy to use,
4. Timely delivery of radiology images with reports to clinicians through the longitudinal electronic patient record.
5. The system's fault tolerance not require 99.999% up time.
6. The installation be at minimal cost

22.3.5 The ePR with Image Distribution Architecture and Workflow Steps

The ePR with image distribution architecture and workflow steps as shown in Figure 22.8 are as follows:

1. Local DICOM images are sent from the PAC and mini-PAC systems to the HA image central archive.
2. The central archive captures images at full resolution for one month with the capacity of 20 TB a year.
3. Images are compressed from 10 to 30 times, using the JPEG 2000 wavelet lossy compression method, into the long-term ePR "reference quality" image archive.
4. The radiology information system (RIS) at each hospital includes a link to the image as part of the radiology report. Radiologists provide remote readings (see blue dotted lines) and also enter the RIS in the report to indicate that their link exists.
5. When the clinician pulls up the radiology report from the ePR Web client WS, an icon indicating that electronic images linkage is available.
6. Clicking on this icon will pull up the corresponding compressed images from the ePR archive.
7. Additional features being developed to be implemented at the PACS WS are (a) the flagging of key images from large studies using the "key object document" feature of the DICOM standard expressly addressing this need, (b) annotating images, (c) 3-D reconstructions or multiplanar reformatted CT images included as key images, (d) storing key images and annotated images into the central archive, and (e) storing key images at the ePR image server in JPEG format.

22.3.6 Implementation Experiences and Lessons Learned

The HA ePR with images following the designed criteria has been on line since late 2006, connecting many of the 10,000 existing WSs in over twelve of the larger HA hospitals. The process of deployment to rest of the 31 of the 43 hospitals is continuing. The following are the implementation experiences and lessons learned:

1. Web-based ePR WS: HA has deployed nearly 10,000 workstations to access the CMS and ePR. The existing workstations vary in their specifications, but almost all meet or exceed the minimum requirements (350 Mhz Pentium II PC with 128 Mb RAM and a 15" LCD screen at 1024 × 768 resolution). Many of them are now using the ePR with image distribution. The 10/100 Base T networks

currently in place seems sufficient for distribution of 10–30:1 compressed images. Consequently it is no need yet for a major upgrade to the networks.

2. Storage: Most of the clinical systems in the HA use very expensive high-end storage area network (SAN) disks, but the lower requirements in the design criteria of the ePR with images mean that lower cost SAN disks, or even network attached storage (NAS) disks can be used (see Fig. 22.8).

3. Lossy image compression: The ePR with images system uses existing clinical WS monitors in the clinical wards, which are generally 15" LCD or CRT monitors. Not only does the quality of these monitors preclude diagnostic grade image reading, but the small monitor size also makes intensive image viewing and manipulation impractical. Thus 10–30:1 wavelet compression images with attached diagnostic reports and annotations displayed on these monitors seem satisfactory for most clinical needs. The high compression ratio images alleviate the demand of high-capacity storage devices.

4. System fault tolerance: There was no attempt to build in sufficient resilience into the system to achieve the 99.999% reliability that is commonly quoted as being a requirement for PACS implementations. The reliability of the system remains a question to verify and justify over several years of clinical operation.

5. Full filmless solution: Due to the success of the ePR with image distribution system, a full filmless solution plan is being contemplated as the next step for HA enterprise operation.

22.4 THE MULTIMEDIA ePR SYSTEM FOR PATIENT TREATMENT

The multimedia ePR system for patient treatment addresses two areas of treatment, namely radiation therapy (RT) planning and treatment, and surgery. In this section we consider the framework of ePR system for patient treatment in general. This is followed by discussion of ePR software structure and the data schema for RT (Section 22.5) and for surgery (Section 22.6), respectively. The ePR for RT and ePR for surgery will be expanded in Chapters 23 and 24.

22.4.1 Fundamental Concepts

Fundamental to the functioning of multimedia ePR in clinical treatment is that the input data from other information systems be not only textual and diagnostic images but also include various patient's forms, 2-D clinical waves, identification pictures and finger prints, surgical video, and so forth, all in their original data formats. Data can come from different clinical and treatment departments including radiation therapy and surgery within the hospital or the entire enterprise. The multimedia ePR captures these data, stores the pointers in the ePR database for immediate and future retrieval, and presents them in proper display format and media. The multimedia functions in the ePR take the system design requirements out of the textual and images boundaries to much broader spectra.

22.4.2 Infrastructure and Basic Components

A general purpose multimedia ePR system is difficult to design, since so much ground has to be covered and considered. However, for a small-scale mission-oriented

Central Archive, ePR with Image Integration, and Workflow Steps

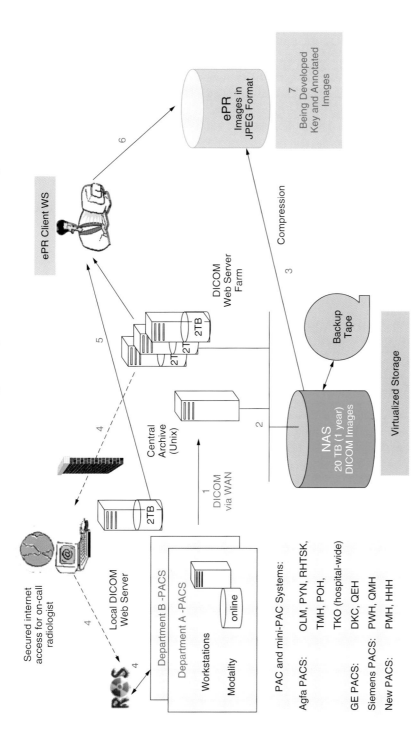

Figure 22.8 Hong Kong Hospital Authority (HK HA) central archive, ePR with image integration, and workflow steps the same as Figure 16.21. This design was based on the existing HK HA clinical information systems shown in Figure 22.7B. (Modified from Cheung et al., fig. 3; courtesy of Dr. Cheung et al).

multimedia ePR system the design can be more manageable. To this end, we restrict the multimedia ePR design to two particular applications, radiation therapy and surgery.

First, once the type of treatment is specified, the goals and boundary of the multimedia ePR can be defined. The ePR is mostly software operated on the well-defined treatment method, operational environment, system hardware, diagnostic systems, treatment devices, and display media. Once all these parameters are clarified and defined, the software can be designed according to the specific treatment. The software infrastructure of the ePR system generally consists of the following components:

1. Software organization
2. Database schema
3. Data model
4. Dataflow model
5. Display

With these components as the base, the next two sections provide the software infrastructure for radiation therapy and surgery, respectively.

22.5   THE MULTIMEDIA ePR SYSTEM FOR RADIATION THERAPY TREATMENT

22.5.1   Background

Comprehensive clinical image data and relevant information is crucial in the image-intensive radiation therapy (RT) for the planning and treatment of cancer. Multiple stand-alone systems utilizing technological advancements in imaging, therapeutic radiation, and computer treatment planning systems acquire key data during the RT treatment course of a patient. Currently the data are scattered in various RT information systems throughout the RT department. Scattered data can compromise an efficient clinical workflow, since the data crucial to a clinical decision may be time-consuming to retrieve, temporarily missing, or even lost. An integrated image-based radiation therapy planning and treatment multimedia ePR system is needed to improve the workflow and efficiency of the RT treatment and therapy process (see also Section 20.4.5).

RT planning and treatment is normal a long-term process requires weeks or several months from the patient to return for multiple treatments. Real-time data acquisition is not necessary but multimedia is essential, and the static multimedia ePR model would fit into this clinical environment.

22.5.2   Basic Components

22.5.2.1   The ePR Software Organization   The purpose that multimedia ePR server for RT is to organize all related images/data from image-intensive RT into one unified ePR system that facilitates longitudinal radiation therapy for a patient. The images used are from both radiological diagnostic imaging systems and from radiation therapy systems.

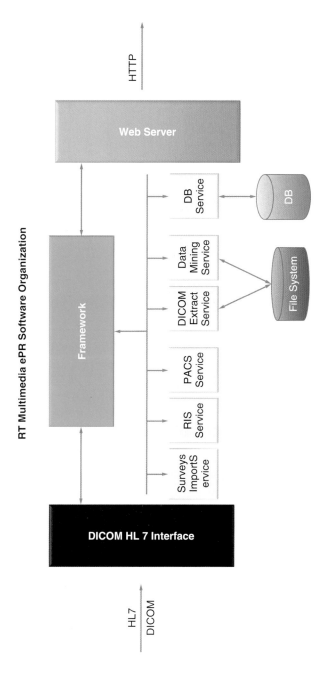

Figure 22.9 RT multimedia ePR software organization. DICOM and HL7 standards are used; the ePR server is Web-based. The yellow boxes are the ePR services.

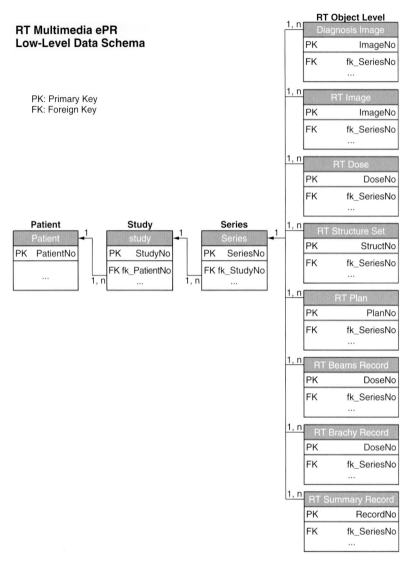

Figure 22.10   RT multimedia ePR low-level data schema. The DICOM data model starts from patient and proceeds to study, series, and RT objects level, which consists of one DCIOM diagnosis image object (top) and seven DICOM RT objects.

The DICOM RT standard is available for the integration all RT objects under one standard. The ePR software organization following the DCIOM RT is shown in Figure 22.9.

22.5.2.2 *Database Schema*   A low-level data schema is depicted in Figure 22.10. From left to right, if follows the DICOM model, starting from the patient, study, series to RT object level in which there are seven DICOM RT objects: RT images, RT dose, RT structure set, RT plan, RT beams record, RT Brachy record, and RT summary. In addition there are the diagnosis images from the diagnostic systems.

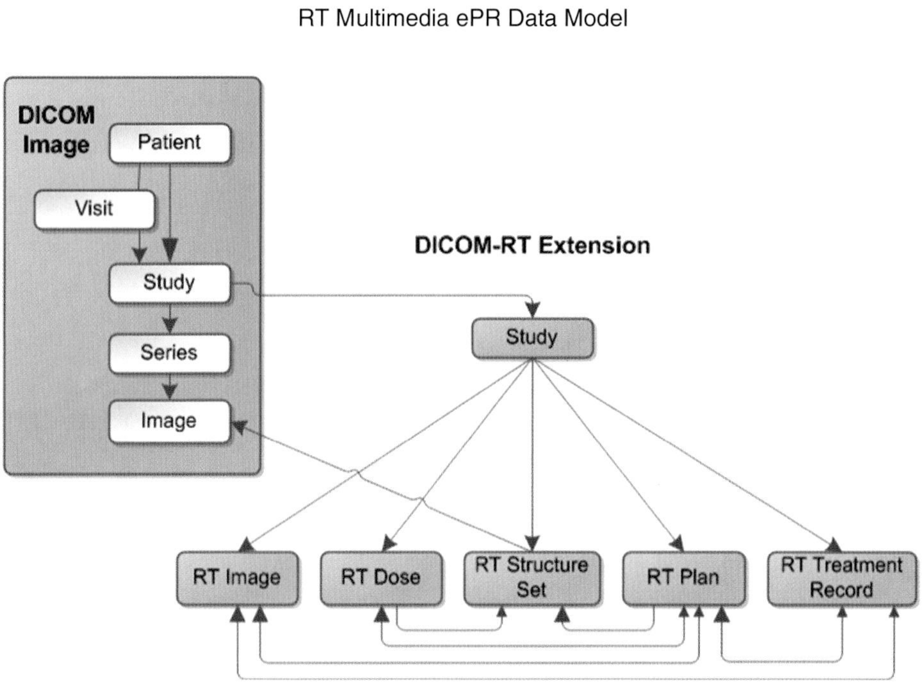

RT Multimedia ePR Data Model

Figure 22.11   RT multimedia ePR data model. The left side shows the DICOM Image, and right side shows the DICOM RT. Only five DICOM RT objects are used in the RT ePR. The sixth is the RT summary, which is a textual file that does not require further processing.

22.5.2.3   *Data Model*   The ePR data model is shown in Figure 22.11 in which the study level consists of seven DICOM RT objects excluding the RT summary and RT Brachy record. The former is a textual file that does not require further processing. The latter is not considered in standard RT planning and treatment.

22.5.2.4   *Data Flow Model*   We delay the discussion of dataflow of the multimedia ePR for RT to Chapter 23. Using a real example to describe the workflow steps would be a clearer way to explain the model.

22.6   THE MULTIMEDIA ePR SYSTEM FOR MINIMALLY INVASIVE SPINAL SURGERY

22.6.1   Background

Image-guided minimally invasive spinal surgery (MISS) is a relatively new branch of neurosurgery that relies on multimodality images for guiding the surgical procedure. The surgical procedure is relatively simple and safe performed by the expert and with a rapid patient recovery time. Despite the overall advantageous and benefits of this type of surgery compared to conventional open surgery, there are challenges to using MISS, including the integration of pre-, intra-, and post-op surgical data

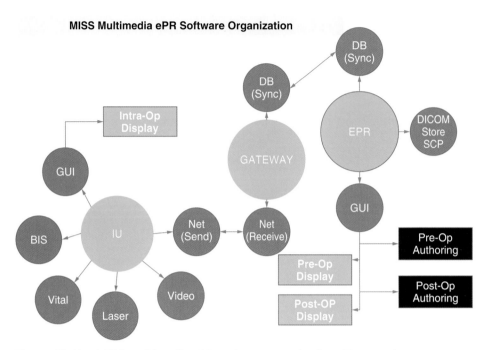

Figure 22.12 MISS multimedia ePR software organization. Three major components are the IU (integration unit), gateway, and ePR server (all in green color). There are three display modules for pre-op, intra-op, and post-op, respectively (yellow), and two data authoring modules, one for pre-op and the second for post-op patient document (dark blue).

from scattered data acquisition systems with some data acquired in real time during the surgery, and improvement of the efficiency of surgical workflow. An integrated multimedia ePR system is needed to overcome these challenges (see also Section 20.4.6).

Since real-time data acquisition of images, waveforms, and surgical video during surgery is necessary to guide the surgical procedure, real-time display and storage of the multimedia data is necessary. Dynamic multimedia ePR is the model of choice.

22.6.2 Basic Components

22.6.2.1 *The ePR Software Organization* The multimedia ePR system is dedicated to collecting pre-, intra-, and post-op surgical multimedia data for (1) improving surgical workflow, (2) obtaining post-op patient report and document, and (3) performing patient outcome studies. DICOM data model is used for the database schema, data model, and dataflow model software development. The ePR software organization is shown in Figure 22.12. Three major components are the integration unit (IU), which collects all real-time patient vital information, the surgical C-arm radiographs, and endoscopic video images and clips. The gateway (GATEW) manipulates all input data and ensures that they are DICOM compliant. The ePR

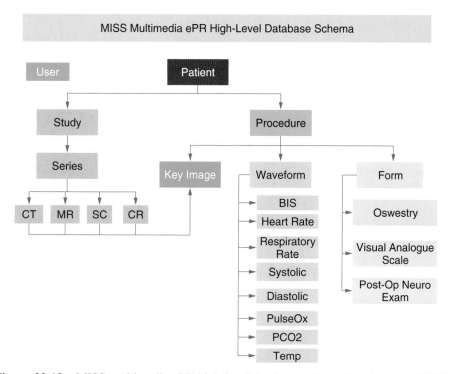

Figure 22.13 MISS multimedia ePR high-level database schema based on the DICOM data model. Left (blue) is the DICOM Image from pre-op. The procedural data consist of key images, waveforms, and patient forms. Key images include presurgical authored images needed during surgery, intra-op images, and video clips. Waveforms are from patient's attached devices measuring vital signs and conditions during intra-op. Patient forms are obtained during pre-op and post-op.

server (EPR) is used to monitor the data workflow. In addition there are three display software for pre-OP, intra-OP, and post-Op surgical data; and two authored packages for pre-Op and post-Op patient documents.

22.6.2.2 Database Schema The high-level database schema followed the DICOM data model is depicted in Figure 22.13. The users are surgeons and personnel in the surgical team. The left-side branch is pre-surgical authored images and data. The right-hand branch is the data obtained during the surgical procedure. Normally surgery on one spinal disc is counted as one procedure. Thus one procedure consists of key images forwarded from pre-op authored images as well as images during surgery, all live patient surgical waveforms (middle column), and digitized surgical forms (right column).

The low-level database schema is shown in Figure 22.14 as well as the DCIOM data model standard used (see Chapter 9).

22.6.2.3 Data Model The data model is depicted in Figure 22.15. Notice the data structure and the data search steps in the database.

MISS Multimedia ePR Low-Level Database Schema

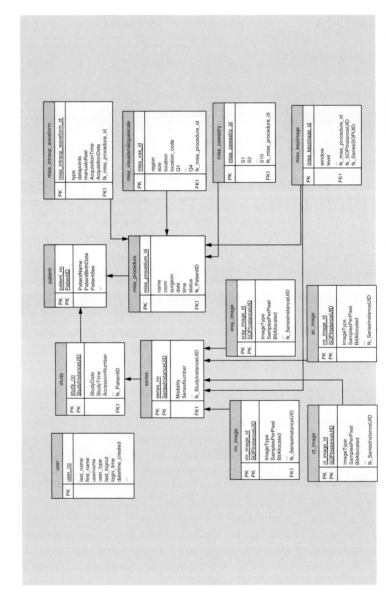

Figure 22.14 MISS multimedia ePR low-level database schema based on the DICOM data model.

MISS Multimedia ePR Data Model

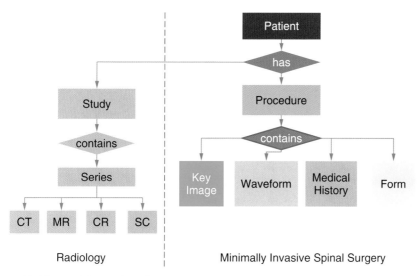

Figure 22.15   MISS multimedia ePR high-level data model based on the DICOM data model (compare color scheme with Fig. 22.13).

22.6.2.4   *Data Flow Model*   Figure 22.16 shows the pre-, intra-, and post-op dataflow that utilizes the DCIOM C-Store, C-Find, and C-Move services. Chapter 24 will present the complete multimedia ePR system for minimally invasive spinal surgery in operation.

22.7   SUMMARY OF THE MULTIMEDIA ePR SYSTEM

Traditional ePR contains mainly textual information. It requires complex software to handle the connectivity among many medical related information systems that contains the pertinent patient information. However, the requirements for connection to various hardware systems, the storage capacity, and network communication speed are rather minimal. The multimedia ePR system on the other hand, not only needs more complex software but also the storage and networks requirements are very demanding. In this chapter we characterize textual ePR, ePR with images, and multimedia ePR systems based on their contents.

Two large-scale ePR with image distribution systems in the U.S. Veterans Affairs Healthcare Enterprise and in the Hospital Authority (HA) of Hong Kong were presented to highlight their specificities, design criteria, and operation. We explain the basic principles of multimedia ePR system, and its software architecture. Two multimedia ePR for treatment, one in radiation therapy and the other in minimally invasive spinal surgery were defined and their software data models were illustrated. These two multimedia ePR systems are the focus of the detailed discussions in Chapters 23 and 24.

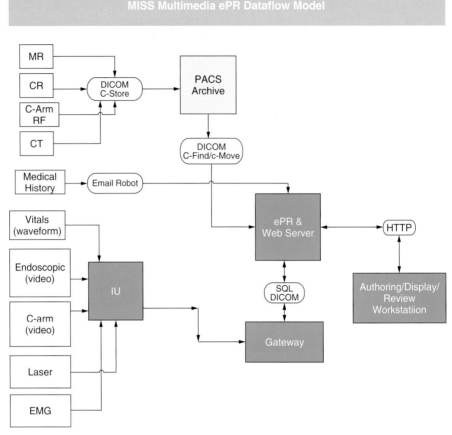

Figure 22.16 MISS multimedia ePR dataflow model. The various clinical devices used during surgery are listed (see Chapter 24 for terminology). Observe the positions of the four major components: IU, gateway, ePR server and display in the workflow (see also Fig. 22.12). The PACS archive (middle top) is the source of the pre-op images.

References

Bergh B, Pietsch M, Schlaefke A, Vogl TJ. Performance of Web-based image distribution: client-oriented measurements, *Eur Radiol* 13(9): 2161–9; 2003.

Cheung NT, Fung KW, Wong KC, Cheung A, Cheung J, Ho W, Cheung C, Shung E, Fung V, Fung H. Medical informatics—the state of the art in the Hospital Authority. *Int J Med Inf* 62(2–3): 113–9; 2001.

Cheung NT, Fung V, Kong JHB. The Hong Kong Hospital Authority's information architecture. Proceedings, M. Fieschi et al (Eds). Amsterdam: IOS Press *MeDINFO*; 2004.

McDonald CJ. The barriers to electronic medical record systems and how to overcome them. *J Am Med Inform Assoc* 4: 213–21; 1997.

Kuzmak PM and Dayhoff RE. The use of digital imaging and communications in medicine (DICOM) in the integration of imaging into the electronic patient record at the Department of Veterans Affairs. *Journal of Digital Imaging* 13 (2 Suppl 1): 133–137; 2000.

CHAPTER 23

Multimedia Electronic Patient Record System in Radiation Therapy

Information in an electronic patient record (ePR) system for radiation therapy (RT) consists of text, images, and graphics. We use the term ePR in this chapter for convenience. To enable the exchange of RT patient information between systems within an institution and across institutions, the DICOM standard should be used. This chapter describes a DICOM RT ePR system for information exchange and sharing. The system is based on Web technology and uses a server as the common platform for archiving all RT related multimedia information and for the distribution and viewing of ePR image/data. The contents of this chapter follow the description of RT multimodality concept and workflow presented in Sections 5.3.2 and 22.5.

Figure 20.9 is reproduced here as Figure 23.1, the center rectangle and the lower ellipse in orange color show the position of, and components involved in, the chapter.

23.1 BACKGROUND IN RADIATION THERAPY PLANNING AND TREATMENT

Radiation therapy (RT) uses radiation for the treatment of diseases that usually are malignant. Before delivering the dose of radiation, careful treatment planning needs to be done. This ensures that the target tumor volume is accurately irradiated while the neighboring normal tissue is spared as much as possible. Such treatment planning results in isodose treatment plans superimposed on CT images illustrating the radiation dose distribution in the irradiated volume, dose volume histograms, treatment parameters, and treatment records. It can be seen that in radiation therapy, not only radiological images are involved, graphics and textual information are generated. For convenience, Figure 5.5 is reproduced here as Figure 23.2 to provide a quick review of the RT workflow which gives a summary of the work and data involved in radiation therapy. We use the DICOM RT standard to integrate all such RT information originated from other RT systems.

The DICOM standard is the cornerstone to the successful implementation of PACS in radiology. Following the implementation of DICOM format, seven DICOM radiotherapy (RT) objects in DICOM format have been ratified by the DICOM Committee for transmission and storage of radiotherapy multimedia information. The seven

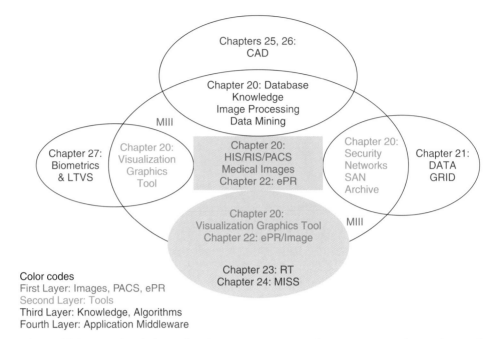

Figure 23.1   Imaging informatics data sources (rectangle), concepts, technologies, and applications (large and small ellipses) as discussed in the chapters of Part IV. Color codes refer to the five-layer informatics infrastructure shown in Figure 20.2. This chapter presents the multimedia ePR system in RT.

DICOM RT objects include RT image, RT plan, RT structure set, RT dose, RT beams treatment record, RT Brachy treatment record, and RT summary record (Fig. 23.3, seven blue boxes).

23.2   RADIATION THERAPY WORKFLOW

External beam radiation therapy (RT) involves treatment planning and treatment delivery. It makes up over 90% or the workload in radiation therapy and is an image and computer graphic intensive process. Patient imaging information is needed in the RT planning process, image registration to identify regions to be treated, and markers to align images to ensure treatment setup accuracy. Multimodality images from projection X-rays, computed tomography (CT), magnetic resonance imaging (MRI), and positron emission tomography (PET) are used for tumor localization and critical organ identification. These include the shape, size, and location of the targets and radiosensitive vital organs. Sometimes images from different modalities need to be fused for better tumor and critical organ identification. From such information, treatment planning generates computer graphics and radiation dose distribution that overlay on the images to ensure the delivery of uniform high dose to target tumors but not to adjacent critical structures. In addition to careful monitoring of treatment, optimization and dose calculation are essential for successful patient treatment outcomes. During all these processes PACS and imaging informatics technologies are

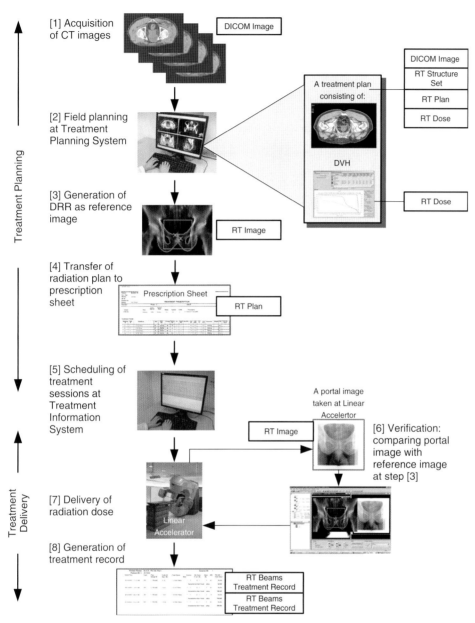

Figure 23.2 Generic external beam radiation therapy workflow, including treatment planning and delivery in the prostate cancer example. RT information is scattered as it is generated. The yellow boxes indicate the RT-related images and data that could be generated in the workflow. Treatment planning steps 1, 2, and 3; and treatment delivery step 6 shown in yellow boxes are described in Section 5.3.2. Step 2 in RT treatment plan with radiation dose distribution involves the superposition of the radiotherapy object: RT plan, RT structure set and RT dose upon the corresponding set CT images. DRR: digital reconstructed radiograph; DVH: dose–volume histogram. (Courtesy of Dr. M Law)

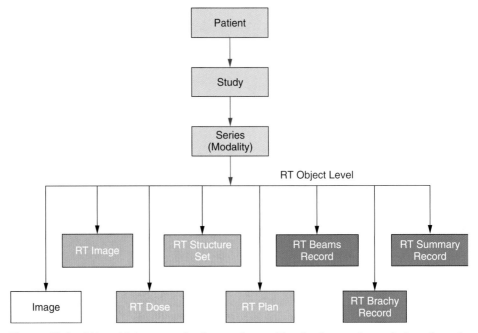

Figure 23.3 RT archive server database schema. The database schema is based on the DICOM data model of the real world. The seven DICOM-RT objects in the blue shaded boxes are integrated within the modality of the series module along with the diagnostic image object (light yellow box) to keep each RT object grouped under a modality similar to the CT or MR. The four light blue boxes are the RT image, RT structure, RT dose, and RT plan. The two upper darker blue boxes are the RT beams and the summary record, the lower one is the RT Brachy record, which is not used for external therapy.

used extensively. Radiation therapy emphasizes the individual patient treatment process and has not taken advantages of utilizing informatics to improve RT workflow and patient treatment outcomes until recently. Figure 23.2 depicts a generic workflow of RT, including treatment planning and delivery using a prostate cancer treatment plan and delivery as an example. In this section we present the multimodalities imaging component of RT treatment planning and delivery, in particular, following the numerals in Fig. 23.2, (1) image acquisition, (2) field planning at the treatment planning system, (3) generation of DRR (digitally reconstructed radiography), and (6) verification by comparing portal image and reference DRR, described in the yellow boxes of the workflow.

23.3   THE ePR DATA MODEL AND DICOM RT OBJECTS

23.3.1   The ePR Data Model

To develop an electronic patient record, a conceptual data model of the clinical department is required and this in turn determines how patient data are physically represented in the database. To develop the conceptual data model, the radiation therapy workflow should first be reviewed from which the data required are defined. At the same time, the views of the users (radiation oncologists, medical physicists, radiation therapists) are collected. From these views, the conceptual data model can be increasingly refined with more details. The model is based on the daily operation mode in a radiation therapy department and the users' requirements. The data in the model are parsed from the DICOM images and DICOM RT objects. When an object is inserted, a link is created at the corresponding location in the table. The output data and the links in the model form the foundation of the design of graphical user interface (GUI) display windows.

23.3.2   DICOM RT Objects

Using a prostate cancer RT planning and treatment as an example, we describe some DICOM RT objects as follows (also refer to Section 5.3.2):

1. RT structure set information object (Fig. 23.4A(a); see also Fig. 5.6A): This object defines a set of areas of significance in radiation therapy, such as body contours, tumor volumes—gross target volume (GTV), clinical target volume (CTV), and planning target volume (PTV)—organs at risk (OARs), and other regions of interest. In a prostate cancer case, the target volume is the prostate gland and the extension of the cancer around the gland. The OARs are the urinary bladder, the rectum, and the heads of the femur. Each structure will be associated with a frame of reference and with or without reference to the diagnostic images.

2. RT plan information object (Fig. 23.4A(b); see also Fig. 5.6B): Treatment planning is a process to determine how best the radiation beam should be placed so that an optimum dose distribution can be delivered. It involves localization of the tumor and OARs, and the design of radiation beams and their dose weighting with respect to the PTV and OARs. A clinical treatment plan may refer to the totality of structures marked on the CT image, the beam positions and beam sizes, and the dose distribution displayed on the image. In the DICOM RT standard, information about the structures are contained in the RT structure set object and the dose distribution in the RT dose object, which requires the coordinates for indication of their positions. Thus the RT plan object only refers to the textual information in treatment plans, whether generated manually, by a virtual simulation system, or by a treatment planning system. Such information includes treatment beam parameters, fractionation scheme, prescription, accessories used, and patient setup in external beam or brachytherapy.

3. RT dose information object (Fig. 23.4A(c); see also Fig. 5.6C): The distribution of radiation dose for a treatment is represented by the isodose lines expressed in percentage or in dose units (gray). The isodose lines can be displayed in relation to the tumor volume and OARs and superimposed on images. This object contains such radiation dose data from TPSs. It allows the transmission of a 3-D array of dose data as a set of 2-D dose planes. Examples are the isodose distribution dose data either in relation to the corresponding CT or MR image or on their own and the DVHs (Fig. 23.4A(d); see also Fig. 5.6D).

4. RT image information object (Fig. 23.4*B*): In contrast to the DICOM Image object, where the different image types are contained in objects for different modalities, the RT image information object specifies the attributes of those images that are "acquired or calculated using conical geometry" in radiotherapy. Examples are projection simulator images, portal images acquired at linear accelerators, or DRRs generated from CT scans at TPSs.

5. RT beams treatment record information object: This object contains mainly textual data that specify treatment sessions report generated by a treatment verification system during a course of external beam treatment or treatment information during treatment delivery. Such information includes machine, radiation type and energy used, date and time of treatment, external beam details, treatment beam accessories, treatment fraction detail, the monitor units (dose), calculated dose, cumulative dose, verification image taken and optional treatment summary. Each treatment is represented by an instance of RT beams treatment record. Figure 23.4*B* provides an example of the RT beam treatment record.

Together with these DICOM RT objects shown in Figure 23.4*A* and *B*; the DICOM RT descriptions of the prostate cancer radiation therapy plan and treatment of a patient's can be defined.

23.4 INFRASTRUCTURE, WORKFLOW, AND COMPONENTS OF THE MULTIMEDIA ePR IN RT

The mission of the ePR system is that all RT-related information of a patient can be viewed within a system (i.e., with the pertinent multimedia information of treatment plans, graphs, images, records and clinician's remarks) from different RT sources to form an electronic patient record with the data standardized in DICOM RT.

23.4.1 DICOM RT Based ePR System Architectural Design

We use the DICOM data model as the base for designing the multimedia ePR system in RT. Figure 23.5*A* shows the general PACS model being used today and Figure 23.5*B* depicts the model of the multimedia ePR system in RT; observe the similarity of both models. The ePR in RT consists of three major components: the DICOM-RT objects input, the DICOM-RT gateway, and the DICOM-RT based ePR system platform (dotted rectangle). The ePR platform consists of three modules, the DICOM RT archive server, the RT Web server and the Web-based client workstations (WSs). Note that the RT Web server has to handle more complex multimedia data than the Web server in PACS (Fig. 23.5*A*).

23.4.2 DICOM RT Objects' Input

The workflow diagram shown in Figure 23.2 identifies all DICOM RT objects. They can come from any RT information systems, treatment planning system, linear accelerator WS, modality simulator, PACS, and in addition pertinent information related to the patient in the hospital information system (HIS) depicted in Figure 23.5*B*.

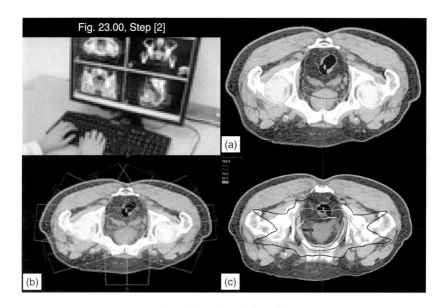

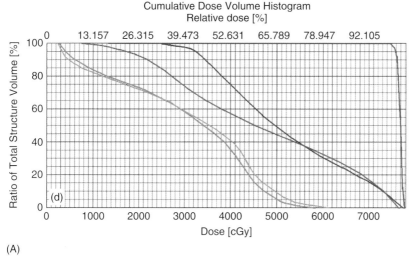

Figure 23.4   (*A*) Three DICOM RT objects: (*a*) RT structure, (*b*) RT plan, and (*c*) RT dose; and (*d*) DVH curves (reproduced from Fig. 5.6) (*B*) The three RT treatment records. These objects include the RT beams treatment record, RT Brachy treatment record, and RT treatment summary record. The figure shows the RT beams treatment record, which records the dose given for each radiation beam at each treatment session (rows). Column 1 shows the date on which the radiation dose was delivered. The other columns show the dose (in monitor units) delivered to Radiation fields 1–11 on a given date. Radiation field number 12–15 show a second phase of treatment that consists of only 4 radiation fields. (Courtesy of Dr. M Law)

Field	1	2	3	4	5	6	7	8	9	10	11	12	13	14	15
Wedge	3RW60	3RW45	4RW45	4RW45	4RW45							3RW30	1VW15		3RW45
Date\MU	128	94	187	47	47	75	15	166	30	15	15	128	67	20	104
2002/6/26	128	94	187	47	47	75	15	166	30	15	15				
2002/6/27	128	94	187	47	47	75	15	166	30	15	15				
2002/6/28	128	94	187	47	47	75	15	166	30	15	15				
2002/6/29	128	94	187	47	47	75	15	166	30	15	15				
2002/7/1	128	94	187	47	47	75	15	166	30	15	15				
2002/7/2	128	94	187	47	47	75	15	166	30	15	15				
2002/7/3	128	94	187	47	47	75	15	166	30	15	15				
2002/7/4	128	94	187	47	47	75	15	166	30	15	15				
2002/7/5	128	94	187	47	47	75	15	166	30	15	15				
2002/7/19												128	67	20	104
2002/7/20												128	67	20	104
2002/7/22												128	67	20	104
2002/7/23												128	67	20	104
2002/7/24												128	67	20	104

(B)

Figure 23.4 (*Continued*)

These systems are connected by Internet and departmental Intranet communication networks. Preselected DICOM and DICOM RT objects are first identified by each system and then either pushed to, or pulled by, the DICOM RT gateway shown in Figure 23.5*B*. Other RT functional requirements (e.g., treatment plan approval by radiation oncologists) in the workflow review in textual format are converted into the system technical details based on the DICOM RT object definitions and the data flow of the objects and entered by radiographic technicians to the gateway also. The DICOM standard service classes such as DICOM storage and query/retrieve are incorporated into each component of the ePR information system.

23.4.3 DICOM RT Gateway

After receiving the RT objects, the DICOM RT Gateway (Fig. 23.5*B*) extracts information from the objects and puts them into the RT data model as required in the DICOM RT archive server. It also converts any nonstandard data objects to the standard required by the DICOM RT server. The outputs of the gateway are packaged DICOM and DICOM RT objects, which are automatically pushed by the gateway to the RT archive server.

23.4.4 DICOM RT Archive Server

Following the DICOM hierarchical structure, a database schema for the DICOM RT archive server (Fig. 23.5*B*) can be constructed. It consists of 4 levels (patient, study, RT series, and RT objects) with 11 modules as represented by the colored boxes in Figure 23.3. The schema follows the DICOM data model of the real world and includes the 7 DICOM RT data objects and the DICOM diagnostic images. It is important to that most current PAC systems not support DICOM RT objects (except DICOM RT image) because of the need to have a more elaborated internal schema for an RT archive server. PACS manufacturers are beginning to incorporate the DICOM RT objects to gradually migrate their PACS server to be compatible with the RT archive server.

In the ePR in RT, the RT server is used mostly for management and storage for RT objects rather than for processing the RT data (attributes) encapsulated in the objects,

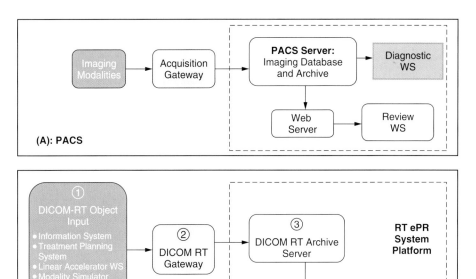

Figure 23.5 Structural similarities between the PACS and the DICOM-RT based ePR system. (*A*) Generic PACS components and data flow; the key PACS components that are successfully utilized today within the radiology workflow. PACS uses diagnostic WS for high-quality viewing, and the PACS Web server and review WS are mostly used for reviewing radiological image studies by referring physicians. (*B*) Multimedia DICOM-RT ePR System components and data flow. Most of the RT components follow the PACS data model (modules 1–3 relate to the imaging modalities, acquisition gateway, and PACS server, respectively, in *A*). The ePR system platform (dotted rectangle) is used to extract information from the DICOM RT server to develop the Web-based ePR system. Note that the RT Web server is more complex in *B* (refer to Fig. 23.6 for detail) when compared to *A*, since the RT data contain more complex Imaging and Informatics data objects, while the Web server in *A* contains only diagnostic image studies and reports. Also there are different Web application pages within the RT Web client workstations utilized by oncologists, radiation therapists, and medical physicist based on their different needs. (Modified from original drawing by Dr. M Law)

which is quite contrast to the functions of the PACS server. Upon receiving DICOM RT objects and images from the DICOM RT gateway, the RT server abstracts only the essential aspects of the entities for the necessary transactions and auto-routes all the data to the RT Web server (Fig. 23.5*B*) to be processed for display on the RT Web client WS.

23.4.5 RT Web-Based ePR Server

While the RT archive server is responsible for storage and transmission of DICOM images and DICOM RT objects, the RT Web server (Fig. 23.5*B*) receives the objects,

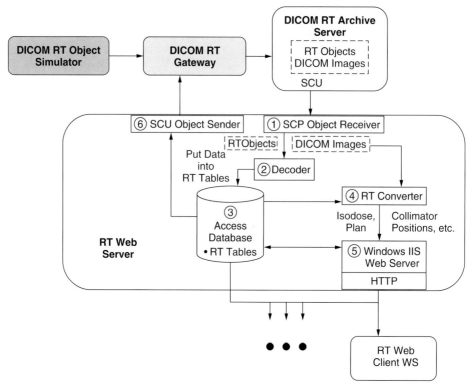

Figure 23.6   Architecture of the RT Web server of the DICOM-RT ePR system. Six key components are shown within the Web server rectangular domain. Note that the RT Web server is more complex than a PACS Web server, since it must handle the multimedia image and informatics data from the seven DICOM RT objects in addition to the DICOM diagnostic images from radiology. SCP: Service class provider; SCU: service class user; HTTP: hypertext transfer protocol.

decodes them to the corresponding position in the RT Web database, and organizes the data into the Web viewing mode for display in the client workstations (Fig. 23.6). In this sense the Web server is the "brain" for the RT multimedia ePR system, since all actions are processed here.

There are six major components in the RT Web server as shown in Figure 23.6. Following the numerals in the figure, the workflow process between the DICOM RT archive server and the RT Web server is as follows:

DICOM-RT objects and DICOM diagnostic images are sent by the DICOM RT archive server through the DICOM SCU (service class user) service (see Chapter 9) to the RT Web server (SCU is a built-in service in the DICOM RT archive server). The images are received by the object receiver (1) using DICOM SCP (service class provider). RT objects are translated by a decoder (2), and the data are arranged in the RT tables and RT database (3). The data from the tables, for examples, RT structures and RT dose, are superimposed on the corresponding positions of the DICOM images by the RT converter (4) and be sent by the Web server (5) to the client workstations using HTTP (hypertext transfer protocol). When the RT Web server has generated the new data needed to update the DICOM RT archive server, for example, a revision in the treatment plan by the oncology, the object sender (6) in the RT Web server will be called upon to perform the task. In this case it uses the DICOM SCU service to send the updated objects to the RT archive server via the DICOM RT gateway for storage. The updated information will be in queue to update the DICOM RT archive server, which completes the data loop.

The DICOM standard has grouped various RT attributes into modules and object IODs (DICOM information object definition). The overall database schema of the RT Web server adopts what is defined by the DICOM data model and consists of 72 tables (in its prototype) to facilitate Web viewing in the client workstations. This information includes key data items such as treatment plan parameters, beam records, isodose curves, region of interests (ROIs) including the tumor volume and organs at risk (OAR) contours, and dose–volume histograms (DVHs) (see Figs. 5.6 and 23.4). These data are parsed from the DICOM-RT objects as needed to be displayed in the Web client WSs.

The data objects from the Web-based server can be used to develop quantified knowledge and metadata which can be added to the database schema. Further outcomes data can also be added to the overall database schema. Therefore it is important to design the database schema to be as flexible as possible to extend it for knowledge base and outcome data that are not part of the DICOM standard.

23.4.6   RT Web Client Workstation (WS)

For the RT Web client WSs (Fig. 23.5*B*), the GUI (graphical user interface) is designed for users to access information within the database according to the functional requirements for radiation therapists, dosimetrists, physicists, and oncologists. Based on the user requirements documentation, all necessary data required are included in the database tables of the Web server. The RT workflow also serves to drive the GUI design. Figure 23.7 depicts the timeline window of a cancer patient's RT planning and treatment overview.

23.5   DATABASE SCHEMA

We have discussed the macro aspect of the multimedia ePR in RT including infrastructure, system components and workflow. In Figure 23.3 the high-level of the ePR database schema was presented. Now let us consider the micro aspect of the ePR, namely the data schema in the RT database. The database schema refers to how data are physically represented. It is concerned with data structures, file organizations, and mechanism for the operation of the system and data storage. From the data flow diagram shown in Figure 23.5*B*, it can be seen that in this ePR system has two databases, one for the RT archive server and the other for the RT Web-based server. The former is for management and storage of DICOM objects (including DICOM RT objects and DCIOM images), and the latter is first for partition of the collected DICOM RT objects data and then the server parses them strategically to be viewed by users at the Web client.

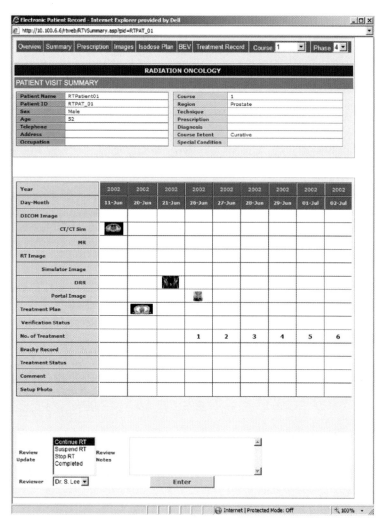

Figure 23.7 Screenshot of a Web client application page on the client WS from the DICOM RT ePR system prototype developed in the Hong Kong Polytechnic University showing the timeline overview of a RT patient's ePR display window. Key data extracted from some DICOM RT objects are displayed as thumbnail representations for users to select and review in more detail using the GUI at the client WS. This patient had a CT scan on 11 June 2002, a dosimetric treatment plan done on 20 June, a DRR generated on 21 June, and portal image produced on 26 June, after which treatment started immediately on 26 June. Six radiation doses were delivered from 26 June to 2 July. GUI: Graphical user interface; DRR: digitally reconstructed radiograph.

23.5.1 Database Schema of the RT Archive Server

The Web-based RT ePR server component can be designed as a three-tier client-server architecture. In the three-tier architecture, a middle tier is added between the user interface client environment and the database management server environment (see the dotted box in Fig. 23.5*B*). For this design, the three tiers are (1) the RT archive server, which provides such functions as managing, archiving, and transferring of the DICOM images and DICOM RT objects; (2) the RT Web-based server focusing on processing RT planning and treatment data of the patient; and (3) the RT Web client that presents the patient's record

DICOM is an object-oriented standard. The external aspects (operation) of an object are separated from the internal details of the data, which are hidden from the outside world (information hiding). This organization allows identification of the object, or any operations on the object first, and delays the implementation of details. Also changes to the internal details at a later stage will not affect the applications that use it, provided that the external aspects remain unchanged. This way the database server only needs to identify what an object is and what it does (the DICOM RT archive server). The internal details or the data structure of an object can be implemented or processed later in the application server (the Web-based RT server). This has been the way that the PACS server was designed; hence it has a simple data model for the operations of its objects. Such a design can also be adopted for the ePR system, that is, the DICOM RT archive server only manages the essential aspects of the RT objects and leaves the implementation of details to the RT Web server. Thus the DICOM RT archive server has only the basic database schema based on the first few levels of the DICOM hierarchical structure (see Fig. 23.3), namely "patient," "study," "series," and its RT objects and diagnostic images.

23.5.2 Data Schema of the RT Web Server

For implementing the details of the DICOM RT objects using the Web-based RT server, a data model different and more elaborated than that of the RT server is required. The basic data structures are given in the DICOM standard documents. How the data are used depends on the actual application at the client WS, which in turn determines how much is included in the data model. From the user requirements collected earlier (see Section 23.3.1), the physical data model for the Web server can be designed and implemented following the DICOM standard as shown in Figure 23.8.

23.6 GRAPHICAL USER INTERFACE DESIGN

The user interface presents the patient's information to the users and is an important part of the ePR. The design of the interface can be based on the survey of the user requirements mentioned in Section 23.3.1. Radiation therapists and oncologists should be involved in the design process. Figure 23.9*A* shows the hierarchical structure of the user interface windows and the functions served by each window. The detail of which can be referred to Figure 23.9*B* (Law, 2005). The user interface can be implemented by using the standard GUI software package, for example, the

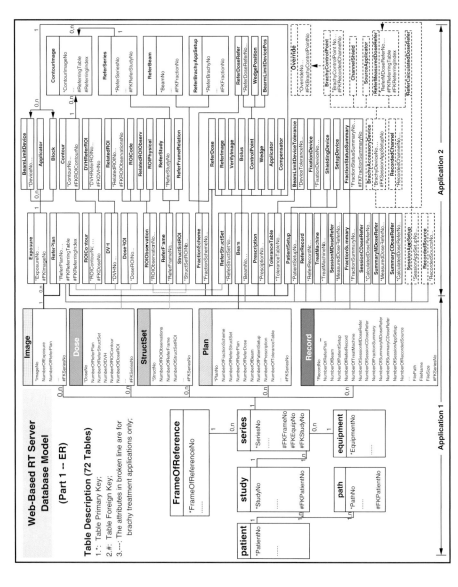

Figure 23.8 Database schema of the RT Web application server based on a multimedia ePR system in RT prototype developed in the Hong Kong Polytechnic University. Although the database schema is generic, it can be modified for other oncology departments with different workflows, treatment plans, and viewing conditions. (Courtesy of Dr. M. Law)

interactive functions of the Visual Basic (VB) scripts embedded in the ASP (active server page), a feature of WIIS (Window Internet Information Server).

23.7 VALIDATION OF THE CONCEPT OF MULTIMEDIA ePR SYSTEM IN RT

23.7.1 Integration of the ePR System

23.7.1.1 The RT ePR Prototype The concept of the multimedia ePR system in RT presented in previous sections was tested by Dr. M. Law at the Hong Kong Polytechnic University, where she has used and developed a prototype ePR system since 2004. The prototype has five major components shown in Figure 23.10, from right to left the RT object simulator, DICOM RT gateway, RT archive server, Web-based RT server, and RT client WS (see Fig. 23.5*B*). In this section we present the prototype system that supports the concept of the multimedia ePR system in RT.

23.7.1.2 Hardware and Software All components in the prototype are PC based except the RT archive server, which is a SUN Ultra 2 computer with SCSI hard disk and 100 MB Ethernet adapter operating under SunOS 5.8. The software includes

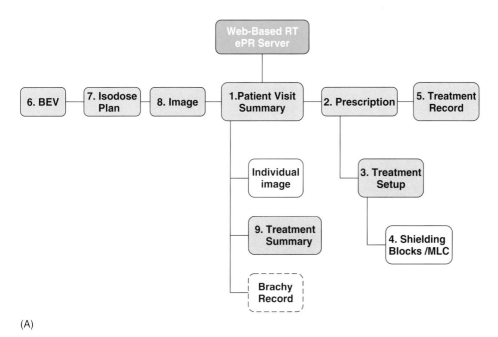

(A)

Figure 23.9 (*A*) Web site hierarchy of a multimedia ePR system in RT prototype developed at the Hong Kong Polytechnic University. Minor modifications may be needed for other oncology centers with different workflows and display requirements from the users. BEV: Beam's eye view; MLC: multileaf Collimator. (*B*) Workflow of the graphical user interface. Minor modifications may be needed for other Oncology Centers with different workflows and display requirements from the users. (Courtesy of Dr. M. Law)

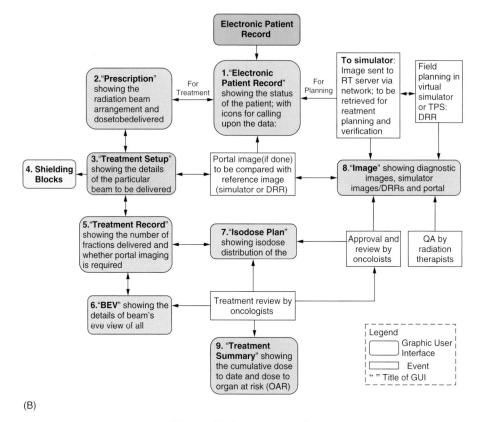

(B)

Figure 23.9   (*Continued*)

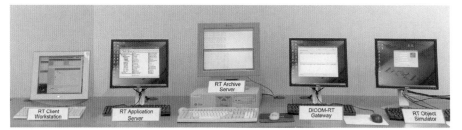

Figure 23.10   Photograph of the multimedia ePR system in RT prototype implemented within the laboratory environment for evaluation of the RT data objects and workflow. Each component represents the conceptual diagram from Figure 23.5*B*. From right to left: (1) RT object simulator for DICOM RT data input; (2) DICOM RT gateway; (3) DICOM RT archive server; (4) RT Web-based server (refer to Fig. 23.6 for RT Web server architecture), and (5) RT client WS. (Courtesy of M. Law)

SUN Workshop Compilers CC++, PACS Programming Library, and Oracle8i release 8.1.7 Database Management System. A Microsoft Access 2000 database was used as the database for the RT web server (see Fig. 23.6). For distribution of RT information, a web server, the Window Internet Information Server (WIIS) was used and the data were sent using the hypertext transfer protocol (HTTP). Microsoft Access 2000 was used for the database.

23.7.1.3 *Graphical User Interface (GUI) in the WS*   The prototype RT Web server system is comprised of a Web-based display and database structure designed in-house. The front end includes the data objects, structure, and communication protocol, and the back end consists of encoding and decoding with open standards (see Fig. 23.9*A* and *B*). The user interface windows for the Web client WS were created with embedded interactive functions. Within the Web application server, graphical illustrations such as dosimetric plans were created, stored, and displayed in the JPEG format. They result from the overlays of the DICOM CT image, RT structure set, RT plan, and RT dose objects. DICOM standard inherently provides cross-referencing among these objects. Decoding and encoding software applications were developed based on the IODs (information object definition) of DICOM. For multiple data items that are required on the same display such as the dosimetric plan, the DICOM objects containing the target volumes, organs at risk, and isodose distribution are decoded to and encoded from the database records of the coordinates in the Web application server based on the definition of the DICOM sequences. Those Web-based displays are achieved by plotting coordinates onto the referenced CT image.

23.7.2 Data Collection

Different types of RT files (DICOM and non-DICOM) were collected from RT vendors and clinical departments. DICOM files include CT and MR images, digitized simulator and portal images, RT plan, RT structure set, and RT dose. Non-DICOM files include treatment planning files and the treatment record in textual format, and the portal image in tiff/bitmap format. The names of patients were anonymized. The non-DICOM files were translated to DICOM format. After testing the files for successful transmission through the laboratory computer components, the DICOM files were grouped into folders to form 10 virtual patients so that their electronic records could be displayed in the Web client. The virtual patients' information was successfully transmitted, stored, and viewed at the RT Web client. Using the user interface windows, we illustrate next the ePR of one of the patients stored in the archive server.

23.7.3 Multimedia Electronic Patient Record of a Sample RT Patient

A patient, whose name is RTPatient01, with a Hong Kong Identity card number (HKID) of RTPat_01, was planned for a course of radiotherapy. He had finished all the earlier treatment planning procedures and is receiving the radiation treatment. He comes back for this treatment. At the reception of the treatment unit, the receptionist or the radiation therapist calls up the patient query page and types in the patient's HKID number or just "RT" against the HKID to search for the patient's detail.

The list of patients beginning with HKID number of "RT" is shown (Fig. 23.11A). In the database only two patients are listed with a beginning "RT," so only two patients' names are shown; RTPatient02 is the other patient. The same page and search procedure can be used when a patient re-visits the department for planning procedures or goes to see a radiation oncologist for review or to receive further radiation treatment.

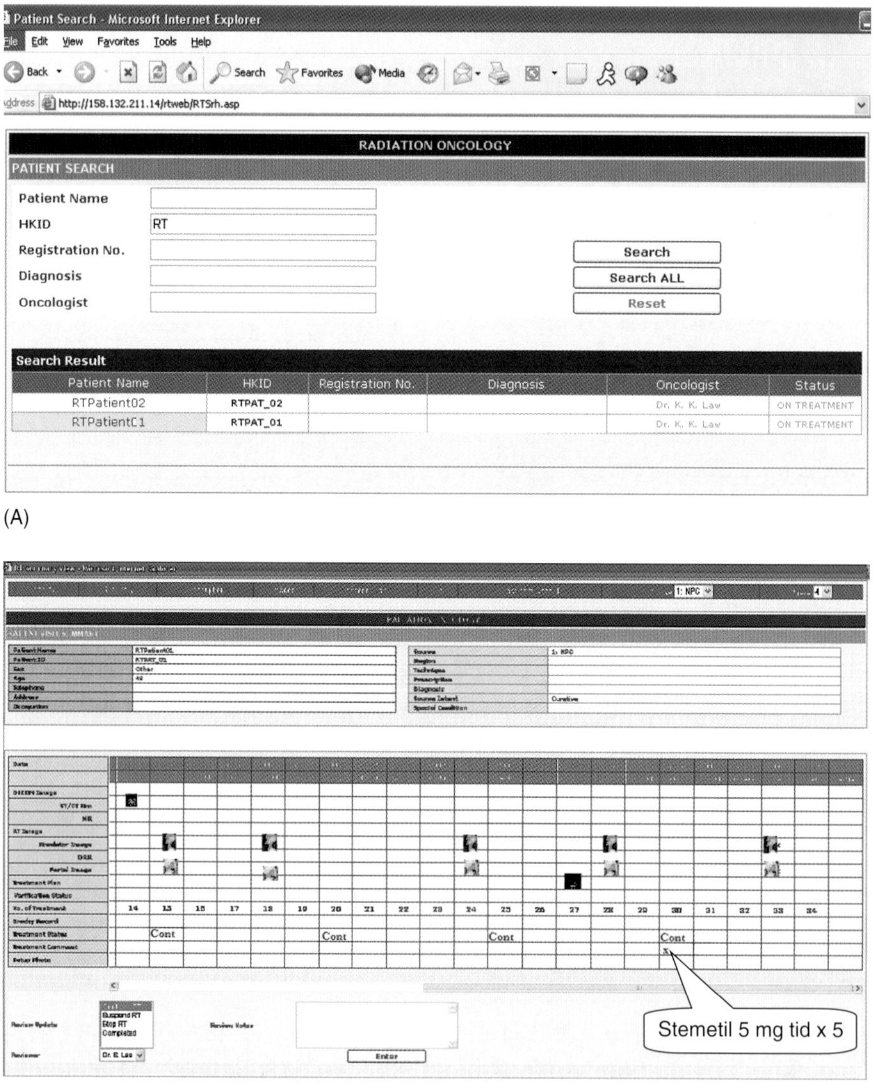

(A)

(B)

Figure 23.11 Sample RT patient record from the multimedia ePR system in which some GUI windows are shown in the RT web client. (A) patient list, stemetil 5 mg tid ×5 (antiemetic medicine, 3 times a day for 5 days.) (B) patient visit summary, (C) prescription page, (D) treatment setup page, (E) shielding block position, (F) treatment record, and (G) treatment summary record. (Courtesy of Dr. M. Law)

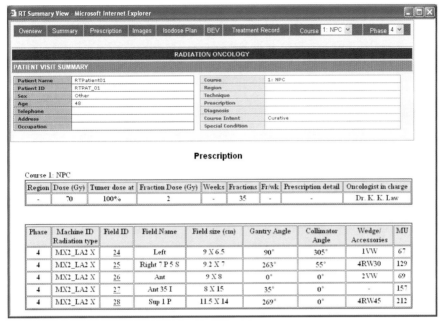

(C)

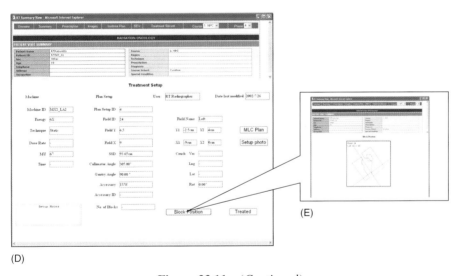

(D)

(E)

Figure 23.11 (*Continued*)

A click on the patient's name, RTPatient01 pops up the patient's visit summary (Fig. 23.11*B*) with all the procedures done. The radiation therapist or the radiation oncologist can then, at a glance, learn the status of the patient. In this case, in the treatment status row, the latest comment from the radiation oncologist is "Cont. RT," meaning to continue with the treatment. If the visit is to consult the oncologist, the same visit summary can be used for the oncologist to add his/her comments about the patient. Pointing at the treatment comment is the balloon containing the oncologist's comments.

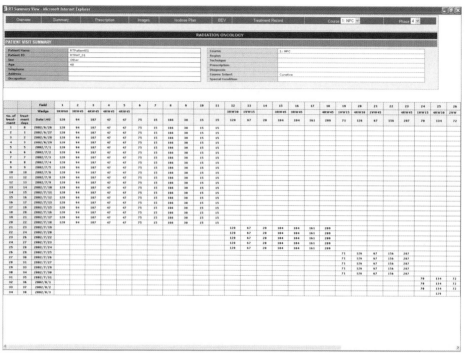

(F)

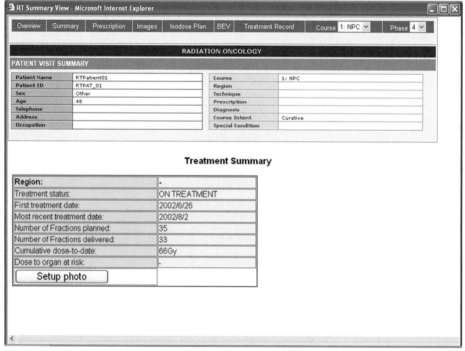

(G)

Figure 23.11 (*Continued*)

To set up the patient for treatment, the radiation therapist needs to refer to the prescription of the patient. In the toolbar at the top of the window is a list of functions the users can click on to switch between pages in searching the information about the patient as needed. One of the function button is "prescription." A click on the "prescription" pops up the prescription page with all the essential details about the treatment prescription (Fig. 23.11C), including the radiation fields to be treated.

Clicking on any of the buttons in the field ID (column 3) leads to the setup details for that radiation field. In this case field 24 is to be treated, the field ID "24" is clicked and that leads to the setup page where greater detail about the treatment plan is provided (Fig. 23.11D). On the treatment setup page, a click on the block position button shows the shielding block as in Figure 23.11E.

Similarly a click to the MLC plan button (right-hand side) will call up the MLC shape. From the recommendation of a clinical radiation therapist, a button is added to link to any photo that is taken related to the setup.

When the radiation dose for a field is delivered, a click on the "treated" button will update the field in the treatment record (Fig. 23.11F). When all the fields prescribed for the day are treated, the cumulative dose in the treatment record will be added and the summary record will also be updated (Fig. 23.11G).

Some buttons of the toolbar at the top of each page provide a link to the stated information. For example, "summary" leads to the treatment summary record window (Fig. 23.11G), "images" leads to all the images of the patient for the particular course, and "isodose plan" leads to the window showing the distribution of radiation dose around the marked target volume and other nearby anatomical structures on the cross-sectional CT images. Examples of some images, isodose plan, and other types of data displayed on the Web WS from other virtual patients are shown in Figure 23.4A and B, and Figure 23.7.

23.8 ADVANTAGES OF THE MULTIMEDIA ePR SYSTEM IN RT FOR DAILY CLINICAL PRACTICE

23.8.1 Communication between Isolated Information Systems and Archival of Information

In a radiotheraphy department, often there are different isolated information systems with only small scope and for single-purpose applications. They usually come with the purchase of individual applications, like one system for brachytherapy, another system for stereotactic radiotherapy/radiosurgery (SRT/SRS). They often stand alone, having little interface with other systems. A BrainLab workstation for SRT/SRS has its own storage for the plans performed at its workstation. For conventional radiotherapy the treatment plans are stored in the conventional treatment planning system (TPS) and the treatment records in another information system. A patient whose treatment involves all three workstations will have treatment information in three different places. Currently such treatment information is normally "linked" by a paper record or folder of the patient. This has not taken into account the hardcopy films of images that are stored separately in the film library, as is very common in radiotherapy departments. Were the paper record lost, then the patient treatment information would be "disintegrated." Using the DICOM and DICOM RT standards, the multimedia ePR system integrates patient information from different systems and a live summary of the patient's treatment record can be displayed as required. This can help archive patient information from different systems and save efforts and time in searching for records and films as well as safeguarding such loss.

23.8.2   Information Sharing

Most hospital information systems and subsystems have been organization-oriented or system-oriented rather than patient-oriented. This means that to query medical information of a patient, one may need to go through several systems. Also patient data collected in these systems are generally not widely available for immediate integration due to the differences in formats between workstations and systems. This situation becomes worse if consultation is required across institutions. The lack of an integrated database causes discontinuities in care and often results in redundant questioning or, worse, clinical decisions based on incomplete data. It also limits the ability to conduct clinical and research queries, including the creation of patient cohorts for prospective or retrospective studies. The multimedia ePR system in RT provides a platform for information sharing.

23.8.3   A Model of Comprehensive Electronic Patient Record

With the DICOM standard, PACS, and IHE (integrating the healthcare enterprise) now having matured, researchers are working toward incorporating medical images such as radiology images, endoscopy images, and microscopy images into the electronic patient records. However, the radiation therapy plans and records have not been taken care of since there does not exist yet a system with a common standard integrating multimedia that includes text, images, and graphics. This is because other than being image-intensive, radiation therapy is highly technical, and its use of radiation also involves radiobiological factors. All these parameters have to be recorded for future reference in the management of cancer patients treated by radiation therapy. Hence, other than textual information, all related treatment plans and images need to go into the patient's record. The DICOM RT standards are now set. It is a matter of implementation and refinement before radiotherapy information can be, like other images, linked to the electronic patient record to make it complete. The integrated concept and prototype system described in this chapter is a starting point to this initiative of completing the comprehensive electronic patient record.

23.9   UTILIZATION OF THE MULTIMEDIA ePR SYSTEM IN RT FOR IMAGE-ASSISTED KNOWLEDGE DISCOVERY AND DECISION SUPPORT

Currently in RT the practical use of imaging informatics tools is limited. DICOM is mostly used for transmitting PACS images to an RT system, and treatment planning systems are limited to dose computations and graphical data displays. Pertinent RT data results do not have a standardized protocol. The concept and prototype of the multimedia ePR system in RT address and can remedy these shortcomings. In addition the ePR system in RT can provide image-assisted knowledge discovery and decision support.

Figure 23.12 shows the overview of the methodology for developing image-assisted knowledge discovery and decision support based on the infrastructure of the

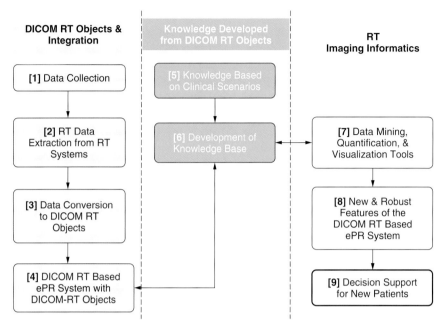

Figure 23.12   Medical Imaging Informatics approach toward development of decision-support tools for the DICOM RT based ePR system. Steps 1–4 were presented in Figures 23.5*B* and 23.6; steps 5–9 appeared in the figure are discussed in text. The long-term results are new and robust features for the ePR system to provide decision support for new patient cases. This methodology can be applied to different cancers as well as different types of RT treatments for prompt response of new decision-support tools. (Courtesy of Dr. B. Liu)

multimedia ePR system in RT. Steps 1 to 4 in the leftmost column of Figure 23.12 refer to the multimedia ePR system. Assuming that RT data objects are integrated and standardized within the ePR, steps 5 and 6 represent the development of knowledge extracted from the standardized RT objects. The knowledge defined is based on clinical RT workflow scenarios where the expert user assesses data to make a decision. Step 7 represents the development of decision-support tools based on the knowledge base. These tools can be data mining, quantification, or visualization tools for the knowledge database and can assist in the decision-making of the expert user within the RT workflow. The end result is represented by steps 8 and 9 where the tools naturally become new and robust features of the ePR and assist in the decision support for new cases once the historical RT data and knowledge are collected. Image-assisted knowledge discovery and decision support using imaging informatics methodology based on the ePR in RT is a current trend of research in radiation therapy.

23.10   SUMMARY OF THE MULTIMEDIA ePR IN RADIATION THERAPY

All radiation therapy vendors are moving toward implementing their information systems from a generated electronic patient record, be it complete or not. Nevertheless, such records are still in vendor-specific formats that may not be readily read in other systems. A major impeding factor is that DICOM RT records are still not implemented in most cases. This chapter provides the concept and framework for integrating all multimedia RT information using the DICOM and DICOM RT standards. Discussed are the image-intensive radiation therapy workflow, the DICOM RT standard, the RT database schema, and the infrastructure and components of the multimedia ePR system in RT. We use in this chapter the prototype multimedia ePR system in RT developed at the Hong Kong Polytechnic University to demonstrate the concept and components in the ePR system. Easy-to-use graphical user interface windows in the Web client workstation are emphasized. Utilization of the multimedia ePR system to perform image-assisted knowledge discovery and decision support tools is the current trend in radiation therapy image informatics research.

We observe in this chapter that RT is image-intensive and requires input from multimedia. However, none of the input is required in real time. The time lag of receiving and integrating the data can be from seconds to minutes, hours, or even days; the importance criterion is data integration. Thus this criterion satisfies the condition of "static multimedia" discussed in Chapter 22. In the next chapter we present the concept of multimedia ePR in surgery, where the criteria are not only data integration but also some data acquisition and integration has to be performed in real time during the surgery. This type of multimedia ePR is classified as "dynamic multimedia."

References

Bidgood WD, Horii SC. Introduction to the ACR-NEMA DICOM Standard. *Radiographics* 12: 345–55; 1992.

Connolly T, Begg C. *Database Systems: A Practical Approach to Design, Implementation, and Management*, 2nd ed. Reading, MA: Addison Wesley; 1998.

Dennis A, Wixom BH, Roth RM. Systems Analysis Design. 3rd ed. Hoboken, NJWiley; 2006.

DICOM in radiotherapy. http://medical.nema.org/dicom/geninfo/brochure/.

DICOM Part 3: Information object definitions. http://medical.nema.org/dicom/2007/.

DICOM Standard 2003. http://medical.nema.org/dicom/2003.html.

DICOM Supplement 11: Radiotherapy objects, 1997.

DICOM Supplement 15: Visible light image for endoscopy, microscopy, and photography.

DICOM Supplement 29: Radiotherapy treatment record and media extensions; 1999.

DICOM Supplement 30: Waveform interchange.

DICOM Supplement 48: Intravascular ultrasound (IVUS).

DICOM Supplement 91: Ophthalmic photography SOP classes.

DICOM Supplement 102: Radiotherapy extensions for ion therapy.

DICOM Supplement 110: Ophthalmic coherence tomography (OCT) storage SOP class.

DICOM Supplement 122: Specimen identification and revised pathology.

Horii SC. Part Four: A nontechnical introduction to DICOM. *Radiographics* 17: 1297–1309; 1997.

Huang HK. *PACS and Imaging Informatics: Basic Principles and Applications*. Hoboken, NJ: Wiley-Liss; 2004.

IHE-Radiation Oncology Technical Framework. Vols. 1–2. Draft for trial implementation. ASTRO Integrating the Healthcare Enterprise, 18 Aug 2007.

Johns ML. *Information Management for Health Professions*, 2nd ed. Australia: Delmar; Albany, NY, 2002.

Kushniruk A. Evaluation in the design of health information systems: application of approaches emerging from usability engineering. *Comp Biol Med* 32: 141–9; 2002.

Kuzmak PM, Dayhoff RE. The use of digital imaging and communications in medicine (DICOM) in the integration of imaging into the electronic patient record at the Department of Veterans Affairs. *J Digit Imag* 13 (2 suppl 1): 133–7; 2000.

Law MYY, Huang HK, Zhang X, Zhang J. DICOM and imaging informatics-based radiation therapy server. *Proc SPIE CD-ROM*, *Med Imag*: 4685, 160–7; 2002.

Law MYY, Huang HK. Concept of a PACS and imaging informatics-based server for radiation therapy. *Comput Med Imag Graph* 27(1): 1–9; 2003.

Law MYY, Zhou Z. New direction in PACS training. *Comput Med Imag Graph* 27 (2–3): 147–56; 2003.

Law MYY, Huang HK, Zhang X, Zhang J. The Data Model of a PACS-based DICOM Radiation Therapy Server. *Proc SPIE on CD-ROM*, *Med Imag*: 5033, 118–29; 2003.

Law MYY. The design and implementation of a DICOM-based integrated radiotherapy information system. PhD thesis. Chinese Academy of Sciences; 2004.

Law MYY, Huang HK, Chan CW, Zhang X, Zhang J. A DICOM-based radiotherapy information system. *Proc SPIE on CD-ROM, Med Imag*: 5371, 118–29; 2004.

Law MYY. A model of DICOM-based electronic patient record in radiation therapy. *J Comput Med Imag Graph* 29: 125–36; 2005.

Law MYY, Liu BJ. DICOM-RT and its utilization in radiation therapy. *Radiographics*: 29: 655–667; 2009.

Law MYY, Liu BJ, L Chan, A DICOM-RT Based ePR (Electronic Patient Record) Information System for Radiation ePR in RadiationTherapy. *Radiographics*: 29: 961–972; 2009.

Nagata Y, Okajima K, Murata R, et al. Development of an integrated radiotherapy network system. *Int J Radiat Oncol Biol Phys* 34: 1105–11; 1996.

Palta JR, Frouhar VA, Dempsey JF. Web-based submission, archive, and review of radiotherapy data for clinical quality assurance: a new paradigm. *Int J Radiat* Oncol *Biol Phys* 57(5): 1427–36; 2003.

Ratib O, Swiernik M, McCoy JM. From PACS to integrated EMR. *Comput Med Imag Graph* 27(2–3): 207–15; 2003.

Schultheiss ET, Coia LR, Martin EE, Lau HY, Hanks GE. Clinical applications of picture archival and communications systems in radiation oncology. *Sem Radia Oncol* 7: 39–48; 1997.

Wasson CS. *System Analysis, Design, and Development: Concepts, Principles, and Practices*. Hoboken, NJ: Wiley; 2006.

CHAPTER 24

Multimedia Electronic Patient Record (ePR) System for Image-Assisted Spinal Surgery

The multimedia electronic patient record (ePR) system for image-assisted surgery consists of text, consent forms, imaged, waveforms, and graphics. We use the term ePR in this chapter for convenience. The criteria in multimedia are not only data integration but also some data acquisition and integration has to be performed in real time during the surgery. This type of multimedia ePR is classified as the "dynamic multimedia." Therefore the real-time component has to be considered rigorously and its handling and managing are different from the static multimedia.

For convenience, Figure 20.9 reproduced here as Figure 24.1, the center rectangle and the lower ellipse in orange color show the position of, and components involved in, the chapter.

In Chapter 23 the static multimedia ePR system in RT was presented as a concept and validated by using a laboratory prototype with 10 virtual patients. In this chapter the dynamic multimedia ePR system for minimally invasive spinal surgery (MISS) will be described. We start from scratch, step by step, to tell what is MISS, why it needs the ePR, how to design based on existing clinical workflow and parameters, implement, and deploy the system for daily clinical operation. The California Spine Institute (CSI) is the clinical partner for developing this system.

24.1 INTEGRATION OF MEDICAL DIAGNOSIS WITH IMAGE-ASSISTED SURGERY TREATMENT

24.1.1 Bridging the Gap between Diagnostic Images and Surgical Treatment

Imaging is traditionally used for diagnosis, from the imaging diagnoses, a treatment plan is then derived. The treatment can be of different methods, or a combination of different methods, like radiation therapy (see Chapter 23), surgery (this chapter), or drug treatment (not discussed in this book). This section discusses the concept of bridging the gap between diagnostic images and image-assisted surgical treatment in the sense that real-time multimodality images are acquired continuously, guiding the surgeon to perform the operation. The left side of Figure 24.2 shows the diagnostic

PACS and Imaging Informatics, Second Edition, by H. K. Huang
Copyright © 2010 John Wiley & Sons, Inc.

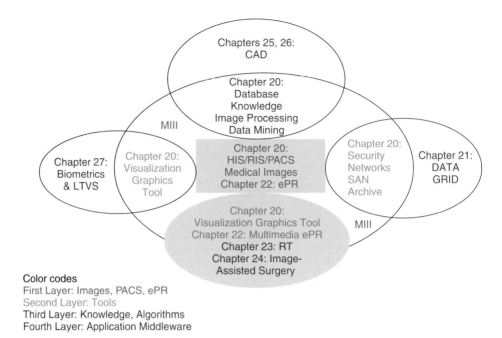

Color codes
First Layer: Images, PACS, ePR
Second Layer: Tools
Third Layer: Knowledge, Algorithms
Fourth Layer: Application Middleware

Figure 24.1   Imaging informatics data sources (rectangle), concepts, technologies, and applications (large and small ellipses) as discussed in Part IV (the largest ellipse) consists of the data sources and fundamental tools used by applications; Data Grid is for fault-tolerance medical image archive; SAN for storage area network; CAD for computer-aided detection and diagnosis; LTVS for location tracking and verification using biometric technologies; surgery for minimally invasive spinal surgery; RT for radiation therapy treatment and planning; HIS/RIS/PACS for medical images, and ePR for color codes refer to the five-layer informatics infrastructure shown in Figure 20.2. This chapter presents multimedia ePR system for image-assisted spinal surgery.

image domain and the right depicts the treatment domain. The arrow in the bottom bridging the chasm between these two domains creates a continuum between diagnosis and treatment in real-time. There are many imaging modalities shown at the left, and different treatment methods shown at the right. To simplify the discussion of the concept of multimedia ePR for surgery, we focus on the image-assisted minimally invasive spinal surgery (MISS). For this particular surgical procedure, in addition to the use of images, forms, waveforms, and textual data for planning the surgery, two real-time imaging techniques (digital fluoroscopic, DF) and endoscope video images (Endo), and more than half a dozen live vital signs of the patient during surgery are needed to assist and monitor the surgery. These data have to be acquired, displayed, and archived as well. The images are shown in blue fonts in both the diagnosis and treatment domains.

24.1.2   Minimally Invasive Spinal Surgery (MISS)

Back and neck pain is the price human beings pay for poor posture, prolonged sitting, lifting, repeated bending, obesity, and injury from accidents. This ailment gives

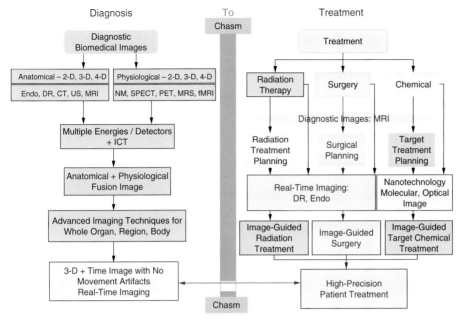

Figure 24.2 Creation of a continuum across the chasm from diagnostic images to treatment. Several years ago a patient was first diagnosed with imaging techniques, and the surgeon performed the surgery based on the diagnostic results; until recently it was rare that the surgeon performed the surgery guided (or assisted) by real-time images. The example in minimally invasive spinal surgery shows the surgeon performing the spinal surgery first based on diagnosis from 3-D MRI images (second row leftmost column under diagnosis, dark blue background box) and then under the guidance and assistance of two real-time imaging techniques. Endoscope and DR (fifth row leftmost column under treatments, light green background box).

the United States a massive economic headache. Approximately 85% of inhabitants of the Western world are afflicted with some degree of back or neck pain at some point in their lives. About 25% of our population has been incapacitated for two weeks or more due to back pain and an estimated 8 to 10 million people have a permanent disability from it. The economic impact is obvious. In most cases simple treatments such as bed rest, exercise, physiotherapy, and pain medication bring relief. Many sufferers are not so fortunate. If one or more of their vertebral discs ruptures and presses on nerve roots, the pain radiating from the back or neck and down the limbs can be incapacitating and severe. Until recently the only treatment was surgical removal of part of the ruptured disc, a major operation that required general anesthesia, the dissection of muscle, removal of bone, manipulation of nerve roots, and, at times, bone fusion. In an effort to overcome the disadvantages of traditional surgical techniques, the scientific medical community began exploring the use of endoscopy (arthroscopy) for minimally invasive spinal surgery (MISS) surgical operation.

An endoscope provides clear visualization and magnification of deep structures in real time. With the advancement of scientific technology and miniaturization, including fiber optics, video imaging technology, laser treatment, and experience gained through minimally invasive spinal surgery, there is a less traumatic disectomy procedure for some patients with disc problems. In the recent years development of image-guided surgery has improved the precision and reduced surgical tissue trauma. Figure 24.3 depicts the cervical, thoracic, and lumbar spines on MRI before (pre-op) and after (post-op) the endoscopic-guided spinal discectomy. The lesion(s) at each spinal region have clearly healed after the surgery.

24.1.3 Minimally Invasive Spinal Surgery Procedure

The patient scheduled for a MISS first went through a pre-op consultation after the surgeon determined the patient was fit for surgery. A pre-op consultation was done and all pertinent patient information and pre-op images were collected, studied, and entered into the patient's surgical file. A surgical team was then assembled, and the team met outside the operation room (OR) to review the MISS plan (Figure 24.4*A*); after the review the team entered the OR and prepared the patient for surgery (Figure 24.4*B*). The OR is shown in Figure 24.5 equipped with all necessary surgical devices including the DF and endoscopic imaging equipment. Notice that the figure shows the OR crowded with equipment, display systems, and personnel. External to the OR setup are the pre-op consultation information and images as well as real-time devices to be connected to the patient for monitoring and assisting in the surgery. Many separate real-time devices each with a separate display and archive are also seen.

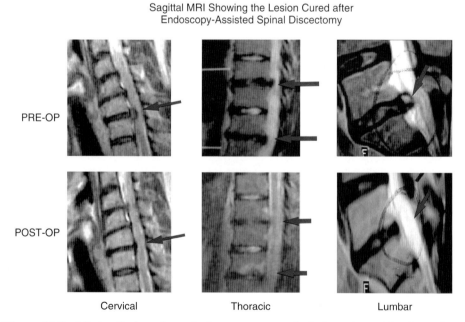

Figure 24.3   Minimally invasive spinal surgery on cervical, thoracic, and lumbar spines. Upper row: Pre-operation arrows show the areas where the disc protrudes the spine. Lower row: Post–endoscopic-assisted spinal surgery shows the lesions have been cured. (Courtesy of Dr. J. Chiu, CSI)

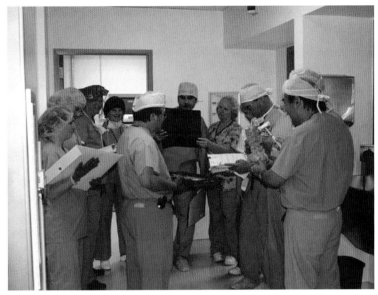

(A)

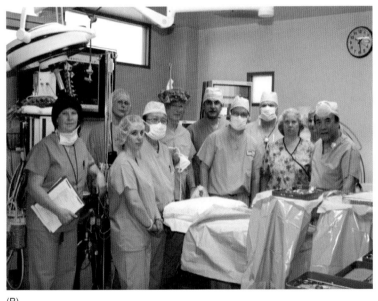

(B)

Figure 24.4 (*A*) Surgical team assembles outside the OR reviewing the surgical plan before the operation. (*B*) Surgical team is inside the OR preparing for the MISS procedure.

As the patient is readied for operation, all necessary live monitoring devices are connected to the patient (Fig. 24.6*A* and *B*). Depending on the type of spinal surgery, the minimally invasive spinal surgery (MISS) procedure is performed with the patient under a local anesthesia or in some situations, a brief general anesthesia. External real-time minimal exposure digital fluoroscopy (DF, Fig. 24.6*C*) is used to guide the

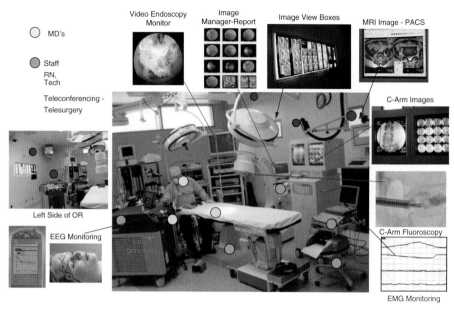

Figure 24.5 Traditional, present-day image-assisted OR suite for MISS operation with endoscopic imaging system and C-Arm digital fluorography for image-assisted operation. Notice the many live monitoring waveform devices scattered around the suite and the surgical video for documentation. In the periphery of the OR are the images, waveforms and other information used during the operation. With the design and implementation of the ePR described in this chapter, today's suite becomes a real-time image-guided MISS OR (see Fig. 24.12). (Courtesy of Dr. J. Chiu)

surgeon and pinpoint the exact location of the damaged disc based on the presurgical evaluation of the MRI's spinal scans. After the location of the problem disc is marked on the skin, a small hollow tube (about 6 mm) is inserted by the surgeon into the disc's space (Fig. 24.7A). An endoscope and a variety of MISS surgical instruments can be inserted through the hollow tube including miniature-forceps, curettes, trephines, rasps, burrs, cutters, and other types of probes (Fig. 24.7B) for disc decompression guided by real-time continuous endoscopic video images (Fig. 24.6D). Lasers are also used to shrink and tighten the disc and to remove portions of the protruded disc (Fig. 24.8). The procedure takes about 30 minutes per disc on average. The discectome, a hollow probe, is used to cut, suction, and remove (Fig. 24.9) small pieces of disc material until enough of the disc is removed to decompress the affected nerve root (Fig. 24.9, bottom right). The supporting structure of the disc is not disturbed. Upon completion, several sutures and a small Band-aid are applied to the external incision. The patient is then relocated to the recovery area for monitoring, and is discharged in about 45 minutes to one hour. This endoscopic procedure is also used currently for bony decompression in spinal stenosis. Based on more than 5000 patient studies in the California Spine Institute (CSI) in Thousand Oaks, California, endoscopic spine surgery has a patient satisfaction score of 91%, and a 94% success rate (for a single level of disc problem). The complication rate is much less than 1%, and the mortality rate directly from spinal disc surgery is zero (Figure 24.10).

24.1.4   The Algorithm of Spine Care

Image-guided minimally invasive spinal surgery (MISS) is a relatively new branch of neurosurgery that relies on multimodality images for guiding the surgical procedure. The surgical procedure is relatively simple and safe when performed by the expert, and with a rapid patient recovery time. The surgical procedure is much less painful, and the patient recovery time is shortened from months to days. Therefore MISS has gradually been replacing many unnecessary open spinal surgeries. Figure 24.11 shows the algorithm of spine care for degenerative and herniated spinal discs, and spinal stenosis; MISS has taken over the treatment of medium spinal disc aliments.

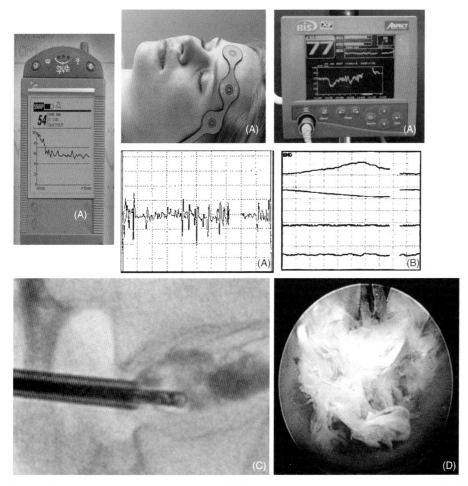

Figure 24.6   (*A*) Continuous conscious EEG monitoring with the computerized SNAP device (SNAP index or BIS Monitor) improves anesthesia and reduces drug requirement. (*B*) Continuous intra-op EMG monitoring prevents undue trauma to the spinal nerve to be decompressed. (*C*) Real-time C-Arm fluoroscopy during surgery for positioning of the endoscopy. (*D*) Real-time digital video endoscopic images, both static images and video clips. (Courtesy of Dr. J Chiu)

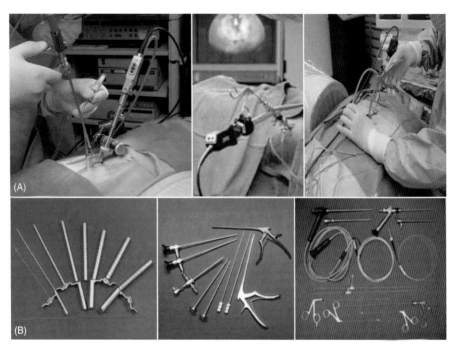

Figure 24.7 Location of problematic disc marked on the skin, with a small hollow tube (about 6 mm) inserted by the surgeon into the disc space (*A*). The location is verified by the C-Arm image. An endoscope (see the endoscopic image shown in the middle above the insertion) and a variety of MISS surgical instruments can be inserted through the hollow tube, including mini-forceps, curettes, trephines, rasps, burrs, cutters, and other types of probes shown in (*B*) during the image-assisted operation. (Courtesy of Dr. J. Chiu)

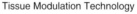

Tissue Modulation Technology

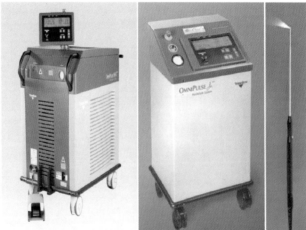

Figure 24.8 Tissue modulation technology, including Holmium YAG laser digital equipment and radiofrequency, among technologies that can be used for thermodisko-plasty. The lasers are used to shrink and tighten the disc and to remove portions of a protruded disc. The figure shows the laser generators and the right angle (side-firing) laser probe. (Courtesy of Dr. J. Chiu)

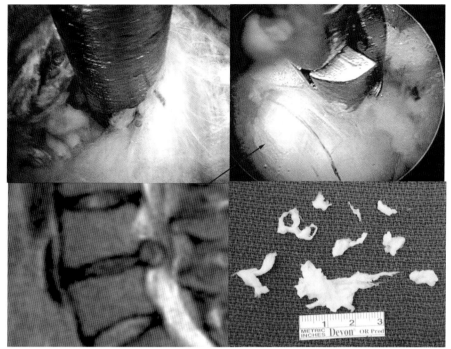

Large extruded L4 disc   Removed extruded disc fragments

Figure 24.9 Lower left: MRI sagittal view showing the large extruded L4 disc. Upper left and right: The lumbar endoscopic posterior lateral approach showing two endoscopic lumbar discectomy images with the lumbar nerve root in close proximity. Lower right: Removed extruded disc fragments.

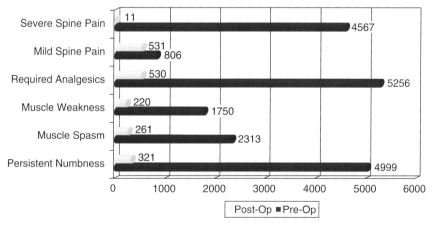

Figure 24.10 Minimally invasive endoscopic spine surgery (MISS) patient surgical outcome (symptomatic improvements) from 5373 patients performed by Dr. J. Chiu at the California Spinal Institute (CSI), Thousand Oaks, California.

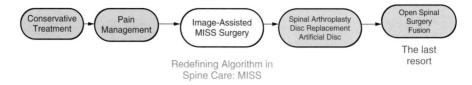

Redefining Algorithm in
Spine Care: MISS

Characteristics:

- Recovering time – 2 to 3 weeks
- Less invasive
- Patient can walk the same day after surgery
- Average of 30 mins/vertebra

Figure 24.11 Algorithm of spine care for degenerative and herniated spinal discs, and spinal stenosis. Before MISS, the spine care ranged from conservative treatment to pain management to spinal arthroplasty disc replacement or artificial disc, and to open spinal surgery fusion. With MISS, there exists an additional option (yellow ellipse) offered before the patient has to choose between the other two extremes.

24.1.5 Rationale of the Development of the Multimedia ePR System for Image-Assisted MISS

Minimally invasive spinal surgery (MISS) will be the method of choice for future spinal surgery to treat cases of herniated lumbar discs, postfusion junctional disc herniation, neural compression, osteophytes, spinal stenosis, vertebral compression fractures, spinal tumor, synovial cysts, and other types of spinal traumas. Over the last few decades its popularity has been gaining as a preferred option of treatment because of the benefits it provides against open surgery. Despite the overall advantages of MISS compared to conventional open spinal surgery, there are challenges remaining in MISS due to (1) the scattered pre-, intra-, and post-op surgical data in data acquisition systems; (2) the difficulty of real-time data collection during the surgery; and (3) some lapses in the efficiency of surgical workflow. An integrated dynamic mode multimedia ePR system promises to be an ideal way to overcome these challenges. It should take MISS to a higher level of excellence by which surgical expertise in minimally invasive spinal surgery is combined with frontier advancements in imaging informatics. The outcomes will benefit those patients who, suffering from spinal pain, may recover much sooner with less cost and enjoy a better quality of life. In return, society benefits as a whole.

24.1.6 The Goals of the ePR

The two clear objectives of ePR are (1) to develop a totally integrated multimedia ePR system for image-assisted minimally invasive spinal surgery and (2) to deploy the ePR at CSI for daily clinical use. Multimedia integration means that all data collected for the patient from pre-op, intra-op and post-op will be acquired, displayed, and archived at each point of the surgical workflow. In intra-op, the data will be acquired, displayed, and archived in real time. Any record in the ePR can be retrieved instantaneously over the life time of the patient.

Figure 24.12 depicts the ePR prototype system running at the MISS OR of CSI, with two large LCDs (liquid crystal display), one for the pre-op consultation

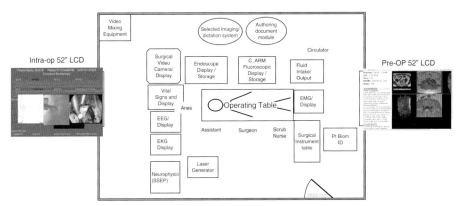

Figure 24.12 Schematic of the dynamic multimedia ePR system for image-assisted MISS. The ePR prototype system is running at the MISS OR of CSI, with two large LCDs, one for the pre-op consultation integrated display and the other for the live intra-op integrated display (compare to the existing OR shown in Fig. 24.5).

integrated display and the other for the live intra-op integrated display (compare to the existing OR shown in Fig. 24.5).

24.2 MINIMALLY INVASIVE SPINAL SURGERY WORKFLOW

24.2.1 General MISS Workflow

The MISS current high-level operation workflow that starts from presurgical consultation, proceeds to pre-operation preparation, intra-operation image, vital signs acquisition and display, and postsurgery documentation, and ends with patient recovery monitoring is shown in Figure 24.13. The workflow can be broken down into three phases: (1) before surgery; (2) during surgery (including the preparation); (3) postsurgery, which will be discussed below.

1. Before surgery (pre-op): Prior to the actual surgical procedure usually the patient presents with a problem and is evaluated by the physician to determine whether MISS is needed and whether it would be helpful to the patient. If this case is true, then a procedure is scheduled. At this stage the surgeon or surgeons in combination with the physician's assistant plan the surgical

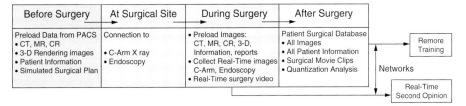

Figure 24.13 General workflow of the MISS procedure showing three different stages: before surgery (pre-op, green), patient preparation at the surgical site and surgical operation (intra-op, blue), and postsurgery (post-op, yellow).

procedure using digital diagnostic images such as CR, CT, and MRI. In addition to the information obtained from the medical studies, the patients fill out a set of questionnaires that determine the level of pain that they feel.

2. During surgery (intra-op): As the surgeon(s) operate on the disc(s) that need to be corrected, there is a significant amount of data being acquired that help monitor the body responses of the patient to the procedure. Video and image data are also acquired with the endoscope. A single vertebrae procedure lasts 30 minutes on average.

3. After surgery (post-op): As the patient recovers from surgery, the patient is continuously monitored in the recovery area to ensure all vitals signs are stable. In addition a set of tests are performed to assess the outcome of the surgical procedure, which includes an additional set of forms that the patient fills out.

The recovery period after surgery lasts from 45 minutes to one hour. The patient is then discharged. Therapy can begin the next day and the patient can go back to work within 2 to 3 days.

We will follow the basic general concept of software organization, high- and low-level database schema, data model, and data flow model presented in Section 22.6.2, to design and implement the multimedia ePR system for image-assisted MISS with the goals set in Section 24.1.6.

24.2.2 Clinical Site for Developing the MISS

The design and implementation has been in collaboration with the California Spinal Institute (CSI) in Thousand Oaks. CSI is a full self-sufficient independent spinal surgery institute and performs between 10 and 20 minimally invasive spinal surgeries per week. It has its own diagnostic imaging facility including conventional X-ray, CT, and MRI services and a commercial PACS. CSI also provides patients with the full in-house services for spinal surgery from pre-op consultation to post-op evaluation, check-up, and therapy. The concept of developing the multimedia ePR system for image-assisted MISS was conceived five years ago, but technologies were not available until recently. The go ahead development decision was made in early 2007.

Many parameters used in the design were based on daily clinical experiences at CSI during the past five years. The ePR system can be modified for MISS operation at other similar healthcare facilities, and image-guided surgery OR (operation room).

24.3 MULTIMEDIA ePR SYSTEM FOR IMAGE-ASSISTED MISS WORKFLOW AND DATA MODEL

24.3.1 Data Model and Standards

The data model of the ePR for MISS was designed to extend the DICOM data model because of its similarities to the existing medical imaging data at CSI utilizing DICOM. The same as the DICOM data model, the ePR for MISS follows the the patient longitudinally, the medical studies, their series, and images as indicated introduced in Figure 22.13. The modified data model utilized for the current ePR presented in this chapter provides additional entities that describe the data required for MISS. These elements are added to the data model to include the surgical procedure type, waveforms, the key image, questionnaires on pain tolerance, and user information on access to the system. The data model shown in Figure 24.14 will be revisited in later sections.

The standards used in the data model include DICOM (Digital Imaging and Communications in Medicine), HTTPS (hypertext transfer protocol secured), JPEG (Joint Photographic Expert Group), GIF (graphics interchange format), PNG (portable network graphics), and VGA (video graphics array, a display standard introduced in 1987 by IBM for use with IBM PC compatible personal computers). RS-232 (Recommended Standard 232) is used as the interface for each waveform device with the integration unit of the ePR.

24.3.2 The ePR Data Flow

The initial data flow utilized by the ePR system is based on the concept of the workflow presented in Figure 24.13 and detailed in Figure 24.15 where each numeral represents a data flow event. The timeline shows three phases: the pre-op image/data module, the intra-op module, and the post-op module. Each of these modules has four components: input module, input gateway, ePR server, and the visualization and display module.

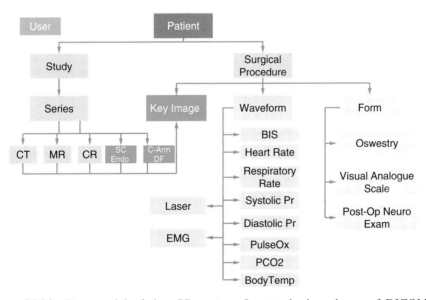

Figure 24.14 Data model of the ePR system. It extends the schema of DICOM to accommodate surgical information, including live waveforms and several standard surgical forms. Additional entities (green) have been augmented to the data model when it was introduced in Figure 22.13.

Data Flow of the Minimally Invasive Spinal Surgery ePR System

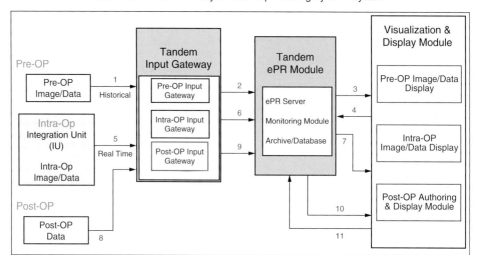

Figure 24.15 Data flow of the ePR system for MISS. There are three time stages—pre-op, intra-op, and post-op—and four operational modules—input units, gateway, ePR server and database, and visualization and display, which forms a 3 × 4 matrix. Each numeral represents one event in the data flow.

24.3.2.1 *Pre-Op Workflow* From Figure 24.15 we have the following workflow:

1. Historical medical imaging studies in DICOM format are acquired from the PACS.
2. The gateway, which is a component of the ePR system, receives the DICOM images and processes them accordingly. The original image is kept in the ePR and a JPEG version is utilized for display purposes via the Web interface of the ePR. All DICOM header information and metadata are extracted and recorded in the database.
3. Pre-op authoring is performed by the surgeon(s) and the physician assistants. The surgical procedure information is entered into the ePR. At this stage the patient's pain questionnaires are also entered into the system. The surgeon selects some key images and makes annotations on the key images that will ultimately be utilized during surgery. The authorized images/data are displayed in the OR utilizing a 52-inch LCD display.
4. Authorized images/data are archived in the ePR server and archive.

24.3.2.2 *Intra-Op Workflow* At steps 5, 6, and 7, the integration unit (IU) is connected to all clinical devices in the OR and continuously gathers live data signals during the surgical procedure. These signals are displayed in real time on a second large 52-inch LCD. At step 6, the gateway server receives the data from the IU and stores the data values and images at the database and the filesystem (see Fig. 24.16) temporarily.

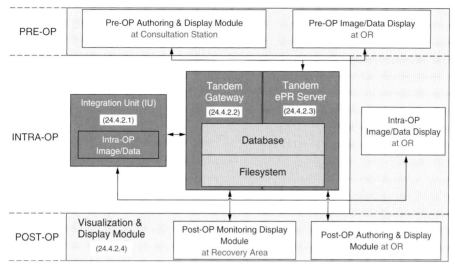

Figure 24.16   ePR system architecture showing three operation phases (first column), pre-op, intra-op, and post-op, as well as four operation modules (partitioned and scattered systematically). Some partitioned modules are bundled up together for ease of data transfer and tandem backup. The arrows show the data flow during the three phases of operation. The outside light gray color side-way U band is the display module backbone (Section 24.4.2.4) with five white rectangular box subunits. Inside the opening of the "U" in dark gray are the integration unit (IU, Section 24.4.2.1), tandem gateway (Section 24.4.2.2), and tandem ePR server (Section 24.4.2.3). Within the gateway and the ePR server, the database and filesystem software are interrelated and shared by both components.

24.3.2.3 Post-Op Workflow

8. While the patient is in the recovery area, the system continues gathering some vital signs that are transferred to the gateway server.

9. The gateway server receives the data and stores the data into the database temporarily.

10. The surgeon uses the post-op authoring module to create a final report out of the data gathered during the pre-, intra-, and post-op stages.

11. The final report will be kept in digital format at the ePR server as the patients' permanent surgical record.

24.4   MINIMALLY INVASIVE SPINAL SURGERY ePR SYSTEM ARCHITECTURE

24.4.1   Overall ePR System Architecture for MISS

Recall Figure 24.15, where the workflow and data flow model of the IG-MISS ePR system was represented by a 3 × 4 dimension matrix model. The three rows are pre-op, intra-op, and post-op workflow process stages, and the four columns are the input data integration unit (IU), input gateway, ePR server, and image/data display.

From the system architecture point of view, the ePR system should be designed for efficiency, effectiveness, and reliability of system operations. For these reasons, although system workflow is separated into pre-op, intra-op, and post-op stages, some modules that handle multiple workflow stages may be combined to share system workload and reliability. For example, the fault-tolerant requirement of each component in the system is better designed to support other existing components of the system for easy system backup and cost containment. Also, although there are four major components and three operational workflow phases in the ePR system, many of the software have similar design backbones, and some software may be bundled together for easier programming effort and faster system execution time. For these reasons the ePR system architecture is reorganized and modified from the data flow shown in Figures 24.15 and 24.16 for better system implementation and operation. Detailed examination of these two figures demonstrates the existence of four components and three operational workflow phases in both. However, some components in Figure 24.16 are bundled together for design and operational convenience. Section 24.4 describes the system design and architecture. Sections 24.5, 24.6, and 24.7 present the detailed technical descriptions of the pre-op, intra-op, and the post-op modules, respectively.

24.4.2 Four Major Components in the MISS ePR System

The four major components in the IG-MISS ePR system are (1) data input integration unit (IU), (2) fault-tolerant gateway server, (3) fault-tolerant ePR server, and (4) visualization and display. Both the input gateway and the ePR server include data storage and archive, system database, system security, system fault tolerance, continuous availability, and failover. The GUI and display module resides within the ePR server. All data input systems like medical imaging, surgical video, vital signs waveform recorders, and textual data recorder generate pre-op, intra-op, and post-op data, and they are all categorized as input data. The imaging and data systems that generate information are existing peripheral surgical supported equipment already within the OR, but they do not belong to the IG-MISS ePR system. However, the ePR system must integrate these systems in order to receive the input data that is acquired before, during, and after surgery to support the surgical procedure.

24.4.2.1 Integration Unit (IU)

Input Data and Archive   The integration unit is responsible for acquiring all data from different peripheral devices that are presented in the OR during surgery (intra-op) and to continuously measure all live vital signs, waveform signals, and surgical related images of the patient undergoing a procedure. The data acquired by the IU from all input devices are synchronized through a master clock and displayed live onto a customized interface using a 52-inch LCD screen (called intra-op live display) in the OR. The data gathered during surgery include the following:

- Digital C-ARM fluorographic images
- Digital endoscopic video images
- Surgical video

- Waveform signals: EMG (electromyography), BIS (bispectral Index), and vitals (blood pressure, heart rate, respiratory rate, pulseOX, body temperature, and partial pressure of carbon dioxide)

The images, videos, and data points mentioned above are transferred automatically and continuously from the various input sources of the different data systems in the OR during operation that are attached to the data input IU. The data are immediately saved in IU memory. The IU software displays the waveforms, images, and streamed videos properly every second (which is a default value) on the large intra-op LCD, and also makes a copy from the memory to the IU local hard drive with 1.5 TB (terabytes) of storage space every five seconds (which is also a default value). These two default values can be adjusted interactively depending on clinical demands.

Normal procedures for a single vertebra surgery takes about 30 minutes on average. The data are sent continuously to the gateway where the images are processed if needed and then placed in a data folder shared with the ePR server where they will be permanently archived. The data values are also extracted and saved to the ePR system database.

Out of Range Input Data Alert Message   In addition to the one second input display described in the last section, the IU features a rule-based alert-software that checks each input waveform for data that is out of the normal range. The IU has a set of rules based on clinical accepted medical practice that determines when a given signal is considered within the normal range for a patient (see Table 24.1). If at any given time during the surgical procedure, a signal falls outside the safe range, the IU will trigger an alert message on the intra-op live display (see Figure 24.22). The alert message prompts the surgeon and key personnel in the OR to take necessary actions during the surgical procedure. The values shown in Table 3.1 are considered normal values within the safe ranges for the signals used in the IU. However, those values might not be considered normal for all patients, so during the pre-op patient consultation time, the default values need to be revised and properly adjusted as necessary.

24.4.2.2 The Tandem Gateway Server   The functions of the input gateway are receiving, staging, managing, and transferring input data during the three workflow stages of the surgery: pre-op, intra-op, and post-op.

TABLE 24.1   **Default values for the safe ranges of the patient's vital signs during MISS operation used as indicators to set off alarms on the real−time intra−op display**

Signal	Lower Value	Upper Value	Units
Blood pressure	80	120	MmHg
Partial pressure	35	45	MmHg
Heart rate	60	100	Beats/minute
Respiratory rate	10	16	Breaths/minute
PulseOX	92		%
BIS	40	70	Score value
Body temperature	36.1	38	Celcius

Pre-Op Stage The gateway receives DICOM images and diagnostic reports from PACS. Once images are received by the gateway, a pre-op script is automatically launched by the gateway to properly extract all the information from the headers of the DICOM files. The data are then saved in the database. This whole process is automated at the gateway and does not require any user intervention.

Intra-Op Stage During intra-op, the gateway receives live data from the IU using an API (application program interface). The transfer protocol used is the HTTPS (hypertext transfer protocol secure) standard. Before any data is sent to the gateway, the IU needs to properly authenticate itself in order to avoid conflict with other possible input devices. Once the data are received by the gateway server, the API will place the data in a specific location in the ePR where a script will be executed to process the data accordingly.

Post-Op Stage During post-op, the patient is kept under observation in the recovery area by a nurse and the surgeon. The vital signs and other monitoring equipment are used to evaluate the patient's post-op condition. For the 45 minutes to one hour observation period, live data of the patient are continuously received and displayed at the bedside monitor by the post-op module.

24.4.2.3 The Tandem ePR Server

The ePR server is the heart of the IG-MISS ePR system, the basic components are shown in Figure 24.17. The ePR server is the front end of the system where the users will login to perform all the necessary tasks during the surgical workflow. The ePR server allows access to the pre-op authoring module, the pre-op display in the OR and the post-op authoring module (see Fig. 24.16). Administrative tasks such as giving the users access to the system, registration of patient information, scheduling, and fingerprint registration and identification are included.

The ePR, by definition, allows the participants to obtain any necessary information about the patient from a single interface, and that information follows the patient. The ePR goes beyond PACS because it not only shows information about the medical examinations for the patients but also any other related data such as clinical history, pain surveys, biometric information, and data acquired during the surgical procedure.

The ePR is developed utilizing PHP (PHP: hypertext preprocessor) as the backend programming language. The data values are stored using a MySQL database. The Web pages are structured with HTML (hyper text markup language), and they are styled using CSS (cascading style sheet). The interfaces are dynamically updated using JavaScript.

Data Storage and Archive and System Database Managing the data acquired by the ePR system is a critical task. A dual-system backup mechanism is implemented as follows (see Fig. 24.17): First, the ePR server has the server hardware, and the gateway has the gateway hardware. Two identical server software packages are implemented, one in the ePR server hardware as the primary and the other in the gateway hardware as the backup. By the same token, two gateway software packages are implemented, the primary package is in the gateway hardware, and the secondary package is in the ePR server hardware as the backup. As shown in the middle row

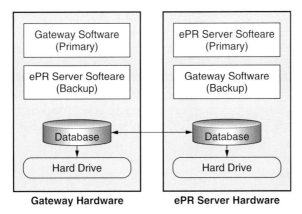

Figure 24.17 Tandem dual-system backup schema with two hardware pieces: gateway hardware and ePR server hardware. Each hardware piece has two softwares—ePR server software, and gateway software—and a tandem database with hard drive for data and metadata archive.

of Figure 24.16, the gateway and the ePR server each has its own hardware, where each hardware piece is housing both the ePR server software and the gateway software; one is the backup of the other. Figure 24.17 depicts the dual-system backup mechanism.

The input data first comes to the gateway hardware, where the gateway software categorizes them by images, live waveform information, and textual information. Images include DICOM images in their original DICOM format as well as in JPEG format for Web display, along with endoscopic videos, endoscopic single frame images, and digital C-arm fluoroscopic images. The metadata in the DICOM images and other data are stored in the database disks. All acquired data and metadata are immediately backed up by the ePR server hardware.

Database Schema   The database schema is another important component of the system; it contains all values and relationships of the data objects that are stored. Figure 24.14 shows the database schema and all relationships among data tables based on the DICOM data model standard. The database schema is supported by the filesystem shown in Figure 24.16 where the images (DICOM, jpeg, gif, etc.), videos, and text files are stored. The database holds all metadata, data values, and pointers to the location of the objects stored in the filesystem as well. This database schema was first introduced for an ePR for radiation therapy for the decision-support purpose discussed in Chapter 23.

System Security   The system security has been considered carefully during the design in order to comply with the HIPAA (Health Insurance Portability and Accountability Act) requirement. Only users who have been granted permission are allowed access to the system. At the same time the privacy of the communications are kept to prevent any unauthorized receiver from obtaining a patient's private information. To guarantee the security of the data, Web access to the ePR is established with HTTPS that encrypts all communication between the server and the clients (Web browsers).

In addition the ePR system handles permissions that allow users to perform different tasks on the system. Different user groups in the system have a different set of enabled permissions, but permission can be overwritten for an individual user by the system manager, if necessary, thus providing a level of flexibility.

Tandem System, Continuous Availability and Fail Over   The information that is kept in the ePR is unique and cannot be obtained from any other source if lost. Even images that were acquired from the PACS become unique once they were annotated in the ePR, so they cannot be found anywhere else. To overcome any possible lost of data, a fault-tolerant solution that replicates the data of the ePR to more than one place has been implemented. The primary gateway serves as the backup for the primary ePR server, and vice versa.

In addition to having the data stored with more than one copy, system redundancy with an automatic failover mechanism has been designed to access the data in case of failure of any component in the system and thus to guarantee system continuous availability.

24.4.2.4 Visualization and Display   The last of the four components in the ePR system is the graphic user interface (GUI) and display. In order to have the ePR system to be utilized as an effective tool that can improve the workflow of the surgery department, it is important to have a user-friendly GUI that presents all the necessary contents for the surgery in an easy-to-use manner. For this reason the ePR system is designed to operate in the three interrelated stages of a surgical procedure: planning (pre-op), surgery (intra-op), and patient recovery (post-op). The interface design between these three stages is critical. The display interface design (see Fig. 24.16) includes the main page, the pre-op display at the patient consultation room, the pre-op display at the OR, the intra-op display at the OR, the post-op at the patient recovery area, the post-op at the OR for surgical documentation, and the administrative pages.

Figure 24.18 shows the main page of the ePR system with the three workflow steps listed. Pre-op lists the surgical patients scheduled to be operated on; intra-op lists the next scheduled procedures of the patient; and post-op records the procedures performed on the patient in intra-op.

24.5 PRE-OP AUTHORING MODULE

The pre-op stage of a MISS procedure is where all necessary information prior to the surgery procedure is collected and organized in a patient e-folder. The pre-op occurs days prior to the surgery and involves querying, interviewing, collecting, and storing of presurgical medical images, patient demographic information, as well as other pertinent data value that can assist the surgery procedure.

24.5.1 Workflow Analysis

The pre-op software module details the following steps:

1. The patient goes to the surgery planning center where proper medical examinations are performed. Usually they are X-ray and MRI exams that are stored in

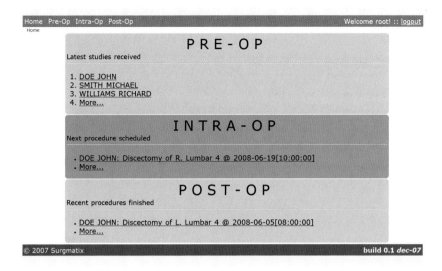

Figure 24.18 The home page of the ePR system showing the three surgical stages pre-op, intra-op, and post-op. The pre-op page shows there are three patients with pre-op consultations; the intra-op and post-op pages show patient John Doe being operated on.

the PACS. These images are then reviewed by a medical specialist to determine the proper treatment course.

2. Once the patient has been recommended for a MISS procedure, the patient visits the surgeon for a consultation session. At this point the patient registers in the MISS ePR system to have his/her fingerprint recorded for biometric verification and authentication. Also the patient fills out all the necessary forms on pain and clinical history, which are later entered into the ePR system.

3. Next the MISS clinical personnel create the surgical procedure planning in the ePR system (Fig. 24.19*A*). The ePR interface allows them to obtain studies from PACS if those images have not yet been downloaded onto the ePR server.

4. After the study is sent from the PACS to the ePR, the key images, including axial and sagittal MRI series images required for the surgical procedure, are selected and annotated by a physician assistant. The key images are labeled to properly identify the surgical region of the body.

5. The pre-op authoring phase is complete once all the necessary image and text information is entered into the ePR system; the information can be reviewed at the pre-op authoring and display module at the consultation workstation.

24.5.2 Participants in the Surgical Planning

The staff members at the MISS clinical site involved in the pre-op authoring module include the following:

1. Receptionists: They register the patient in the ePR system by entering the patient demographics, such as name, date of birth, sex, gender, patient ID, and

Pre-Op Consultation Procedure Information

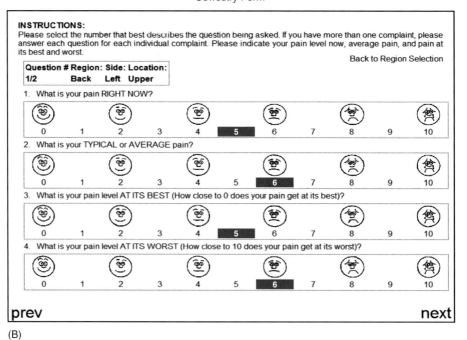

(A)

Oswestry Form

INSTRUCTIONS:
Please select the number that best describes the question being asked. If you have more than one complaint, please answer each question for each individual complaint. Please indicate your pain level now, average pain, and pain at its best and worst.

Back to Region Selection

Question # Region: Side: Location:
1/2   Back   Left Upper

1. What is your pain RIGHT NOW?

0 1 2 3 4 **5** 6 7 8 9 10

2. What is your TYPICAL or AVERAGE pain?

0 1 2 3 4 5 **6** 7 8 9 10

3. What is your pain level AT ITS BEST (How close to 0 does your pain get at its best)?

0 1 2 3 4 **5** 6 7 8 9 10

4. What is your pain level AT ITS WORST (How close to 10 does your pain get at its worst)?

0 1 2 3 4 5 **6** 7 8 9 10

prev   next

(B)

Figure 24.19 **A.** Based on the patient exam, history and recommendation, a physician assistant creates the surgical procedure planning in the ePR system pre-op module. **B.** Oswestry disability index, a survey to identify how the pain in the back or legs is affecting the patient in his/her daily activities.

the accession number, as well as the pain questionnaire results. They also take a fingerprint of the patient for biometric registration (used later at the OR for patient identification). They are in charge of scheduling the procedures and making sure there are no time conflicts.

2. Physician assistants: They retrieve presurgical PACS images of the patient using a query/retrieve function in the pre-op authoring and display module of the ePR system. After the images of the patient have been transferred to the ePR system, they select the key images that are to be used during the intra-op stage. At the display module they create the surgical procedures by entering annotations that would be later displayed with the images in the Pre-Op large LCD display monitor (52-inch) in the OR.

3. Surgeon: The surgeon approves the pre-op contents prior to display on the pre-op monitor in the OR. The surgeon works closely with the physician assistants to determine which images should be included in the procedures.

4. Administrators: They are in charge of assigning user access rights to the ePR system.

24.5.3 Significance of Pre-Op Data Organization

24.5.3.1 Organization of the Pre-Op Data
Traditionally surgeons have relied on their memory for locating the body region where the procedure is to be performed. They review the MRI and X-ray images the day before surgery and study the approach to be taken during the procedure. These images are also brought to the OR for reference. But they are displayed in hardcopy in an unorganized fashion scattered throughout the OR. The next few paragraphs focus on the organization of the pre-op patient information that requires the preparation process described earlier. This process is not done on the day of surgery; the information is saved days in advance with the display streamlined and organized for efficiency purposes.

24.5.3.2 Surgical Whiteboard Data
In addition to the input data described earlier, one type of pre-op data that is critical during surgery is the handwritten whiteboard information located at the entrance of the OR that contains a very short summary of the patient such as name, gender, age, weight, height, any allergies, comorbidity, and pain. The pre-op authoring module described has been designed to integrate the whiteboard information onto the same pre-op screen for display in the OR during the surgery. The following survey measures are included:

1. Visual analog scale (VAS): This a psychometric response scale to describe the amount of pain a patient is feeling from a specific part of her/his body.

2. Oswestry disability index: This is based on the patient's responses to the pain survey used to identify how the pain in the back or legs is affecting the patient in his/her daily activities (Fig. 24.19B).

24.5.4 Graphical User Interface

The ePR system is designed to be user-friendly but effective at the same time. So a criterion of the user interface is to minimize the number of mouse clicks needed to perform a certain task and to aggregate information adequately into a single interface whenever possible. The current pre-op authoring module is a self-contained interface where the users can download, edit, add, and delete the contents as needed. The pre-op has two major interfaces, one for editing and one for display in the OR.

24.5.4.1 Editing

To Create a Procedure   The interface allows the users to create the surgical procedures by first selecting the key images as well as adding annotations to those key images as shown in Figure 24.20*A*. On this screen the PACS image and surgical procedures are combined into one display in the pre-op module. Image studies related to the surgical procedure are shown on the left-hand side based on the surgical data model (see Fig. 24.20*A*). To view an image in a study, the users can either drag

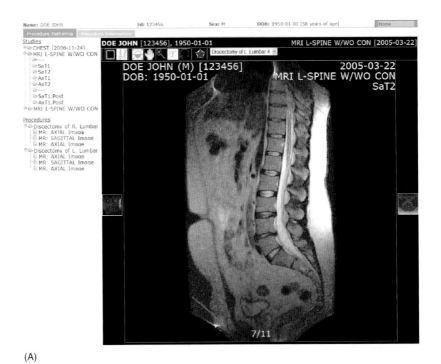

(A)

Figure 24.20   (*A*) Pre-op authoring module page. The upper left-hand text list depicts the surgical data model showing the studies and procedures. After the user clicks on an item in the list, the proper image, in this case, a sagittal MRI, is shown on the right. (*B*) The neuronavigator tool allows the correlation of the position of the lesion in the sagittal (left) and the axial view (right). The red lines are the two corresponding sagittal and axial sections. (*C*) The pre-op display organized during patient consultation as seen on the pre-op display monitor in the OR during intra-op. Top left: Whiteboard information; Bottom left: Extracted patient history summary. Right: Images and annotation during pre-op consultation (see Fig. 24.12, right) (*D*) Method of extracting pertinent and concise clinical history information by highlighting (yellow) the full report during pre-op editing (compared to (*C*), left). The extracted concise information is for display with the whiteboard information shown in (*C*) during intra-op.

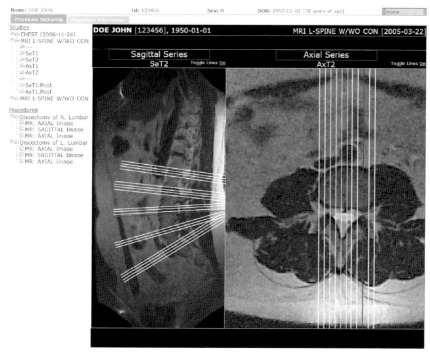

(B)

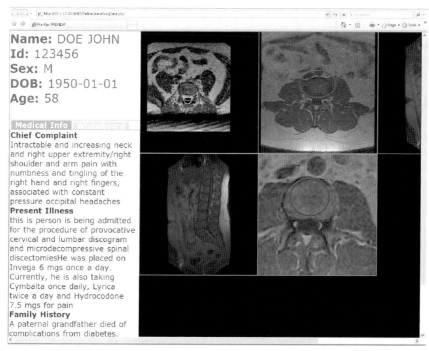

(C)

Figure 24.20 (*Continued*)

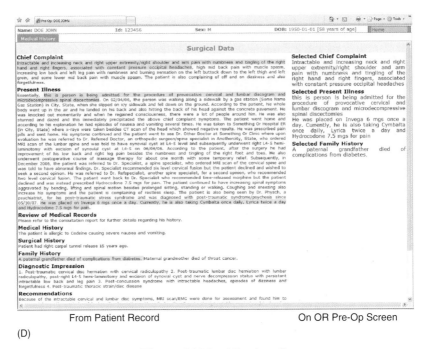

From Patient Record   On OR Pre-Op Screen

(D)

Figure 24.20 (*Continued*)

the study shown in the list at the left to the viewing pane on the right-hand side or double-click on the study from the list at the left. Figure 24.20*A* displays a sagittal MRI image with patient's ID above the image. The toolbar with icons at the top of the viewing pane allows the users to perform certain tasks accordingly to the current status of the editing module.

To Perform Editing

1. To view images in a study: The two icons on both the right and the left sides allow the user to preview images in the study series.

2. To perform image manipulation: The toolbar for the pre-op includes some basic image manipulation tools such as window/level, pan, and zoom. With this functionality, the images can be displayed optimally at the exact location of the lesion.

24.5.4.2 The Neuronavigator Tool for Image Correlation   During a MISS operation the axial view has to be correlated with the corresponding sagittal view of an MRI. The neuronavigator tool in the pre-op module allows such correlation through the display, as shown in Figure. 24.20*B*.

24.5.4.3 Pre-Op Display   A MISS surgical procedure requires multimedia data during the pre-op stage, including patient history, images, and consultation results. These data should be organized and displayed in the pre-op display during surgery. An example is shown in Figure 24.20*C*, which depicts the whiteboard information outside of the OR (top left), the extracted clinical history of the patient (bottom left),

as well as the key images selected from the MRI study with their annotations during consultation (right). The term that is used for this display is the pre-op display since the pre-op authored data is actually displayed during the intra-op workflow stage.

24.5.4.4 Extraction of Clinical History for Display   Figure 24.20*C* depicts the extracted clinical history of the patient from a detailed report for display purpose during the intra-op. Figure 24.20*D* illustrates the method of extraction by highlighting (yellow) the full report during the pre-op editing (compared to Fig. 24.20*C*).

24.6 INTRA-OP MODULE

24.6.1 The Intra-Op Module

The intra-op stage is defined by the time that it takes for the surgical procedure is accomplished by the surgeon in the OR. All information collected during the pre-op are displayed in the pre-op monitor in OR. In addition live data from different input devices during the surgery are collected by the integration unit (IU) and displayed on the intra-op monitor. Before the surgery starts, the patients' fingerprint is captured in the OR and verified with the biometric data acquired during the pre-op stage. This is an important step toward reducing error and ensuring correct patient identification prior to surgery.

24.6.2 Participants in the OR

In addition to their standard assigned surgical tasks, the surgical personnel involved in the ePR intra-op module include:

1. Surgeons and medical staff: The chief surgeon operates on the patient and makes decisions based on the ePR pre-op and intra-op displays while the procedure is taking place. Other surgeons and medical staff would alert the chief surgeon based on alert messaging on the intra-op display. Thus the ePR system facilitates their multiple tasking by displaying any relevant information in an organized and efficient easy-to-view way.
2. Anesthesiologist: He/she provides anesthesia to the patient and monitors the vital signs during the procedure.
3. Nurses and technicians: Each has assigned tasks to perform during the surgery. In particular, these are activating the pre-op ad intra-op displays, verifying the identity of the patient by biometric means, turning on and off DF and endo imaging systems.

24.6.3 Data Acquired during Surgery

During surgery, while the surgeon is operating, all important live data are automatically acquired and saved by the IU (see Fig. 24.16) as follows:

1. BIS (bispectral index system): BIS signals comes from an array of electrodes that are attached to the patient's forehead and monitor the patient consciousness. The value that comes out is in the range of 0 to 100, where zero means

no brain activity and 100 is full consciousness. The safe range is considered to be between 40 and 70. Currently the output data from this device is obtained from a serial port (RS232).

2. Vital signs: The data obtained from the vital signs device include the respiratory rate, the heart beat rate, the temperature, the blood pressure, the pulseOX and the CO_2 respiratory emission levels of the patient (see Table 24.1 for other possible data). Currently the data output from this device is obtained from a serial port (RS232).

3. EMG: The electromyography (EMG) device monitors the electrical activity of the muscles and nerves through a set of small needles inserted into the patient's body with the goal of preventing damage to the spinal cord while the surgeon is operating with the endoscope. Currently the real-time output data from this device is obtained from an Ethernet connection.

4. C-arm fluoroscopic images: The C-arm imaging device takes X-ray images that assist the surgeon to pinpoint the exact position of the spinal column where the lesion is located in real-time with respect to endoscopic probes. These images are also encapsulated in a DICOM file and sent to the ePR.

5. Endoscopic images and video: The MISS procedure is performed using an endoscope through a small incision (6 mm) made on the patient's body. The video stream of the camera inserted in the endoscope is displayed continuously on the intra-op live display and is also saved in the IU for later review. At the same time the IU takes snapshots of the endoscopic video and saves them as images at the same pre-assigned default time interval as the other live data being acquired. The resolution of the video and images can vary from vendor to vendor; currently the ePR system is acquiring the output in the VGA (video graphics array) standard with a resolution of 640×480 pixels. The output data from this device is obtained from an S-video port.

6. Laser: The laser is inserted in the endoscope and is used to cauterize a wound inside the body for both cutting and healing purposes, but its usage depends on the type of treatment. The current available output from this device is from a serial port (RS232).

24.6.4 Internal Architecture of the Integration Unit (IU)

Figure 24.21 shows the interconnectivity between the existing input devices presented in the OR during surgery (see Fig. 24.15 workflow step 5). The left-hand side shows the data inputs or sources, as explained in the previous section; the middle is the IU, and the right-hand side depicts the connectivity between the IU and the intra-op live display monitor. The pre-op display shown at top right (yellow) also presents in the OR. The current setup allows the IU to support the available input devices at the implementation site at CSI, but the IU has been designed to be flexible enough to support various vendors' input devices using different interfaces (serial ports, VGA, Ethernet, etc.).

As seen in the figure, there is an interactive input device called the surgeon keypad that permits surgeons to manage some functionality of the IU. With this keypad the surgeon can take a screenshot of all the data and images any time during the surgery, and it can also be used to have a side-by-side freeze frame display of the endoscopic

Intra-Op Workflow of the Integration Unit (IU)

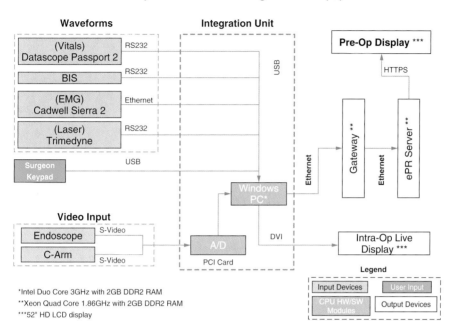

Figure 24.21   Hardware and software interconnectivity diagram for a MISS procedure using the ePR system. During Intra-op live data are continuously displayed on the intra-op monitor. A system default allows the live intra-op data to be acquired at a specific time interval. The surgeon has an option to acquire additional data during the entire course of operation by pushing the surgeon keypad (green). The IU in the middle column accepts different input devices and sends them to the intra-op live display (lower-right, yellow).

video with a prior endoscopic screenshot for comparison purposes. This feature will facilitate the surgeon to obtain patient documentation during post-op patient reporting.

24.6.5 Interaction with the Gateway

During the surgery, the IU saves all the data acquired temporarily from different connected devices in its hard drive; after completion of the surgery, the IU connects and sends all data to the gateway server. The protocol used to send the data is HTTPS. If the primary gateway is down, the IU will try to connect to the secondary gateway, which is the ePR server for failover (see Fig. 24.17 for the data backup schema). To reduce the total sending time, the data are compressed and combined in a single zip file. Once the data are correctly received by the gateway server, the fill is then uncompressed and processed accordingly.

24.6.6 Graphical User Interface

Figure 24.22 shows the intra-op live display of a patient with waveforms and images. The horizontal axis is time. There are eight groups of waveforms: six vital signs with heart rate, blood pressure, respiratory rate, pulse oxygen concentration, $pCO2$, plus

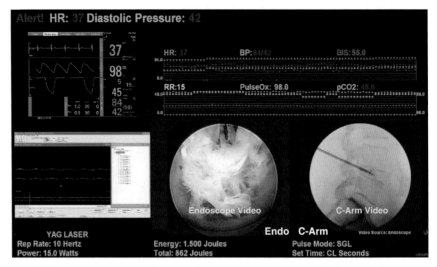

Figure 24.22   Example of the intra-op live display as seen on the intra-op large monitor in OR (see Fig. 24.12, left). (Top row) Eight waveforms of six vital signs, plus BIS, and IVF with digital values. Alert message on low HR & Diastolic pressure; the horizontal axis is time. (Middle row from left to right). Waveform of EMG, endoscopic images, and fluoroscopic image; (bottom row): Laser output values.

temperature, and BIS, IVF (intravenous fluid). Every dot in the waveform represents a data point over a one second interval. Also displayed the C-Arm fluoroscopic (right) and the endoscopic video images (middle), and EMG waveforms at the left. Last, laser energy is given in joules shown in the bottom row. The video is updated on the intra-op live display with a frame rate of 30 per second (a default value).

24.6.7 Rule-Based Alert Mechanism

If a signal falls outside its safe range, a three stage mechanism will alert personnel in the OR about that situation.

1. Warning mode: If a numeral falls outside the safe range, it will change color to red (as seen with the pulseOX and blood pressure in Fig. 24.22).
2. Emergency mode: If the condition falls to a value greater or lower in 25% of the safe range then the intra-op live display will place an alert message at the top of the screen.
3. Critical mode: If the data signal value is either greater or lower in 50% to the values in the safe range, then the alert message will cover the whole screen.

24.7 POST-OP MODULE

24.7.1 Post-Op Module

The post-op stage takes place after the completion of the surgical procedure. There are three time substages: (1) patient in the recovery area and then discharged, (2) the surgeon documents the surgical results, and (3) follow-up pain questionnaires.

24.7.2 Participants in the Post-Op Module Activities

The personnel involved in the post-op module activities include the following:

1. Surgeons: The chief surgeon reviews the patient's ePR record, including pre-op, intra-op, and post-op files and images, and then dictates the surgical report. He/she also determines which images from the ePR should be included in the report. They are ultimately responsible for the contents of the report.
2. Physician assistants: They assist the surgeon in creating the surgical report.
3. Nurses and front-desk personnel: They perform follow-up surveys several times after the surgery, and enter the pain data from patient questionnaires into the ePR system as a follow-up on the progress of the patient.

24.7.3 Patient in the Recovery Area

While the patient is in the recovery area, some of the patient's vital signs (pulseOX, heart rate, and blood pressure) are still being recorded with the Vitals devices and can be displayed on the recovery monitor within the recovery area (see Fig. 24.16). In addition the patient is questioned by a nurse about immediate pain levels before being discharged, as a follow-up monitoring of the surgery's effectiveness. These data are entered into the ePR post-op module for statistical outcome studies in the patient recovery record.

24.7.4 Post-Op Documentation — The Graphical User Interface (GUI)

The surgeon performing the post-op documentation can retrieve information from the post-op module pertinent to the surgery using the GUI. This process involves four major steps:

1. Finding the patient from the ePR system: The correct patient can be found from the ePR by clicking the first line of the bottom block section of GUI (Fig. 24.18).
2. Selecting images: From this GUI, the surgeon can select endoscopic images that will be included in the final report by clicking on the star at the top left-hand corner of the viewing pane. In Figure 24.23 that image is selected for the final report.
3. Selecting waveforms: The waveforms are displayed at the bottom of the GUI (Fig. 24.23). They can be dynamically selected by clicking on their corresponding boxes at the upper right-hand side of the interface.
4. Data synchronization: A blue slider at the bottom of the graph (Fig. 24.23) allows for synchronized viewing of all the image and waveform data being displayed.

Figure 24.23 presents a documentation page that has been authored by the surgeon from the ePR system using the post-op GUI. The data displayed and documented include an endoscopic image, heart rate, diastole and systole blood pressures, respiratory rate, BIS score value, oxygen pressure, partial pressure of CO_2, and temperature.

Live Intra-Op Data Saved in Real Time in the ePR during Surgery for Post-Op Patient Document

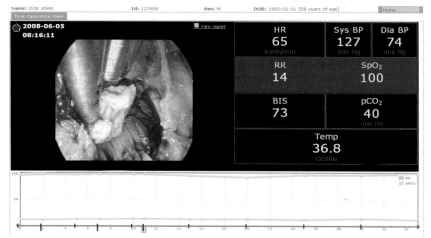

Figure 24.23   Post-op authoring module displaying a post-op document showing data acquired during the surgery. This page can be synchronized by the surgeon's post-op dictation. It is in PDF format for easy insertion into the report. The red time marks at the bottom are default intra-op data capture. Blue marks are additional data the surgeons saved during the surgery. The green mark represents the time frame when this page was captured.

There are also two curves shown in the bottom (respiratory rate and pulseOX); these are waveforms obtained from another intra-op device.

During the documentation the surgeon also dictates the report, which will be synchronized with the authorized image and waveform paged.

24.7.5 Follow-up Pain Surveys

Nurses and front-desk personnel take pain surveys several times after the surgery and enter the survey data into the post-op module of the ePR system as a follow-up of the progress of the patient. The collective information can be used for future patient outcome analyses.

24.8 SYSTEM DEPLOYMENT AND USER TRAINING AND SUPPORT

The prototype system was deployed in August 2008 to the California Spine Institute (CSI) located in Thousand Oaks, California, which is the only clinical site in southern California that performs MISS. This section summarizes the highlights.

24.8.1 System Deployment

24.8.1.1 Planning and Design Phase   The ePR system for MISS was developed at the IPILab, Department of Radiology, USC, IPI and CSI have had close collaboration for more than five years. There are three phases of the implementation.

First, to test the functionality of the ePR system, a prototype for each of the ePR components was developed and integrated at the CSI research facility; in addition mock-up data were collected at CSI that included an intra-op signal simulator for the IU device. Second, once the system was tested fully in the laboratory environment, it was deployed in the OR to obtain user feedback and clinical evaluation. The hardware and software components consisted of the gateway server, the ePR server, the IU, and fingerprint readers. Other software packages included the ePR Web pages, the IU application, the fingerprint application, the database, and the Web server.

The final stage of the clinical implementation was to deploy the ePR system in the OR. This stage was challenging. Since the OR was continuously in use for MISS, both the clinical team and the engineering team have to work together to circumvent the clinical schedule, and minimize the risk of any possible disruption of the clinical service, through coordinating of various tasks among the team members. This was especially difficult in the final stage of implementation, when the ePR was commandeered for some regular duties usually handled by the traditional surgical method.

24.8.1.2 Hardware Installation   The ePR and gateway servers were installed at CSI on a rack at their server room. Figure 24.24*A* shows the installation in progress

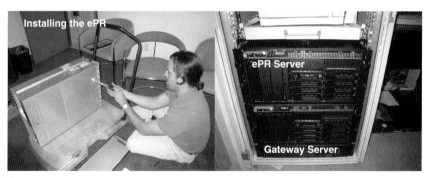

(A)

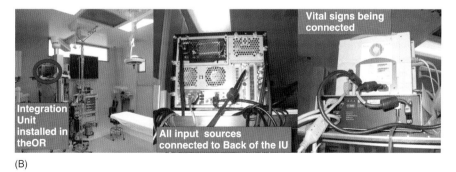

(B)

Figure 24.24   (*A*) ePR server installation at the server room of CSI. Dr. J. Documet is shown installing the servers. (*B*) Left: Integration unit (IU, inside the red ring) installed in the OR and connected to different input sources. Middle: Input units cables are connected to the back of the IU. Right: Vital signs of device is being connected.

and the final location of the servers. In addition to these two servers, the IU was also installed in one of the ORs at CSI. Recall that the IU needs to be connected to all required peripheral devices that are presented in the OR for monitoring the real-time patients' response during the clinical procedure. The IU, located in the OR, and its connection to input devices are shown in Figure 24.24*B*.

24.8.1.3 Software Installation   Once the servers were installed at the clinical facility, the next step was to configure all necessary software components of the ePR system. Those components included:

1. ePR server: A Web application that provides the user interface for the pre-op and post-op authoring module and the pre-op display (during surgery) as well. In addition this server requires the installation of the Web server (Apache) and the database (MySQL).
2. Gateway server: A listener software that receives incoming DICOM studies sent from the PACS and a set of scripts to extract the metadata information and store it at the database. This server also receives the real-time surgical data, including live images and waveforms collected during a surgical procedure, which are sent by the IU using an API.
3. Integration unit: It acquires the surgical data in the form of data points, images, and videos from the surgical peripheral devices at the OR. A program developed in C++ is utilized to make low-level system calls to the different interfaces, depending on performance requirements to display real-time data in the OR.
4. Fingerprint module: The registration and identification of patients at the clinical facility is performed during the pre-op stage and the identification and verification at the intra-op stage. This module makes use of a fingerprint SDK (Software Development Kit) from CrossMatch.

24.8.1.4 Special Software for Training   Training the users of the ePR system was a primary objective during deployment, Section 7.3 explains this task in more detail. Training software was installed that allowed the users to be trained more effectively and efficiently.

24.8.2 Training and Supports for Clinical Users

The following users were among those trained on the use of the ePR system:

1. Surgeons: Training was provided on the pre-op and post-op authoring modules (post-op was demonstrated using mock-up data), on how to use them by adding, editing, and deleting contents. In addition surgeons were taught how to interpret the two large pre-op and intra-op LCD displays.
2. Physician assistants: Both group and individual training sessions were held on the pre-op authoring module, including query/retrieve functionality, image manipulation, key image selection, procedure management, and annotations for key selected images.

3. Nurses: Nurses were trained how to enter information related to the patient's whiteboard data and survey forms.

4. Front-desk assistants: Front-desk assistants received training on the scheduling of surgical procedures, input of pain surveys for pre-op and post-op stages as well as patient registration, which included registration of patients' fingerprints.

5. Technicians: The training given to technicians included verifying the patients' identity at the OR using the fingerprint module. In addition they were instructed on how to read the data presented on the LCD monitor displays at the OR.

6. Administrative staff: Administrative personnel were given training on how to add or remove a user from the ePR system and how to manage the consent documents for different procedures.

The engineering team provided three months on-site training on the ePR system and assisted the duty staff in preparing the pre-op module. Figure 24.25 shows both the group and individual training for pre-op and intra-op. As for the post-op, the module has been released to the surgeons and physician assistants for clinical use, system refinement for report authoring in continuing.

24.8.3 Experience Gained and Lessons Learned

Much of the experience gained and the many lessons learned in developing the multimedia ePR for image-assisted MISS are similar to those of earlier times when PACS was developed and deployed in radiology departments, and later to hospitals. However, there are some differences, since the ePR users are mostly local and not at large enterprise type hospitals. Some issues encountered are listed below with comments on the differences and similarities between them whenever appropriate.

1. *Lack of standards from peripheral data and imaging devices used in the OR.* A major obstacle during the implementation phase was that many vendors sold peripheral devices to ORs where no data format or communication standard compliance was required. Different vendors export their data in different ways, adding complexity to the mechanisms for data retrieval and limiting the interoperability to certain vendors and products. In imaging, most ORs still use pre-op hardcopy for reference during surgery. For image-assisted surgery, the intra-op endoscopic and C-Arm radiographic images are for assisting the surgeon during the surgery, and there is no requirement for keeping hard or soft copies for surgical documentation. The multimedia ePR system for MISS, on the other hand, keeps all live data during the surgery in the database, and so will be selected by the surgeon to include in the patient report during post-op authoring. Therefore a major challenge in acquiring data came from real-time peripheral devices, and also from endoscopic images and C-Arm radiography in the OR during surgery. In the PACS installation, similar problems occurred in the imaging modalities connectivity, but this issue was resolved by the mandated compliance to DICOM standard in almost all the purchases in imaging systems and PACS in the late 1990s. The development of the integration unit (IU) in the ePR system prototype is the first step toward all devices being integrated. Several years down the road, surgical OR may see the advantages

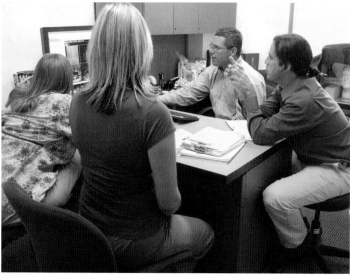

(A)

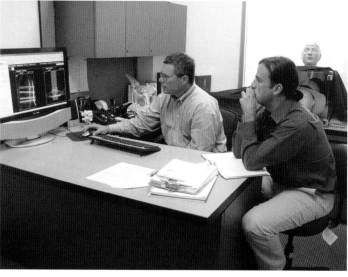

(B)

Figure 24.25 Training of the ePR system for the clinical staff at CSI. (*A*) Group training in pre-op authoring at the consultation room. (*B*) One-to-one training at the consultation room on GUI. (*C*) Training of the integration unit (IU) at the OR for input devices connectivity. The engineer is behind the IU.

of data integration in the ePR and enforce vendors to output data with certain standards.

2. *Different clinical environment was from the laboratory environment.* When the ePR prototype was moved from the laboratory environment to the clinical site, the engineering team encountered a culture shock. In the laboratory, the

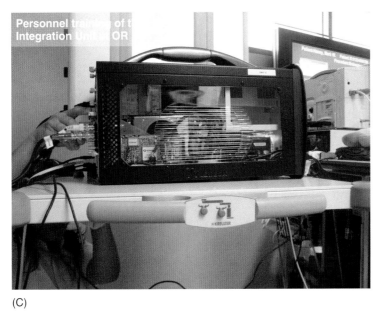

(C)

Figure 24.25 (*Continued*)

environment was under control and debugging and modifications could be performed easily. In the clinic, the reality of the real world sank in, and it was very difficult to make modifications for two reasons: (1) once the ePR was installed, clinical use of the system was given the highest priority, and any modifications were of secondary interest; (2) users were reluctant to continuously adopt new changes. Unlike the PACS installation, which had long passed its R&D mode, nowadays a prototype system should rarely be installed in a clinical site without extensive testing at the manufacturer's site first.

3. *Clinical institution not always in control of its computer and ICT (information and communication technology) equipment.* Installing new applications in clinical computers might sometimes require administrative privileges. In addition, configuring and adding new servers to CSI might need to be performed by a third party IT (information technology) team, which can cause implementation issues. This was the case with many PACS installations as well.

4. *Users acceptance.* Whenever a new application in the ePR was implemented at CSI, users were reluctant to fully embrace the new application. This is because the new application would temporarily disrupt their normal routine clinical workflow even though they knew that the system would improve their clinical workflow in the long run. User acceptance is easier in PACS now, since the healthcare community has gained more than 15 years of experience.

5. *Graphical user interface challenging for new users.* When a new application is developed, training is crucial for users not familiar with the interface and functionality. This issue is 100% the same as with PACS for a first-time user or when a new PACS or new GUI is installed.

24.9 SUMMARY OF DEVELOPING THE MULTIMEDIA ePR SYSTEM FOR IMAGE-ASSISTED SPINAL SURGERY

We have taken a step-by-step approach to introducing the development of a multimedia cPR system for imaging-assisted minimally invasive spinal surgery (MISS). We started by introducing MISS, the three stages of MISS workflow in pre-op, intra-op, and post op. The ePR architecture was developed using a (three time modules) × (our hardware and software components) model. The three time modules are the pre-op, intra-op, and post-op, and the four components are the input integration unit, fault-tolerant gateway server, fault-tolerant ePR server, and the visualization and display component. A prototype was then built and deployed to a MISS clinical site with user training and supports for daily use. The special experience gained in the clinical setting provided valuable lessons on developing the system and on how the multimedia ePR methodology can be extended to other image-assisted minimally invasive surgery.

References

Apache Web server. Apache Software foundation. http://httpd.apache.org.

Blum T, Padoy N, Feussner H, Navab N, Workflow mining for visualization and analysis of surgeries. *Int J CARS* 3: 379–86; 2008.

Chiu JC. The decade of evolving minimally invasive spinal surgery (MISS) and technological considerations. *Internet J Mini Invasive Spinal Technol* 2(3); 2008

Chiu J. Technological developments for computer assisted endoscopic minimally invasive spinal surgery (MISS). *Proc Comp Asst Rad Surg* 20th International Congress, Osaka, Japan, 28 Jun–1 Jul; CARS, Elsevier, Amsterdam, Netherland 2006.

Chiu JC, Savitz MH. Operating room of the future for spinal procedures. In: Savitz MH, Chiu JC, Rauschning W, Yeung AT, eds. *The Practice of Minimally Invasive Spinal Technique*. New York: AAMISS Press, 645–8; 2005.

Chiu JC, Savitz MH. Multicenter Study of Percutaneous Endoscopic Discectomy. In: Savitz MH, Chiu JC, Rauschning W, Yeung AT, eds. *The Practice of Minimally Invasive Spinal Technique*. New York: AAMISS Press, 622–6; 2005.

Chiu JC, Savitz MH. Use of laser in minimally invasive spinal surgery and pain management. In: Kambin P, ed. *Arthroscopic and Endoscopic Spinal Surgery: Text and Atlas*, 2nd ed. Totowa, NJ: *Humana Press*, 259–69; 2005.

Chiu J. Anterior endoscopic cervical microdiscectomy. In: Kim D, Fessler R, Regan J, eds. *Endoscopic Spine Surgery and Instrumentation*. New York: *Thieme Medical*, 48–58; 2004.

Chiu J. Endoscopic lumbar foraminoplasty In: Kim D, Fessler R, Regan J, eds. *Endoscopic Spine Surgery and Instrumentation*. New York: *Thieme Medical*, 212–29; 2004.

Chiu J, Clifford T, Greenspan M. Percutaneous microdecompressive endoscopic cervical discectomy with laser thermodiskoplasty. *Mt Sinai J Med* 67: 278–82; 2000.

CrossMatch Technologies, Inc. http://www.crossmatch.com.

Huang HK. The role of imaging informatics in MISS. *Proc 21st CARS Intern Congress in Comp Asst Rad Surg*, Berlin, Germany, 27–30 Jun; 2007.

Huang HK. March, 2004. *PACS and Imaging Informatics: Principles and Applications*. Hoboken, NJ: Wiley; 2004.

Huang HK. PACS, informatics, and the neurosurgery command module. *J Mini Invasive Spinal Technique* 1: 62–7; 2001.

Jensen M, Brant-Zawadzki M, Obuchowski N, et al. Magnetic resonance imaging of the lumbar spine in people without back pain. *N Engl J Med* 331: 69–116; 1994.

Liu BJ, Law YY, Documet J, Gertych A. Image-assisted knowledge discovery and decision support in radiation therapy planning, *Comput Med Imag Graph*, 31(4–5): 311–21; 2007.

MySQL AB, Sun Solaris Microsystems Inc. http://dev.mysql.org.

Vallfors B. Acute, subacute and chronic low back pain: clinical symptoms, absenteeism and working environment. *Scan J Rehab Med* 11(suppl): 1–98; 1985.

Computer-Aided Diagnosis (CAD) and Image-Guided Decision Support

Chapters 25 and 26 cover computer-aided detection and diagnosis. Chapter 25 discuses computer-aided diagnosis (CAD) and image-guided decision support with examples. Chapter 26 focuses on the integration of CAD with PACS for daily clinical use. In these two chapters, we use the terms aided, assisted, and guided loosely, but detection to only mean detect, and diagnosis to mean detection followed by diagnosis. For convenience, Figure 20.9 is reproduced here as Figure 25.1 showing how these two chapters (in orange purple color) correspond to other chapters in the domain of image informatics research.

25.1 COMPUTER-AIDED DIAGNOSIS (CAD)

25.1.1 CAD Overview

Computer-aided detection (CADe) and computer-aided diagnosis (CADx), or just in general, computer-aided diagnosis (CAD), research started in the early 1980s and has gradually evolved as a clinically supported tool. In mammography, CAD has in fact become a part of the routine clinical operation for detection of breast cancers in many medical centers and screening sites in the United States. In addition various CAD schemes are being developed for detection and classification of many different kinds of lesions obtained with the use of various imaging modalities because the concept of CAD is broad, and also for assisting radiologists by providing the computer output as a "second opinion." The usefulness and practicality of CAD, however, depend on many factors, including the availability of digital image data, computer power, and high-quality display and image-archiving systems. So it is apparent that CAD needs to be integrated into a part of PACS to be effective for clinical practice. Image-based knowledge discovery and decision support by use of CAD are a new trend in research that translates CAD diagnostic results to assist in short- and long-term treatments. PACS was developed more than 20 years ago and has become an integral part of daily clinical operations. Integration of CAD with PACS would take advantage of the image resources in PACS and enhance the value of CAD. CAD applications could therefore emerge into mainstream image-aided clinical practice.

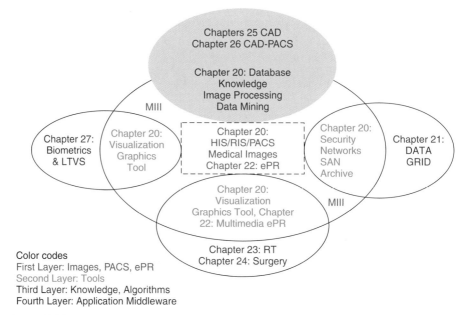

Figure 25.1 Imaging informatics data sources (rectangle), concepts, technologies and applications (large and small ellipses) as discussed in the chapters of Part IV. Color codes refer to the five-layer informatics infrastructure shown in Figure 20.2. CAD and CAD–PACS integration to be discussed in Chapters 25 and 26 are in orange color.

Computer-aided diagnosis has become one of the major research subjects in medical imaging informatics and diagnostic radiology. With CAD, radiologists use the computer output as a "second opinion" and make the final decisions. CAD is a concept that was established by taking into account equally the roles of physicians and computers, whereas automated computer diagnosis is a concept based on computer algorithms only. With CAD, the performance by computers does not have to be comparable to or better than that by physicians, but needs to be complementary to that by physicians.

25.1.2 CAD Research and Development (R&D)

We loosely divide CAD R&D into five categories based on its research methods and clinical use:

1. CAD algorithms research and development. This category covers general CAD algorithms development in chest radiography, mammography, MR breast imaging, thin-slice CT nodules, and multidimensional medical imaging in organs and diseases. The algorithm development is mostly for general purpose applications. This category attracts most CAD R&D interests. Doi reviewed these works extensively, among them are recent advances that merge CAD with other technologies, as shown in Figure 25.2*A*, *B*, and *C*: multi-view chest radiographs, temporal subtraction of nuclear medicine bone scans, and database search for separating a benign versus malignant mass in mammograms.

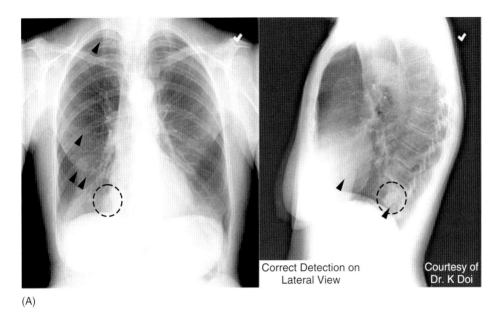

Correct Detection on
Lateral View

Courtesy of
Dr. K Doi

(A)

Figure 25.2 (*A*) Demonstration of multi-view CAD. The relatively large, but very subtle lung nodule (dotted circles) located in the right mediastinum region was correctly marked by CAD (triangles) on the lateral view of a chest radiograph but was not marked by CAD on the PA view. (*B*) Temporal subtraction image obtained from previous and current nuclear medicine bone scan images. One cold lesion (white solid circle) and two hot lesions (dark dotted circles) on the subtraction image were correctly marked by CAD method. The temporal subtraction image for successive whole-body bone scans has the potential to enhance the interval changes between two temporal images. (*C*) Image matching from collected nodules in the PACS/MIII or imaging informatics nodule database (see also Fig. 20.8). Comparison of an unknown case of a mass in a mammogram in the center (blue) with two benign masses on the left and two malignant masses on the right, which may be retrieved from the PACS database. Most observers were able to visually identify the unknown case correctly as being more similar to malignant masses (right, orange) than to benign ones (left, green). (Courtesy of Dr. K. Doi)

2. Target CAD applications. This category focuses on CAD application for a specific aliment on a specific imaging modality under a certain clinical environment. In other words, the CAD method may not be necessarily developed for a general clinical setting, but it is used for assisting the healthcare provider at the critical moment in a particular time and space to obtain a more accurate and timely diagnosis. An example is computer- aided-detection of small acute intracranial hemorrhage (AIH) on brain CT, which has been developed for patients in the emergency room suspecting of non-penetrating brain injury when a neuroradiologist may not be readily available to read the CT images.

3. Decision support. Decision support means that the CAD method developed contributes to a component of a larger CAD system for achieving a common goal. The goal could be an assessment process or contribution to decision

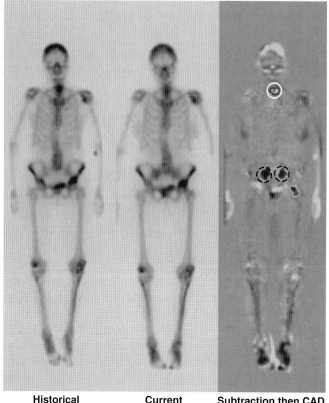

Historical   **Current**   **Subtraction then CAD**

(B)

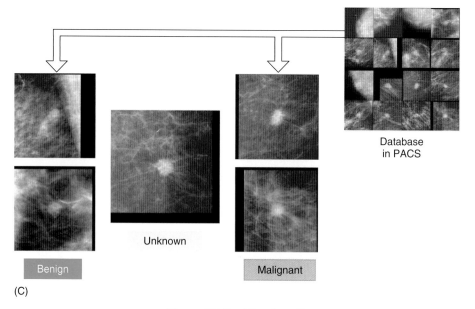

(C)

Figure 25.2   (*Continued*)

support toward a final diagnosis or a treatment plan. An example is in bone age assessment of children using CAD on a hand radiograph. In this case the bone age assessment is based on multiple CAD algorithms on three different regions of the hand, the phalangeal, carpal bone, and the wrist joint region.

4. CAD system and evaluation. This category considers a complete CAD system that contains several CAD algorithms, one for each part of the body anatomy for a local decision support. Each algorithm can be a CAD algorithm mentioned in category 3. Together they form a CAD system for achieving a common diagnostic or assessment goal. In the case of bone age assessment the combination of phalangeal, carpal, and wrist joint bone results is assembled using a fuzzy logic method to derive the final bone age.

5. Security and CAD-PACS integration. Integration of CAD and PACS requires the consideration of data security and the method of integration. Data security is necessary to ensure the integrity of images sent to the CAD algorithm for processing, and the integrity of the CAD output data sent back to the workstation for reading and archiving in the PACS environment. The method of integration considers how to transfer images from PACS to CAD for processing and return the CAD results to PACS most efficiently.

Doi has tracked the CAD R&D progress since 2000 as shown in Tables 25.1*A* and *B* based on the RSNA (Radiological Society of North America) annual presentations in this field of study. The progression in the table shows the increasing interest and the acceptance by the radiological community through the years in using CAD for assisting clinical diagnosis in various body regions. It is commonly agreed that the integration of CAD with PACS will lead to the emergence of CAD applications into mainstream image-aided clinical practice in both diagnosis and treatment.

25.2 COMPUTER-AIDED DETECTION AND DIAGNOSIS (CAD) WITHOUT PACS

25.2.1 CAD without PACS and without Digital Image

The computer-aided detection or diagnosis engine can stand alone as a PACS-based application server, or it can be organized as a MIII resource. The purpose is to

TABLE 25.1*A* **Topics and numbers of CAD related presentations at the RSNA meetings, 2000 to 2008**

	2000	2001	2002	2003	2004	2005	2006	2007	2008
CAD	55	86	134	191	161	165	167	192	227
Digital mammograms	12	15	20	25	27	22	34	44	31
Lung cancer screening	6	12	19	21	17	7	18	10	10
CR/DR/FPD*	14	20	14	25	18	16	27	24	9

RSNA: Radiological Society of North America, Annual Meeting Chicago, IL.
*CR/DR/FPD: Computed radiography/digital radiography/flat-panel detector

TABLE 25.1*B* **Number of CAD presentations at the RSNA meetings, 2003 to 2008**

	2003	2004	2005	2006	2007	2008
Chest	94	70	48	62	72	73
Breast	37	48	49	47	39	51
Colon	17	15	30	25	32	24
Brain	10	9	17	12	13	20
Liver	9	9	9	8	8	22
Skeletal	9	8	5	7	11	6
Vascular, and other[a]	15	2	7	6	17	31
Total	191	161	165	167	192	227

[a]Cardiac, prostate, pediatric, dental, PACS.

use image postprocessing to derive additional parameters to aid the physician as a second reader to improve diagnostic performance. Traditional CAD is performed off line in the sense that an image set of a patient is acquired from a given modality either through a peripheral device or network transmission, from which image processing is performed to extract relevant parameters. These parameters are then used to provide additional information to pinpoint sites of potential pathology in the image set to alert the physician. The derived parameters are not appended to the images for later retrieval. These procedures are performed without taking advantage of the PACS resource.

An example of a film-based CAD is the one used in mammography. In this film-based CAD (Fig. 25.3), screen/film mammograms are digitized, subsampled, and fed to a processor that contains the CAD algorithms for detection of micro calcification, masses, and other abnormalities. Results from the CAD are superimposed on the subsampled digitized mammogram and display (see Fig. 25.3, red color) on a specific CAD workstation (WS) with a standard set of monitor(s), whcih may not be in the quality of making primary diagnosis on digital mammogram. An expert radiologist with mammography training displays the film mammogram on the light box viewer (see Fig. 25.3, blue color) to visually compare it with the subsampled digitized mammograms with detected lesions on the WS. This off-line CAD method is a two-step process requiring special hardware and software to accomplish the detection process. Such a CAD system consists of a film digitizer, a workstation, a CAD processor, and a mammography film light box viewer for comparing the CAD result with the original film mammogram.

CAD can be integrated in a PACS or MIII (medical imaging informatics infrastructure) environment by taking advantage of the existing resources in its storage, retrieval, communication networks and display components. Figure 25.3 depicts the data flow in film-based CAD mammography.

25.2.2 CAD without PACS but with Digital Image

CAD without PACS can use either direct digital input or film with a digitizer. In either case, CAD is an off-line isolated system. Table 25.2 lists the procedure in performing CAD in such a system. The film-based CAD system for mammography shown in Figure 25.3 is an example.

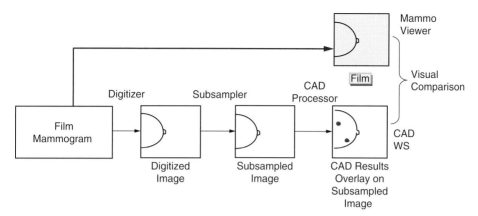

Figure 25.3   Data flow in film-based CAD mammography. Only a single monitor and singlae light box viewer are shown in the diagram.

TABLE 25.2   CAD without PACS and with or without digital input

- Collect films or digital images based on patient's record
- Digitize films or develop an interface program to read digital images
- Input images to the CAD workstation (WS)
- CAD algorithm
- Return results to CAD WS

25.3   CONCEPTUAL METHODS OF INTEGRATING CAD WITH DICOM PACS AND MIII

Integration of CAD with DICOM PACS or MIII can have four approaches. In the first three described below, the CAD is connected directly to the PACS. The fourth approach is a separate CAD server that can be connected to either the PACS or the MIII, or both.

25.3.1   PACS WS Q/R, CAD WS Detect

In this approach, the PACS workstation (WS) queries and retrieves (Q/R) images from the PACS database and the CAD WS performs the detection. Table 24.3*A* and Figure 25.4*A* illustrate the steps for the CAD. This method involves the PACS server, the PACS WS, and the CAD WS. A DICOM C-store function must be installed in the CAD WS.

25.3.2   CAD WS Q/R and Detect

In this approach the CAD WS performs both query and retrieve and then the detection. This method only involves the PACS server and the CAD WS. The function of

TABLE 25.3A   CAD with DICOM PACS: PACS WS Q/R, CAD WS detect

At the PACS server

- Connect CAD WS to PACS
- Register CAD WS (IP address, port number, application entity [AE]) title to receive images

At the PACS WS

- Use DICOM query/retrieve to select patient/studies/images
- Use DICOM C-get to select images from PACS server which pushes the images to CAD WS

At the CAD WS

- Develop DICOM storage class provider (SCP) to accept images
- CAD
- Develop database to archive CAD results

TABLE 25.3B   CAD with DICOM PACS: CAD WS Q/R and detect

At the PACS server

- Connect CAD WS to PACS
- Register CAD WS (IP address, port number, AE title) at PACS

At the CAD WS

- Develop DICOM Q/R client and storage class to select/accept patient/study/images
- CAD
- Develop database to archive CAD results

TABLE 25.3C   CAD with PACS: PACS WS with CAD software

- Install CAD software at PACS WSs
- PACS WSs Q/R Patient/Study/Images
- Establish software linkage in WS for CAD software to access DICOM images
- Develop DICOM format decoder to convert images to CAD format
- CAD at PACS WS
- Develop CAD database in the WS to archive CAD results

TABLE 25.3*D*   **Integration of CAD server with DICOM PACS and/or MIII**

- Connect CAD server to PACS and/or MIII
- CAD server performs Q/R Patient/study/images from PACS
- Archive in CAD server
- DICOM format decoder
- Distribute images to CAD WS

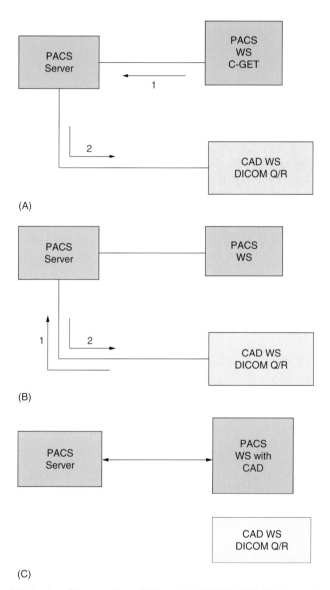

Figure 25.4   Methods of integrating CAD with DICOM PACS (see also Table 25.3). (*A*) PACS WS query/retrieve, CAD WS detect (C-GET is a DICOM service); (*B*) CAD WS query/retrieve and detect; (*C*) PACS WS has CAD software; (*D*) integration of CAD server with PACS and/or MIII.

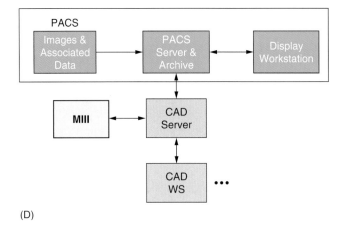

(D)

Figure 25.4 (*Continued*)

the PACS server is almost identical to that of the last method. The only difference is that the last method uses the PACS WS for Q/R images, whereas in this method the CAD WS performs the Q/R. For this reason DICOM Q/R must be installed in the CAD WS. Table 25.3*B* and Figure 25.4*B* describe the steps.

25.3.3 PACS WS with CAD Software

The next approach is to install the CAD software in the PACS WS. This will eliminate all components in the CAD system and its connection to the PACS. Table 25.3*C* and Figure 25.4*C* show the steps involved.

25.3.4 Integration of CAD Server with PACS or MIII

In this method the CAD server is connected to the PACS server. This server can also be attached to the MIII as a computational resource. The CAD server is used to perform CAD for PACS and MIII WSs. This concept is similar to the distributed, Web and computational grid servers described in Sections 20.4.1, 21.1, and 21.2. Table 25.3*D* and Figure 25.4*D* describe the steps involved.

25.4 COMPUTER-AIDED DETECTION OF SMALL ACUTE INTRACRANIAL HEMORRHAGE (AIH) ON COMPUTER TOMOGRAPHY (CT) OF BRAIN

Starting from problem definition and going to rationale, methods, data collection, validation, and system evaluation, in this and next section we develop an application of the CAD method. To be concise in covering every step, we select a small-scale CAD method in a target CAD application of computer-aided detection of a small acute intracranial hemorrhage (AIH) on a brain CT. With CAD it is possible to distinguish genuine intracranial hemorrhage from mimicking normal variants or artifacts based on image features and anatomical information, because detection is accomplished by construction of a coordinate system that incorporates positional information of normal brain structures. Once it is integrated with the PACS, such a system can benefit patient care especially in emergency situations and critical environments when timely management decisions need to be made by acute care physicians.

The discussion will focus on the imaging informatics approach and not on the development of the algorithm per se. In this example the integration of CAD with PACS is not discussed; the topic is left to Chapter 26 where we also introduce the CAD-PACS Integration toolkit.

25.4.1 Clinical Aspect of Small Acute Intracranial Hemorrhage (AIH) on CT of Brain

Acute intracranial hemorrhage (AIH) is a recent ($<$ 72 hours) bleeding inside the skull. It can result from a stroke or be a complication of a head injury. The presence or absence of AIH requires different treatment strategies and its identification is of immediate importance for triage of patients presenting an acute neurological disturbance or a head injury. However, it is well recognized that clinical findings cannot accurately differentiate between symptoms of AIH and of other neurological emergencies. Therefore neuroimaging is essential for immediate decision making. CT has been the modality of choice for evaluating suspected AIH cases because it is widely available, quick to perform, and compatible with most life support devices. On CT images, acute blood clot shows higher X-ray attenuation than normal brain parenchyma. The contrast between AIH and the adjacent structures depends on (1) intrinsic physical properties of blood clot including the density, volume, and location; (2) relationship to surrounding structures; and (3) technical factors including scanning angle, slice thickness, and windowing. Although diagnosis of AIH on CT is usually straightforward, identification of the demonstrable AIH on CT can become difficult when the lesion is inconspicuous, so small (≤ 1.00 cm) as to be masked by normal structures, or when the reader is inexperienced.

In most parts of the world outside the United States, acute care physicians, including emergency physicians, internists, and neural surgeons, are left to read the CT images at odd hours when radiologists' expertise is not immediately available. This is not a desirable arrangement because the skill of acute care physicians in interpreting brain CTs has been shown to be imperfect. Even radiology residents can, albeit infrequently, overlook a hemorrhage on a brain CT. Therefore a CAD system was developed that identifies a small AIH can help in the management of patients presenting an acute neurological disturbance or a head injury in an emergent setting.

25.4.2 Development of the CAD Algorithm for AIH on CT

25.4.2.1 *Data Collection and Radiologist Readings*   To develop the CAD for AIH on CT brain, extensive data collection was required. There were two data collection phases used for (1) working out the algorithm and validating the CAD system's effectiveness and (2) a performance evaluation of CAD detection compared with radiologists' and physicians' readings. Phase one involved 186 brain CT studies, 62 cases of which were confirmed to be AIH (note that a single case can have multiple contiguous AIH volumes). The 124 cases showing no AIH were retrospectively retrieved from the PACS archive. All studies had used the CT scanner (HiSpeed

CT, GE Medical Systems, Milwaukee, Wisconsin). All images were axial images obtained parallel to the orbito-meatal line (OML), at 120 kV and 80 to 200 mA. These cases were divided into 120 for training and 66 for validation.

The radiological diagnoses in all the cases were established by the consensus of two radiologists, one with 7 years and the other with 11 years of experience in reading brain CTs. In addition, dimensions, locations, and type of individual disjoint AIH volumes were measured. Altogether there were 123 contiguous volumes of small AIH, 77 in the training cases and 46 in the validation dataset, with well-represented samples of each different type of AIH and different sizes (≤ 1.0 cm).

25.4.2.2   *The CAD System Development*   The dataflow of the CAD algorithm is illustrated in Figure 25.5. The image processing and analysis methods used in the scheme are listed in Table 25.4. All image processing methods were readily available in Mat-Lab Software Library (The Math Works, Inc., Natick, Massachusetts). The numerals in the figure correspond to the numerals in the table.

Segmentation of Brain (Fig. 25.5, 1)   The skull, by virtue of its exceptionally high X-ray attenuation values, can be removed using global thresholding. A

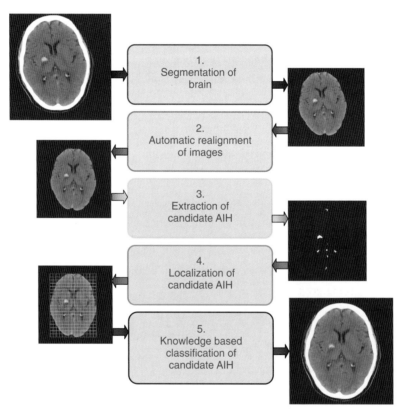

Figure 25.5   Schematic of the CAD system. Intermediary outputs of an image showing right basal ganglia hemorrhage illustrate the effect of individual steps. Details of individual steps are outlined in Table 25.4. (Courtesy of Dr. T. Chan)

TABLE 25.4 Details of individual image processing and analysis steps of in the CAD for AIH algorithm as outlined in Figure 25.5

Steps	Methods	Purposes
1A. Segmentation of intracranial contents	Global thresholding and morphological operations	Remove bones of skull and face
	Remove structures not contiguous with the main central bulk of intracranial contents	Remove scalp, orbits, and other head and neck soft tissues
1B. Preprocessing of intracranial contents	Median filtering	De-noising
	Adjustment of intensity according to distance from the skull	Correct for CT cupping artifacts
2. Automatic realignment of images	Automatic localization of limits of brain, ventricles, floor of anterior intracranial fossa, mid-sagittal plane	Align the brain into the normal position
3. Extraction of candidate AIH	Top-hat view transformation	Highlight local high-density regions
	Subtraction between the two sides	Extract asymmetrically high-density regions
4. Localization of candidate AIH	Registration of the brain in question against a normalized coordinate system	Render the candidate AIH anatomical information
5. Knowledge based classification of AIH	Rule-based system with inputs of image features and anatomical coordinates of the extracted candidates	Distinguish genuine AIH from false positives resulting from noise, artifacts, and normal variants

morphological opening algorithm is used to remove connections that may remain between the intracranial contents and the scalp. Afterward the scalp and other extrinsic structures become separated from the centrally located intracranial contents by regions of void that represent the removed bones. The intracranial contents can subsequently be segmented by selectively removing elements that are not contiguous with the central component.

The segmented intracranial contents undergo preprocessing steps that include median filtering for noise reduction and adjustment for CT cupping artifacts. This produces a more homogeneous background against which abnormalities become more conspicuous.

Realignment of Images (Fig. 25.5, 2)   The brain is realigned into the conventional orientation after automatic localization of mid-sagittal plane and boundaries of the whole series of images. This is necessary as images obtained in an emergent clinical setting are often not optimally positioned. Figures 25.6 and 25.7 depict the process and the results of these operations.

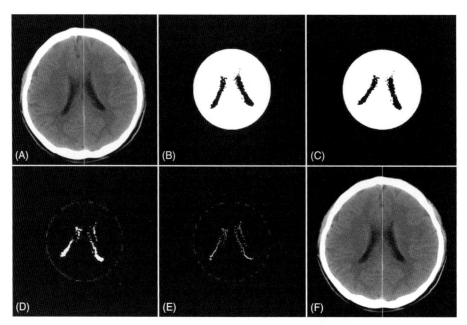

Figure 25.6   Angle of the mid-sagittal plane obtained by finding the line of symmetry of the body of lateral ventricles. The section containing the body of lateral ventricles (*a*) is automatically selected as described in text. The central portion of the image is binarized with threshold at CSF attenuation. It is rotated over a range of angles. The differences between the rotated image (*b*) and its mirror image (*c*) are obtained (*d*). The angle that gives the least difference (*e*) is the angle of the mid-sagittal plane (*f*). (Courtesy of Dr. T. Chan)

Extraction of AIH Candidates (Fig. 25.5, 3)   High attenuation components are next segmented as candidate AIHs from each of the axial sections. The segmentation is based on combined (1) top-hat view transformations, essentially selecting pixels of higher attenuation than those in their vicinity, and (2) subtraction between the two sides of the brain about the midline, which highlights regions of higher attenuation than the contralateral anatomical region. The parameters are adjusted so that a good number of AIH candidates are generated to avoid missing any small lesions. The processes are shown in Figures 25.8 and 25.9.

Localization of AIH Candidates (Fig. 25.5, 4)   The many image features of the AIH candidates, including mean and variation of attenuation, area, long- and short-axis diameters, and relative orientation, are quantified. In addition the candidate AIHs are given anatomical context by registration against a special coordinate system. This coordinate system is conceptually similar to the commonly used Talairach coordinate system in anatomy but is different in that it can be readily applicable for relatively thick section axial images obtained using ordinary clinical protocols.

Coordinates on the coordinate system have their own anatomical label as a result of a normalization procedure using axial brain CT normal subjects obtained using a clinical protocol. Through the registration process between the study in question and the normalized coordinate system, each pixel location of the brain in question

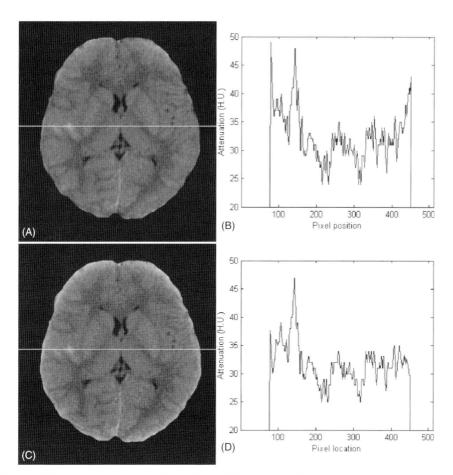

Figure 25.7   Original image with artifactual increase in signal intensity toward the brain skull interface (*a*). Horizontal line indicating the position from where the intensity profile (*b*) is obtained. Image after correction of cupping artifacts (*c*). Intensity profile along the same horizontal line (*d*). It can be appreciated by comparison of (*b*) and (*d*) that the peak intensity at the pixel position of around 140 due to AIH is more prominent after correction of cupping artifacts. (Courtesy of Dr. T. Chan)

is correlated with a coordinate location of the normalized brain and its embedded anatomical label.

Knowledge-Based Classification of AIH Candidates (Fig. 25.5, 5)   The image features and coordinates of the AIH candidates provide the input for the rule-based classification system (Table 25.5), which primarily reduces false positives caused by normal variants and artifacts. The classification is possible because genuine AIH or normal variants tend to follow certain patterns at some typical anatomical locations.

The algorithm's output is displayed as images with red overlays at perimeters of the AIHs determined by the system (Fig. 25.10). The original images and the corresponding CAD output images are displayed side by side, one axial section at a

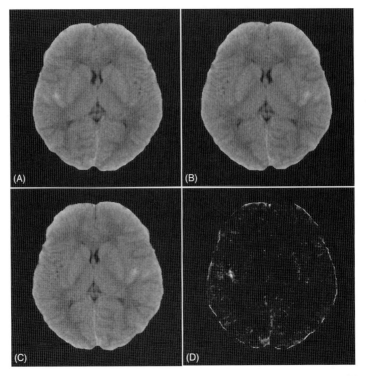

Figure 25.8 Procedure of highlighting asymmetrical high-density region illustrated by the intermediary outputs of the CAD scheme. Original is shown in (*a*). Flipped image (*b*) is elastically transformed to reduce the normal structural asymmetry between the two sides of the brain (*c*). Difference between (*a*) and the morphological closing transformation of (*c*) indicates that AIH within the right Sylvian fissure is of higher signal than CSF in the left contralateral Sylvian fissure (*d*). (Courtesy of Dr. T. Chan)

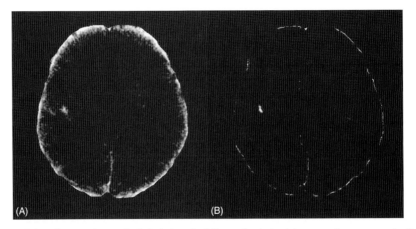

Figure 25.9 Comparison of global thresholding of original image after removal of skull and extracranial tissues (*a*), and thresholding of the combined processing steps including correction of cupping artifacts, image top hat transformation, and left-right comparison (*b*). Notice that the result of (*b*) is much cleaner and manageable for subsequent processing. (Courtesy of Dr. T. Chan)

TABLE 25.5   Sample rules used in the knowledge base classification in the CAD system for AIH on CT brain

Anatomy Rules (P)[a]	Imaging Feature Rules (Q)[a]	Interpretation	Probability of AIH
Low probability of AIH for candidates presenting calcifications or normal high-density structures			
Mid-sagittal plane, supracranial fossa	Vertically aligned, ↑ attenuation, ↑ eccentricity, ↑ long axis length, ↓ short axis length	Falx calcification	↓
Mid-sagittal plane, supracranial fossa Periphery	Intermediate attenuation, Intermediate eccentricity, ↓ convex hull	Superior sagittal sinus	↓
Medial portion of basal ganglia	↑ Attenuation (↑ if area ↑), ↓ area (↑ if symmetrical), Symmetrical	Basal ganglia calcification	↓
Central portion of cerebellum	↑ Attenuation (↑ if area ↑), ↓ area (↑ if symmetrical), symmetrical	Dentate nuclei calcification	↓
Low probability of AIH for candidates presenting artifacts			
Posterior cranial fossa	↑ Eccentricity, ↑ long axis length, ↓ short axis length	Beam hardening artifact	↓
Above anterior cranial fossa Above temporal bone Periphery near vertex	↑ Attenuation ↓ area beyond adjacent bone in contiguous section	Partial volume averaging	↓
High probability of AIH for candidates presenting particular type of AIH			
Sylvian fissure	Vertically aligned, intermediate attenuation, ↑ eccentricity, intermediate long axis length, ↓ short axis length	Sylvian fissure subarachnoid hemorrhage	↑
Periphery	Perpendicular to perimeter of brain, ↓ long axis length, ↓ short axis length	Sulcal space subarachnoid hemorrhage	↑

[a] The rules that incorporate anatomical and imaging features information take the following form:

$$P \rightarrow Q$$

$$Q \rightarrow \Delta \text{ probability of AIH}$$

Sample rules used in the knowledge base classification system. P are the set of rules used to check for the anatomical locations and Q are the rules used to evaluate the imaging features appropriate for some particular anatomical positions. A candidate AIH is first checked for the anatomical position. If the position is one that satisfies a particular P, the corresponding Q will be invoked to evaluate the image features of the candidate AIH. If an appropriate pair of P and Q is satisfied, the probability of AIH for the candidate is adjusted accordingly.

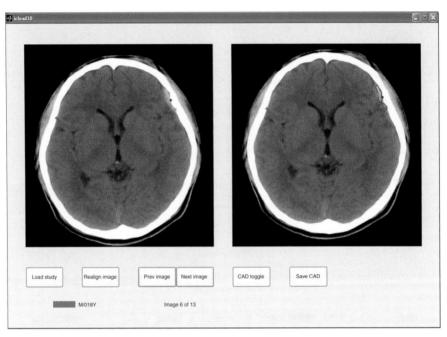

Figure 25.10 Screen capture of the CAD system graphical user interface. Original images are displayed at the left window while the output images with the overlays of outlined AIH are displayed at the right. Original and output images are displayed in stripe mode and linked such that they can be scrolled together for review of the whole image series. (Courtesy of Dr. T. Chan)

time in the CT stack mode. The user can scroll through the whole series of synchronized original images and corresponding CAD output images. This arrangement is to facilitate comparison between the original and the CAD output images.

Some Difficult AIH Cases   It is believed that the CAD system for AIH can detect lesions that are difficult to find by acute care physicians or even radiology residents. Some such lesions are shown in Figure 25.11. In the evaluation study to be discussed in the Section 25.5, such cases were included in a study that found emergency physicians and radiology residents to have missed them, whereas CAD could make the correct diagnosis using anatomically related lesion characteristics in accord with the knowledge-based rules discussed in the previous section.

Training and Validation of the CAD System   Training of the CAD system involved using known clinical cases to improve the performance of the CAD; validating of the CAD, on the other hand, meant studying different known cases to validate the trained CAD method. There were two distinct sets of data and they could not be overlapped.

The system was trained with 40 AIH cases and 80 without AIH, and the validation used 22 positive cases and 44 controls, all obtained from the first phase of data collection. Some of the cases were not used in the collected data for CAD training or validation for various reasons, among these being cases used in training the human

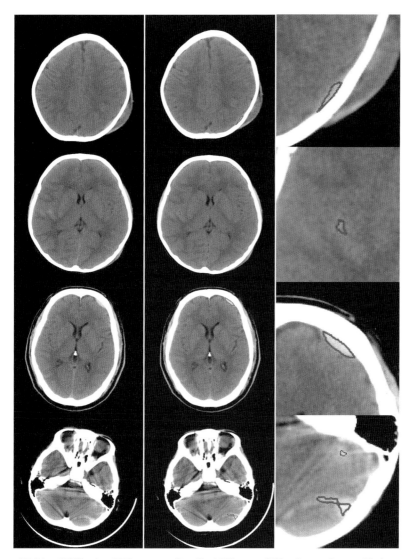

Figure 25.11 Difficult AIH cases. Small AIH are difficult to detect if they are of similar attenuation as adjacent structures or confused with normal variants and artifacts. Examples of some difficult cases (the left column) with their CAD results (the middle column) and magnified views (the right column) are shown. The system identifies AIH by red perimeter outlines. High-density regions that are segmented but subsequently classified as unlikely to be AIH are identified by blue perimeter outlines. (Courtesy of Dr. T. Chan)

observers and cases where the AIH was larger than 1.00 cm. Table 25.6 shows the training and validation results. From the table, it can be seen that on a per patient basis, the sensitivity and specificity were 95% (38/40) and 88.8% (71/80), respectively, for the training cases. The system achieved sensitivity of 100% (22/22) and specificity of 84.1% (37/44) for the diagnosis of AIH for the validation cases.

TABLE 25.6   CAD results based on training data and validation data

	Validation Positive	Validation Negative
A. Summary of CAD results on a per patient basis for training cases		
AIH present	38	2
AIH absent	9	71
Sensitivity = (38/40) 95.0%		
Specificity = (71/80) 88.9%		
Accuracy = 90.8%		
Positive predictive value = 80.8%		
Negative predictive value = 97.3%		
B. Summary of CAD results on a per patient basis for validation cases		
AIH present	22	0
AIH absent	7	37
Sensitivity = (22/22) 100.0%		
Specificity = (37/44) 84.1%		
Accuracy = 89.3%		
Positive Predictive Value = 75.9%		
Negative Predictive Value = 100.0%		

The speed of the current system was not optimized during the validation stage. It takes on average approximately 15 seconds per image to produce the output. But the time can variy substantially, depending on number of image and number of candidate AIH introduced to be evaluated by the classification system.

25.5 EVALUATION OF THE CAD FOR AIH

25.5.1 Rationale of Evaluation of a CAD System

The CAD system is evaluated after the system had been trained and validated. A new data set (see Section 25.4.2.1, phase 2 of data collection) is then collected to use in comparing the performance of the CAD with the human observers' performance, or to study if the CAD can help the human observers improve their performance.

In the AIH case, after the CAD algorithm was validated, the next step involved testing its performance by different healthcare providers who would use the CAD in a clinical situation or by physicians interested in improving their diagnostic skills. A CAD system can be useful if it proves to be beneficial to the human observer in making precise diagnoses. In other words, the CAD system should identify lesions that may otherwise be missed by the human observer. As opposed to early unsuccessful attempts to replace radiologists by computers in the 1960s and 1970s, current CAD schemes now aim to assist readers in making diagnoses by providing quantitative analyses of radiological images. Therefore investigations of possible human–computer interaction such as the receiver operating characteristic (ROC) studies are necessary.

For this purpose the MRMC (multiple-reader multiple-case receiver operating characteristic) ROC (receiver operating characteristic; see Section 6.5.4) paradigm has been used in the evaluation of CAD systems. The MRMC is not only efficient in terms of resource requirement (i.e., fewer readers and cases are required for a specified precision), but it also produces results that can generalize to the populations of readers and cases from which the samples were drawn. In the case of CAD for AIH on CT, the comparison is between CAD and emergency room physicians, attending physicians, radiology residents, fellows, radiologists, and neuroradiologists. The goal is to evaluate the effectiveness of CAD by way of MRMC ROC to potentially assist clinicians' performance in detection of small acute intracranial hemorrhage.

25.5.2 MRMC ROC Analysis for CAD Evaluation

25.5.2.1 Data Collection   The second phase of data collection was for the CAD evaluation study. All the readers and cases were recruited from a 1200 bed acute hospital in Hong Kong. Institute review board (IRB) approval was obtained for this study.

Sixty sets of axial brain CT images, of thicknesses between 5 and 10 mm, made up the test cases used in the observer performance study. All were emergency brain CTs performed on a single detector CT scanner (HiSpeed CT, GE Medical Systems, Milwaukee, Wisconsim). All images were axial images obtained parallel to the orbito-meatal line (OML), at 120 kV and 80 to 200 mA. Thirty cases showed AIH, the radiological diagnosis being established by consensus of two experienced neuroradiologists who did not participate in the observer study. In 26 of the cases, the presence of AIH was considered unambiguous by the radiologists. In the other 4, the diagnoses were concluded with a follow-up CT/MRI. AIHs of different types, including intracerebral hemorrhage (ICH), intraventricular hemorrhage (IVH), subarachnoid hemorrhage (SAH), subdural hemorrhage (SDH), and extradural hemorrhage (EDH), were included.

All intracerebral hematomas included in this study were smaller than 1.00 cm in the long-axis diameter, while all extraaxial hematomas were thinner than 1.00 cm. Only small hematomas were included because detection of large hematomas is straightforward and unlikely to be problematic for clinicians. The other 30 cases revealed either normal findings or pathology other than hemorrhage, which included acute and chronic infarct, ischemia, and tumor.

25.5.2.2 ROC Observers   Seven emergency physicians (EP) with 5 to 9 years (average 6.4 years) of experience in emergent brain CT interpretation, 7 radiology residents (RR) with 1 to 4 years of experience (average 2.3 years), and 6 board certified radiology specialists (RS) with 7 to 30 years of experience (average 17.8 years) were invited to participate in the evaluation of the CAD system. One of the specialists (subject 5) is a fellowship trained neuroradiologist with 12 years of experience.

25.5.2.3 ROC Procedure   The readers were provided with the original images and a graphical user interface (GUI) specifically implemented for this study, as shown on Figure 25.12. One axial section was displayed at a time. The readers could scroll through the images of a particular case back and forth, a total of 60 (with and without AIH cases with mixed orders) in the study. The experiment was conducted in a radiologist's reporting room, where ambient light was low. They were allowed to adjust the brightness of the screen to suit their individual needs, but image windowing has not been provided because this on its own could be considered one

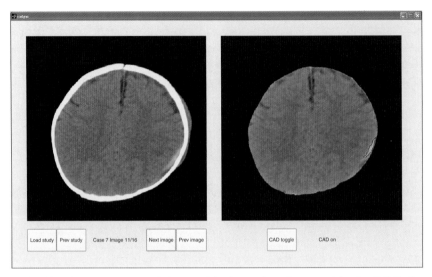

Figure 25.12 Screen capture of the graphical user interface used in the ROC observer study. The original images are displayed at the left window in stack mode. The second reading's, output images of CAD are displayed at the right window. An output image that contained the segmented and realigned intracranial contents, and AIH, is outlined. The original and CAD output images are scrolled at the same time. (Courtesy of Dr. T. Chan)

form of diagnostic aide. In particular, it was conceivable that pre-windowing could bias against people less familiar with its use, especially emergency physicians. The readers were instructed to record their confidence in detecting AIH on a scale from 1 (absolute absence of AIH) to 10 (absolute presence of AIH). Readers were also instructed to interpret the score of 5 and 6 as indeterminate, with 5 erring on the side of absent AIH and 6 otherwise.

Immediately after they had finished all 60 cases and recorded the results, they could re-read the images, now with the CAD output images displayed side by side with the corresponding original images (see Fig. 25.12). Both the original and the CAD output images would scroll together in synchrony. They again recorded their confidence levels in the same way.

The readers were informed that during the CAD training and validation tests, the CAD had produced sensitivity of 80–85% on a per lesion basis and a false positive rate of less than 1 in 3 cases in earlier tests, but performance for individual case might depend on size and contrast difference of lesion(s) it contains. They were also reminded that the accuracy of the CAD output in the sample cases during the ROC study that they were going to read might be better or poorer than the quoted figures reflecting difference in case selection.

25.5.2.4 ROC Data Analysis The recorded data were subject to MRMC ROC analyses using the freely available software DBM MRMC developed by the University of Chicago. The program was based on the Dorfman–Berhaum–Metz method, which allows generalization to the population of readers and cases. The ROC curve was obtained by a maximum likelihood estimation of the binormal distributions that best fit the rating data of the readers.

Since it was believed by many, including most of the participants in the test, that the diagnosis of AIH was an all or none question, it was also desirable to present the results in some conventional indicators that were more familiar to clinicians and were based on a yes/no type of response. The scores were placed into two categories of 1–5 and 6–10 that dichotomized the results into absence/presence of AIH. The sensitivity/specificity pair and positive/negative predictive values were calculated accordingly.

In addition the frequency by which the use of CAD resulted in a change of diagnosis during the experiment, as opposed to mere change in confidence of one particular diagnosis or another, was examined. The diagnosis of absence/presence of AIH for individual case was determined based on the aforementioned method of dichotomizing the score ratings. The frequency of change in diagnosis and the correctness of such changes were recorded. This information reflected the impact that use of CAD might have in actual clinical practice where altered diagnostic decisions would affect management options.

25.5.3 Effect of CAD-Assisted Reading on Clinicians' Performance

All the results quoted in subsequent sections refer to those calculated on per case or per patient basis.

25.5.3.1 Clinicians Improved Performance with CAD   The Az values (area under the ROC curve) scored by individuals before and after CAD are presented in Figure 25.13*A* and *B*. Figure 25.13*A* presents individual performance before and after using the CAD. Only 1 of the 20 observers (observer 4) scored marginally lower Az after CAD. The other 19 people all attained a variable increment after use of CAD. Figure 25.12*B* depicts the three ROC curve pairs, each pair shows the group's (RS in green, RR in red, and EP in blue) performance to have improved (from a lighter to a darker color) with the aid of CAD.

Significantly improved performance is observed in the EP (emergency physician) average area under the ROC curve (Az), which increased from 0.8422 to 0.9294 ($p = 0.0107$) when the diagnosis was made without and with the support of CAD. Az for RR (radiology resident) increased from 0.9371 to 0.9762 ($p = 0.0088$). Az for RS (radiology specialist) increased from 0.9742 to 0.9868 ($p = 0.1755$) but was statistically insignificant. The results are shown in Figure 25.13*B*.

It was clear that the performance of the EP with support of CAD approached that of the RR without CAD. The performance of the RR with CAD was close to that of RS in this experimental condition, since the readers were limited to viewing images without the benefit of windowing or tiling images. This result signifies that the CAD can improve reader performance as well as reduce variability among different clinician groups.

25.5.3.2 Sensitivity, Specificity, Positive, and Negative Predictive Values
The sensitivity, specificity, positive, and negative predictive values were calculated for each reader both before and after use of CAD (Table 25.7). It was demonstrated that both sensitivity and specificity improved for each group. The gain was the most remarkable for the EP whose average sensitivity/specificity improved from 73.3/81.4% to 80.5/90.5%, and less for the RR, which was from 86.2/88.1% to 93.8/92.9%, and least for the RS, which was from 92.2/93.3% to 95/94.4%.

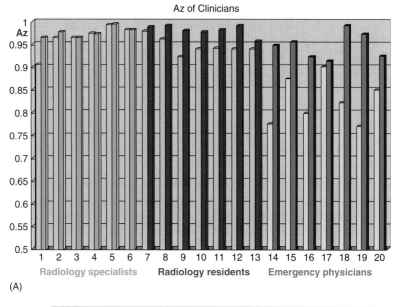

(A)

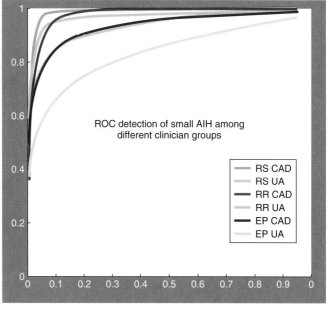

(B)

Figure 25.13 (*A*) ROC detection of AIH among different clinician groups. EP for emergency physicians; RR for radiology residents; RS for board certified radiology specialists. The lighter colored bars are unaided reading mode; the darker colored bars are CAD-assisted reading mode. Notice that among the 20 readers, all but reader 4 improved their performance with CAD-assisted reading. (*B*) Area Az under the ROC curves of all six curves. CAD can be used to improve the readings, which are the ROC Az values, in all three physician groups. Compare each of the three color groups: green, red, and blue. The lighter colored curves represent UA (unaided reading mode); the darker colored curves represent CAD–assisted reading mode.

TABLE 25.7   Average performance indicators included are sensitivity, specificity, positive predictive value, and negative predictive value for different clinician groups with and without CAD support

	Emergency Physicians		Radiology Residents		Radiology Specialists	
	Unaided	CAD	Unaided	CAD	Unaided	CAD
Sensitivity	73.3	80.4	86.2	93.8	92.2	95.0
Specificity	81.4	90.5	88.1	92.9	93.3	94.4
Positive predictive value	80.0	89.5	88.4	93.0	93.3	94.5
Negative predictive value	75.7	82.5	86.7	93.8	92.6	95.1

Note: All indicators in all clinician groups are improved after use of CAD.

Again, it was clear that the EP results with support of CAD approached that of the RR without CAD, and the results of the residents with CAD approached those of the specialists without CAD.

After the use of CAD, the positive predictive values improved from 80.1% to 89.5% for EP, from 88.4% to 93.0% for RR, and from 93.3% to 94.5% for RS. The negative predictive values also improved from 75.7% to 82.5% for ER, from 86.7% to 93.8% for RR, and from 92.6% to 95.1% for RS.

Again, it was clear that these conventional indicators of diagnostic accuracy for the EP with support of CAD approached that of the RR without CAD, and the results of the RR with CAD approached those of the RS without CAD.

25.5.3.3 Change of Diagnostic Decision after CAD Assistance   When the diagnostic decision for each case was considered, it was found that use of CAD corrected the diagnosis far more frequently than misled the readers to a wrong diagnosis. For the EP, use of CAD led to 46 correct changes (beneficial effect) in diagnosis and 12 wrong changes (detrimental effect) out of the maximum number of possible change of 420 (7 readers × 60 cases). For the RR, the figures were 29 versus 3 out of 420. For the RS, the figures were 7 and 0 out of 360. Thus use of CAD is associated with change in diagnosis in decreasing order of relative frequency from EP (13.8%), to RR (7.0%), to RS (1.9%). On the other hand, the relative frequency of correct change versus incorrect change shows an increasing trend from 79.3%:20.7% for EP, to 90.6%:19.4% for RR, to 100%:0% for RS (Table 25.8).

25.5.3.4 Some Clinical Considerations

How and Where Should CAD Be Used for AIH on CT   The previous section confirms that CAD for AIH can improve the diagnostic performance of all three types of physicians: emergency clinicians, radiology residents, and radiology specialists, and especially for the former two categories under the given environment and conditions. Unlike tumor detection in mammography, chest radiography, and CT, expert radiologists can diagnose AIH at very high accuracy. But this does not preclude the current system from becoming a clinical useful tool. It is because a patient's emergency brain CT often needs to be interpreted by acute care physicians to make an immediate judgment about the course of action when radiologists are not readily available to do the reading. The acute care physicians, however, cannot be expected

TABLE 25.8 Cases in which clinicians change their diagnostic decision after CAD

	Emergency Physicians	Radiology Residents	Radiology Specialists
Correct change (% of actual number that change)	46 (79.3%)	29 (90.6%)	7 (100%)
Incorrect change (% of actual number that change)	12 (20.7%)	3 (9.4%)	0 (0%)
Frequency of change in decision	58	32	7
Change in decision/total possible change	13.8% (58/420)	7.6% (32/420)	1.9% (7/360)

Note: The proportion of correct change relative to incorrect change increased from EP to RR to RS. The total and relative number of change decreased from EP to RR to RS.

to have honed the interpretation skills of a radiologist and thus to expertly detect small or difficult AIHs, or to distinguish a genuine AIH from a mimicking variant or artifact. For these reasons the CAD system can be usefully implemented into daily clinical practice in the emergency room and other critical care environments. In the event of natural disasters the CAD system can be depended on to distinguish patients suffering from minor neurological disturbance from patients suffering head injury. After the CT is performed, clinicians can read the images with help from the CAD system. If AIH can be excluded, then the patients may be safely observed for a shorter period of time without the admission to the neurological unit before discharge.

Integration CAD with PACS   CAD for AIH is different from most current CAD systems designed for routine clinical screening like in breast imaging, for which speed is of less concern. For urgent care applications, immediate availability without significant time delay is of critical importance, and AIH is one such critical area of application. Ways of integrating CAD for AIH may include an application server connected with the PACS system (see Section 25.3), or better still, direct incorporation of the system into clinical PACS. How to integrate the CAD into the workflow of acute care physician or the emergency room will be addressed in Chapter 26.

Further Evaluation   How do we confirm that the CAD for AIH can perform as well in other clinical environments and different patient populations? How about when it is used on images from different CT scanners and scanning protocols like slice thickness or the 3-D CT data set? We will address these questions in the next section.

25.6 FROM SYSTEM EVALUATION TO CLINICAL PRACTICE

25.6.1 Further Clinical Evaluation

We raised some questions in the last section that how will the CAD for AIH perform in other clinical environments with different patient populations, and how will it work on images from different CT scanners and scanning protocols. To address these issues, we need further evaluation studies.

Acute intracranial hemorrhage is often associated with head trauma, and it is a precipitant of acute neurological disturbances. Identification of AIH is of paramount clinical importance as the nature of its presence dictates distinctive management and treatment strategies. In many parts of the world, emergency department physicians, internists, or neurosurgeons are the first to read emergent CT studies of a patient suffering head trauma, particularly when a radiologist's expertise is not immediately available. The purpose of a CAD system for AIH is to provide a clinical decision-support tool for clinicians, organizations confronting high volumes of potential AIHs, and resource-limited institutions. Up to this point we had completed the first step in creating such a system, used the data collected from Hong Kong, trained, validated, and evaluated the CAD system with these data. The next step is to address the questions raised above.

A large-scale retrospective study is being performed of 300 cases with matched normals from the Emergency Department (ED) at the Los Angeles County +, University of Southern California Hospital (LAC+USC) comprising patients who had been previously diagnosed with AIH. Compared to the hospital in Hong Kong where the validation and evaluation data were collected, LAC+USC is an entirely different clinical environment, serves different patient populations, and utilizes CT scanners from various manufacturers with different clinical protocols. For the questions raised above, the interim results are very promising, with 85% sensitivity and a little bit lower in specificity. Further improvement is expected.

25.6.2 Next Steps for Deployment of the CAD System for AIH in Clinical Environment

After the evaluation described in Section 25.6.1 is completed, the next logical step in the evolution of the system is actual integration of the CAD into a normal radiology infrastructure and workflow. It is important to implement the system such that future enhancements can readily be tested within a true clinical environment rather than in the isolation of a development or test environment. This next step will allow fine-tuning aspects of the system design that must be optimized before a CAD system can be truly effective.

The CAD system must be integrated into the existing systems architecture to automatically run in real time, intercepting new studies and running prior to or in parallel with other existing workflow processes. Furthermore the results of the CAD system must be stored as distinct files, preserving the original studies but remaining immediately accessible within the existing client software. Integration must therefore occur ahead of PACS or integrated with the PACS system.

Existing radiology and emergency department workflow must be altered to take advantage of the presence of the CAD system. However, acceptance testing of the CAD system within a clinical environment requires stringent confirmatory steps to ensure that no treatment decisions are made wholly based on the CAD system until such time that the CAD system has been validated within the clinical environment. This specifically applies to clinicians who must be instructed to consult with a radiologist despite the presence of CAD output during this next phase of development. Radiologists must also be recruited to facilitate validation in the clinical environment by modifying their existing workflow to reference CAD output and by assisting in documenting the successes and failures of both the algorithm and the system. Most important, the system enhancements based on user input, from both clinicians and radiologists, is an essential next step in the evolution of the CAD system. Factors like processing time, output visualization, accessibility, reporting, and logging, which may not have been primary drivers in the development and testing environments, become more important aspects of a production environment and must be developed and enhanced to deliver a complete CAD solution. Figure 25.14 summarizes these steps involved in the iterative process of clinical evaluation.

Once these nonalgorithmic elements are established, future iterations of the CAD system can be focused on enhancement of the core algorithm and/or minor systems-related enhancements within the overall systems architecture. Figure 25.15 shows

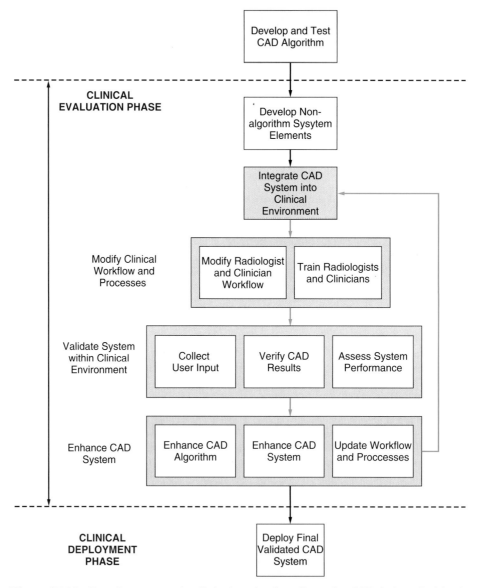

Figure 25.14   Iterative process in clinical evaluation. Once the CAD is installed in the clinical environment for evaluation, it goes through several phases of iterative processes, shown in green arrows. With this iterative process is completed, the CAD system can be deployed for clinical use. (Courtesy of Dr. R. Lee)

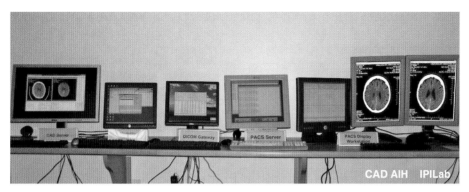

Figure 25.15 CAD-PACS integration prototype in the laboratory environment showing two systems: the CAD server for AIH, and the PACS simulator. The leftmost component is the CAD server running an AIH case study. Other components are the PACS simulator (see Chapters 7 and 28). The PACS simulator has all the essential components of a real PACS, including a modality simulator, DICOM gateway, PACS server, and PACS WS. It is used for PACS training and for testing the functionality of CAD-PACS integration. The PACS WS is located at the rightmost position with the same AIH case shown on the monitor of the CAD server. A physician reads the case at the PACS WS with and without the CAD-assistance.

the prototype of the CAD-PACS integration in the laboratory environment before its deployment to the clinical environment for evaluation.

A second CAD system on bone age assessment of children, which will be discussed in Chapter 26, has passed many of the stages discussed above. This system is presently being evaluated clinically in pediatric radiology by integrating the CAD and radiologists' readings.

25.7 SUMMARY OF COMPUTER-ASSISTED DIAGNOSIS

In this chapter we present the essentials of medical image-based computer-aided detection and diagnosis (CAD). We start with a brief review of the growth of CAD over the last 10 years. We discuss CAD not in a mathematical algorithm context but from a medical imaging informatics perspective. Conceptual methods of CAD-PACS integration are described that will lead to the CAD-PACS integration toolkit to be discussed in Chapter 26.

A self-contained CAD method for acute intracranial hemorrhage(AIH) detection on CT is given to illustrate that CAD is not necessarily to be used for large-scale screening and daily radiological report generation, but also for particular clinical environments like the emergency room or in environments where a radiologist specialist may not be readily available. CAD may be able to assist in making a timely diagnosis to treat a patient with AIH. A step-by-step approach is used to illustrate all the basic ingredients, from the CAD problem definition, to algorithm development, data collection to training the CAD, validation of the CAD system, evaluation of CAD performance compared with human observers, and to deployment of the CAD for daily clinical use.

For CAD to be really useful to healthcare providers on a daily base, it has to be integrated with PACS. This chapter lays down the CAD basic foundation that will be picked up in Chapter 26 where we explain CAD-PACS system integration.

References

Alberdi E, et al. Effects of incorrect computer-aided detection (CAD) output on human decision-making in mammography. *Acad Radiol* 11(8): 909–18; 2004.

Ardekani BA, et al. Automatic detection of the mid-sagittal plane in 3-D brain images. *IEEE Trans Med Imag* 16(6): 947–52; 1997.

Bagley LJ. Imaging of neurological emergencies: trauma, hemorrhage, and infarction. *Semin Roentgenol* 34(2): 144–59; 1999.

Barrett JF, Keat N. Artifacts in CT: recognition and avoidance. *Radiographics* 24(6): 1679–91; 2004.

Beiden SV, et al., Independent versus sequential reading in ROC studies of computer-assist modalities: analysis of components of variance. *Acad Radiol* 9(9): 1036–43; 2002.

Broderick JP, et al. Guidelines for the management of spontaneous intracerebral hemorrhage: a statement for healthcare professionals from a special writing group of the Stroke Council, American Heart Association. *Stroke* 30(4): 905–15; 1999.

Chan T. Computer Aided Detection of Small Acute Intracranial Hemorrhage on Computer Tomography of Brain, *J Comput Med Imag Graph* 31: 285–98; 2007.

Chan T, Huang HK. Effect of a computer-aided diagnosis system on clinicians' performance in detection of small acute intracranial hemorrhage on computed tomography. *Acad Radiol* 15(3): 290–9; 2008.

Cohen W, Wayman L. Computed tomography of intracranial hemorrhage. *Neuroimag Clin N Am* 2: 75–87; 1992.

Diehl JT, CT scanning in traumatic and emergency patients. *Comput Tomogr* 2(3): 183–7; 1978.

Doi K. Current status and future potential of computer-aided diagnosis in medical imaging. *Br J Radiol* 78(1): S3–S19; 2005.

Doi K. Computer-aided diagnosis in medical imaging: Historical review: current status and future potential, *J Comput Med Imag Graph* 31: 198–211; 2007.

Doi K, Huang HK. Computer-aided diagnosis (CAD) and image-guided decision support. Editorial. *J Comput Med Imag Graph* 31: 195–7; 2007.

Dorfman DD, Berbaum KS, Metz CE. Receiver operating characteristic rating analysis: generalization to the population of readers and patients with the jackknife method. *Invest Radiol* 27(9): 723–31; 1992.

Ducan J, Ayache N. Medical image analysis: progress over two decades and the challenges ahead. *IEEE Trans Pattern Anal Mach Intell* 22(1): 85–106; 2000.

Erickson BJ, and Bartholmai B. Computer-aided detection and diagnosis at the start of the third millennium. *J Digit Imag* 15(2): 59–68; 2002.

Gertych A, Zhang A, Sayre J, Pospiech-Kurkowska S, Huang HK. Bone age assessment of children using a digital hand atlas. *Comput Med Imag Graph* 31(4–5): 322–31; 2007.

Goto H, et al. CAD system in the emergency medical care for abdominal and head trauma, presented at the 91st Scientific Assembly and Annual Meeting Radiological Society of North America (RSNA) Chicago; 2005.

Gur D, ROC-type assessments of medical imaging and CAD technologies: a perspective. *Acad Radiol* 10(4): 402–3; 2003.

Hodgson R, et al. CAD system for detecting haemorrhage in CT of stroke presented at the 90th Scientific Assembly and Annual Meeting at *RSNA*. Chicago; 2004.

Huang HK. Utilization of medical imaging informatics and biometric technologies in healthcare delivery. *Intern J Comp Asst Rad Surg* 3: 27–39; 2008.

Huang HK. *PACS and Imaging Informatics: Principles and Applications*. Hoboken, NJ: Wiley; 2004.

Huang HK, Zhang A, Liu BJ, Zhou Z, Documet J, King N, Chan LWC. Data Grid for large-scale medical image archive and analysis. *Proc 13th ACM Int Conf Multimedia*, 1005–13 Association for Computing Machinery, NY, NY; 2005.

Jagoda AS, et al. Clinical policy: neuroimaging and decisionmaking in adult mild traumatic brain injury in the acute setting. *Ann Emerg Med* 40(2): 231–49; 2002.

Junck L, et al., Correlation methods for the centering, rotation, and alignment of functional brain images. *J Nucl Med* 31(7): 1220–6; 1990.

Kobayashi T, et al. Effect of a computer-aided diagnosis scheme on radiologists' performance in detection of lung nodules on radiographs. *Radiology* 199(3): 843–8; 1996.

LABMRMC. http://xray.bsd.uchicago.edu/krl/KRL_ROC/software_index.htm.

Lev MH, et al. Acute stroke: improved nonenhanced CT detection—benefits of soft-copy interpretation by using variable window width and center level settings. *Radiology* 213(1): 150–5; 1999.

Liu BJ, Law YY, Documet J, Gertych A. Image-assisted knowledge discovery and decision support in radiation therapy planning, *Comput Med Imag Graph* 31(4–5): 311–21; 2007.

Mader TJ, Mandel A. A new clinical scoring system fails to differentiate hemorrhagic from ischemic stroke when used in the acute care setting. *J Emerg Med* 16(1): 9–13; 1998.

Maldjian JA, et al. Automated CT segmentation and analysis for acute middle cerebral artery stroke. *Am J Neuroradiol* 22(6): 1050–5; 2001.

MEDIC. http://medic.rad.jhu.edu/download/public/.

Metz CE. Fundamental ROC analysis. In: B. J., K. H.L., and V.M. R.L., eds. *Handbook of Medical Imaging*. Vol 1. *Physics and Psychophysics*, Bellingham, WA: SPIE Press, 751–69; 2000.

Metz CE. Some practical issues of experimental design and data analysis in radiological ROC studies. *Invest Radiol* 24(3): 234–45; 1989.

Minoshima S, et al. An automated method for rotational correction and centering of three-dimensional functional brain images. *J Nucl Med* 33(8): 1579–85; 1992.

Mullins ME, Modern emergent stroke imaging: pearls, protocols, and pitfalls. *Radiol Clin North Am* 44(1): 41–62, vii–viii; 2006.

Norman D, et al. Quantitative aspects of computed tomography of the blood and cerebrospinal fluid. *Radiology* 123(2): 335–8; 1977.

Panagos PD, Jauch EC, Broderick JP. Intracerebral hemorrhage. *Emerg Med Clin North Am* 20(3): 631–55; 2002.

Partain CL, et al. Biomedical Imaging Research Opportunities Workshop II: report and recommendations. *Radiology* 236(2): 389–403; 2005.

Perry JJ, et al. Attitudes and judgment of emergency physicians in the management of patients with acute headache. *Acad Emerg Med* 12(1): 33–7; 2005.

Pietka E, Gertych A, Pospiech S, Cao F, Huang HK, Gilsanz V. Computer assisted bone age assessment: image processing and epiphyseal/Metaphyseal ROI extraction. *IEEE Trans Med Imag* 20: 715–29; 2001.

Pietka E, Pospiech-Kurkowska S, Gertych A, Cao F, Huang HK. Computer-assisted bone age assessment: image analysis and fuzzy classification. *Radiology* 225(P): 751; 2002.

Pietka E, Pospiech S, Gertych A, Cao F, Huang HK, Gilsanz V. Computer automated approach to the extraction of epiphyseal regions in hand radiographs. *J Digit Imag* 14: 165–72; 2002.

Pietka E, Gertych A, Pospiech-Kurkowska S, Cao F, Huang HK, Gilzanz V. Computer assisted bone age assessment: graphical user interface for image processing and comparison. *J Digit Imag* 17(3): 175–188; 2004.

Pietka E, Gertych A, Witko K. Informatics infrastructure of CAD system. *Comput Med Imag Graph* 29(2–3): 157–69; 2005.

Ruttimann UE, et al. Fully automated segmentation of cerebrospinal fluid in computed tomography. *Psych Res* 50(2): 101–19; 1993.

Schriger DL, et al. Cranial computed tomography interpretation in acute stroke: physician accuracy in determining eligibility for thrombolytic therapy. *JAMA* 279(16): 1293–7; 1998.

Soille P. Morphological image analysis: principles and applications, 2nd ed; 2003.

SPM 5. www.fil.ion.ucl.ac.uk/spm/.

Talairach J, Tournoux P. *Co-planar Stereotaxic Atlas of the Human Brain. 3-Dimensional Proportional System: An Approach to Cerebral Imaging*. Stuttgart: Thieme Medical, viii, 122; 1988.

Wagner RF, et al. Assessment of medical imaging and computer-assist systems: lessons from recent experience. *Acad Radiol* 9(11): 1264–77; 2002.

Weiss KL, et al. Clinical brain MR imaging prescriptions in Talairach space: technologist- and computer-driven methods. *Am J Neuroradiol* 24(5): 922–9; 2003.

Wysoki MG, et al. Head trauma: CT scan interpretation by radiology residents versus staff radiologists. *Radiology* 208(1): 125–8; 1998.

Yang GL, et al. A practical computer-aided diagnosis system for intracranial hemorrhage detection in acute stroke presented at the 91st Scientific Assembly and Annual Meeting Radiological Society of North America (*RSNA*). Chicago; 2005.

Zhang A, Gertych A, Liu BJ. Automatic bone age assessment for young children from newborn to 7-year-old using carpal bones. *Comput Med Imag Graph* 31(4–5): 299–310; 2007.

Zhang A, Sayre, JW, Vachon L, Liu BJ, Huang HK. Cross-racial differences in growth patterns of children based on bone age assessment. *J Radiol*, 290(1): 228–235; 2009.

Zheng Z. Huang HK, Liu BJ. Lossless digital signature embedding methods for assuring 2-D and 3-D medical image integrity. In: Dhawan AP, Huang HK, Kim DS, eds. *Principles and Advanced Methods in Medical Imaging and Image Analysis* Singapore: World Scientific Publications, 573–98; 2008.

CHAPTER 26

Integration of Computer-Aided Diagnosis (CAD) with PACS

In this chapter we present two CAD applications that accomplished their ultimate goal of becoming integrated into daily clinical practice. The two CAD applications are for detection of multiple sclerosis on brain MRI with informatics output, and bone age assessment of children from hand radiographs. The rationale behind the CAD system's development and the validation and evaluation processes will be reviewed, the same as in Chapter 25, but with an additional important component not discussed in Chapter 25, which is its integration with PACS for daily operation. For convenience, Figure 20.9 is reproduced here as Figure 26.1 to show how this chapter (in orange color) corresponds as well to other chapters of Part IV.

CAD-PACS integration requires new concepts and additional technical background. Hence we introduce in this chapter DICOM screen capture and structured reporting framework, some specific IHE (integrating the healthcare enterprise) workflow profiles, and CAD-PACS toolkit.

26.1 THE NEED FOR CAD-PACS INTEGRATION

The main purpose in integrating CAD with PACS for daily clinical operation is to utilize CAD as a second reader. To recap our discussion in Chapter 25, CAD software can be implemented within a stand-alone CAD workstation (WS), a CAD server, or be integrated in PACS as PACS-based CAD. Currently several PACS and CAD companies have successfully integrated their CAD applications within the PACS operation, but these applications are either in a CAD-specific WS or in a closed PACS operation environment using proprietary software. For example, in mammography, CAD has become an integral part of a routine clinical assessment of breast cancer in many hospitals and clinics across the United States and abroad. However, the value and effectiveness of CAD applications are compromised by the inconvenience of the dedicated stand-alone CAD WS or server. The daily use of DICOM, PACS, and IHE technologies in the clinical environment may offer a clue as to how to work around these obstacles. The CAD–PACS integration has many distinct advantages:

PACS and Imaging Informatics, Second Edition, by H. K. Huang
Copyright © 2010 John Wiley & Sons, Inc.

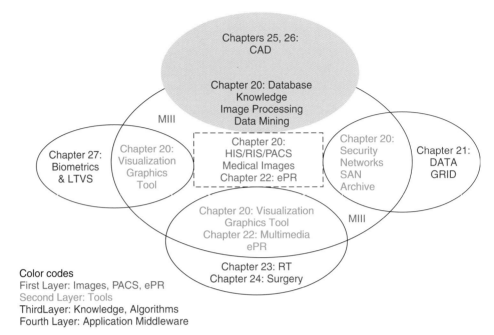

Figure 26.1   Imaging informatics data sources (rectangle), concepts, technologies, and applications (large and small ellipses) as discussed in the chapters of Part IV. Color codes refer to the five-layer informatics infrastructure shown in Figure 20.2. CAD–PACS integration is in orange color. CAD basic presented in Chapter 25 and integrated of CAD with PACS in this chapter are in orange color.

1. PACS technology is mature. Integrating CAD with its powerful computers and high-speed networks dedicated to the storage, retrieval, distribution, and presentation of clinical images would facilitate the daily operations of health-care providers.
2. PACS-based easy query/retrieve tools provide the user with images and related patient data obtained from CAD workstations.
3. The DICOM structured reporting (SR) and IHE workflow profiles can be readily applied to facilitate the CAD–PACS integration.
4. CAD–PACS integration results can be directly viewed and utilized at the PACS WS together with the PACS database.
5. The very large, dynamic, and up-to-date PACS database can be used by CAD to improve its diagnostic accuracy.

Clinical examples that illustrate the importance and usefulness of the CAD-PACS Toolkit will be discussed in detail in Sections 26.4.2, 26.6, and 26.7.

26.2   DICOM STANDARD AND IHE WORKFLOW PROFILES

CAD–HIS/RIS/PACS integration requires certain basic ingredients from HL7 (heath level 7) standard for textual data, DICOM (Digital Imaging and Communications in

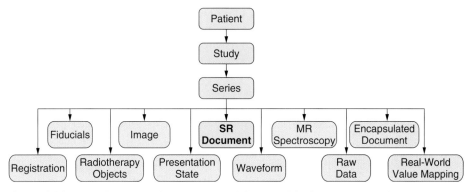

Figure 26.2   DICOM SR objects in the DICOM model of the real world. The green SR document is located in the DICOM data module (green box), which is at the same level as the DICOM Image.

Medicine) standard for image, and IHE (integrating the healthcare enterprise) work-flow profiles in order to comply with the HIPAA (Health Insurance Portability and Accountability Act) requirements. Among the DICOM standard and IHE workflow profiles, DICOM structured reporting (DICOM-SR), and IHE key image note (KIN), simple image and numeric report (SINR), and postprocessing workflows (PWF) are important in CAD–HIS/RIS/PACS integration.

26.2.1 DICOM Structured Reporting (DICOM SR)

The scope of DICOM SR is the standardization of structured reporting (SR) documents in the imaging environment. SR documents record observations made for an imaging-based diagnostic or interventional procedure, particularly information that describes or references images, waveforms, or specific regions of interest (ROI). DICOM SR was introduced in 1994 and achieved major recognition when Supplement 23 was adopted into DICOM standard in 1999 as the first DICOM SR for clinical reports (see Chapter 9). The DICOM Committee has initiated more than 12 supplements to define specific SR document templates. Among these supplements, two relate to capturing CAD results—the Mammography CAD SR (Supplement 50, 2000) and Chest CT CAD SR (Supplement 65, 2001)—have been ratified. In practice, the use of structured forms for reporting is known to be beneficial in reducing the ambiguity of natural language format reporting by enhancing the precision, clarity, and value of the clinical document.

DICOM SR is generalized by using DICOM information object definitions (IODs) and services for the storage and transmission of structured reports. Figure 26.2 provides a simplified version of the DICOM model of the real world showing where DICOM SR objects reside. The most important part of an SR object is the SR document content, which is an "SR template" that consists of different design patterns for various applications. In Section 26.5 we provide a step-by-step summary on how to generate a SR using the clinical example shown in Section 26.6.

Once the CAD results with images, graphs, overlays, annotations, and text have been translated into an SR template designed for this application, the data in the specific template can be treated as a DICOM object stored in the worklist of the data model (see Fig. 26.2 boxes with light green background), and it can be displayed for review by a PACS WS with the SR Display function. The viewing requires the original images from which the CAD results were generated so that the results can be overlaid onto the images. The SR display function can link and download these images from the PACS archive and display them as well on the WS.

26.2.2   IHE Profiles

Three IHE profiles are useful for CAD-PACS integration:

1. Key image note (KIN) profile: This profile allows users to flag images as significant (for referring, for surgery, etc.) and add a note.
2. Simple image and numeric report (SINR) profile: This profile specifies how diagnostic radiology reports (including images and numeric data) are created, exchanged, and used.
3. Postprocessing workflow (PWF) profile: This profile provides a worklist, status and result tracking for post-acquisition tasks, such as computer-aided detection or image processing.

26.3   THE CAD–PACS© INTEGRATION TOOLKIT

CAD software can be in a stand-alone CAD WS, CAD server, or integrated within the PACS as PACS-based CAD (see Section 25.3). Regardless where the CAD software is installed, the goal is to have CAD results integrated with the daily clinical PACS operation. In this section the CAD workflow in current practice is first described, followed by a presentation of the CAD–PACS integration toolkit for extending the CAD workflow to the PACS environment. The CAD–PACS toolkit is a software package that was developed in 2006 at the Image Processing and Informatics Laboratory (IPILab). The CAD–PACS integration application was presented at the RSNA Annual Meetings in 2006 and 2007.

26.3.1   Current CAD Workflow

Figure 26.3 depicts the PACS environment (blue box) and a CAD WS/server location (red box) that is outside the realm of PACS. These two systems are usually disjoint. When an image is needed for CAD processing (see numbers in Fig. 26.3), the workflow that occurs is as follows:

1. CAD processes the exam ordered through RIS, or directly from its modality.
2. A technologist or radiologist transmits the original images from the PACS server or PACS WS to CAD WS for processing. Results are stored within the CAD domain, since the CAD WS or server is a closed system and clinicians need to physically go to the CAD WS to view results.
3. The CAD–PACS toolkit (purple box), which can integrate with the PACS server, PACS WS, and the CAD server/WS together via the DICOM standard

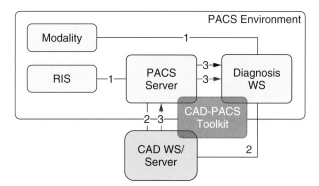

Figure 26.3 CAD workflow (orange) in the PACS environment (blue) with the CAD–PACS toolkit (purple). See the color code used in Figure 26.4.

and IHE profiles, passes the CAD results to the PACS server for archiving and the PACS WS for viewing; and query/retrieve original images from PACS server to PACS WS to be overlaid with the CAD results. In addition it can automatically pass images directly from the PACS server or PACS WS to the CAD WS for processing.

26.3.2   Concept

CAD-PACS© is a software toolkit using the HL7 standard for textual information; the DICOM standard for various types of data formats, including images, waveforms, graphics, overlays, and annotations; and IHE workflow profiles described in the aforementioned section for the integration of CAD results within the PACS workflow. This CAD software toolkit is modularized and its components can be installed in five different configurations: (1) in a stand-alone CAD workstation; (2) in a CAD server; (3) in a PACS workstation; (4) in a PACS server; or (5) in a mix of the previous four configurations. In general, a CAD manufacturer would be more comfortable with the first two approaches because there is very little collaboration needed for the PACS software, which is too complex for most CAD manufacturers. On the other hand, a PACS manufacturer would prefer to use an in-house CAD or acquire the CAD from outside and integrate it with its own PACS with the latter three approaches.

26.3.3   The Infrastructure

The CAD–PACS© toolkit has three editions: DICOM-SC^{TM}, first edition; DICOM–PACS–IHE^{TM}, second edition; and DICOM–CAD–IHE^{TM}, 3rd edition; and five software modules: i-CAD-SC^{TM}, i-CAD^{TM}, i-PPM^{TM}, Receive-SR^{TM}, and Display-SR^{TM}. Each edition contains some or all of the software modules. Figure 26.4 shows the architecture of the toolkit.

The toolkit is classified into three editions for the different levels of PACS integration requirements. Table 26.1 compares the three integration approaches. The first edition shows a simple screen capture output, and the CAD data are not stored for

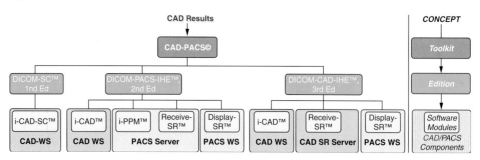

Figure 26.4 Rightmost: The concept of four level CAD-PACS Integration toolkit. CAD–PACS Integration toolkit (purple), three CAD–PACS© editions (green), the five distinct software modules (yellow), CAD components and results (red/orange), and PACS components (blue). Left: The CAD–PACS© toolkit first edition DICOM-SC™ utilizes DICOM screen capture service to view CAD results. This edition is easy to integrate, but the CAD output is not in a database for future retrieval. Middle: The second edition DICOM-PACS-IHE™ is utilized for integration with a full PACS. It consists of four CAD–PACS software modules, and allows a PACS manufacturer to integrate an existing CAD into its own PACS. Right: The third edition DICOM-CAD-IHE™ is utilized for integration with the CAD server. This component is independent from the PACS manufacturer as long as the PACS workstation is DICOM SR Compliant. The CAD results can then be viewed at a PACS WS. It is favored by the CAD manufacturers or research laboratories for integration. The three modules i-CAD™, Receive-SR™, and Display-SR™ are the same in both DICOM-PACS-IHE™ and DICOM-CAD-IHE™ editions. PPM (postprocessing manager) allows the integration of CAD results with the PACS server that are PACS specific and would require PACS vendor's assistance for implementation. In the lower level components, in either PACS or CAD, proper toolkit software modules can be installed in the corresponding system components for CAD–PACS integration.

TABLE 26.1   Comparison of the three CAD–PACS integration editions

Specifications	DICOM-SC 1st Edition	DICOM-PACS-IHE 2nd Edition	DICOM-CAD-IHE 3rd Edition
Using secondary captured Image to store CAD results	✓		
Using DICOM SR		✓	✓
PACS without SR support	✓		✓
PACS with SR support		✓	
Display referenced image	✓	✓	✓
Toggling between image and annotation		✓	✓

future use. The second edition is for full CAD–PACS integration requiring elaborate collaboration between the CAD developer and the PACS manufacturer. The third edition does not require the elaborate integration efforts of the two parties, and proper use of the CAD-PACS toolkit is sufficient, which favors the independent CAD developer.

26.3.4   Functions of the Three Editions

26.3.4.1   DICOM-SC^{TM}*, 1st Edition*   The first edition utilized the i-CAD-SC^{TM} software module, which relies on the DICOM screen capture (SC) service. Its design is simple to implement but has limited use in clinical research because it uses screen capture to store CAD results for viewing purposes only.

26.3.4.2   DICOM–PACS–IHE^{TM}*, 2nd Edition*   The second edition consists of four software modules: i-CAD^{TM}, i-PPM^{TM}, Receive-SR^{TM}, and Display-SR^{TM}. It utilizes the DICOM structured reporting (DICOM-SR) service and several IHE workflow profiles; its methodology is elegant but requires installation of the four modules within the PACS server. The i-PPM^{TM} module (postprocessing manager) requires thorough understanding of the entire PACS workflow, and would need intensive collaboration with the PACS manufacturer during integration. The integration could test the patience and perseverance of the integrator because of the protective culture of the PACS business.

26.3.4.3   DICOM–CAD–IHE^{TM}*, 3rd Edition*   The third edition is comprised of three software modules: i-CAD^{TM}, Receive-SR^{TM}, Display-SR^{TM}. This edition utilizes DICOM-SR and the key image note IHE profile, a method that reduces the necessity of altering the current PACS server, but CAD results are stored in the CAD server and not in PACS. DICOM SR links PACS image/data and CAD results for viewing. This edition is favored by CAD manufacturers because they have the ability to install the toolkit in their CAD server and integrate CAD results with the PACS clinical workflow without the complexity of the previous edition. DICOM SR provides the data format, allowing CAD results, text, images, graphics and annotations to be directly archived within the DICOM SR compliant CAD server.

The second and the third editions provide the correct methods of integrating CAD with PACS. The availability of direct CAD results in the daily clinical workflow would enhance the PACS operation as well as future PACS research possibilities.

26.3.5   Data Flow of the Three Editions

26.3.5.1   DICOM-SC^{TM}*, 1st Edition*   The data flow within the DICOM-SC^{TM} is simple and straight forward. The PACS WS sends the image to the CAD WS or CAD server. Results are captured on screen by the i-CAD-SC residing in the CAD WS as a DICOM image object and sent to the PACS server for archiving. This object can be viewed by the PACS WS. In this edition, results can only be viewed, and data cannot be used for other purposes. The display quality is marginal.

26.3.5.2   DICOM–PACS–IHE^{TM}*, 2nd Edition*   Figure 26.5 shows the workflow of this edition. Four software modules (yellow) must be installed in the appropriate PACS and CAD components, if those PACS components do not have the required

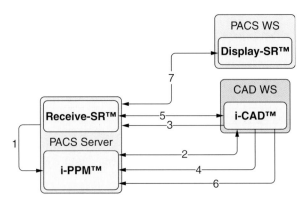

Figure 26.5 Data flow of the DICOM-PACS-IHE^{TM} second edition and locations of the four modules (yellow) of DICOM-PACS-IHE^{TM} in the CAD and PACS components (see also the color code used in Fig. 26.4). Numbers represent data flow steps during the integration. (1) CAD requests; (2) query CAD worklist, work item claimed; (3) retrieve images for CAD; (4) worklist purpose procedure step (PPS) in PPM in the process; (5) CAD results; (6) work item PPS completed; (7) retrieve images/CAD results.

functions. The challenge of this version is that the CAD developer has to collaborate closely with the PACS server manufacturer to fully understand the PACS workflow, which is different from the CAD–PACS integration workflow. To integrate CAD results with the PACS workflow using i-PPM^{TM} is an elaborate task.

26.3.5.3 *DICOM–CAD–IHE^{TM}, 3rd Edition* Figure 26.6 shows the data workflow. In this edition the CAD has two components, the CAD WS and CAD SR server. The latter takes care of monitoring and archiving of CAD results, and retrieving original images and data from PACS.

26.4 INTEGRATING USING THE CAD–PACS TOOLKIT

26.4.1 Cases of DICOM SR Already Available

This section presents two cases where CAD results were integrated into a PACS clinical environment using the CAD–PACS integration toolkit. In both cases CAD outputs had been converted by the manufacturers to the DICOM SR format, which is required by the CAD–PACS toolkit as the CAD output format for integration of the exchange object. Furthermore we can assume that the original images from which the CAD results were obtained had already been stored in PACS. Both cases use similar toolkit components to integrate the CAD system with the PACS system.

In order to have seamless integration between the CAD and PACS systems the following steps and components from the toolkit are required: (1) assign a DICOM node for the SR server, (2) establish connections between PACS and the SR server for image query and retrieval, (3) activate the CAD WS/server and the SR server to receive DICOM SR objects, and (4) set up Display-SR at the PACS WS.

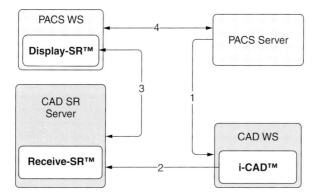

Figure 26.6 Data flow of the DICOM-CAD-IHE^{TM} third edition shows the locations of the three software modules (yellow) in the CAD SR server and PACS, respectively (see also the color code used in Fig. 26.4). The data flow steps are (1) PACS server pushes the CT images to CAD WS for CAD process; (2) CAD WS pushes the DICOM SR CAD results to CAD SR server, which consists of the Receive-SR^{TM} module with a SR database for archiving CAD results; (3) Web-based Display-SR^{TM} at PACS WS queries/retrieves DICOM SR CAD results from CAD SR server; (4) the Display-SR automatically queries and retrieves original images referenced in the DICOM SR CAD results in the PACS server for reviewing both original images and SR. In this edition, CAD SR server also keeps all CAD results in SR format.

26.4.2 Integration of Commercial CADs with PACS

The first case concerns CAD detection of lesions on chest CT images used by a PACS manufacture (General Electric Medical Systems, Milwaukee, Wisconsin), and the second case concerns CAD diagnosis of breast cancer on mammograms developed by a CAD manufacturer (R2/Hologic, Inc. Bedford, Massachusetts). In both cases the available CAD outputs had already been converted to a DICOM SR format by both manufacturers, and the original images were stored in PACS. The objective was to demonstrate that with the given CAD results in DICOM SR format stored in a CAD WS, the toolkit can integrate the CAD WS with a PACS for receiving and displaying the CAD results on the PACS WS. The CAD–PACS integration can be summarized by these steps: (1) the CAD WS or server completes the CAD process and sends the DICOM SR document containing the CAD results to the SR server (CAD–PACS toolkit); (2) the SR server utilizes the Receive-SR module (toolkit) to store the DICOM SR CAD results and automatically prefetches reference images from PACS; (3) CAD results are ready for viewing on a PACS WS using the Display-SR module (toolkit).

Figures 26.7 and 26.8 show the screenshots of a chest CT CAD and a mammogram CAD results in DICOM SR format displayed on a PACS WS, respectively. These images in the PACS WS can be manipulated as DICOM images. The top of each image shows the patient information, the left side displays the structured report, and the right side the DICOM images with nodule/lesion identified by overlaid annotations.

As shown in Figure 26.7, the location of the chest nodule is identified from DICOM SR object and sent to the Display-SR module to display as annotations (red

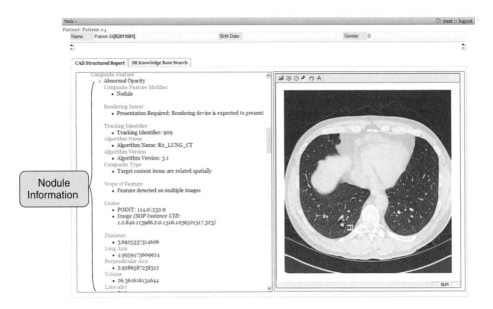

Figure 26.7 Manufacturer's chest CAD report already in DICOM SR format (left) with referenced image and annotation (right). Annotation (red circle) in the DICOM SR allows the user to toggle it on or off. (Case materials courtesy of R2/Hologic, Inc.)

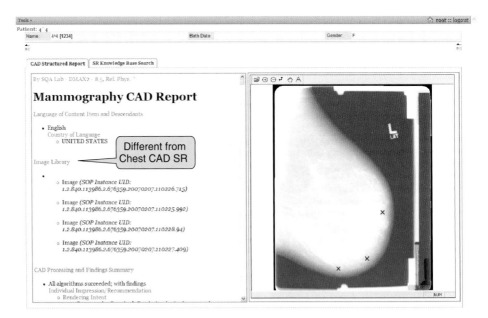

Figure 26.8 Manufacturer's mammography CAD report already in DICOM SR (left) with referenced image and annotation (right). Note that the DICOM-SR format is different from that in the CAD on CT (red fonts). Annotation (blue crosses) in the DICOM-SR allows the user to toggle it on or off. (Case materials courtesy of R2/Hologic, Inc.)

circle) on top of the original CT image stored in PACS. This information is stored separately from the DICOM images and allows annotation to be toggled on/off from the original image that is displayed. The same is true for the mammography CAD shown in Figure 26.8, in which the locations of the breast lesions are indicated by blue crosses. The differences between the chest CT CAD and the mammography CAD are that (1) the two CAD algorithms are different, and (2) the structures of the two DICOM SR objects are also different (see rectangular box annotation on the left of each figure). For example, the chest CT CAD SR does not reference the whole CT chest study but only those few CT images (red fonts) with nodules detected, whereas the mammography CAD DICOM SR object includes all four images (red fonts) in a screening mammography study. One reason is that a CT study has many images and the SR should only reference those images where the lesions were detected. Therefore each CAD algorithm or CAD for a different body region should have a different SR template to present complete and precise CAD results.

26.5 DICOM SR AND THE CAD–PACS INTEGRATION TOOLKIT

In the last two cases we discussed, the CAD results were converted to DICOM SR format. When the CAD results are not in DICOM SR format, they have to be converted first so that the results comply with the CAD–PACS toolkit standard. The last two cases were easy to integrate with PACS because the CAD was developed by manufacturers that had already converted the CAD results to DICOM SR format, compared to the examples we will see in Sections 26.6 and 26.7 whose results are required to be converted to DICOM SR format first before the integration. Table 26.2 summarizes the integration requirements of CAD with PACS for the last two cases, lesions on chest CT and breast cancer on mammogram. CAD for multiple sclerosis (MS) on MRI and for bone age assessment are described in Sections 26.6 and 26.7. This In the CAD of multiple sclerosis case study we present the method of data format conversion.

26.5.1 Multiple Sclerosis (MS) on MRI

Multiple sclerosis (MS) is a progressive neurological disease affecting myelin pathways in the brain. Multiple lesions in the white matter can cause paralysis and severe motor disabilities of the affected patient. Symptoms are changes in sensation, visual problems, muscle weakness, and depression. Currently MRI T1 and FLAIR pulse sequences are used for radiological diagnosis. In these images MS appears as multiple white lesions in the white matter area of the brain. MRI is also used to follow up and monitor the progress of the disease and the effectiveness of therapy after the patient is treated with drugs. Since MRI provides excellent delineation of MS, it is fairly easy for radiologists to make the diagnosis. However, due to the possibility of a large number of multiple lesions in the MRI 3-D volume set of the brain, it is tedious and time-consuming to identify the 3-D aspect of each lesion and quantify the number and size of these lesions. Moreover the quantitative reproducibility through human observers is poor. Augmenting CAD with imaging informatics methods, a 3-D CAD MS package would facilitate the physician's timely diagnosis, improve accuracy, and assess quantitatively the progress of therapy treatment.

TABLE 26.2 Tasks and requirements for integrating CAD with PACS systems in the three examples

CAD Systems	CAD Algorithm	CAD Output Format	Integration Tasks
1. Commercial CAD: lesions on Chest CT and breast cancer on mammogram	Developed proprietary	DICOM SR document	Store SR files in SR server and display SR on PACS WS
2. CAD for multiple sclerosis (MS) on MRI	Developed proprietary	Text or XML, images (DICOM/bitmap)	Create SR template and SR files Store SR files in SR server and display SR on PACS WS
3. CAD for bone age assessment	Developed proprietary	Text or XML, images (DICOM/bitmap)	Create SR template and SR files Store SR files in SR server and display SR on PACS WS

Figure 26.9 shows the most common data obtained from 3-D CAD results. The data includes the original 3-D MRI data set, Figure 26.9*a* shows an MRI FLAIR image, CAD detected multiple lesions (Fig. 26.9*b*), radiologist identified lesions (Fig. 26.9*c*, normally not shown in the results, depicted here only for comparison purposes); the detected MS lesions are color coded on each 2-D image (Fig. 26.9*d*, one slice; Fig. 26.9*e*, two slices; and Fig. 26.9*f*, all 26 slices). Figure 26.9*g* gives the quantitative result of all lesions detected by CAD. Figure 26.9*h* gives three 2-D oblique views of the brain overlaid with 26 MS lesions. The CAD results were generated through collaboration between IPILab, USC and the Guardian Technologies, Inc., Dulles, Virginia.

Currently these results can be shown only on the specialized MS detection CAD WS but cannot be linked or viewed in the daily clinical PACS WS. The PACS database does not contain these results as DICOM objects, and the CAD WS or database does not know what other data the patient might have within the PACS. Sections 26.5.2 and 26.6 demonstrate how the CAD–PACS integration would allow such to happen, that is, to receive the CAD results from the CAD WS and display them on the PACS WS.

26.5.2 Generation of the DICOM SR Document from a CAD Report

To convert the CAD results from a text file, like the one shown in Figure 26.9, into DICOM SR format, a special CAD template is first tailored to satisfy the specific need for presenting complete results. Figure 26.10 shows a SR template for the MS application. The template is similiar to the two ratified CAD SR templates for mammography and chest CT in the DICOM standard shown in Figures 26.7 and 26.8. A new MS DICOM SR object for this application based on the tree structure is defined, designed, and implemented. This design, which utilizes the DICOM Standard Supplement 23 and computer science terminologies, has a document root MS CAD (see Fig. 26.10) that branches into four parent nodes (detections, analyses, summary,

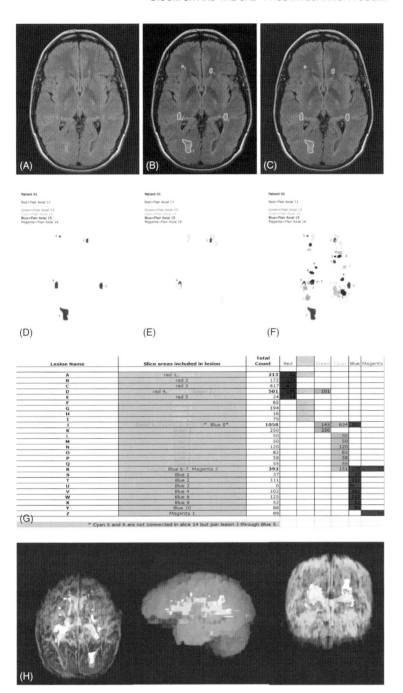

Figure 26.9 Commonly obtained data from 3-D multiple sclerosis (MS) CAD results. The data include the original 3-D MRI data set: (*A*) MRI FLAIR image; (*B*) CAD detected multiple lesions; (*C*) radiologist identified lesions (normally not shown in the results, depicted here for comparison purpose only); (*D*) color-coded MS lesions on a 2-D image; (*E*) on two slices; (*f*) on all slices; (*G*) quantitative results of all 26 lesions detected by CAD; (*H*) three oblique views of 2-D images with all 26 MS overlaid. Green color shows the ventricles. (Data: courtesy of Drs. A. Gertych and B. Guo; and Guardian Technology, Inc.)

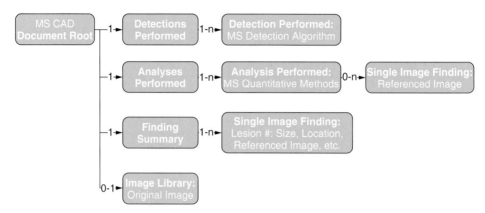

Figure 26.10 Multiple sclerosis (MS) CAD SR template. The SR template is designed following a tree structure starting from the Document Root, which branches into four parent nodes; each parent node branches to $(1 - n)$ child nodes.

and image library). Within this context the detections performed can have one or more child nodes, detection performed $(1 - n)$, with various detailed algorithms used for lesions detection. By the same token, the analyses performed parent node describes one or more methods of quantitative analysis performed on each lesion. Each analysis performed can be further branched to one or multiple $(1 - n)$ grandchild nodes, single image finding. The finding summary parent node is the most important part of an SR, which includes CAD results. This node can branch into multiple child nodes $(1 - n)$, each containing the name of the detection and analysis methods together with detailed results of each lesion on each single image finding. The detailed results include number, size, location, and referenced image. The image library parent node is optional; however, in the MS SR, it is used to reference original images where the CAD was performed on. The data structure format of each child can be obtained directly from the DICOM Standard, Supplement 23.

26.6 INTEGRATION OF CAD WITH PACS FOR MULTIPLE SCLEROSIS (MS) ON MRI

26.6.1 Connecting the DICOM SR with the CAD–PACS Toolkit

After the SR template is defined and designed, integrating the CAD with PACS can be implemented by using the toolkit. The first step is to use a PACS simulator to verify the data flow, as shown in Figure 26.11. The PACS simulator has been used since 2000 in the IPILab, USC as a training tool for PACS and imaging informatics research and development, and to verify the HIPAA compliance; the PACS simulator is currently utilized as a research tool in CAD–PACS integration.

The integrating steps can be summarized as follows (see numerals in Fig. 26.11): (1) the i-CAD module is configured with the MS SR template and all data (measurements, nodule images, and summary) to create the DICOM SR object; (2) the CAD WS is configured to run the CAD application automatically after receiving DICOM images from modality simulator or PACS simulator; (3) based on the SR template,

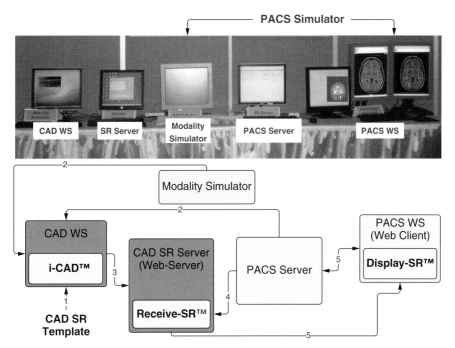

Figure 26.11 Use the PACS simulator to verify the data flow between the integrated PACS and CAD systems. Top: PACS simulator displayed at RSNA Annual Scientific Exhibit annually from 2000 to 2004. Bottom: Workflow of CAD–PACS integration: PACS simulator components (blue); CAD components (red); CAD–PACS toolkit modules (yellow). The integration steps in numerals are described in the text. The PACS WS (the rightmost compoent) displays the original image (middle) from PACS where the CAD results (right) were obtained. The left monitor shows the CAD–SR (see also Fig. 26.12.)

i-CAD module automatically starts to create an SR upon completion of the CAD process, and the results are sent in DICOM SR format to Receive-SR for storage; (4) the SR server prefetches the referenced images from the PACS server; and (5) the CAD results are ready for viewing on PACS WS.

In this case study, the CAD generates results as shown in Figure 26.9, among which are a number of lesions, 3-D coordinates of the lesions, the volume of each lesion, and their 2-D presentations in each detected MR slice at various oblique angles. These 2-D presentations can be used for 3-D viewing on a 2-D monitor.

26.6.2   Integration of PACS with CAD for MS

Figure 26.12 gives a screen shot of the CAD MS results at the PACS WS. The example shown is an of MS DICOM SR object with one 3-D view of multiple oblique 2-D images obtained by DICOM SC (See Figure 26.9H). Although, this example only displays the 2-D oblique images, theoretically the DICOM SR specification should include image references and CAD results that can be used to display real-time 3-D rendered images.

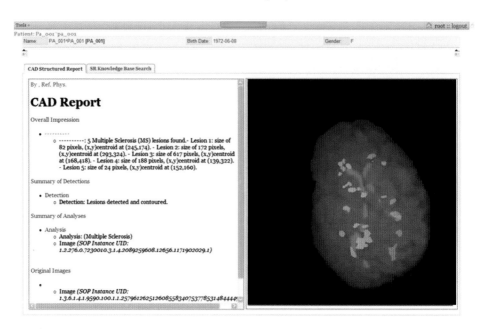

Figure 26.12   Multiple sclerosis CAD report in DICOM SR format (left) and a 2-D oblique image (right). Refer to Figure 26.9 for original images and CAD results.

26.7   INTEGRATION OF CAD WITH PACS FOR BONE AGE ASSESSMENT OF CHILDREN – THE DIGITAL HAND ATLAS

In this section we provide step-by-step guidelines to develop a CAD method for bone age assessment of children on a hand and wrist radiograph with relevance to the clinical standard, a rationale to create a more comprehensive Digital Hand Atlas, Institutional Review Board (IRB) approval data collection and use of the data, patient anonymity, CAD development, CAD validation and evaluation, and HIPAA compliance of the CAD evaluation in clinical environment. These guidelines are the standard procedure for developing a CAD method from incubation of a concept, to CAD development and productization, and finally to clinical site deployment.

26.7.1   Bone Age Assessment of Children

26.7.1.1   Classical Method of Bone Age Assessment of Children from a Hand Radiograph   Bone age assessment (BAA) is a clinical procedure in pediatric radiology to evaluate the stage of skeletal maturity based on a left hand and wrist radiograph through bone growth observations. The determination of skeletal maturity ("bone age") plays an important role in diagnostic and therapeutic investigations of endocrinological abnormality and growth disorders of children. In clinical practice the most commonly used bone age assessment method is atlas matching by a left hand and wrist radiograph against the Greulich & Pyle (G&P) atlas, which contains a reference set of normal standard hand images collected in 1950s with subjects exclusively from middle and upper class Caucasian populations. Figure 26.13

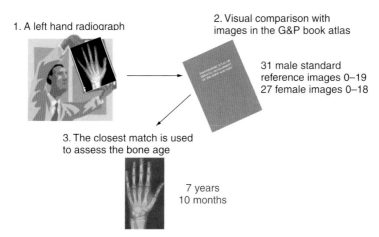

1. A left hand radiograph

2. Visual comparison with images in the G&P book atlas

31 male standard reference images 0–19
27 female images 0–18

3. The closest match is used to assess the bone age

7 years
10 months

Figure 26.13 Procedure of current clinical practice in bone age assessment for children that is based on comparing the child's hand radiograph with the G&P atlas (blue) with data over 70 years old.

depicts the BAA method using the G&P atlas. The atlas has been used for BAA round the world for more than 50 years.

26.7.1.2 Rationale for the Development of a CAD Method for Bone Age Assessment
Over the past thirty years many studies have raised questions of the appropriateness of using the G&P atlas for bone age assessment of contemporary children. In 1975 Roche showed that the average child in the United States was less mature than the 1959 standards of G&P. And Ontell in 1996 examined the applicability of the standards to diverse ethnic origin of children. However, these studies along with others did not provide a large-scale and systematic method for validation. Thus, to meet our objective to replace the out-of-date G&P we (1) collected up-to-date data on normal and healthy children to create a digital hand atlas (DHA), (2) used the DHA to evaluate, on the basis of the G&P atlas method, racial differences in skeletal growth patterns of Asian, African American, Caucasian, and Hispanic children in the United States, and (3) developed a CAD method to assess bone age of children based on the data collected in the DHA.

26.7.2 Data Collection

The protocol of the retrospective data collection was approved and has been renewed annually by the Institutional Review Board of our institutions; written informed consent was obtained from all subjects or their legal guardians. This study was compliant with the Health Insurance Portability and Accountability Act (HIPPA). Patient anonymity was achieved by replacing the patient name and other traceable information with a data encryption method.

26.7.2.1 Subject Recruitment
Over the past 10 years (May 1997–March 2008), with support from the National Institutes of Health (R01 LM 06270 and R01 EB 00298), the digital hand atlas (DHA) we developed contains 1390 hand and

wrist radiographs of healthy and normal Asian, African American, Caucasian, and Hispanic boys and girls. All subjects (age range, 1 day to 18 years) were recruited from public schools in Los Angeles County, California, starting in the late 1990s.

26.7.2.2 Case Selection Criteria Before the hand was examined with radiography, a physical examination was performed to determine the health and the Tanner maturity index of the subject to ensure that he or she was healthy and that his or her skeletal development was normal. Height, trunk height, and weight were measured and used to calculate the body mass index (BMI).

26.7.2.3 Image Acquisition Each radiograph of the hand and wrist was obtained with a strict data collection protocol. The radiographs were made using an X-ray generator (Polyphos 50; Siemens, Erlangen, Germany) at 55 kVp and 1.2 mAs (Figure 26.14A). The radiation dose delivered per image was less than 1 mrem, which is equivalent to approximately one day of natural background radiation. The hand was adjusted to an exact position that required the subject to keep the fingers apart and maintain hand straightness as much as possible (Figure 26.14B); no hand jewelry was worn. The distance between the X-ray tube and the image cassette was 40 inches. The hand of a normal child is less than 1 inch thick; therefore the magnification factor was approximately 1.

26.7.2.4 Image Interpretation After a radiograph of the hand was acquired from each subject, two experienced pediatric radiologists (each with more than 25 years experience in bone age assessment) performed independent readings based on the G&P atlas standards. During the reading, radiologists were blind to the subject's chronologic age, racial group, and other identifying information.

The subject's bone age, as determined by the radiologist was compared with the subject's chronologic age. The image was selected and accepted to the DHA only if the difference between subject's bone age, as determined by the radiologist and the subject's chronologic age was less than 3 years. The acceptance rate was higher than 90%.

26.7.2.5 Film Digitization For data analysis, Web-based image and data distribution, and communication in the clinical environment and public domain, each accepted radiograph (subject name and identification were covered with black tape) was digitized into a Digital Imaging and Communication in Medicine (DICOM) format by using a laser film digitizer (Model 2905, Array Corporation, Tokyo, Japan); each subject's information (excluding the subject's name, as well as any other traceable identification data) was put in the DICOM header. The scanner parameters used were 12 bits per pixel, optical density 0.0 to 4.0, and 100 micron pixel spacing. The size of the image corresponded to the size of the original radiograph (Fig. 26.14A). An example is given in Table 26.3 of the pertinent information on four 14-year-old boys of different races, the corresponding radiographs of their hands are shown in Figure 26.15.

26.7.2.6 Data Collection Summary There were two cycles of data collection, each with eight categories (Asian girls, Asian boys, African-American girls, African-American boys, Caucasian girls, Caucasian boys, Hispanic girls, and Hispanic boys).

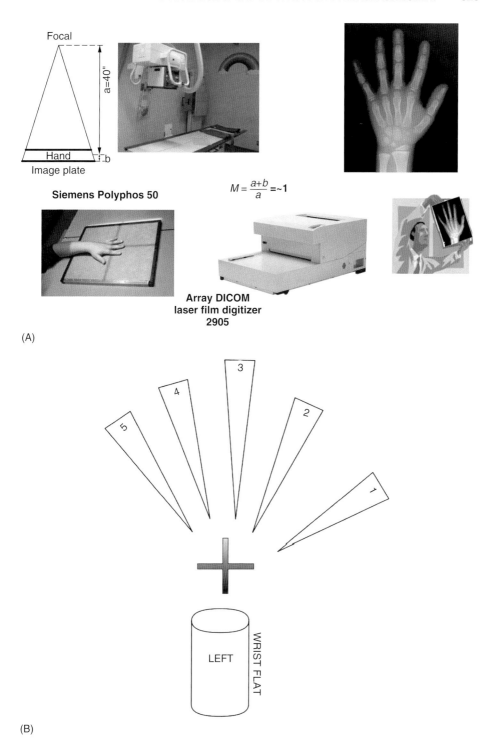

(A)

(B)

Figure 26.14   (*A*) Procedure of obtaining a hand radiograph and converting it to a digital image. (*B*) The protocol used to obtain the hand raiograph, the figure shows where the five fingers and the wrist joint should be placed. 1 represents the thumb. (Courtesy of Dr. P. Moin's drawing)

TABLE 26.3. Pertinent Information in four 14-year-old boys of different races

Subject	Race	Sex	Birth Date	Exam Date	Chronological Age (year)	Tanner Materity Index	Height (cm)	Trunk Height (cm)	Weight (kg)	Reader 1 (year)	Reader 2 (year)
a	AS	M	May/26/1987	July/12/2001	14.13	5	170.00	88.90	55.50	15.75	15.50
b	AA	M	July/18/1981	Dec/3/1995	14.46	3.5	168.00	82.55	49.30	13.25	14.00
c	CA	M	July/5/1979	Apr/19/1994	14.79	4	169.00	86.70	56.00	14.00	14.50
d	HI	M	Sept/13/1983	May/6/1998	14.64	5	168.40	83.82	51.60	15.00	15.00

Note: The DICOM header of each case includes subject's demographic and health-related information and two radiologists' readings. These data along with the corresponding image can be retrieved from the Web-based digital hand atlas. AS = Asian; AA = African American; CA = Caucasian; HI = Hispanic.

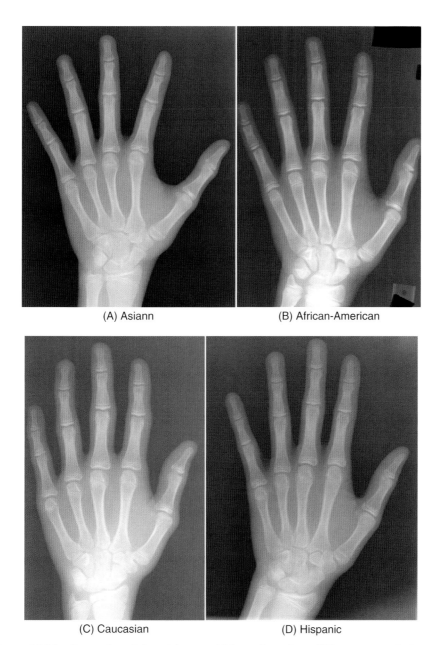

Figure 26.15 Examples of four 14-year-old boys from four different races, their corresponding demographic data and two radiologists' readings are included in the DICOM image header shown in Table 26.3. (*A*) 14.13-year-old Asian boy; (*B*) 14.46-year-old African-American boy; (*C*) 14.79-year-old Caucasian boy; (*D*) 14.64-year-old Hispanic boy.

Each category contains 19 age groups (one for subjects younger than 1 year and 18 sets at 1-year intervals for subjects aged 1–18 years). The two pediatric radiologists independently read all images obtained in each cycle. Cycle 1 consisted of 1103 digitized hand images with demographic data. Five cases for each younger age group (1–9 years) and 10 cases for each older age group (10–18 years) were included. The sample sizes were chosen to achieve a precision of approximately 0.20 for all age groups with 95% confidence interval when using the digital hand atlas to compare bone age with chronologic age. Precision is defined as the confidence interval width divided by the estimated mean value of the chronologic age. Subjects younger than 1 year were considered infants, and their data were not used for the analysis.

In order to study the active growth period in children aged 5 to 14 more closely, data were collected in 287 subjects during the second cycle after the first cycle had been completed. Thus a total of 1390 cases were included in the DHA. The breakdown of cases is as follows: 167 Asian girls, 167 Asian boys, 174 African-American girls, 184 African-American boys, 166 Caucasian girls, and 167 Caucasian boys. 183 Hispanic girls, and 182 Hispanic boys. These 1390 cases, shown in Table 26.4, were used to derive the results described in this study.

26.7.3   Methods of Analysis

26.7.3.1   *Statistical Analysis*   Statistical analyses was performed using computer software (SPSS, version 15.0 for Windows, SPSS Inc., Chicago, Illinois). Graphs were generated by third-party software groups (KaleidaGraph 3.5, Synergy Software, Reading, Pennsylvania). Two types of analyses, paired-samples *t*-test and ANOVA (analysis of variance), were conducted using the chronologic age as the reference standard. Age 0 group was not used for analysis. Two-cycle data were combined for each race and a given gender with the entire ages ranging from 1 to 18; then paired-samples *t*-tests were performed case by case to find the mean difference between the average of two readings and the chronologic age. The results were eight categories for comparison: Asian girls, Asian boys, African-American girls, African-American boys, Caucasian girls, Caucasian boys, Hispanic girls, and Hispanic boys (ASF, ASM, AAF, AAM, CAF, CAM, HIF, and HIM) each depicting the overall view of differences between the radiologists' average bone age reading against the chronologic age for subjects of each race and sex.

On the basis of the effects of growth factor and sexual hormones, as well as our observations from phalangeal, carpal, and wrist joint regions, we divided the entire growth age ranging from age 1 year to 18 years into four age subsets, shown in Figure 26.16 (right column). These subsets were used to study the differences in growth patterns of children of different races for a given subset. ANOVA (analysis of variance) was used to study the cross-racial comparisons for a given subset of growth range based on the differences between chronologic age and bone age.

26.7.3.2   *Radiologists' Interpretation*   Table 26.5 shows the mean difference in age between the average bone age reading by two radiologists and the chronologic age for each of the eight categories by race and sex. Since we collected data in children with normal skeletal development, the differences, shown with asterisks in Table 26.5, are within two standard deviations between the normal chronologic age

TABLE 26.4. Images and data contained in the digital hand atlas

	Cycle 1								Cycle 2							
	AS		AA		CA		HI			AS		AA		CA		HI	
Age Group /Category	F	M	F	M	F	M	F	M	Age Group /Category	F	M	F	M	F	M	F	M
00	1	2	4	5	3	3	1	4									
01	5	5	5	5	5	5	5	5									
02	5	5	5	5	5	5	5	5									
03	5	5	5	5	5	5	5	5									
04	5	5	5	5	5	5	5	5									
05	5	5	5	5	5	5	5	5	05	3	4	4	4	2	5	5	4
06	5	5	5	5	5	5	5	5	06	2	1	4	2	2	3	5	4
07	5	5	5	5	5	5	5	5	07	2	2	4	4	3	4	5	5
08	5	5	5	5	5	5	5	5	08	4	0	5	5	4	5	4	5
09	5	5	5	5	5	5	5	5	09	2	2	4	5	3	2	5	5
10	10	10	10	10	10	10	10	10	10	5	4	2	5	2	1	4	2
11	10	10	10	10	10	10	10	10	11	2	5	0	5	3	4	5	4
12	10	10	10	10	10	10	10	10	12	4	5	5	5	4	3	5	5
13	10	10	10	10	10	10	10	10	13	5	5	5	5	4	2	5	5
14	10	10	10	10	10	10	10	10	14	3	2	2	4	1	0	4	4
15	10	10	10	10	10	10	10	10									
16	10	10	10	10	10	10	10	10									
17	10	10	10	10	10	10	10	10									
18	10	10	10	10	10	10	10	10									
Subtotal	136	137	139	140	138	138	136	139	Subtotal	31	30	35	44	28	29	47	43

Note: Cycle 1 totaled 1103 cases with two readings per case; cycle 2 totaled 287 cases with four readings per case.

829

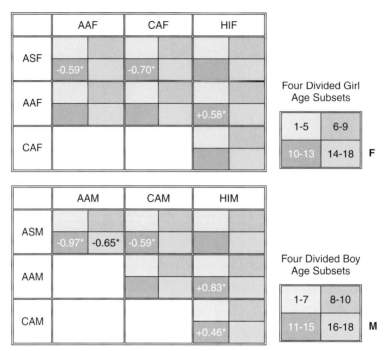

Figure 26.16 Right column: Small charts show the four divided age subsets for (F) girls and (M) boys. These charts provide a road map for use in the study of racial differences during different growth periods. (F) Green indicates 1 to 5 years of age; blue: 6 to 9 years; purple: 10 to 13 years; orange: 14 to 18 years. (M) Green indicates 1 to 7 years of age; blue: 8 to 10 years; purple: 11 to 15 years; orange: 16 to 18 years. Left column: Large charts show cross-racial comparison for (F) girls (upper chart), and (M) boys (lower chart). Data are shown only if differences are significant ($P \leq 0.05$). Each racial block was divided into the four age groups described. The plus and minus signs indicated under- and overestimation of bone age, respectively, by radiologists in comparing rows with columns. ASF = Asian girls, ASM = Asian boys, AAF = African-American girls, AAM = African-American boys, CAF = Caucasian girls, CAM = Caucasian boys, HIF = Hispanic girls, and HIM = Hispanic boys.

and the average bone age (see the Case Selection Criteria section) and may not be important from a clinical perspective, However, we were able to conclude that the radiologists had a slight tendency, which was statistically significant, to overestimate bone age in the Asian and Hispanic populations as a whole.

26.7.3.3 Cross-racial Comparisons The cross-racial differences assessed with analysis of variance among the four races in the four divided age subsets (see Figure 26.16, right column) are presented in the left column of Figure 26.16.

Figure 26.16*F* (upper row) shows that in girls, significant mean differences of average reading between races were observed in the third age subset (10–13 years, purple). Radiologists overestimated bone age in Asian girls in comparison with their African-American and Caucasian peers by approximately 0.59 year and 0.70 year, respectively. Similarly radiologists overestimated bone age by 0.58 year in Hispanic

TABLE 26.5   Mean difference between bone age as assessed by radiologists and chronologic age according to race and sex

Characteristics	Asian Girls (F)	Asian Boys (M)	African-American Girls (F)	African-American Boys (M)	Caucasian Girls (F)	Caucasian Girls (M)	Hispanic Girls (F)	Hispanic Boys (M)
Mean difference between bone age assessed by radiologists and chronological age	0.24^a	0.41^a	0.03	-0.02	-0.15^a	0.01	0.24^a	0.30^a
Number of Cases[b]	166	165	170	179	163	164	182	178

[a] Indicates that mean difference between bone age assessed by radiologists and chronological ages was significant ($p \leq 0.05$).

[b] Infants (children younger than 1 year) were excluded from the analysis.

girls when compared with African-American girls. Figure 26.17 shows the plots of bone age versus chronologic age in Asian girls versus Caucasian girls, Asian girls versus African-American girls, and Hispanic girls versus African-American girls. In each comparison the figure at the left covers the entire age range (1–18 years), whereas the figure at the right shows a close-up of the third age subset (10–13 years).

Similar patterns were observed in boys (Fig. 26.16*M*, chart in the lower row). In the third age subset (11–15 years, purple) significant over-estimation of bone age of 0.97 year and 0.83 year was observed in Asian and Hispanic boys, respectively, when compared with African-American boys. Overestimation of 0.65 year continued until fourth age subset (16–18 years, orange) when Asian boys were compared with African-American boys. Furthermore comparison of Caucasian boys with Asian boys and Hispanic boys in the third age subset (11–15 years) resulted in significant overreading of 0.59 year and 0.46 year, respectively. Figure 26.17 shows bone age versus chronologic age in four racial pairs: (1) Hispanic boys versus African-American boys, (2) Asian boys versus African American boys, (3) Asian boys versus Caucasian boys, and (4) Hispanic boys versus Caucasian boys.

26.7.3.4   *Development of the Digital Hand Atlas for Clinical Evaluation*

To recap, an up-to-date digital hand atlas (DHA) for four ethnic group was developed with 1390 hand and wrist radiographs obtained in Asian, African-American, Caucasian, and Hispanic boys and girls with normal skeletal development aged between 1 day and 18 years. Each case was read by two pediatric radiologists working independently on the basis of the Greulich and Pyle (G&P) atlas standard. The normality and consistency of the data were ensured by radiologists' readings plus a rigorous quality assurance data collection protocol. Hand radiographs were digitized and stored in DICOM format, which facilitates image viewing and transmission in the clinical environment for training and image-assisted daily clinical operation.

Previous studies have been performed in which researchers examined the applicability of G&P atlas for use in contemporary children. Mora et al.

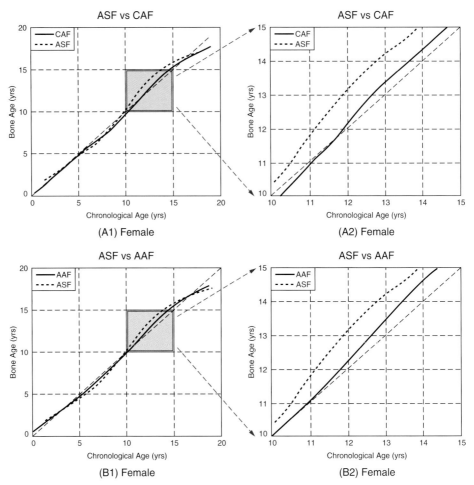

Figure 26.17 Graphs show comparisons of three racial pairs. The *x*-axis shows the chronologic age, the *y*-axis shows the average bone age, and the 45° dotted line shows the normal standard comparison in (A1) Asian girls (ASF) versus Caucasian girl (CAF), (B1) Asian girls versus African-American girls (AAF), and (C1) Hispanic girls (HIF) versus African-American girls. The graphs on the left show the plots or the entire age (1–18 years) range, whereas the graphs on the right (A2, B2, C2) are close-up plots for the third age subset (10–13 years).

examined 534 children of European and African descent, and Ontell et al. collected data in 765 trauma patients of four races. Both studies are close to our study in that they involve use and evaluation of the G&P atlas in each of the racial groups. However in neither study did the authors compare cross-ratio differences. In creating the digital hand atlas, we observed differences in readings of two pediatric radiologists in subjects of four races on the basis of the G&P atlas standard, and we recorded these differences systematically. Our results show the cross-racial differences between skeletal growth patterns of Asian and Hispanic children and skeletal growth patterns of Caucasian

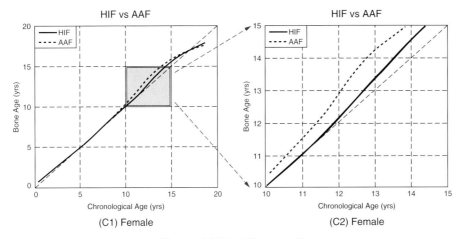

Figure 26.17   (*Continued*)

and African-American children. Radiologists assessed the bone age that was relatively close to the chronologic age of African-American and Caucasian children.

The DHA provides an up-to-date standard with which to classify normal bone growth and development in children. Currently the DHA is accessible from the World Wide Web for on-line learning and teaching. As of now, we can conclude that it is difficult to collect normal hand radiographs with supporting growth data from childern and that there are deficiencies of using the G & P atlas to assess bone age of children.

26.8   INTEGRATION OF CAD WITH PACS FOR BONE AGE ASSESSMENT OF CHILDREN — THE CAD SYSTEM

26.8.1   The CAD System Based on Fuzzy Logic for Bone Age Assessment

A fully automatic computer-aided-diagnosis (CAD) method for bone age assessment of children based on the DHA has been modeled for the boys and girls of the four races. The CAD method is a fuzzy logic system applied to several regions of interest of the hand and wrist radiograph. A three-compartment model was used for the image analysis results, which included the phalangeal bones, carpal bones, and the distal radius. The three compartment model was arranged in a modular and extensible fuzzy system integrating phalanges, carpals, and the distal radius for bone age assessment (BAA). The DHA formed the knowledge base of the fuzzy system, under the assumption that bone age is equal to chronologic age since the normality of children was ensured for each case during data collection of DHA. The fuzzy logic concept is derived from the imprecise phenomena that commonly occur in real-world situations such as in biological growth and incorporates a simple rule-based approach, thus making it suitable for the application of bone age assessment. To

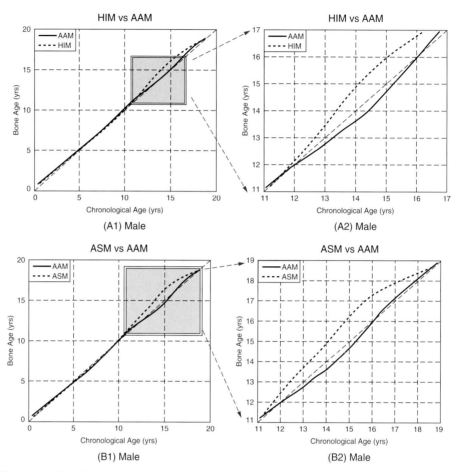

Figure 26.18 Comparisons (as in Fig. 26.17) of (A1) Hispanic (HIM) versus African-American boys (AAM), (B1) Asian (ASM) versus African American boys, (C1) Asian versus Caucasian boys (CAM), and (D1) Hispanic versus Caucasian boys. Left: entire age range (1–18 years). Right: third age subset (11–15 years) (A2, C2, D2) and third and fourth age subsets (11–18 years) (B2).

address the imprecise nature of the relationship between bone growth and bone age, a rule-based fuzzy inference system was developed to provide alternative options for a set of unresolved issues in the current G&P atlas matching method. The system was trained using the DHA to adapt to an individual's ethnicity and gender. To avoid subjectivity, two measurements were taken in sequence. First, a degree of membership was used to express the intermediate bone age from individual regions with quantitative measures. The final bone age was then aggregated from multiple regions and defuzzified. The results obtained from the fuzzy system were validated using normal subjects in the digital hand atlas and evaluated with subjects in clinical environments. For details of the fuzzy logic concept, refer to references at the end of this chapter.

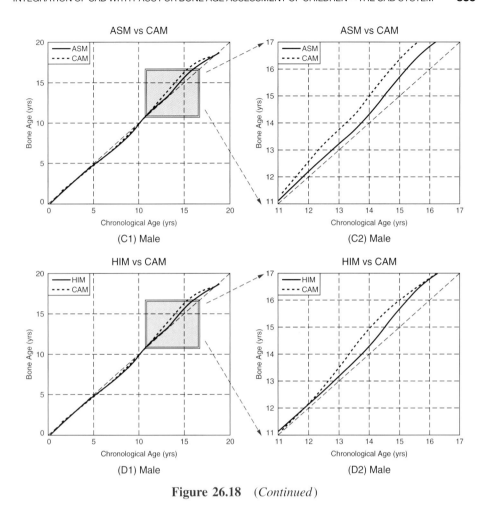

Figure 26.18 (*Continued*)

26.8.2 Fuzzy System Architecture

26.8.2.1 *Knowledge Base Derived from the DHA*   The CAD system is based on three regions of interest: the phalanges, carpals, and distal radius. Table 26.6 summarizes the clinical reliability of using these three regions of interest (ROI) for bone age assessment. Based on this clinical knowledge, the CAD method's parameters were extracted from these regions. Phalangeal analysis is most reliable from late childhood to early adolescence, both in epi-metaphysis segmentation and the ability of extracted features to predict the bone age. During this range of ages, as carpal bones ossify, they overlap beginning at age five in females and age seven in males. Thus the use of carpal bones in the determination of bone age is most sensitive during infancy and early childhood. Prior to complete ossification and overlap in the anteroposterior projection, carpal bone analysis has proved to be very reliable in both carpal bone segmentation and the use of the morphology of the segmented bones to predict the bone age for young children. For adolescents, the phalangeal and carpal regions lose a significant degree of sensitivity in the characterization of skeletal growth while the wrist region, specifically the distal radius, provides more

TABLE 26.6   Clinical reliability of using three ROIs for bone age assessment in different age groups

Age Group	Phalangeal ROIs	Carpal ROI	Distal Radius ROI
0 – 5 (female) 0 – 7 (male)	Feature analysis of epi-metaphysis - NOT reliable	Size and shape analysis of carpal bones - Reliable	
6 – 13 (female) 8 – 15 (male)	Feature analysis of epi-metaphysis - Reliable	Degree of overlapping of carpal bones - NOT reliable	
14 – 18 (female) 16 – 18 (male)	Feature analysis of epi-metaphysis - NOT sufficient		Feature analysis of epi-diaphysis - Reliable

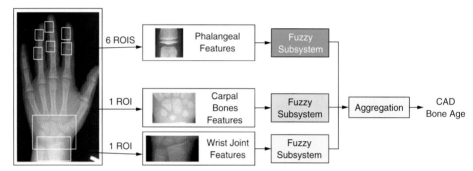

Figure 26.19   BAA fuzzy logic CAD algorithm workflow consists of eight regions of interest (ROIs): six phalangeal, one carpal bones, and one wrist joint. All regions are automatically detected by the CAD. There are three fuzzy logic systems; the aggregation of the three systems gives the CAD bone age of the child.

reliable growth information. These image analyses are further discussed in literature listed at the end of the chapter.

Figure 26.19 shows the CAD algorithm workflow. After image preprocessing, three regions of interest (ROIs)—carpal bones (see left, large white rectangle), wrist joint (large white rectangle), and the phalangeal region, which has six sub-regions (six white rectangles)—are automatically located and extracted as shown in the figure. Anatomical features are then extracted from the segmented osseous structures from each of the ROIs and inputted into the respective fuzzy subsystems. The results from the three regions are then aggregated to determine the final bone age. The following subsections describe fuzzy system development (see the four color boxes in Figure 26.19). For each subsystem, the generation methodology for membership functions and fuzzy rules refer to the references at the end of the chapter.

26.8.2.2 Phalangeal Fuzzy Subsystem

The middle and distal epimetaphyseal regions of the second through fourth digits were localized and extracted from each hand radiograph. A total of six phalangeal subregions of interest were thus isolated and acquired in the phalangeal ROI. Through image segmentation and feature extraction, 8 quantitative size and shape features for those 0 to 12 years of age and

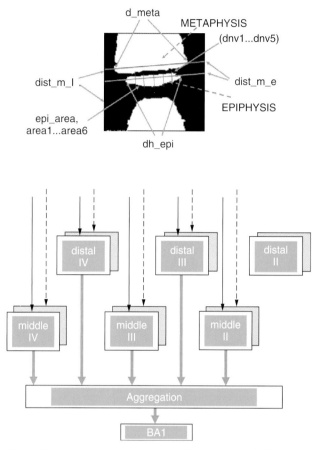

Figure 26.20 Top: Features extracted from a phalangeal sub-ROI segmentation from which features are extracted. Bottom: Phalangeal fuzzy subsystems, consisting of six components, each with a module for shape and size features (solid lines), and wavelet features (dash lines). The aggregation of all features from six sub-regions yields the bone age, BA1, of the phalangeal.

10 wavelet features for children of 10 to 18 were obtained from each phalangeal sub-ROI. As summarized in the top of Figure 26.20, size and shape features segmented and extracted, among these, the following features were found to contribute most to the bone growth: metaphsyeal diameter, epiphyseal diameter, epiphyseal-metaphyseal distance, horizontal epiphyseal diameter, and the distance between the more distal phalangeal metaphysis and the more proximal phalangeal epiphysis; these are the features also used for bone age assessment. These features are then inputted into the fuzzy subsystem, which consists of six components in the fuzzy logic for phalangeal epimetaphyseal subregions (Fig. 26.20, bottom). Each component includes two modules, one for shape and size features and another for wavelet features. The fuzzy bone age is assessed in two stages. First, each of the six components yields an intermediate output. Then, the six outputs are aggregated by finding their mean to obtain the fuzzy BA1 as shown in the base of Figure 26.20.

Carpal Bone ROI Analysis

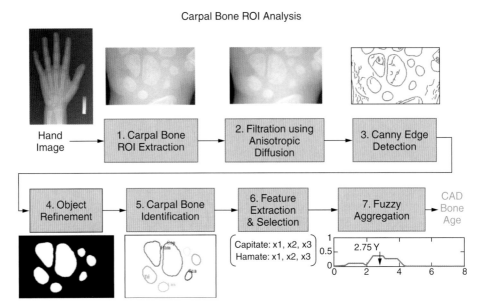

Figure 26.21 Example of using the carpal bones region alone to determine the bone age. Steps 1 to 7 describe the total procedure. Capitate (Cap) and Hamate (Ham), are the two bones provided sufficient information to assess the bone age; each with three features: one size (x1), and two shape, eccentricity (x2) and triangularity (x3). In this case, the bone age, BA2 is 2.75 years.

26.8.2.3 *Carpal Bone Fuzzy Subsystem*

The carpal fuzzy subsystem consists of two components, the capitate (Cap) and the hamate (Ham). After the carpal bones are segmented, the carpal ROI is extracted from the hand image as shown in Figure 26.21. The capitate and the hamate, the first two bones to ossify in the carpal region during development, are identified using a knowledge-based model and used to assess the carpal bone age. One size ($\times 1$) and two shape features, eccentricity ($\times 2$), and triangularity ($\times 3$) features, are then extracted from both the capitate and the hamate. Hence a total of six features are inputted into the carpal bones fuzzy subsystem for BAA. The fuzzy bone age determined by the carpal bone region is assessed in two stages. First, each of the two carpal bones yields an intermediate output. Then, the two intermediate outputs are aggregated by finding their mean to obtain the fuzzy BA2.

26.8.2.4 *Wrist Joint Fuzzy Subsystem*

The goal of wrist joint analysis is to yield higher accuracy for older children (girls: 14–18; boys: 16–18) based on the growth plate development and its separation from the radius. To perform wrist region assessment, the radius is first segmented based on the anatomical location, shape, and structure of the radius. The growth plate region is located and extracted. Wavelet features are obtained and then passed through the wrist joint fuzzy logic system to obtain the fuzzy BA3 as shown in Figure 26.22. It should be noted that the wrist region does not need an aggregate result because it is a single region of interest, unlike the six regions of the the phalangeal subsystem and the two regions in the carpal subsystem. To obtain good features from the wrist joint, positioning

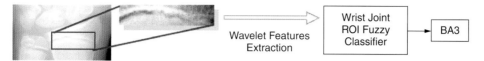

Figure 26.22 Result of wrist region analysis and growth plate segmentation, and the workflow of converting wavelet features into bone age BA3.

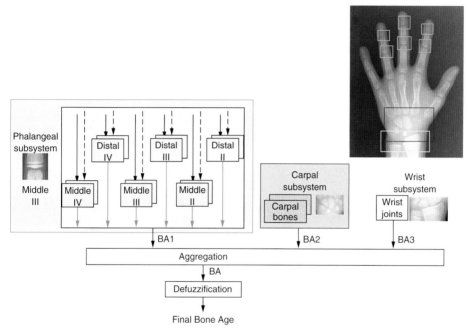

Figure 26.23 Fuzzy integration of eight ROIs, phanlangeal (6), carpal bones (1), and wrist (1), for the final bone age assessment.

of the hand while taking the radiograph has to adhere to the protocol shown in Figure 26.14*B*.

26.8.3 Fuzzy Integration of Three Regions

The final bone age assessment (BAA) is determined by three fuzzy bone ages from the phalangeal subsystem (BA1), carpal subsystem (BA2), and distal radius subsystem (BA3). These three fuzzy output membership functions were aggregated into the final fuzzy bone age as shown in Figure 26.23.

A final bone age is then obtained through defuzzification, the conversion of fuzzy output from the integration procedure to a precise bone age. The center of gravity method is used.

The completed BAA program with a three-region analysis and the corresponding fuzzy logic classifiers is applied to the digital hand atlas cases to obtain a computer-aided bone age assessment.

26.8.4 Validation of the CAD and Comparison of the CAD Result with the Radiologists' Assessment

26.8.4.1 Validation of the CAD In Section 26.7, we presented the cross-racial comparisons of radiologists' assessment of bone age of children contained in the digital hand atlas (DHA) on the basis of the G&P atlas standard. In the comparisons we discovered that for girls between 10 and 13 years, radiologists overestimated the bone age of Asian compared to Caucasian, Asian compared to African-American, and Hispanic compared to African-American. For boys, radiologists also overestimated the bone age of Hispanic compared to African-American, Asian compared to African-American, Asian compared to Caucasian, and Hispanic compared to Caucasian in the age group of 11 to 15 years. The overestimated bone ages extended from 11 to 18 years for Asian compared to African-American. The knowledge gained from the DHA was incorporated in the design of the CAD fuzzy logic system for bone age assessment. The validation of the CAD bone age assessment as performed uses all data contained in the DHA.

The CAD fuzzy logic system described in Section 26.8 was utilized to assess the bone age of all subjects contained in the DHA. An easy-to-use graphical user interface (GUI) was designed to cross-plot these results for comparison. The results are shown in Figure 26.24.

26.8.4.2 Comparison of CAD versus Radiologists' Assessment of Bone Age Figure 26.24 shows comparisons of the radiologists' and the CAD method's assessments of bone age for the four racial pairs. The four pairs are Asian, Caucasian, Hispanic, and African-American, *A*:girls; *B*:boys. In each plot the dotted curve is the radiologist's assessment, which as was used to derive the results presented in Section 26.7 and plotted on Figures 26.17 and 26.18. Each solid curve of Figure 26.24 is a plot of the results obtained by the CAD method. The plots of the cross-comparisons between the radiologists and the CAD assessments were obtained from the GUI of BAA CAD system.

The results shown in Figure 26.24 are for visual comparison. The rigorous statistical analysis we performed in determining the overestimation of radiologists in bone age assessment based on the G&P atlas, as shown in Figures 26.17 and 26.18, is still a work in progress. Nevertheless, certain patterns can be observed in these plots:

All Subjects Combined in the DHA

1. When combining all subjects in the DHA, CAD (solid line) underestimates subjects older than 8 to 10 years and overestimate subjects younger than 8 to 9 years, compared to radiologists' assessment.

2. CAD underestimates all subjects combined, all girls, and all boys over 16 to 18 years old, compared to radiologists' assessment. This may be because the wrist joint bone assessment is more difficult for the CAD to perform due to the fact that radius joint separation requires good image quality to distinguish the joint space and obtain wavelet measurements.

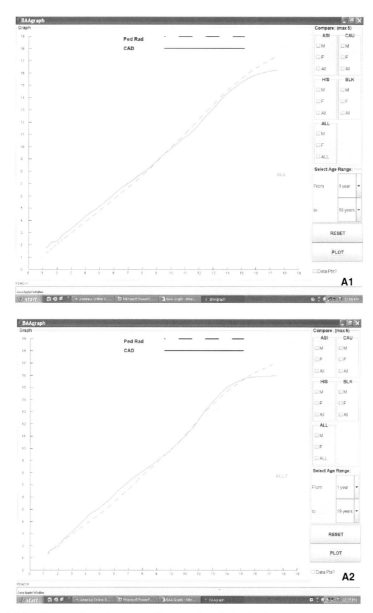

Figure 26.24   Comparison between CAD and radiologists' assessment of bone age. (*A*) Girls (F); (*B*) Boys (M). Each sex group shows six comparisons (1–6): all subjects contained in the digital hand atlas (ALL), all girls contained in the DHA (ALLF), Asian (ASI), Caucasian (CAU), Hispanic (HIS), and African-American (BLK). Each screenshot shows the GUI of the display component (www.IPILab. Org/BAAgraph) of the CAD system. The user clicks proper icons on the screen (right) to specify the data in the DHA, and format to be plotted. Dotted line: Radiologists average reading, solid line: CAD assessment. Note that A1 and B1 are identical.

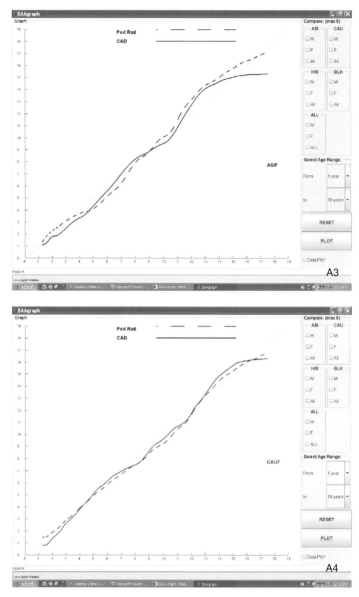

Figure 26.24   (*Continued*)

Girls Only, Compared to Radiologists' Assessment

1. When combining all girls in the DHA, CAD overestimates the 2 to 9 years group, and the 13 to 15 years group.
2. For all girls in each race the two plot-pairs, namely CAD versus radiologists' assessment crosses each other several times through different age groups. Among these, it seems that CAD versus radiologists exhibits the smallest differences in bone age assessment in Caucasian and African-American children, and overestimates all girls older than a 3-year-old Hispanic.

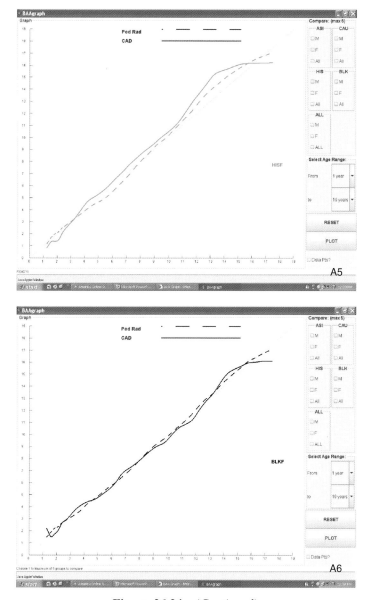

Figure 26.24   (*Continued*)

Boys Only, Compared to Radiologists' Assessment

1. When combining all boys in the DHA, CAD overestimates the 2 to 5 years group, and underestimates the 10 to 18 years group, compared to radiologists' assessment.

2. For all boys in each race, CAD underestimates all four races of subjects older than 10 years, compared to radiologists' assessment. For under 10 years old, there are slight overestimations in Asian and Caucasian, and underestimate in Hispanic, and a very close match with African-American.

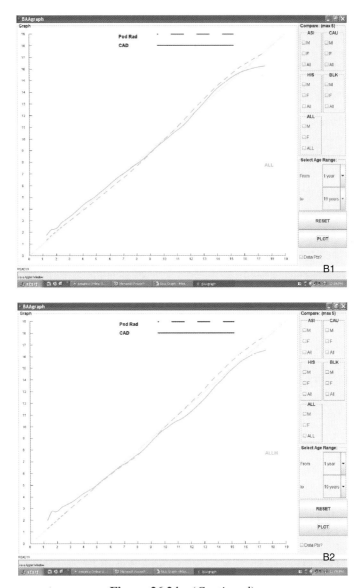

Figure 26.24   (*Continued*)

26.8.5   Clinical Evaluation of the CAD System for Bone Age Assessment

26.8.5.1   BAA Evaluation in the Clinical Environment   The next step after the validation is to bring DHA and BAA CAD system into a clinical setting for evaluation. The goal is to assist radiologists in their daily practice using the CAD results. To do that, a Web-based client-server system was designed with such a novel clinical implementation approach for on-line and real-time BAA. The digital hand atlas is already available on line in JPEG format at http://www.ipilab.org/BAAweb. The clinical validation system includes a stand-alone CAD workstation that is connected with the clinical PACS, a Web-based graphical user interface (GUI) at the

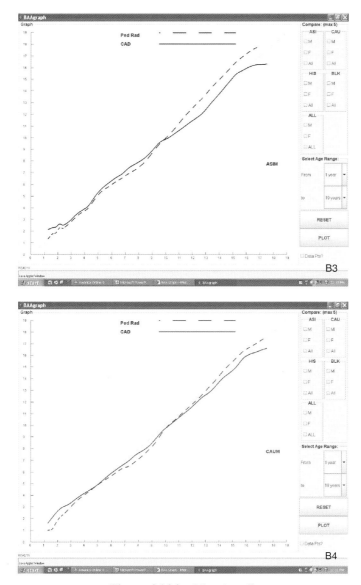

Figure 26.24   (*Continued*)

CAD workstation, and a CAD workflow designed specifically for the clinical environment. The system is integrated at the radiology department of Los Angeles County Hospital (LAC), and cases are collected both in real time and retroactively to analyze the CAD system's performance. In addition images in the G&P hand atlas were digitized and stored in the G&P atlas database for easy comparison.

26.8.5.2 Clinical Evaluation Workflow Design   The clinical workflow of BAA CAD had been previously designed by IPILab, USC and tested within the laboratory environment. Figure 26.25 shows the clinical workflow diagram simulated as if it was in clinical environment.

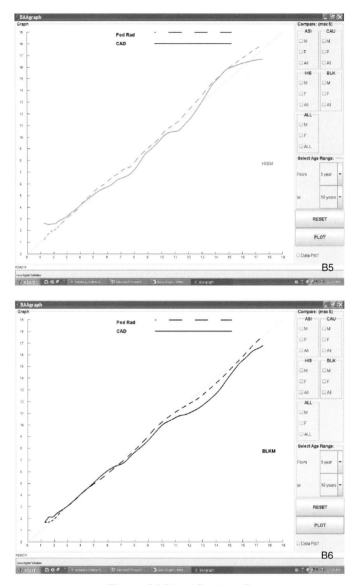

Figure 26.24 (*Continued*)

The workflow has six steps, the first three steps include conventional PACS workflow in radiology and the last three steps detail how data is transmitted in the presence of a CAD workstation:

1. Hand image is sent from the modality simulator (which simulates a CR, DR, or film scanner) to the acquisition gateway
2. Acquisition gateway transmits the image into the PACS storage server
3. PACS workstation queries and retrieves the hand image from PACS and display the image on the PACS WS

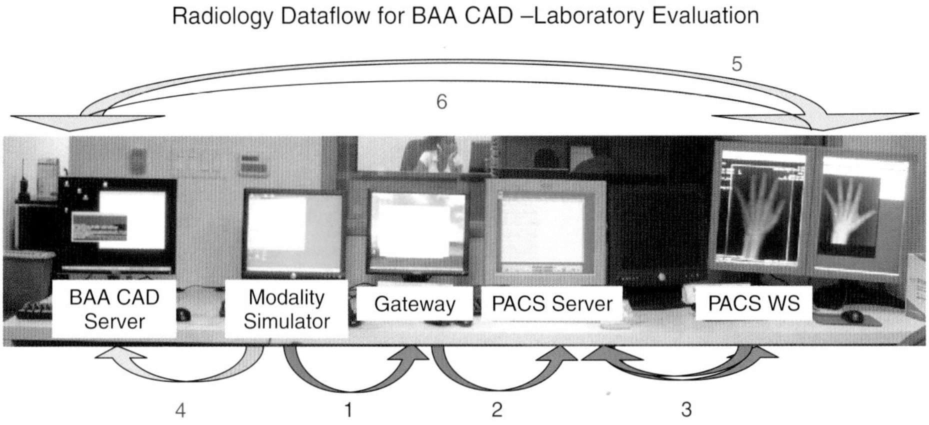

Radiology Dataflow for BAA CAD –Laboratory Evaluation

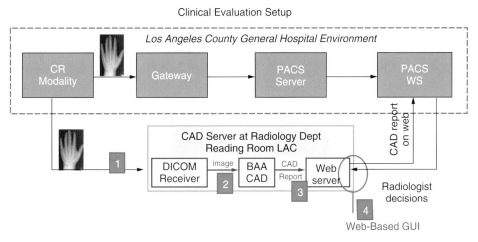

Figure 26.25 Simulated clinical workflow diagram of the BAA CAD system using the PACS simulator.

Clinical Evaluation Setup

Figure 26.26 Clinical evaluation of the BAA CAD system. The workflow was implemented in Los Angeles County Hospital with the clinical PACS and the CAD server.

4. The modality sends a second copy of the hand image to the CAD workstation/server. The server processes CAD results.
5. CAD server sends CAD results to the PCAS WS. Radiologists review both the case and CAD results on the PACS WS.
6. Readings by radiologists are captured and send back to CAD server for storage

After the laboratory validation the BAA CAD system and WS were installed for clinical evaluation at the radiology department of Los Angeles County Hospital (LAC), where the CAD WS can access the county's PACS and CR (computed radiograph) images. The actual clinical validation workflow is presented by Figure 26.26.

The implemented workflow largely corresponds to the proposed workflow:

1. CR sends a copy of the hand image to the CAD server located in the radiology reading room.
2. CAD program receives the image, performs BAA and records results in the server database.
3. Web server searches the database to locate the original image in PACS and links up with BAA results from the BAA database, as well as the best-matched DHA image (determined by the CAD bone age assessment, see Fig 26.27*B* and *C*. Another method is to use the average image described in Section 20.4.3 and Fig. 20.8).
4. GUI in the WS displays the original image and best-matched image (see Fig. 20.8), and guides radiologists through validation steps.

26.8.5.3 Web-Based BAA Clinical Evaluation System

The BAA CAD server has three components: a CAD server that performs automated BAA, a Web server that serves as a database manager, and a graphical user interface for display and a walk through of the clinical validation process.

CAD Server   The BAA CAD program is written in MATLAB® and then converted to an executable file for better integration and compatibility. The DICOM receivers and other necessary functions are handled by open-source DICOM Toolkit DCMTK®.

Web Server   The Web server is set up such that the CAD results and the validation procedures can be accessed remotely via TCP/IP. A standard Apache® Web server is used, and the Web user interface is designed in PHP. The database is handled by MySQL.

Graphical User Interface (GUI)   The Web user interface guides the radiologist through the validation process, which is separated into three steps. Figures 26.27*A*, *B*, and *C* are screenshots showing how the GUI works.

During step 1, the GUI displays the list of patients waiting to be evaluated. CAD results have already been stored (not displayed here). Each patient is anonymized, and patients' genders and ethnicities are displayed. Since ethnicities are not stored in the DICOM header, radiologists have to manually input patients' ethnicities. The radiologist clicks on a patient ID to continue the evaluation process. For example, in Figure 26.27*A*, the user can select patient "00002" from the work list.

Continue to step 2, the GUI displays the patient's hand image as well as the scanned hand images from G&P hand atlas (Fig. 26.27*B*). The purpose of this stage is to let radiologists make an unbiased diagnosis using the current G&P standard. After the best-fit G&P atlas image is selected by the radiologist, the result is saved into the database when the user clicks on the link to go to step 3.

During step 3, following Figure 26.27*C*, the GUI displays the patient's original hand image (left), the G&P atlas hand image selected in step 2 (middle), and the best-matched digital hand atlas image determined by CAD bone age (right). The CAD textual result is displayed on the right top corner, as well as a normality graph that

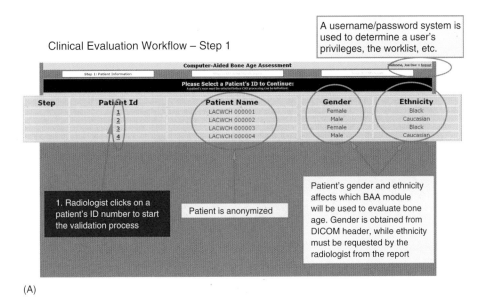

(A)

(B)

Figure 26.27 BAA CAD clinical evaluation Web GUI as shown on the PACS WS monitor. (*A*) Step 1. Retrieve a patient's hand image from PACS, and link it with the CAD results in the CAD server database. (*B*) Step 2. Compare the original image (left) with the best matched G&P atlas image (right). The match criterion is to use the patient's chronologic age to search the G & P atlas, in the order of race, sex and age, for the image which has the closest age, which is defined as the best matched image in the G & P atlas. (*C*) Step 3. Compare the original image (left), with the best matched G&P atlas image (center), and the best-matched DHA image (right). The chronologic age, bone age, and the matched DHA age are shown at the top right of the screen within the green ellipse. The CAD accessed child bone age (red dot) compared to the children in the normal range in the DHA is shown in the plot.

GUI – Step 3

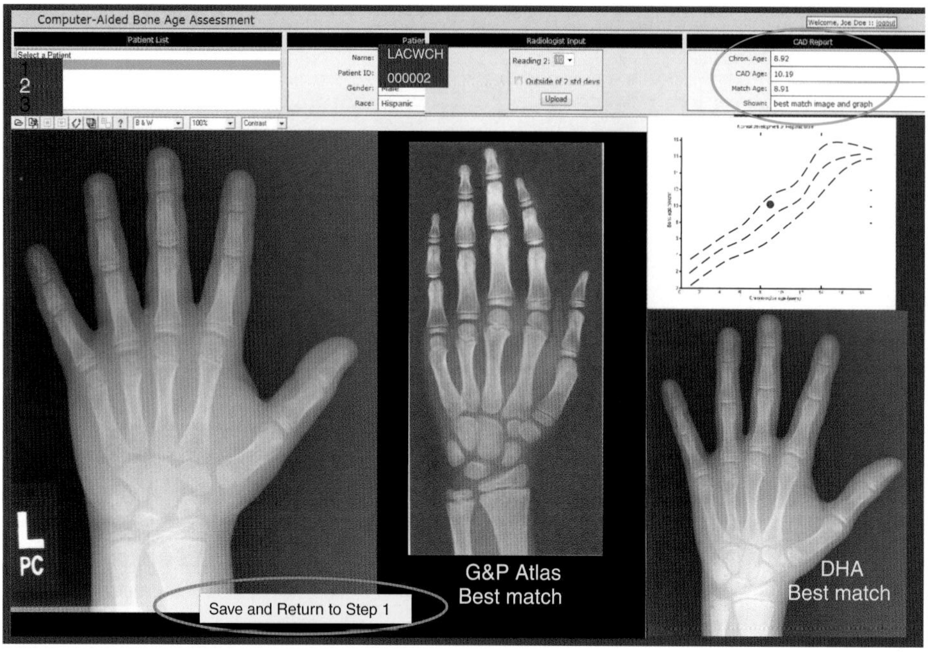

(C)

Figure 26.27 (*Continued*)

shows if the patient's BA falls within the range of normal determined by the mean and two standard deviations from the G&P atlas. Here the radiologist can choose if the original diagnosis with G&P atlas is more accurate or if the CAD result is more accurate. When the radiologist clicks the "Save and Return to Step 1" link at the left bottom corner of the GUI, the evaluation of this patient is complete and ready for the next patient.

Integration with Los Angeles County General Hospital   The CAD system was installed in LAC Women and Children's Hospital in February 2008. A DICOM receiving node was created such that the CR system on site can send copies of acquired left-hand images to the CAD server. As of November 2008, the Los Angeles County Hospital has been moved to a new location, and thus the system has to be reinstalled and integrated with PACS. The CAD validation in the clinical environment is still in progress as of today.

26.8.6 Integrating CAD for Bone Age Assessment with Other Informatics Systems

Up to this subsection, we have a step-by-step description of current clinical practice in bone age assessment (BAA) for children and its drawbacks, the rationale why CAD should be developed, a method of data collection and analysis, background on the CAD system development and its validation to clinical evaluation. So far we have also presented many imaging informatics concepts and technologies, including computing and data grid, multimedia ePR, ePR for special clinical applications in radiation therapy and surgery, CAD DICOM structured reporting (SR), and CAD-PACS integration. In this subsection, we extend the CAD BAA to the imaging informatics application level by integrating it with computing and Data Grid, and DICOM (SR).

26.8.6.1 DICOM Structured Reporting
In Sections 26.5 and 26.6 we presented the concept of DICOM SR and a clinical example using multiple sclerosis (MS) on how to develop the SR format from a text file CAD report to the SR format, overlay the contents in SR on the original image, and display it on the PACS workstation (WS). In the BAA CAD similar procedure can be used to convert the BAA CAD report to the DICOM SR and display it on PACS WS. The five Integration steps are as follows:

1. Create DICOM SR:
    a. Design the BAA SR template (each type of CAD should have its own template to accommodate specific requirements).
    b. Convert patient hand image in the DHA and the matched image in the G&P atlas (JPEG format) to DICOM SC images (a built-in module in the DICOM-SC edition of the CAD-PACS© integration toolkit).
    c. Configure i-CAD© in the CAD-PACS integration toolkit with the defined BAA SR template applied on all available data (text file, plots, three DICOM images, i.e., the original image, the best-matched image from the DHA, and the best-matched image from the G&P atlas to create the DICOM SR).
2. Configure SR-server to run i-CAD© automatically when the CAD application finishes the CAD process.
3. Send DICOM SR to SR-server (without user intervention).
4. Store DICOM SR, query and retrieve referenced images in DICOM format from the two atlases for PACS WS display.
5. CAD results are ready for viewing at PACS WS.

Figure 26.28 shows the BAA DICOM SR template. Figure 26.29 depicts a patient CAD SR report (left) along with some contents in the SR as a plot of the CAD result (right) shown before in Figure 26.27C.

26.8.6.2 Integration of Content-Based DICOM SR with CAD
In Chapter 21, we mentioned that Data Grid technology is the preferred method for reliable image data storage. Data Grid can also be integrated with DICOM SR, which is content-based, for (1) improving the storage reliability of the DCIOM SR data and (2) utilizing the DICOM SR for multiple site-access data mining applications. In order to integrate, the following steps are needed to be implemented in the Data Grid:

1. Support CAD structured reports in the DICOM services layer of the Data Grid.
2. Extend Data Grid's database for CAD SR contents within a DICOM data model schema.

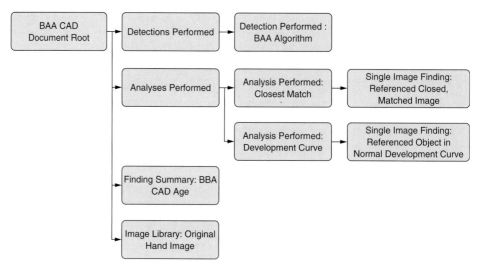

Figure 26.28 DICOM SR template for BAA CAD. The SR template is designed based on the types of output radiologists require to review.

3. Design a recursive algorithm to extract specific contents of interest from CAD structured reports using a knowledge-based approach combined with the DICOM standard.
4. Implement Web-based client interfaces to allow remote data mining from the structured reports and link images archived in the Data Grid by quantitative retrieval method, rather than patient identifiers or study UIDs. The workflow of these steps is illustrated in Figure 26.30.

26.8.6.3 Computational Services in Data Grid

Computational Services Architecture in the Data Grid   Data Grid uses the Globus Toolkit 4.02. Although in Data Grid for storage we use mostly data transfer and storage services, other computational services in the Globus Toolkit are readily available. In the Grid environment an application component in computing can be implemented in different source files, each complied to run in a different type of target architecture. Exact replicas of the executable file can be stored in many locations, which helps reduce execution time. Data files can also be replicated in various locations. Each file has a description of its contents in terms of application-specific metadata. The Metadata Service, including Catalog Service (see Figure 21.5, user-level middleware), responds to queries based on application-specific metadata and returns the logical names of files containing the required data, if they already exist. Given a logical file name that uniquely identifies a file without specifying a location, the Replica Location Service (RLS) (Fig. 21.5, core middleware) can be used to find physical location for the file on the Grid.

Figure 26.31*A* shows the operation architecture of the computational services in the Grid environment. First, the client requests resources from MDS (monitoring and discovery system) server in the core middleware (Fig. 26.31*A*, step 1), which manages the resources and distributes the jobs to the computational services. The index

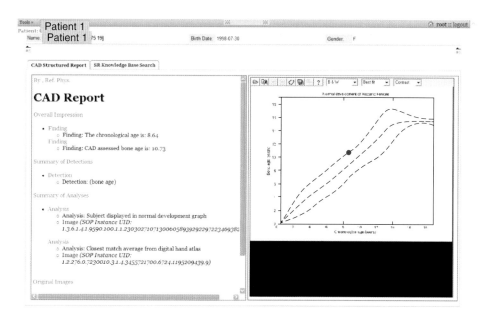

Figure 26.29 Integrating bone age assessment CAD with DICOM SR. Left: CAD report in DICOM SR format based on the design of the SR template as shown in Figure 26.28. Right: A component in the DICOM SR that is a plot of the CAD BAA results of a patient (red dot) compared with the normals and ± two standard deviations in the digital hand atlas (see also Fig. 26.27*C*).

service in MDS finds resources appropriate to the requirements of application components and notifies the client to send the application to the Grid Resource Allocation and Management (GRAM) service (right), step 2. The GRAM service acknowledges MDS after it receives the application, step 3. After the GRAM service receives the application, jobs that completely specified for execution are sent to schedulers that manage the resources and monitor execution progress. Execute acknowledges MDS server, the completion of the job in step 3, which in turn notifies the client, step 4.

Utilization of Data Grid Computational Service for Bone Age Assessment for Children When BAA CAD becomes a daily clinical tool, many centers in pediatric radiology will use it as a method of subjective BAA for children. BAA CAD does require extensive computing that fits into the domain of Data Grid for storage and computational services in the Globus for image processing. Following the discussion on bone age assessment (BAA) of children using the CAD, we model the computational aspect of the CAD BAA based on the Data Grid architecture as shown in Figure 26.31*B*, which subdivides the entire hand image into multiple regions of interest, including six epi-metaphyseal ROIs from three phalanges, the carpal bones ROI, and the wrist joint ROI. These ROIs are processed by remote grid resource nodes; all results are merged together through the Data Grid MDS server. For a child hand image submitted to the Data Grid computational service, the overall

Integration of CAD DICOM SR with Data Grid

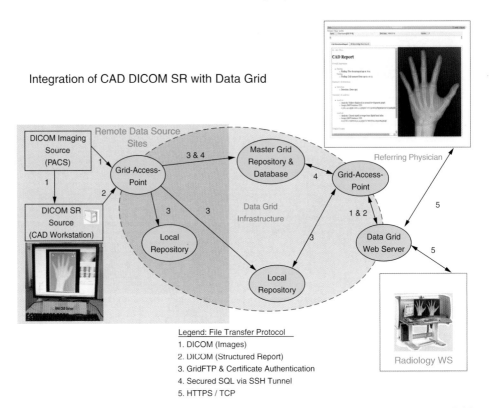

Legend: File Transfer Protocol
1. DICOM (Images)
2. DICOM (Structured Report)
3. GridFTP & Certificate Authentication
4. Secured SQL via SSH Tunnel
5. HTTPS / TCP

Figure 26.30 Workflow steps of integrating the CAD DICOM SR with the Data Grid. Color code: Data sources and CAD (light blue); Data Grid infrastructure (pink); referring physician and radiology WS (blue); workflow processes (green). There are a Data Grid Web server (right) and multiple grid access points (GAPs). Data flow: Input to the Data Grid—Images (1) and CAD results in DICOM SR format (2) move across from left to right through the GAP (left), secured SQL via SSG tunnel requests data to be transmitted using GRIDFTP service for certificate authentication and stored in multiple local repositories (3), and metadata in master grid repository and database (3, 4). Output—Multiple sites referring physicians and radiologists view images and DICOM SR results from WSs by requesting the Data Grid Web server through the GAP (right), which fetches images, and CAD DICOM SR data (3, 4), and perform data mining using either HTTPS or TCP communication protocol (5). Data Grid provides both reliability and redundancy of images and DICOM SR, and allows secured multiple user-accesses. SSG: Service Selection Gateway.

operation workflow of bone age assessment is as shown in sequences 1, 2, and 3 in Figure 26.31C.

26.9 RESEARCH AND DEVELOPMENT TRENDS IN CAD–PACS INTEGRATION

Currently CAD and PACS are two separate independent systems with only minimal communications between them. In this chapter we describe a CAD–PACS toolkit as

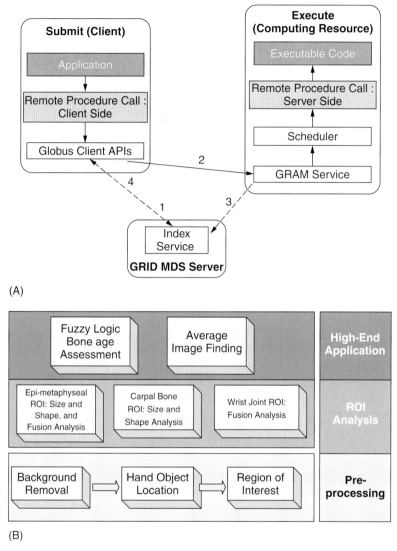

(A)

(B)

Figure 26.31 (*A*) Operation architecture of a computational grid. Numerals represent the workflow. (*B*) Three-layer procedure of BAA CAD. (*C*) Operation workflow of BAA computational services. The MDS allocates the computation requirements according to the available resources in the Data Grid. Numerals represent the workflow.

a universal method to integrate CAD results with PACS in daily clinical environment. The toolkit utilizes HL7 standard for textual data and the DICOM standard for imaging so that it follows the industrial standard for data format and communications. The method needs the DICOM structured reporting (DICOM SR) standard to reformat CAD results into an SR template so that they can be integrated as a component in the DICOM data mode for viewing on the PACS workstations. It also uses three IHE workflow profiles: key image note (KIN), simple image and numeric

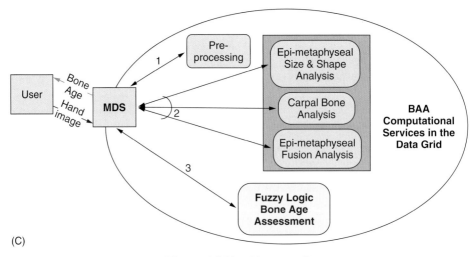

Figure 26.31 (*Continued*)

report (SINR), and postprocessing workflow profiles (PWF) to facilitate data trans-mission and communication in clinical workflow. We have shown CAD examples to illustrate explicitly how to integrate existing CAD results into PACS daily clinical operation.

PACS is a mature healthcare technology that continues to accumulate tremendous amount of imaging data daily. Unfortunately, the vast majority of this data in PACS is hardly utilized except for daily clinical service.

There are many other advantages for the integrating CAD results with PACS. CAD is a growing field, its applications range from chest to breast, colon, brain, liver, skeletal, and vascular. Doi, in his 2008 survey, reports that the number of presentations in CAD at the Annual RSNA (Radiological Society of North America) Scientific Assembly increased from 59 in 2000 to 227 in 2008. From the view point of a CAD developer, PACS has tremendously large databases that can help improve further the research and development of the new CAD methods. Integrating CAD results adds to these databases by providing quantified results that were previously unavailable through the standard DICOM image of a PACS study.

Because of the rich contents in the DICOM SR, it benefits CAD developers to produce a comprehensive and standardized results findings and quantitative values in DICOM SR format. The DICOM standard and template can guide the CAD developers in applying their knowledge to building high-quality and valuable reports for many other purposes.

Postprocessing of medical images generated by the imaging modalities is often done to enhance their diagnosis values. Postprocessing of medical images is different from CAD in the sense that it produces some form of display, some quantitative mea-surements, but does not provide detection nor diagnosis. To this day there are new technologies available for quantitative measurements obtained from postprocessing or CAD that still reside within the postprocessing workstation or the CAD server in the clinical environment. There has been some collaboration between postprocessing and CAD manufacturers with PACS manufacturers to improve PACS workflow by providing an integrated PACS workstation. However, the integration has resulted in poor image quality performance and a return to stand-alone postprocessing worksta-tions. With the introduction of the CAD–PACS toolkit, even these results could be converted to the DICOM SR format and be made readily available for direct query by PACS WS, and thus revolutionizing clinical workflow from single-event patient-based queries to longitudinal-based queries on valuable metadata and quantitative measurements.

The trend of CAD and PACS integration is to incorporate CAD findings and DICOM key image referencing into its DICOM-compliant databases and services in the form of DICOM SR data objects. By way of DICOM SR, content-based query/retrieval of DICOM imaging studies can be performed based on quantitative findings rather than patient identification and/or disease category. Query/retrieval of content-based imaging data can be advantageous for medical imaging research and clinical practice.

26.10 SUMMARY OF CAD–PACS INTEGRATION

In this chapter we emphasize the rationale and methods of CAD–PACS integration. The CAD–PACS toolkit in three editions is introduced as a cookbook for integration. The workflow and components of the toolkit based on the DICOM standard and IHE workflow are described in detail. The first edition provides for a quick and easy DICOM screen capture method; in essence, it is what you see from the display monitor is what you get. Postprocessing is not possible and the display quality is minimal. The second edition introduces integrating CAD with full PACS. It is an elegant but tedious way to integrate, and extensive collaboration is required between the CAD vendor and the PACS manufacturer. The third edition does not require full knowledge of PACS operation, only the understanding and know how that comes from using the CAD–PACS toolkit. The CAD results do not reside in the PACS server and storage; instead they are in the CAD server. PACS images needed by the CAD are link with the CAD results so that both images and CAD results in DICOM format can be display on the PACS WS. This edition is recommended to CAD vendors for integrating their CAD results with the PACS.

We use a clinical case in multiple sclerosis (MS) on MRI as an introduction to the advantage of imaging informatics for clinical practice. In general, physicians can easily diagnose MS, but it can be difficult for them to evaluate the effectiveness of a certain drug treatment to the MS patient without informatics tools. This is because the number of MSs on MRI are sometime too many to keep track of and account for in obtaining precise quantitative measurements. Imaging informatics teamed up with CAD can be an effective way to handle this situation. We also use this case to introduce the combination of CAD results with DICOM SR; with the CAD results in SR format, they can be overlaid on DICOM images and be displayed on PACS WS.

We use the CAD bone age assessment for children as a comprehensive way to guide the reader from A to Z on why and how to develop the CAD, and how to validate it in the laboratory and perform the evaluation in the clinical environment. The chapter concludes with some CAD–PACS research work in progress, including the total integration of CAD, DICOM SR, and Data Grid with computational ser-vices, which represents the current state-of-the-art in medical imaging informatics development.

References

Cao F, Huang HK, Liu B, Zhou Z, Zhang J, Mogel G. Fault-tolerant PACS server, InfoRAD Exhibit. *Radiol Soc N Am 87th* Scientific Assembly and Annual Meeting, 25–30 Nov, p. 737; 2001.

DICOM Standard. Supplement 23: Structured Reporting Object; 1999.

DICOM Standard. Supplement 50: Mammography CA; 2000.

DICOM Standard. Supplement 65: Chest CAD SR SOP Class; 2001.

DICOM Standards; 2008. http://medical.nema.org/medical/dicom/2008

Doi K. Computer-aided diagnosis in medical imaging: Historical review, current status and future potential. *Comput Med Imag Graph* 31(4–5): 198–211; 2007.

Gertych A, Zhang A, Sayre J, Pospiech-Kurkowska S, Huang HK. Bone age assessment of children using a digital hand atlas. *Comput Med Imag Graph* 31: 323–331; 2007.

Greulich WW, Pyle SI. *Radiographic Atlas of Skeletal Development of Hand Wrist*. Stanford: Stanford University Press, 1–36, 190, 194–5; 1959.

Health Level 7; 2008. http://www.hl7.org/.

HHS, Office of Civil Rights, HIPAA; 2008. http://www.hhs.gov/ocr/hipaa.

Hologic R2 Home. http://www.r2tech.com/main/home/index.php.

Huang HK, Doi K. CAD and image-guided decision support. *Comput Med Imag Graph* 31(4–5): 195–7; 2007.

Huang HK, Cao F, Liu BJ, Zhou Z, et al. PACS simulator: a standalone educational tool. InfoRAD Exhibit. *Radiol Soc N Am 86th Scientific Assembly* and Annual Meeting, 26 Nov–1 Dec, p. 688; 2000.

Huang HK. *PACS and Imaging Informatics: Basic Principles and Applications*. Hoboken, NJ: Wiley, 44, 504–7; 2004.

IHE; 2008. http://www.ihe.net.

Le A, Mai L, Liu B, Huang HK. The workflow and procedures for automatic integration of a computer-aided diagnosis workstation with a clinical PACS with real world examples. *Proc SPIE Med Imag* 6919: 1–7; 2008.

Le A HT, Liu B , Huang HK. Integration of computer-aided diagnosis/detection (CAD) results in a PACS environment using CAD-PACS toolkit and DICOM SR, *Intern J. Comp Asst Rad & Surg*, 4: 317–329; 2009

Lee J, Le A, Liu BJ, Huang HK. Integration of content-based DICOM-SR for CAD in the medical imaging informatics Data Grid with examples in CT chest, mammography, and bone-age assessment. Education Exhibit. *Radiol Soc N Am 94th Scientific Assembly* and Annual Meeting, 30 Nov–5 Dec, p. 912; 2008.

Mamdani EH. Application of fuzzy algorithms for control of simple dynamic plant. *Proc IEEE* 121: 1585–8; 1974.

Mora S, Boechat MI, Pietka E, Huang HK, Gilsanz V. Skeletal age determinations in children of European and African descent: applicability of the Greulich and Pyle standards. *Pediat Res* 50(5): 624–8; 2001.

Ontell FK, Ivanovic M, Ablin DS, Barlow TW. Bone Age in Children of Diverse Ethnicity, *American Journal of Roentgenology*, 167: 1395–1398; 1996

Pietka E, Gertych A, Pospiech S, Cao F, Huang HK, Gilsanz V. Computer assisted bone age assessment: image processing and epiphyseal/Metaphyseal ROI extraction. *IEEE Trans Med Imag* 20: 715–29; 2001.

Pietka E, Pospiech S, Gertych A, Cao F, Huang HK, Gilsanz B. Computer automated approach to the extraction of epiphyseal regions in hand radiographs. *J Digit Imag* 14: 165–172; 2001.

Pietka E, Pospiech-Kurkowska S, Gertych A, Cao F, Huang HK. Computer-assisted bone age assessment: image analysis and fuzzy classification. *Radiology* 225(P): 751; 2002.

Roche AF, Roberts J, Harnill PV. Skeletal maturity of children 6–11 years: racial, geographic area and socioeconomic differentials, In: *National Health Survey*, Rockville MD: Health Resources Administration, National Center for Health Statistics, 1975: 1–38.

Ross T. *Fuzzy Logic with Engineering Applications*, 2nd ed. Hoboken, NJ: Wiley; 2004.

Zadeh LA. Fuzzy logic. *Computer* 1(4): 83–93; 1988.

Zadeh LA. Fuzzy sets and systems, in Zadeh LA, Fu KS et al ed. Information and Control. 8: 338–53; 1965.

Zhang A, Gertych A, Liu BJ. Automatic bone age assessment for young children from newborn to 7-year-old using carpal bones. *Comput Med Imag Graph* May; 31: 299–311; 2007.

Zhang A, Uyeda J, Tsao S, Ma K, Vachon L, Liu B, Huang HK. Web-based computer-aided diagnosis (CAD) system for bone age assessment (BAA) of children. *Med Imag* 2008: PACS and Imaging Informatics. Vol 4919; 2008.

Zhang A, Zhou Z, Gertych A, Liu B, Zheng X, Huang HK. Integration of bone age assessment CAD results with the PACS diagnostic workflow utilizing DICOM structure report. *Scientific Poster*, RSNA; 2006.

Zhang A, Sayre JW, Vachon L, Liu BJ, Huang HK. Cross-racial differences in growth patterns of children based on bone age assessment. *J Radiol*; 290, 1, 228–235; 2009.

Zhou Z, Huang HK, Liu BJ, Cao F, Zhang J, Mogel G, Law M. A RIS/PACS simulator with Web-based image distribution and display system for education. *Proc SPIE* 5371: 372–81; 2004.

Zhou Z, Huang HK, Cao F, Liu BJ, et al. An educational RIS/PACS simulator with Web-based image distribution and display system. InfoRad Exhibit, *Radiol Soc N Am 89th Scientific Assembly* and Annual Meeting, 30 Nov–5 Dec, p. 796; 2003.

Zhou Z, Law M, Huang HK, Cao F, Liu B, Zhang J. An educational RIS/PACS simulator. InfoRAD Exhibit. *Radiol Soc N Am 88th Scientific Assembly* and Annual Meeting, 1–6 Dec, p. 753; 2002.

Zhou Z, Le A, Liu B, Huang HK. PACS-CAD toolkit for integrating an independent CAD workstation to diagnosis workflow. *Proc SPIE Med Imag* 6516: 1–8; 2007.

Zhou Z, Liu BJ, Huang HK, Zhang J. Educational RIS/PACS simulator integrated with the HIPAA compliant auditing (HCA) toolkit. *Proc SPIE* 5748: 491–500; 2005.

Zhou Z, Liu BJ, Huang HK, Zhang J. Educational RIS/PACS simulator integrated with HIPAA compliant architecture (HCA) for auditing. InfoRad Exhibit. *Radiol Soc N Am 90th Scientific Assembly* and Annual Meeting, 28 Nov–3 Dec, p. 827; 2004.

Zhou Z, Liu BJ, Le A. CAD-PACS integration tool kit—based on DICOM screen capture (SC) and structured reporting (SR) and IHE workflow profiles. *J Comput Med Imag Graph* 31(4–5): 346–52; 2007.

Location Tracking and Verification System in Clinical Environment

Imaging informatics related to the topics we discuss in Part IV—Data Grid with computational services, multimedia ePR and its applications in radiation therapy and minimally invasive spinal surgery, image-based CAD and CAD–PACS integration all derived from medical images and HIS/RIS/PACS data and their supported resources—will continue to grow with advances in research and development in basic and applied clinical research. In this chapter, we take a different direction and present imaging informatics R&D in the sense that we take advantage of the already or being developed technologies from other fields and modify them for well-defined and needed clinical applications. Figure 20.9 is reproduced here as Figure 27.1 showing how this chapter corresponds to other chapters in the domain of image informatics R&D. In this chapter, we describe a location tracking and verification system (LTVS) that integrates biometric technologies with HIS/RIS/PACS data in the MIII core infrastructure (see Fig. 27.1) to automatically monitor and identify staff and patients in a healthcare image-based environment as a way to partially conform to HIPAA (Health Insurance Portability and Accountability Act) requirement. Biometric technologies used in LTVS include facial features recognition and fingerprint recognition. The HIS/RIS/PACS data utilized are not patient history, diagnosis, treatment, and outcomes as described in previous chapters, but the time stamps of patient registration, procedure workflow, examination, and patient discharge. Visualization and graphic tools are heavily utilized.

27.1 NEED FOR THE LOCATION TRACKING AND VERIFICATION SYSTEM IN CLINICAL ENVIRONMENT

27.1.1 HIPAA Compliance and JCAHO Mandate

With the explosion of digital imaging and medical records, more and more medical data are managed and stored electronically in different medical information systems. Recall the examples discussed previously: hospital information systems (HIS), radiology information systems (RIS), and picture archive and communication systems (PACS), various multi-media ePR (electonic patient record) systems, and CAD results with linkage to PACS. To protect the privacy of personal health

PACS and Imaging Informatics, Second Edition, by H. K. Huang
Copyright © 2010 John Wiley & Sons, Inc.

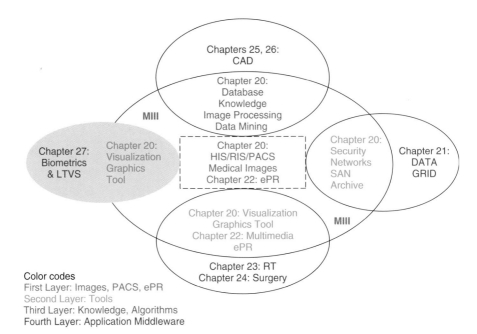

Figure 27.1   Imaging informatics data sources (rectangle), concepts, technologies, and applications (large and small ellipses) as discussed in the chapters of Part IV. Color codes refer to the five-layer informatics infrastructure shown in Figure 20.2. Biometrics and location tracking and verification system (LTVS) presented in this chapter are in orange color.

information, HIPAA privacy rules regarding national standards were published on April 11, 2003, and mandated on April 11, 2006. Great care should be taken to protect patient confidentiality to meet partial HIPAA requirements. Moreover, in an ever-increasingly complex and dynamic clinical environment, mis-identification of patients is a common problem in health facilities.

In the United States, the Joint Commission on Accreditation of Healthcare Organizations (JCAHO) processed root cause analysis information on 126 cases of wrong site surgery between 1998 and 2001. Seventy-six percent of cases involved surgery on the wrong body part or site, 13% surgery on the wrong patient, and 11% the wrong surgical procedure. JCAHO has identified the factor that human error such as misuse of addressograph labels, mishearing, misspelling, and misfiling may lead to mis-identification. In addition patient experience with long waiting time for scheduled appointments is another widespread problem within healthcare. Visitors to U.S. hospital emergency departments (ED) wait an average of 222 minutes, or 3.7 hours, before being seen by a provider, according to a new state-by-state study released by Press Ganey Associates, *USA Today* reports. The study, which examines wait times at ED's across the nation, is based on 1.5 million patient questionnaires filled out in 2005. Most healthcare facilities nowadays struggle with protecting medical data privacy, mis-identification of patients, and long patient waiting times.

For these reasons every healthcare prvoider has to conform to the HIPAA compliance and to abide by the JCAHO mandate during their accrediation visits.

27.1.2   Rationale for Developing the LTVS

To address these issues, a location tracking and verification system (LTVS) was designed and developed using wireless technology for tracking the location of patients, and facial biometric technology for automatically identifying staff and patients. By integrating these two technologies with existing healthcare information resources in the prescribed healthcare environment, LTVS system provides:

1. a simple yet systematic solution to monitor and automatically identify staff and patients in order to streamline the patient workflow,
2. protection against erroneous examinations, and
3. a security zone to prevent and audit unauthorized access to patient healthcare data.

These characteristics satisfiy the criteria for partial compliance of the HIPAA requirements as well as the JCAHO mandate.

27.2   CLINICAL ENVIRONMENT WORKFLOW

27.2.1   Need for a Clinical Environment Workflow Study

To perform a workflow study in clinical environment is mandatory before the LTVS is designed. A workflow study can help system designers better understand the existing clinical working environment and to design the system that best suits the operation at mininal cost. The workflow study includes passive observation, interview with personnel and patients, and active participation in hourly and daily walk throughs with staff members and patients. During this time period, workflow bottlenecks are defined and solutions obtained. Potential problems like the radiation protection walls and structural obstacles in the building are identified and methods of circumvention are considered. In the following subsection we identify a particular clinical workflow study on whose results is based a LTCS design.

27.2.2   The Healthcare Consultation Center II (HCC II)

To best understand the rationale and data collection in a workflow study, an actual clinical environment is used to describe the steps. The workflow study was performed to observe the physical location and movement of patients and staff at the Healthcare Consultation Center II (HCC II), which is a new, stand-alone fully digitalized outpatient imaging center with integrated HIS/RIS/PACS/VR (voice recognition) located in the University of Southern California (USC) Health Science Campus. The facility has one computed tomography (CT) scanner, two magnetic resonance imaging (MRI) scanners, two ultrasound scanners (US, one with biopsy capability), two computed radiography (CR) units, and one special procedure room (fluoroscopy/angiography). There are a total of 31 clinical personnel including 8 technologists, 7 support staff, and 16 rotating radiologists who cover several radiology departments at USC.

A four-week observation period was performed at HCCII. Workflow at the CT, MRI, US, and CR modalities included interaction with the integrated HIS/RIS/PACS/VR (voice recognition) systems, and access to the patient registration

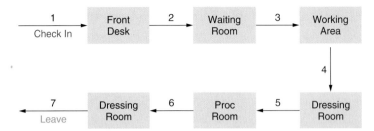

Figure 27.2   General outpatient tracking location workflow at the Out-patient Imaging Center, Healthcare Consultant Center (HCC II), University of Southern California (USC), Los Angeles.

and waiting area and to radiology reading rooms. The workflow of the special procedure room was not observed because the room was not yet in clinical operation during the time of the workflow study.

Figure 27.2 shows the general patient tracking location workflow, which involves seven steps:

1. Patient is scheduled at the registration desk with RIS.
2. Patient waits in the waiting room before the technologist verbally calls his/her name.
3. Patient is taken to the working area based on the modality type of examination.
4. Patient is asked to change clothes in the dressing room.
5. When patient is ready, technologist escorts patient into the procedure room and takes the exam.
6. When exam is completed, patient returns to the dressing room and changes back into his/her own clothes.
7. Patient is released by the technologist and leaves the radiology department.

From the workflow study described above, there can be identified some related concerns for a patient undergoing a radiological examination:

1. Extensive patient time spent in the waiting room. The overall length of patient waiting time was calculated from the time when the patient was registered in the RIS to the time that the technologist started the procedure, which was recorded as time stamp in the RIS. Based on the records, the average patient waiting time was 17.3 minutes for CR, 50.4 minutes for CT, and 65.6 minutes for MRI exaimantion.
2. Unsecured exit doors and reading area rooms at HCCII. There is always a risk of an unauthorized patient easily accessing patient information at a workstation of the reading area without permission.
3. Potential mis-identification of a patient at the working area before the patient enters the procedure room.

To address these issues, a LTVS system was designed and developed using wireless technology for tracking the location of patients, and facial biometric technology for automatically identifying staff and patients.

27.3   AVAILABLE TRACKING AND BIOMETRIC TECHNOLOGIES

27.3.1   Wireless Tracking

LTVS uses a wireless tracking system utilizing Wi-Fi-based positioning technology. This sophisticated real-time tracking system of wireless and portable devices utilizes the concept of radiofrequency signal fingerprinting where three or more access-point signals are detected by a portable Wi-Fi device (wireless fidelity, a trademark of the Wi-Fi Alliance, founded in 1999 as Wireless Ethernet Compatibility Alliance [WECA]) and used to calculate location and movement on an xy plane. The system has already served many purposes ranging from healthcare, to manufacturing, to industry. Figure 27.3 shows the assorted radiofrequency ID products available in terms of their strengthns and weaknesses. The decision to integrate Wi-Fi technology over infrared, passive RFID, and other technologies was made because of its tracking capabilities, user-definable tags, relatively low cost, and scalable setup, since it utilizes any existing wireless network infrastructure. These are key benefits to selecting the clinical tracking system, namely some LTVS include a design that is extensive and modular. Although much initial effort was invested in achieving optimum tracking calibration with the system, its basic wireless access point dependency enabled more mobility during the prototype development stage at various testing locations, conferences, and finally, the clinical environment in comparison with other more permanent and costly systems.

27.3.2   Biometrics Verification System

There are several commercially available biometric verification systems, including facial recognition, fingerprint scanning, voice recognition, and iris scanning biometirc system. For the LTVS many factors were considered in selecting an appropriate design, among them were total system cost, patient static or dynamic environment, user characteristics, speed, reliability, and ease of use. As a result only two products types could be considered, facial biometrics and the fingerprint scanning. For the

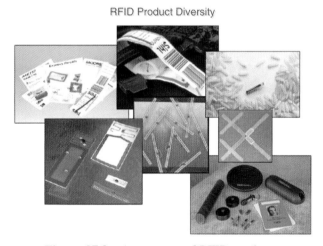

RFID Product Diversity

Figure 27.3   Assortment of RFID products.

prototype LTVS, we selected the facial biometrics becasue it was readily available in the design laboratory during the design phase and was already a popular identity verification technology. With the new HIPAA security standards mandating higher healthcare protection of digital information, facial biometric verification seemed to be the best means of protecting against unauthorized use or disclosure. In the case of surgical patient identification, as discussed in Chapter 24, because a patient is in static mode most of the time, finger print scanning is the method of choice. This example will be revisited in a later section.

Many of facial biometric verification algorithms rely on the special relationship between "nodal points" on the face such as eyes, nose, mouth, chin, and others. The facial biometrics recognition software uses an advanced software that calculates and analyzes landmark positions and features on a face to verify a person's identity (Fig. 27.4). We used a prepared database photo gallery of healthcare staff members and pre- or on-site patient regiatration images, as the facial biometrics recognition system can identify the person detected on the distributed video cameras system in the clincial environment.

LTVS uses a software development toolkit (SDK) (Nevenvision, Inc., San Diego, CA) integrated into the application that can register multiple-photo galleries of people and perform facial biometric verification simultaneously at multiple clinical workstations using simple PC webcams. To keep the image galleries and processing on a single protected LTVS server, each client workstation utilized image-capturing software that would send real-time images from satellite workstations back to the LTVS server for display or processing. Using a PC-based webcam and small image transfer software, clinical workstations already within the clinical environment can be utilized as LTVS client workstations that can perform robust matching of facial images with medical record numbers prior to authorizing access or treatment. Figure 27.4 depicts the SDK system to identify a person based on facial relationship between nodal points to identify a person with a pre-established gallery.

27.4 LOCATION TRACKING AND VERIFICATION SYSTEM (LTVS) DESIGN

27.4.1 Design Concept

The design of the LTVS prototype in the outpatient radiological imaging center of the Healthcare Consultation Center II (HCCII), Radiology Department, USC is based on the workflow study results shown in Table 27.1.

27.4.2 System Infrastructure

The LTVS design centers around a modular architecture that can easily be modified to accommodate other future more advanced tracking and identity verification technologies such as radiofrequency identification and digital fingerprinting. Although the entire LTVS architecture subsides on a single server, its multi-level branching software design allows only the necessary individual modules to be changed rather than having to modify an entire system. Furthermore, although other potential technologies vary in methodology and may arise as better options in the future, LTVS

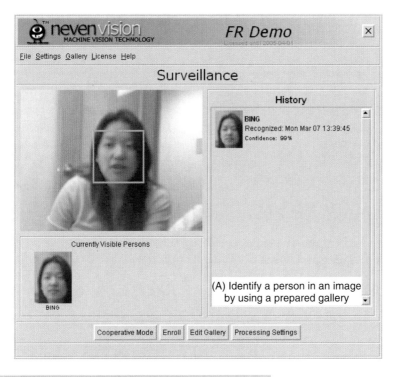

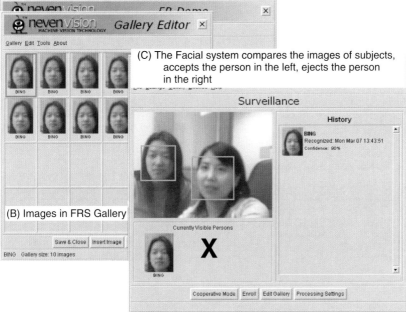

Figure 27.4 Facial recognition biometric system identifying a person in an image. (*A*) Subject is registered in the gallery of the facial biometric system. (*B*) The gallery of this subject. (*C*) Images of two subjects are presented to the database, which selects the one "Bing" who had previously registered.

TABLE 27.1   Features of location tracking and facial verification system (LTVS)

1. Real-time Identification of the movement of patients and selected staff in a hospital environment
2. Proper staff located and contacted quickly
3. Warning provided to department personnel if a particular patient has been in one location (e.g., waiting room) beyond the time limit
4. Patient identity can be verified (e.g., prior to an examination to minimize errors of misidentification)
5. Information security zone created within a given subunit
6. Access right of the patient to vital clinical information by a health provider is verified

modules implement universal and standard parameters that further broaden the scope of capable technological systems that can be integrated.

The LTVS server has two major components: (1) a wireless tracking system using standard IEEE 802.11b or a wireless network technology, and (2) a facial biometric system for verification, as shown in Figure 27.5.

The central LTVS server utilizes the Apache2 Web server to interact with the users in addition to the tracking and facial recognition modules. The application modules for these two systems perform the background processes for LTVS. The facial recognition module uses an application programming interface (API) that is able to maintain its own image database, whereas the tracking systems API requires the creation of a database to manage and communicate device tracking information to the LTVS user. As shown in the infrastructure diagram of Figure 27.6, the tracking

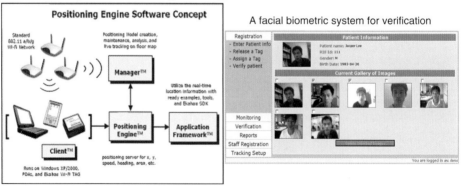

Figure 27.5   Two major components in the location tracking and facial verification system (LTVS). Left: Wireless tracking; right: facial biometrics verification, the patient information window for managing the gallery is shown (Section 27.4.3).

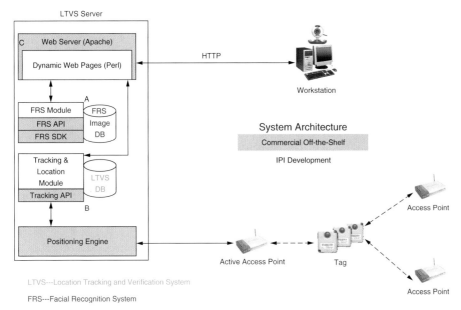

Figure 27.6 Location tracking and facial verification system (LTVS) architecture. Gray: Commercial off-the-shelf; yellow: in-house development. The FRS and LTVS databases are in-house developments. The system architecture shows the LTVS server, which consists of a Web server application that runs the Web-based graphical user Interface (GUI). (*a*) Facial biometrics verification module with cameras; (*b*) wireless location tracking module with tags; (*c*) Web server with GUI for clients to access. Perl = practical extraction and report language; FRS = Facial biometric recognition system; API = application programming Interface.

module's API can only provide real-time data of device information and locations, so the LTVS tracking application and a PostGreSQL database are left to manage both static and dynamic information for the entire LTVS tracking system.

From the figure it can be seen that the LTVS server is the location of most of the processing components—the Web-based application, the facial recognition module, and facial image database, and the tracking module with LTVS database. The Web-based application is written in Perl with dynamic Web pages that interact with the external users at the clinical workstations as well as internally with the facial recognition module and tracking module through the LTVS database. It allows clinicians to register, track, and verify patients and staff by assigning them tracking devices while taking a facial photograph.

In addition to the server, some external hardware pieces are required for the actual tracking and facial recognition functions to work. The Wi-Fi tracking technology uses numerous wireless access points to track devices, which periodically send signal strengths back to the positioning engine so exact locations and movement can be calculated. Also the clinical workstations need to be equipped with webcams and an image capturing/transfer application in order to view real-time images through the LTVS application besides provide images for the facial recognition functionality. Table 27.2 lists the hardware and software components of the LTVS system.

TABLE 27.2   Hardware and software components of LTVS

Hardware	Software
<ul><li>Dedicated LTVS server (on network)</li><li>Clinical workstations equipped with webcams (640 × 480 or higher)</li><li>Wi-Fi positioning technology:<ul><li>Wireless access point</li><li>Wireless tracking devices</li></ul></li></ul>	<ul><li>LTVS GUI Web application Apache2 Web server</li><li>LTVS tracking API<ul><li>Post-GreSQL database with pgAdmin III</li><li>Wi-Fi positioning engine</li></ul></li><li>LTVS facial verification API Image-capturing software (workstations)</li></ul>

27.4.3   Facial Recognition System Module: Registering, Adding, Deleting, and Verifying Facial Images

The facial recognition module is a program written in C++ that utilizes a facial recognition API to perform facial image biometrics. The facial recognition API has an internal database called the "gallery" in which it stores historical facial images with defined facial features as the key to a face's identity. The facial image of a new person will be used to compare corresponding facial features in the gallery to perform facial biometric identification. Under controlled conditions this biometric system has proved in the laboratory to recognize new and existing facial images. In Figure 27.7, the graphical user interface (GUI) of LTVS is seen displaying a sample person's information and picture. In the figure it also depicts windows of the the GUI with applications features shown in the left.

The facial recognition module is the main mechanism that enables LTVS to (1) register new or (2) verify facial images in the database. When the user clicks on either

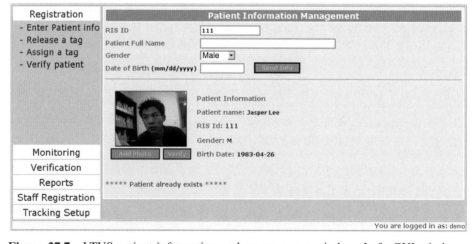

Figure 27.7   LTVS patient information and management window. Left: GUI windows; middle: facial image.

of these two options, the module software compares the new images with the existing gallery. While images are constantly being sent to the LTVS server from all the clinical workstations equipped with webcams, the server doesn't actually call upon the facial recognition module unless the user wants to add or verify a photo. When one of the two options is selected, the file name of the temporary image is sent as a parameter to the facial recognition module where a facial biometric measurement is made and then compared in the image gallery.

There are three possible results from this measurement and comparison: (1) no face found, (2) new face, or (3) existing face. The facial recognition module's API does most of this processing, but the module portion determines what the response is for LTVS. If, for example, the user asks to add a new patient into the image gallery, then the API will return the response of finding a new face that does not yet exist in the image gallery. The module would proceed to tell the API to create a new file for this patient in its gallery. For LTVS, the images for each patient are kept in one permanent image folder with up to 10 images per person in the gallery. Each image file is chronologically numbered and contains the patient or staff's unique identification number within the file name.

Following the same example, if the user wants to add a new image to the gallery, the new image is still compared in the image database. The image is only added if it returns an identification number that matches and if there aren't already 10 images that already contain that person's ID number. In the LTVS, this identification number is a three-digit RIS (radiology infromation system) ID (111) seen in Figure 27.7, in the first line at the middle of the screen shot. The LTVS is tightly coupled with the RIS to receive correct information on the paitent. Figure 27.8 summarizes the basic workflow of the LTVS facial biometric processing.

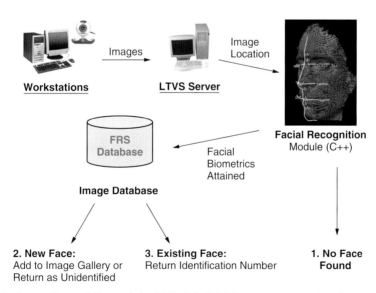

Figure 27.8 Basic workflow of the LTVS facial biometric processing. There are three possibility after a new image is captured: (1) no face found, (2) a new face found, and (3) an existing face found. FRS = facial recognition system.

Images in a gallery can also be removed as seen in the screen shot below. The facial recognition module performs this task by working with the LTVS application in determining which images are to be removed from the API's image gallery. This delete function is necessary to LTVS because more images does not mean higher biometric fidelity (see Fig. 27.5, right).

27.4.4 Location Tracking Module: Design and Methodology

The LTVS tracking application was developed in Java to receive data from the location tracking system API and tailor it to the needs of LTVS. It acts as a listening module that receives tracking device carried by the person that updates on location and movement from the positioning engine through the API. This allows real-time tracking information from the Wi-Fi (wireless fidelity) tracking system to be sent through the API to the listening LTVS tracking module where each device's information can then be processed. Each device carries a unique MAC (media access control in the data link level) address that the LTVS tracking module and database use to identify it by. The processing of all the devices include maintaining a list of available and assignable tags, removing lost devices from both the patient and device lists, processing logical area restrictions according to each tag's assigned status, and, last but not least, maintaining a record log of all tracking events. Updating the database with the status of each device on whether it is assigned or available is crucial to tracking efficiency. The updating involves the coordination of the tracking system and LTVS because there are different scenarios that formulate the final device availability. Table 27.3 describes the possible combinations of tracking device status.

Notice that only activated devices are available for assignment and only assigned devices that have a status of patient or staff qualifies for location and message updating. Whenever a device is assigned or released from a patient or staff, the table of devices (*ltvs_device*) must be updated to reflect its availability, the patient or staff who is assigned the device must have the MAC address added to its information in *ltvs_patient* or *ltvs_staff*, and last, the device must be added or removed from the *ltvs_current* table from which the GUI queries to display all its devices being tracked.

Once a device in the *ltvs_device* changes status to being assigned, it is automatically tracked, meaning data sent in from the positioning engine regarding this device's logical area and xy coordinates is processed by the tracking module. The LTVS tracking application's main job is to keep the *ltvs_current* table in the database

TABLE 27.3 Possible combinations of Wi-Fi tracking device status

TTVS Tracking Device Status	Tracking System Found	LTVS Task	Status for Patient/Staff
Off	False	Nothing	Not available
Activated	True	Add to list of devices	Not assigned
Assigned	True	Update LTVS database	Patient or staff
Released	True	Update LTVS database	Not available
Off or lost	False	Remove from list of devices.	Not available

Note: Five devices were used to test the prototype LTVS prototype system.

updated with the newest real-time device locations on all the assigned devices, but it also performs automated services such as updating the tracking history log every time a location changes and generating alert messages if restricted areas are breached by the assigned device owner.

As seen from the LTVS infrastructure (Fig. 27.6), the LTVS application communicates with the tracking system through the LTVS database. The database is built in PostGreSQL and holds multiple tables of information. Some tables are dynamic interfaces for LTVS GUI to communicate and transmit data. Others are static definition tables from where tracking variables and GUI menus can be queried. Note that static tables are controlled via the LTVS Tracking Setup page, which can be seen farther down in the GUI discussion in the several figures and tables. Table 27.4 gives a list of functions that have been created for the LTVS database.

The design of the LTVS tracking module is complex in design but simple in operation. It is a self-sufficient background program that works seamlessly to bring tracking capabilities to the clinical environment. The thoroughness of the device management rules are intended to increase clinical security and awareness of

TABLE 27.4 Dynamic and static tables in LTVS database

	Function
Dynamic Tables	
ltvs_current	Location information of all actively assigned devices
ltvs_device	All devices that are detected by EPE, identified by MAC
ltvs_log	Periodic log of the number of devices found
ltvs_patient	Relevant patient information from RIS or HIS (i.e., name, age, sex, exam appointment, medical record number, assigned device MAC)
ltvs_staff	Relevant staff Information from RIS or HIS
ltvs_tracking_history	Tracking history log with time stamps of all LTVS device activity including device assignments, change in patient or staff locations, breached restricted areas, unassignment or lost of devices, and when the tracking module is stopped or restarted
Static Tables	
ltvs_area	List of areas defined in the positioning engine
ltvs_allowed_area	Patient areas allowed based on exam type
ltvs_exam	Clinical exams to determine allowed patient areas
ltvs_menu	Static table for GUI application display
ltvs_message	List of alert messages available to the tracking module ("Patient entered restricted area," "Patient waiting for longer than 30 minutes," "Device lost while assigned," etc.)
ltvs_variable	LTVS tracking parameters (frequency in which ltvs_current is updated, frequency of a periodic forced update of all devices, etc.)

human access within its compounds, but the monitoring of staff and patients also serves to improve clinical efficacy in finding its resources and clients in a bustling environment.

27.4.5 LTVS Application Design and Functionality

27.4.5.1 Application Design   The design of the LTVS application was based on the clinical workflow study that was performed at HCCII. The GUI developed for the application has a menu column on the left of the screen that lists the LTVS functions available—registration, monitoring, verification, reports, staff registration, and tracking setup (see Fig. 27.7, right). Each of these menus has various submenues to perform more specific tasks, but the general procedure of entering patients in the clinical environment starts by entering their RIS ID or any other form of medical identification number implemented by the clinic or hospital. Once a patient ID number is entered into the system, access to device-assignment and facial biometric registration and verification are available in the submenues of the GUI. Shown in Figure 27.7 is the first page of the LTVS GUI application entered by a clinical person using a factious RIS (radiology information system) ID. If patients are not registered in the LTVS, the entered patient information will be added to the ltvs_patient database automatically. We use an example to illustrate various functions of the LTVS major funcitons in the following subsections.

The components for the LTVS consists of a facial biometric or a fingerprint recognition module, and in this example the facial biometric is used (Fig. 27.6*A*) in a Wi-Fi (wireless fidelity) based tracking module (Fig. 27.6*B*) integrated into a Web-based application (Fig. 27.6*C*). The facial biometrics recognition module (Fig. 27.6*A*) uses software that calculates and analyzes landmark positions and features on a face to verify a person's identity. High-resolution USB video cameras are used for identity verification purpose. The facial biometrics recognition module has a database for image storage. The tracking module (Fig. 27.6*B*) consists of a wireless radiofrequency solution that utilize IEEE 802.11 b/g access points and Wi-Fi tags to track the current and historical location of patients and staff stored in the LTVS database, which is a local database located at HCCII. LTVS can be connected to any Wi-Fi network, so it complies with the IEEE 802.11 b/g network standard described above. In addition to location information, the integrated Web-based application (Fig. 27.6*C*) stores data inputs into the LTVS database from the facial biometric recognition module as well as other data in the tracking module.

The LTVS application can be installed in any standard PC workstation with a Web browser. A Web-based browser capable personal digital assistant (PDA) can also be utilized as a mobile application for users to monitor patient and staff and verify patient and staff identities. Based on the workflow, the system integration design and the graphical user interface (GUI) allows healthcare providers to extract real-time location information and verify the identity of the patient and staff. The tracking and biometrics module runs independently and synchronously using the Windows 2000 Professional operating system. The design of the LTVS server is modular in design to facilitate any improvements and replacements in the future. The system was demonstrated at the InfoRAD Exhibit, 91st Scientific Assembly and Annual Meeting of the Radiological Society of North America Conference 2005 and received Certificate of Merit Award.

27.4.5.2 LTVS Operation

Patient Registration   First, a patient photo is captured at the registration desk by the video camera, and then correlated with patient information from RIS/HIS and stored in the database of the LTVS.

Tag Assignment   The patient is assigned a Wi-Fi tag that links the patient information, such as the patient name and patient birth date. It is important to include a passive biometric ID because tracking devices can be easily lost or stolen, or they can be used to impersonate a patient or staff in order to gain access to the environment.

Patient Tracking   Once the tags have been assigned to patients or staff, the system allows the staff to access patient location records, including when, where, and who. It also provides the ability to locate patients on a real-time location tracking page in the graphic user interface (GUI) window. In addition the application provides a warning message to the staff if a particular patient has been in one location (e.g., waiting room) beyond the time limit.

Information Security   The system can trigger an alert if an unauthorized person enters a pre-defined restricted area (e.g., a reading room). These pre-defined rules are set not only for areas within the system coverage but also distinguish between authorized and unauthorized access. For example, a technologist would be allowed within the reading room, but a patient would not. Pre-defined rules can be re-configured within the LTVS to reflect such restrictions.

Patient Safety   In order to prevent patient mis-identification, before the patient enters the procedure room for an exam, the technologist can verify the identity of the patient by capturing the patient's facial image, and the software verifies and confirms the patient information including the patient ID, name, and original photos.

27.4.5.3 LTVS User Interface Examples

In Figures 27.9, 27.10, 27.11, and 27.12 four examples of LTVS uses are shown, each with a pair of images. The first image is the screen shot of the GUI of the management WS, and the second image is the corresponding floor activity in the radiology outpatient imaging department as recorded by the LTVS. Each set of images representing a function of the LTVS in real-time during the system evaluation phase. The four examples are as follows:

1. Monitoring page showing the real-time locations of patients and technologists.
2. Reporting page depicting the alert sent by the system to service the patient who has been waiting at the waiting room for over 25 minutes.
3. Alert page presenting a patient who has wandered into a restricted area and the administrator is escorting the patient back to the clinical area.
4. Verification page where a patient is being verified that she is the correct patient to be examined with CT.

Since the LTVS has over 30 functions, these 4 are only for illustration of the clinical usefulness of the system.

27.4.6 Lessons Learned from the LVTS Prototype

27.4.6.1 Address Clinical Needs in the Outpatient Imaging Center   Technical features of the LTVS that meet certain clinical needs are given in Table 27.5. The applications are shown to be robust, flexible, and accessible from any standard PC workstation with a Web browser. In addition the applications can be accessed from a personal digital assistant (PDA) with add-on features. Major key technical features and system workflows of the LTVS were developed to address these clinical needs based on the clinical workflow shown in Table 27.5.

27.4.6.2 Some Clinical Evaluation Results   Table 27.6 shows a two-day clinical summary. There were fifteen sample cases collected, including different type examinations in radiography and CT from HCCII. Clinical testing shows that there

LTVS Real-Time Monitoring Page

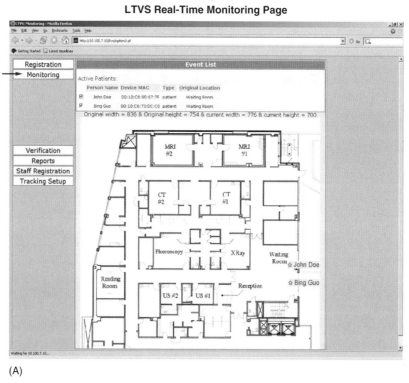

(A)

Figure 27.9   (*A*) LTVS administrative WS GUI display and the corresponding (*B*) real-time floor activities. (*A*) The GUI display window is marked "Monitoring" (left red arrow) page. The GUI shows a window of the floor plan of the clinical evaluation site, USC Healthcare Consultation Center II (HCC II). The "Report" page provides multiple choices for querying the report from the database (see left column). This example depicts two patients John Doe 1 and Bing Guo, each assigned a Wi-Fi tracking tag. Their names, tag accession number Mac address, status, and physical location are shown in event list table above the floor plan. (*B*) The corresponding floor shows two patients (blue) are in the waiting room and three technologists are nearby.

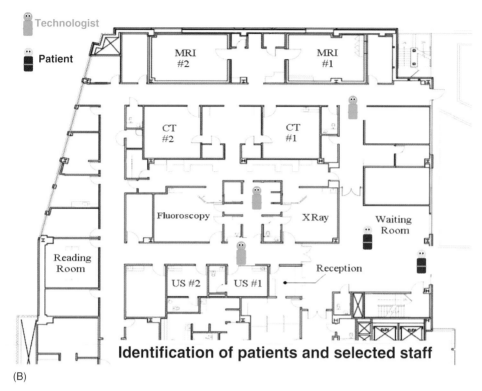

Identification of patients and selected staff

(B)

Figure 27.9 (*Continued*)

were five patients in two days who had CT exams with overall waiting time of more than 30 minutes; there are no recorded incidents of patients who had an X-ray exams waiting time of more than 30 minutes, since the procedure time for X-raying is much faster than the CT modality. The identity of patient was verified by the LTVS system at HCCII during the test period. There were no unauthorized warning messages received during the test period, which seems reasonable since HCCII was a relatively controlled and secure facility.

27.5 BENEFITS OF LTVS

Based on the HCCII prototype system, LTVS demonstrates the following benefits:

1. A patient can be clearly identified and tracked through the course of radiological examinations if the patient, with a photograph taken during the registration, carries a Wi-Fi location tag. It also allows the office administrator to understand the operational bottlenecks at the clinical site and recommend improved workflow.

2. Healthcare providers can know the patient location and the overall time a patient spent during the examination. Prompts can be put in place when the patient has remained in the waiting room for more than a specific amount of

time to decrease the waiting period as to track workflow inefficiencies throughout the time the patient is within the department (see Fig. 27.10*B*, lower right).

3. From a security standpoint, facial recognition will provide instantaneous and highly reliable biometric identity information, and ascertain that the examination being performed is on the right patient. It helps to prevent mis-identification of patients undergoing a radiological procedure.

4. LTVS improves the overall clinical management of policies and procedures in a clinical environment in order to partially fulfill HIPAA requirements for patient electronic data security.

27.6 COST ANALYSIS

The prototype LTVS for a clinical environment was designed and developed within the Image Processing and Informatics laboratory (IPI), USC for the radiology department outpatient imaging center, with an area of 13,000 square feet located at the

LTVS Reporting Page

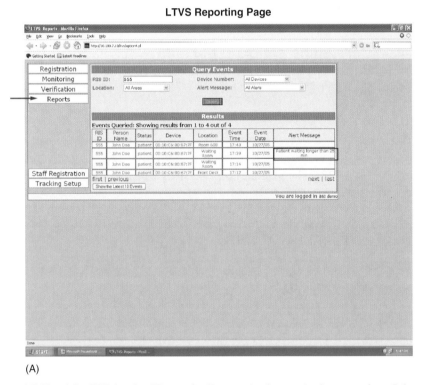

(A)

Figure 27.10 (*A*) GUI in the "Reporting" page (red arrow) shows patient John Doe was tracked starting from the front desk at 17:12 and is still in the waiting room at 17:39. Because of the long delay, an "Alert" message: "Patient waiting longer than 25 minutes" shows up in the administrative display. (*B*) The corresponding floor activity shows that following the "Alert" message, a technologist (green) goes to take the patient to the exam room.

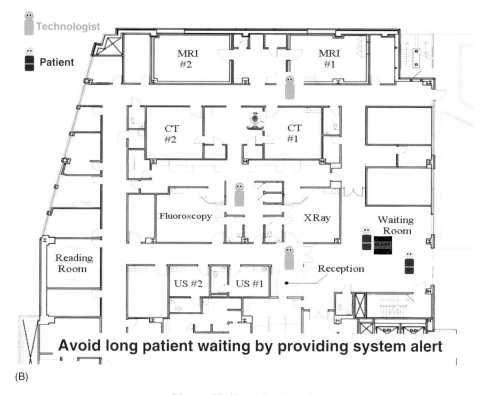

(B)

Figure 27.10   (*Continued*)

Healthcare Consultation Center II (HCCII). The LTVS prototype was then evaluated with the results described in Sections 27.4.6 and 27.5. This section presents the cost analysis. Table 27.7 shows the cost of the LTVS prototype, including hardware and software installed at HCCII but excluding system design, software devlopment, implementation, and evaluation time. The cost of LTVS also includes the annual license fees for facial identification biometric system; purchased hardware and software are at an education discount price.

27.7 ALTERNATIVE IDENTIFICATION DEVICES

27.7.1 System Design

To address the biometric verification component and determine which biometric system is the best for given applications in the complex clinical environment, the fingerprint scan system was added on the LTVS to run parallel with the facial recognition systems. Each solution was evalutated and documented for the advantages and pitfalls in the clinical environment.

Figure 27.13 is a slight modification of Fig. 27.6 in whcih the fingerprint scanning system is added onto the FRS (facial recognition system) to become FRSS (facial and fingerprint recognition system). Because of the modular design of the LTVS, such a mdoifccaiton was not difficult to accomplish.

27.7.2 Operation Procedure

27.7.2.1 Facial Image and Fingerprint Image Registration
A patient photo is captured at the registration desk by the video camera, correlated with patient information from RIS/HIS or input manually by front desk staff, such as the patient name and patient birth date, and stored in the database of the LTVS. It is important to include a biometric ID because tracking devices can be easily stolen and used to impersonate the patient in order to gain access or to sabotage. After patient photo is registered, the fingerprint enrollment step is started by a system message that says "Place finger on sensor." The fingerprint biometric module requires an initial five-time enrollment action in order to complete the registration step and obtain enough fingerprint data samples for verification. The system shows a message "Enroll complete" to notify the user that enrollment process is complete.

27.7.2.2 Facial Recognition and Fingerprint Recognition
In order to prevent patient mis-identification, before the patient enters the procedure room for an exam, the technologist verifies the identity of the patient by capturing the patient's facial image as described previously. This step can be replaced by the fingerprint scan.

LTVS Alert Page

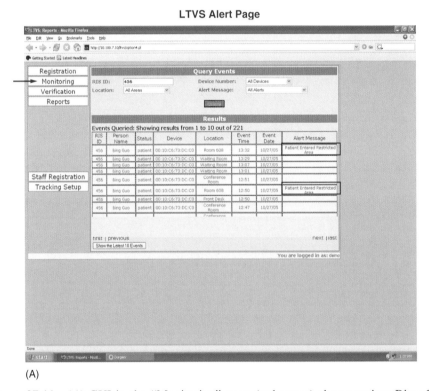

(A)

Figure 27.11 (A) GUI in the "Monitoring" page (red arrow) shows patient Bing Guo was tracked from 12:47 until 13:32, the patient entered the restricted area twice at 12:50 and 13:32. (B) The corresponding floor activity shows the "Stop" message, with the administrative manager escorting the patient away from the reading room.

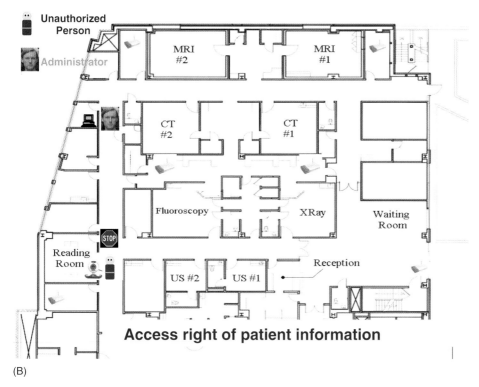

Figure 27.11   (*Continued*)

Figure 27.14*A* and *B* show that both the fingerprint and facial biometric verification technologies in the LTVS are in use. The patient registration page shows how to register a new patient into the LTVS. Observe that both facial verification and fingerprint verification systems are in the menu shown in the left column.

27.7.3 Performance and Accuracy

The accuracy of face recognition, and many biometric verification systems, varies depending on the degree and type of error allowed by the particular environment/client. Although humans have little trouble recognizing thousands of faces, algorithms that perform the same function are much more sensitive to factors such as illumination, camera view/orientation, facial expressions, aging, and accoutrements. We found that the facial biometric recognition system worked best in well-lit rooms using webcams with a minimum resolution of 640×480 or higher. Also the patients or staff having their facial biometric image taken had to be sitting within a certain distance of the webcam to yield sufficient biometric values. Although attaining webcams with the 640×480 resolution was feasible, it was difficult to achieve proper lighting and seating in certain rooms such as the radiology reading room and hallways where the workstation required the user to be standing.

Fingerprint recognition is the oldest and most widely used biometric system; it is also most susceptible to counterfeit possibilities. The disadvantage of the fingerprint biometric system is that silicon duplicates can be easily made, either with cooperation of its owner or by lifting fingerprints left behind on surfaces. Some of the more advanced fingerprint scanners attempt to reconcile this by testing for additional factors such as temperature, conductivity, heartbeat, relative dielectric constant, and blood pressure.

27.7.4 Individual's Privacy Concern

The patients agreed to the surveillance because we explained to them about the purpose of this project before we enrolled their photos and fingerprint images with personal information into the system. In addition all the information in the database was deleted after the testing period. At this point the photographs and fingerprint images of the patients in the LTVS were provided on a voluntary basis, since LTVS we used was a system prototype.

27.7.5 Cost Analysis

The cost of the facial biometric system, including hardware and software, we installed at HCCII was nearly six thousand dollars. The potential additional cost of a facial recognition biometric system runs about five thousand dollars in annual license fees.

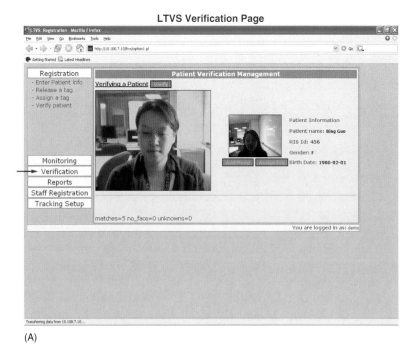

(A)

Figure 27.12 (*A*) GUI in the "Verification" page (red arrow) shows patient Bing Guo is being verified at a camera workstation the correct patient to be examined with the CT scanner. (*B*) The corresponding floor activity shows patient Bing Guo is being verified.

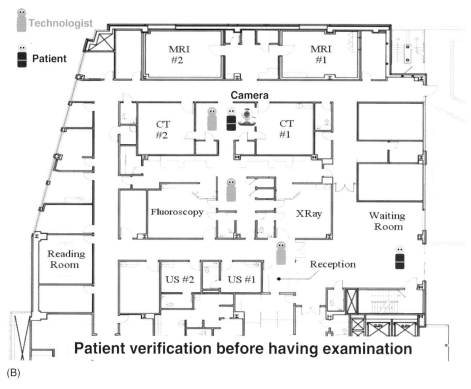

Technologist

Patient

MRI #2

MRI #1

Camera

CT #2

CT #1

Fluoroscopy

XRay

Waiting Room

Reading Room

US #2   US #1

Reception

Patient verification before having examination

(B)

Figure 27.12   (*Continued*)

TABLE 27.5   **Sample cases collected in two days with tracking status for radiography and CT from LTVS at Healthcare Consultation Center II during the evaluation**

Clinical Issues	System Technical Features
Lost patients in the department	Real-time identification of the movement of patients
Patient waiting too long	Warning provided to department personnel if a particular patient has been in one location (e.g., waiting room) beyond the time limit
Patient mis-identification	Patient identity verified biometrically through facial recognition at the exam site
Security for protection and privacy of patient information	Information security zone created within a subunit; biometrically verified access rights to vital clinical information for authorization by the healthcare provider

TABLE 27.6 Fifteen sample cases with tracking status for X ray and CT from LTVS at Healthcare Consultation Center II during the testing over two given days

Case Number	Date	Enter Department	Start Procedure	Waiting Time (min)
X-ray 1	November 7, 2005	8:38 am	8:54 am	16
X-ray 2	November 7, 2005	9:00 am	9:13 am	13
X-ray 3	November 7, 2005	9:39 am	9:48 am	9
X-ray 4	November 7, 2005	9:43 am	10:03 am	20
X-ray 5	November 7, 2005	10:05 am	10:28 am	23
X-ray 6	November 8, 2005	9:08 am	9:37 am	29
X-ray 7	November 8, 2005	10:50 am	11:02 am	12
X-ray 8	November 8, 2005	11:04 am	11:27 am	23
X-ray 9	November 8, 2005	1:02 pm	1:17 pm	15
X-ray 10	November 8, 2005	1:21 pm	1:34 pm	13
CT-1	November 8, 2005	8:44 am	9:52 am	68[a]
CT-2	November 8, 2005	10:05 am	10:43 am	38[a]
CT-3	November 8, 2005	10:49 am	11:43 am	54[a]
CT-4	November 8, 2005	1:06 pm	1:48 pm	42[a]
CT-5	November 8, 2005	2:29 pm	3:19 pm	50[a]

[a]Waiting time more than 30 minutes.

TABLE 27.7 Cost of location tracking and verification system (LTVS) evaluated at HCCII

Item	Quantity	Unit Cost	Subtotal
Hardware			
Wireless access points	6	$35	$210
Active tags	15	$80	$1200
FRS cameras	6	$80	$480
Server (computer)	1	$700	$700
Software			
Web server (Apache)		Free	Free
Database (PostGreSQL)		Free	Free
Facial recognition SDK			$5,000 license fees per year
Wireless location tracking			$5,000 for 15 tags
Total			$12,590

Note: Costs included hardware and software but excluded design, software development and implementation.

With the fingerprint identification device, the cost of the LTVS is relatively cheaper than the facial biometrics system because it does not require annual license fees. The cost of the fingerprint recognition biometric system is nearly three thousand dollars.

27.7.6 Current Status

No one form of biometric identification is universally superior to another; the specific environment or application ultimately defines which system is most effective.

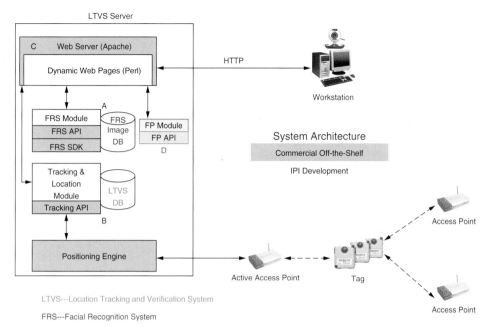

Figure 27.13 Combining facial and fingerprint verification systems in the LTVS; see Figure 27.6 for the original LTVS infrastructure. The fingerprint scanning system (FP) is added to the infrastructure as shown in D (red). The FRS becomes FFRS.

An outpatient radiology facility has several requirements upon which the systems can be evaluated. First, hospital patients would not need to be identified en masse; the purpose here is to use biometrics to verify a single individual's identity rather than locate him or her in a crowd. Thus facial recognition's exclusive attribute of scanning a large group of people is not applicable here. As mentioned earlier, face recognition systems are sensitive to factors such as aging, illumination, accoutrements, and camera orientation. The error rate for using face recognition on the diverse population expected in a clinical setting would be so high that the system might prove to be more of a hindrance than an asset. Therefore fingerprint scanning would be more appropriate than face recognition. In addition the cost of the fingerprint recognition biometric system is much lower than that of the facial recognition biometric system.

With regard to the technical requirements of the two systems, neither demands cumbersome hardware and both systems can be easily integrated into existing computer setups in a clinical setting. However, to be effective in a clinical setting, the biometric verification equipment must easily accommodate patients regardless of age, height, or state of consciousness. Facial recognition requires a great deal of user participation because imaging must be done at close range. This may present obstacles to patients who are unconscious, confined to wheelchairs, or for some other reason cannot physically access the camera. Because fingerprint scanners are so portable and versatile, physical access to the equipment is not an issue. Also, because of its history and ubiquity, fingerprint scanning is most likely to be viewed by the public as a less invasive procedure than a facial recognition system.

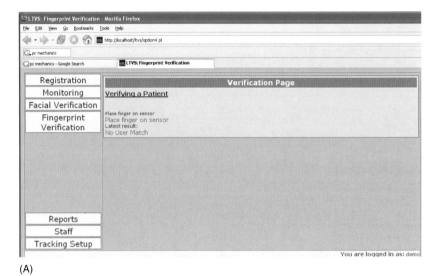

(A)

(B)

Figure 27.14 Combined fingerprint and facial biometric verification technologies in the LTVS. The patient registration page shows how to register a new patient into the LTVS system. First, a patient photo is captured by the video camera and correlated with patient information. After the patient photo registration, the fingerprint enrollment step starts by a system message that says: "Place finger on sensor." The system shows a message "Enroll complete" to notify the user that enrollment process is complete. Observe that both facial verification and fingerprint verification systems are in the menu shown in the left column. (*A*) The message "Place finger on sensor" notifies the user that the verification process starts. (*B*) The system matched the fingerprint placed on the sensor with the patient ID "123" in the database. As a result patient information, including photo image, is displayed on the verification page.

While both systems have their unique strengths and weaknesses, fingerprint scanning is the most appropriate biometric verification system for clinical settings, especially in the static clinical environment where the patient mobility may not be possible, such as during surgery. Also fingerprinting is more user-friendly and has a proven track record. Therefore, based on these criteria, fingerprint recognition is the recommended solution for a clinical environment unless the patient visual image is abolutely necessary. In the next section we present a fingerpinrt scanning system as an add-on patient verifiation step in minimally invasie spinal surgery ePR system discussed in Chapter 24.

27.8 FINGERPRINT SCAN AS AN ADD-ON SUBSYSTEM TO THE MISS ePR FOR VERIFICATION OF SURGICAL PATENT

In the minimally invasive spinal surgery (MISS) ePR system we discussed in Chapter 24, there was no patient identification component to verify the person is the actual

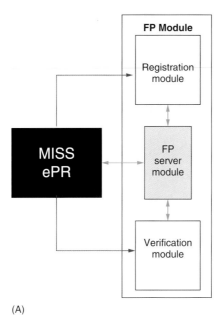

(A)

Figure 27.15   Integration of the fingerprint module with the minimally invasive spinal surgery (MISS) ePR system for patient identification and verification (see Section 24.4, and Figures 24.12 and 24.16 for MISS ePR infrastructure). (*A*) The FP (fingerprint) software module has three components: FP server module, registration module, and verification module. The MISS ePR requests both the verification and the registration modules for specific tasks, and the results are sent to the FP server module where it forwards to the MISS ePR. (*B*) The registration module registers a new patient using the FP scanner. The registered result is forwarded to the ePR patient database for archive. The verification and identification module verifies the patient before surgery starts. After the verification, OR staff trigger the MISS ePR to download both pre-op and intra-op patient information to the two large-screen LCD monitors (see Fig. 24.12). (Courtesy of Dr. J. Documet)

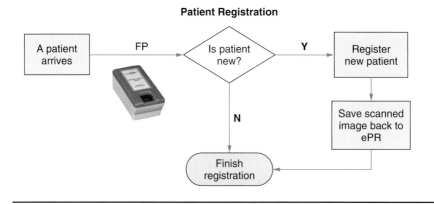

Figure 27.15 (*Continued*)

patient to be operated on. After the MISS ePR had been in clincal evaluation for several months, the surgery in charge suggested that a patient verification system be integrated with the ePR system. Since a surgical patient is mostly immobile, there was no advantage to using the facial verification system, so we decided to use the fingerprint scanning method. We learned a great deal about the fingerprint scanning method, not only its characteristics but also the method of integration with a larger imaging informatic system, during the latter part of the LTVS development. In the previous environment the fingerprint method had been developed as the second patient verificatin system in additon to the facial verification method. So it was not difficult to add this module to the the existing minimally invasive spinal surgery (MISS) ePR. This section summarizes the development, operation procedure, and the current status.

27.8.1 Why the Need to Have Fingerprint Verification in MISS

There are two aims of integrating a fingerprint verification system in the MISS. First, by utilizing the fingerprint in the ePR, the system helps avoid patient mis-identification. Second, one of the main goals of implementing an ePR for MISS is to improve the overall workflow of surgical procedures by increasing efficiency. Thus, once the patient has been identified as the correct patient by the fingerprint module, surgical personnel can download all pertinent information of the patient from the pre-op ePR module to the big LCD screen in the OR. Then the surgery can immediately commence.

27.8.2 System Description

27.8.2.1 The Fingerprint Verification Module   The fingerprint verification module helps reduce any possible patient mis-identification at the time of operation while improving the overall time to load patient related information into the OR pre-op display and intra-op live display. The fingerprint module is composed of two submodules: the patient registration and the verification. The former takes place when the patient visits the consultation offices prior to surgery. The latter happens right before the surgical procedure occurs.

27.8.2.2 Integration of the Fingerprint Verification System into the MISS Operation   The fingerprint module is an add-on module to the MISS ePR and is integrated as a pre-registration step during consultation prior to pre-op stage, and as a mechanism to verify patient's identity at the OR right before the intra-op stage.

27.8.2.3 Software Architecture and Its Connection to the MISS Overall Software   The fingerprint module is composed of three components as shown in Figure 27.15: the registration submodule, the verification submodule, and the server component. The server component is in charge of storing the fingerprint database in terms of images and fingerprint templates, where also the extracted features of the scanned fingerprints are stored. The registration module takes care of scanning a new fingerprint image and sending it back to the MISS ePR (where the server module resides). The verification module is in charge of scanning a fingerprint and comparing that newly image with the current database to verify the patient's identity.

27.8.3 Operational Procedure

The fingerprint module is used at two different occasions of the complete MISS workflow. The first time is when the patient arrives at the clinic for consultation. At this time the patient is fingerprinted by a front-desk assistant, and the image is saved in the ePR database. The finger scanned will be used as the same one for the scan during second occasion. The first order of choice is the right hand: thumb, index, middle, ring, pinky. If the right hand cannot conveniently be scanned, the left hand is used. This step is important because the same order of choice fingers needs to be scanned at the OR to ensure the right person is identified; otherwise, the module will not be able of recognizing the patient.

The second time the patient's fingers are scanned is right before the operation procedure starts. The same finger that was used for registration is used. If the finger matches a previously saved fingerprint, the ePR system will request the person in charge of the patient setup to proceed and load the pre-op data to the pre-op monitor in the OR. Otherwise, a second attempt will be made to identify the person. In the case where the person cannot be recognized by the ePR system, the fallback mechanism is a manual selection from a list of scheduled patients of the day. The reason of the failure will be recorded as well.

27.8.4 Current Status

The registration module was installed four months after the MISS ePR was in clinical evalutaion, and it has been functioning since. Patient fingerprints are scanned and stored in the ePR database.

27.9 SUMMARY OF THE LOCATION TRACKING AND VERIFICATION SYSTEM IN CLINICAL ENVIRONMENT

In this chapter we discuss imaging informatics by taking advantage of other existing information technologies (IT) not necessary in medical imaging, and integrating them with medical imaging advances. In particular, we present a location tracking and verification system (LTVS) in clinical environment. Although technologies used in the LTVS are not necessary in the cutting edge of medical imaging and in IT, the combination of these technologies can help resolve patient workflow and patient protection issues in the clinical environment that have been discussed in the imaging informatics community for many years.

We start the presentation by defining what LTVS is and why we need it. Currently available tracking, identification, and verification technologies are introduced. We give a step-by-step modular system integration of the LTVS—from the prototype design and development, to implementation and clinical evaluation of the prototype in an outpatient imaging center, and to cost analysis. The prototype was used to track the movement of the patients and personnel to improve the efficiency in imaging procedure workflow, and safeguard patients in the clinical environment. We conclude with a discussion of a fingerprint scanning module for surgical patient identification and verification to ensure that the person is the right patient to be operated on.

References

Authentec, Inc. http://www.authentec.com/getpage.cfm?sectionID=3, accessed January 2007.

Brennan TA, et al. Incidence of adverse events and negligence in hospitalized patients: results of the Harvard Medical Practice Study. *Qual Saf Health Care*, 13: 145–152; 2004.

Ekahau Inc.; 2006. http://www.ekahau.com/.

Garcia ML, Centeno MA, Rivera C, DeCario N. Reducing time in an emergency room via a fast-track. *Proc Winter Simulation Conf*, pp. 1048–1053; 1995.

Guo B, Documet J, King N, Liu BJ, Huang HK, Grant EG. Patient tracking and facial biometrics integrated in a clinical environment for HIPAA security compliance. *Radiol Soc N Am, Int Conf*, RSNA Chicago, 27 Nov–2 Dec, p. 873; 2005.

Guo B, Jorge D, Jasper L, et al. A tracking and verification system implemented in a clinical environment for partial HIPAA compliance. *Proc SPIE* 6145: 184–91; 2006.

Guo B, Jorge D, Nelson K. Patient tracking and facial biometrics integrated in a clinical environment for HIPAA security compliance. Presented at the 91st *Scientific Assembly and Annual Meeting of RSNA*. Inforad Exhibit; 2005.

Guo B, Documet J, Lee J, Liu B, King N, Shrestha R, Wang K, Huang HK, Grant EG, Experiences with a Prototype Tracking & Verification System Implemented within an Imaging Center, *Journal of Academic Radiology*, 14(3): 270–278; 2007.

HIPAA. http://www.cms.hhs.gov/hipaa/hipaa2/general/background/p1104191.asp.

HIPAA; 2006. http://www.hhs.gov/ocr/hipaa/.

History of biometrics. http://ntrg.cs.tcd.ie/undergrad/4ba2.02/biometrics/history.html, accessed Jan 2007.

Jain A, Hong L, Pankanti S. Biometric identification. *Comm ACM* 43(2): 91–8; 2000.

Joint Commission on Accreditation of Healthcare Organizations (JCAHO); 2006. http://www.jointcommission.org/.

Joint Commission on Accreditation of Healthcare Organizations (JCAHO). http://www.jointcommission.org/, accessed Jan 2007.

Murphy MF, Kay JDS. Patient identification: problems and potential solutions. *Vox Sanguinis* 87(suppl. 2): 197–202; 2004.

NevenVision; 2006. http://www.nevenvision.com/.

Phillips PJ, Martin A, Wilson CL, Przybocki M. An introduction to evaluating biometric systems. *Computer* 33(2): 56–63; 2000.

Thomas P, Evans C. An identity crisis? Aspects of patient misidentification. *Clin Risk* 10: 18–22; 2004.

van der Putte T, Keuning J. Biometrical fingerprint recognition: don't get your fingers burned. Proceedings of the *Fourth Working Conference on Smart Card Research and Advanced Applications*. Dordrercht: Kluwer Academic 289–303; 2000.

Vissers JMH. Patient flow-based allocation of inpatient resources: a case study. *Eur J Ope Res* 105: 356–70; 1998.

CHAPTER 28

New Directions in PACS and Medical Imaging Informatics Training

The picture archiving and communication system (PACS) is an imaging information system that is now widely used in daily clinical practice. For its successful implementation, training of users has been found to be necessary. A review of PACS training thus far shows that the major emphasis in training has been placed on the use of display workstations (WSs). Although training on the use of the WS is indispensible to clinical and other healthcare users who will utilize the system, PACS as an integrated information system with many components and capabilities also requires that the user understand how the system works and how to utilize many hidden capabilities in addition to reviewing images and making clinical diagnoses. For example, the wealth of data in the PACS database has stimulated many nonradiology physicians and allied healthcare providers, physicists and biologists, and engineers to use the data for applications in their respective fields of expertise, as well as for collaborative research and development with radiologists. The majority of these groups of PACS users may not be as proficient as radiologists in reading and assessing images from the WS, but their combined efforts and results have propelled radiology as a field to higher scientific importance as demonstrated in the proliferation of imaging informatics development over the last five years. These user groups may also need to learn about PACS WSs, although this is not as critical as for radiologists; they should also learn other aspects of PACS in order to treasure hunt in the PACS database. With all the potential for further research and development in imaging informatics using PACS related databases, a more comprehensive education and training program on PACS and imaging informatics is called for. The concept of the PACS simulator as a stand-alone training and research tool not interfering with the daily clinical PACS operation is necessary to be introduced.

In this chapter we first discuss the PACS training, and then expand the methodology to include medical imaging informatics training. Five topics are presented: new directions in PACS and imaging informatics education and training, the concept of the PACS Simulator, training of interdisciplinary specialists, PACS training under interactive media-rich learning environments, and distance learning of PACS. Figure 28.1, repeats Figure 20.3 to show the crossover between PACS and imaging informatics that leads to the training methodology

PACS and Imaging Informatics, Second Edition, by H. K. Huang
Copyright © 2010 John Wiley & Sons, Inc.

28.1 NEW DIRECTIONS IN PACS AND MEDICAL IMAGING INFORMATICS EDUCATION AND TRAINING

28.1.1 PACS as an Integrated Medical Imaging Information Technology System

A PACS is an image information technology (IT) system for the transmission, storage, and display of medical images, as shown in Figure 28.1 (top). After 20 years of development, PACS has been integrated in various hospitals' information systems for daily clinical use. The PACS is an IT system of components with a clinical focus: no one person can claim expertise in all of these components. A review of the history in hospital information technology development demonstrates that the culture's segregation of expertise between health professionals and IT professionals was a hurdle to be overcome during PACS implementation. Health professionals did not have enough IT knowledge to maintain the daily running of the PACS or to communicate with the IT specialists, and IT-based engineers lacked the knowledge and experience in radiology departments and hospital environments to provide efficient workflow for the clinical operations. After some years we come to the awareness that for a successful PACS implementation and operation, a team effort consisting of radiologists, radiological technologists, hospital administrators, radiological clerks, nurses, and IT specialists is required, and hence more comprehensive training of PACS is necessary. Not only radiologists or radiological technologists (radiographers) need the training but also others like IT personnel, system engineers, radiological administrators/clerks, and hospital administrators.

Above all, the team requires a PACS manager or administrator who takes the ownership of the PACS, coordinates a team, services and maintains the day-to-day operation of the PACS; as well as training different groups of staff to use and service the system. This section reviews training methods of PACS during the past years.

28.1.2 Education and Training of PACS in the Past

The history of PACS training can be divided into two periods. The first period started from the time clinical PAC systems were used in the early 90s until five years ago, and the second period is during the past five years.

28.1.2.1 PACS Training until Five Years Ago
In the beginning during the early 80s, PACS was much discussed in scientific meetings. Refresher courses on PACS were offered in the annual meetings of the Radiological Society of North America (RSNA).Various manufacturers organized special private workshops by application specialists, but the emphasis of such training was on how to retrieve images and diagnostic reports from the server and display them on the review WSs, and how to use the tools in the WSs to enhance the image for interpretation. The participants of such training were radiologists, physicians, technologists, and radiographers.

At about the same time, special modality mini PAC systems such as CT PACS, MR PACS, US PACS, and CR PACS were sold to radiology departments as PACS. The training packaged with such purchases consisted of special workshops for technologists and radiologists organized by vendors. The training provided was on the use of the modality, archiving images in the local database, and display images on WSs.

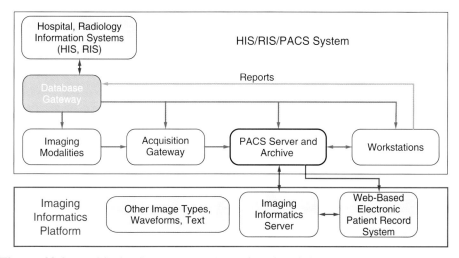

Figure 28.1 PACS dataflow (top) and the imaging informatics platform (bottom). DICOM images and related data are transmitted from the clinical PACS server to the imaging informatics server as well as the Web-based ePR system. Data from the imaging informatics server can be linked but not necessary directly transmitted back to the PACS archive server; from the medical imaging informatics platform processed data can be retrieved by and displayed on PACS workstations using the DICOM structured reporting.

28.1.2.2 PACS Training during the Past Five Years In the last five years similar training has continued while changes had evolved. Instead of didactic refresher courses, special hands-on workshops had been offered by major vendors under the auspices of the RSNA during the annual meetings on how to use their respective viewing WSs. The hands-on sessions usually last one hour, occasionally with a second hour for "advanced PACS," for customizing the display workstations to the users' preference. Interfacing of the PACS with RIS is also demonstrated. The target audience is radiologists or physicians, but any participants of the meetings can enroll into the workshops if they are interested.

The Integrating the Healthcare Enterprise (IHE), an initiative launched since 1998 with the goal of encouraging integration of information systems within the health care enterprise (http://www.rsna.org/IHE/participation/index.shtml 2001–2002), has organized seminars and demonstrations during RSNA annual meetings and HIMSS (Healthcare Information and Management System Society) to showcase the data integration capabilities among manufacturers with the aim of improving workflow and information sharing in support of better patient care. Over 20 manufacturers have participated at each RSNA meeting since 2001 (see Chapter 9).

28.2 CONCEPT OF THE PACS SIMULATOR

28.2.1 Problems with the Past and Current Training Methods

Past training efforts have demonstrated the benefits of PACS and thus attracted professionals to consider implementing PACS in their respective departments. However, the transition from film to digital has been a challenging task for all professionals who used to work with films. To use a WS to review images requires converting many traditional hardcopy viewing procedural steps, from film development to image interpretation. For this reason training on how to use the WS has received the major emphasis. Although the most important and frequently used component in PACS is for clinical care, the WS is still one component among many in PACS. Queries and retrievals from WSs become simple tasks if every other component runs smoothly. Nevertheless, a smooth workflow can never be guaranteed by PACS, since many other factors can cause problems to the system. The single point of failure (SPOF) in a PACS might be in the network, the server, the archive, and the RIS–PACS interface, which can suspend the system and cause users agony. These SPOFs can be minimized if the user understands and learns how to circumvent them before a failure happens. Merging past and current images can result in "loss" of images in some modalities, and this problem can be avoided if the users understand the DICOM data model. Below are some frequently raised questions by clinical professionals:

- How can images be sent to another workstation or a remote site?
- Why can some images shown in the worklist not be read if I had read it already?
- Why a new modality cannot be connected to the PACS although it claims to be DICOM compliant?
- How can I know there is no image loss in the transmission of the whole exam?
- Where is the bottleneck when multiple workstations query/retrieve simultaneously?
- How can we troubleshoot when the workstations cannot query/retrieve image from the PACS archive server?
- How can we make a clinical PACS archive server continuously available?
- How can I access images for teaching purposes?
- What should I do with the PACS during "downtime"? What will happen to my images?

These are hiccups that may or may not be related to the workstations. Of course, if there are on-site IT engineers, solutions to these problems can be immediately addressed. However, these are very practical clinical events that the IT engineer may or may not be able to help with. Moreover few manufacturers provide such a level of support except for the first few weeks of the operation of new modalities. Although remote manufacturer support may be available, it cannot replace the services of a full-time PACS administrator or manager.

These examples demonstrate that existing training on viewing WSs can serve the needs of many clinical professionals to review and make diagnoses from the images; it is not adequate for many others who have the responsibility of implementation and daily operation of the PACS to support the system. PACS training is usually conducted at the clinical site. However, scheduling the training sessions in a clinical department during working hours is not easy: the radiologists, physicians, or technologists are busy or the WSs are being used for clinical purposes. Stability of the system as well as security and privacy of the patients' data are added to the concerns.

28.2.2   The New Trend: Comprehensive Training Including System Integration

Unlike an imaging modality, which is usually a stand-alone unit, PACS involves integration of tens to hundreds of components, including all imaging modalities and WSs and other information systems such as RIS or HIS. The difficulties of its installation have been depicted in the literature. For PACS implementation, knowledge of the department/hospital requirements (in terms of workload and efficiency), workflow, networking infrastructure, as well as the budget are prerequisites. Strategy development, market survey, system specification requirements, involvement of users in planning, technical supports, and training staff to utilize the PACS to its full potential are essential factors to success.

Although how to use the WS is ranked the most important for training clinicians, technologists, nurses, and clerks to use the PACS, past field experience indicates that a comprehensive training that includes system integration in radiology/hospital workflow is the new direction for equipping users, IT personnel, and administrators of the PACS so that they can handle the day-to-day operation of the system. The trend of PACS installation demonstrates that more PACS managers and IT personnel are needed to be educated with a comprehensive training program. Depending on the individual's level of responsibilities, the trainees should possess in-depth knowledge in areas such as WSs, clinical workflow, IT, networking, and data management.

28.2.3   The New Tool — The PACS Simulator

Comprehensive training can be conducted in a clinical radiology department where a PACS has been installed. However, as mentioned above, finding a time slot for the training is never easy in most busy radiology departments because PACS is a 24/7 clinical system. Also it is difficult to provide hands-on experience with PACS in a hospital environment because of network stability and security requirements. A PACS simulator in a laboratory environment with noninvasive one-way transmission of clinical images from PACS to the simulator can provide a more comfortable setting for a more basic understanding of PACS concept and providing practical experience to the trainees under a more controlled and relaxed environment. A generic PACS simulator consists of eight components as shown in Figure 28.2.

28.2.3.1 *Functions of Each Component*   The PACS simulator consists of two simulators, RIS and acquisition modality, and six other components:

1. ***RIS simulator*** randomly generates a pseudopatient registration and examination order and sends the order to the acquisition modality simulator.
2. ***Acquisition modality simulator*** (AMS) simulates the clinical imaging modalities. It inputs thousands of images of various types (CT, MR, CR, US) randomly each day from the clinical PACS (patient's name and ID are anonymized first, and a pseudoname and ID are then assigned) to simulate the production of digital images in a clinical department. The AMS simulates the generation of DICOM exams based on the RIS simulator order and sends the exams to the DICOM gateway automatically or manually.
3. ***DICOM gateway*** receives various modality images from the modality simulator and automatically sends them to the PACS simulator server. It verifies the

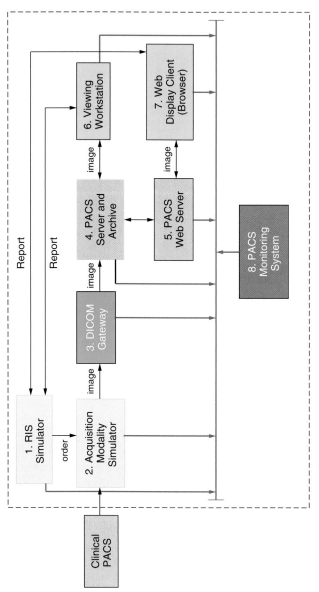

Figure 28.2 Generic PACS simulator of eight components with a non-invasive connection to the clinical PACS for data input to the modality simulator.

image format and reformats non-DICOM images into DICOM formats. More important, it verifies the successful transmission of images. In other words, it guarantees no loss of images. If the server is at fault in receiving images, the DICOM gateway will keep the images until the PACS server resumes its normal function.

4. ***PACS server and archive*** is the heart of the PACS simulator (see Chapter 7). In addition to receiving and archiving DICOM images from the gateway, it is responsible for the automatic or on-demand distribution of images to the PACS Web server and PACS WSs.

5. ***PACS Web server*** is a PACS application server that converts DICOM images to Web-based format images (see Chapter 14) for distribution and retrieval by Web clients. It preserves the image quality as well as the DICOM standard format of the image.

6. ***PACS viewing workstations (WSs)*** are for the viewing of PACS DICOM images. The workstations are where physicians and radiological technologists can query and retrieve images for viewing or for quality assurance. The images can be sent automatically or queried by the WS. There are several WSs of similar quality as a clinical PACS WS, and with good graphical user interface (GUI) and image processing tools that are incorporated to facilitate radiologists' reading and reporting. Several WSs can mimic some leading PACS manufacturers' WS to read their PACS images. A pseudodiagnostic report can be generated for the exam and sent back to the RIS simulator for archive.

7. ***Web clients*** can retrieve images from the Web server in Web-based image format and perform the DICOM image format display.

8. ***PACS monitoring system*** is connected to all components in the PACS simulator. It monitors the workflow and data flow of each component. Normal operations or artificial interruptions of the simulator are recorded and can be reviewed at the system monitor for tracing the work flow or sources of error.

28.2.3.2 *What Trainees Can Learn from the PACS Simulator*   Trainees can acquire the following knowledge from the PACS simulator:

1. *Observe the clinical PACS operation, component by component.* DICOM compliant images triggered by the RIS simulator are generated and manually sends by the trainee to the DICOM gateway at the acquisition modality simulator (AMS). On receiving the images from the AMS, the DICOM gateway automatically sends them to the PACS server. Once the PACS server receives the images, it parses the DICOM image into two parts, the metadata from the DICOM header, which is stored in the database, and the image data, which is stored in the archive. It also distributes the images to the Web server and PACS WSs, either automatically or by query/retrieve. The Web server and viewing workstations put the image metadata into their respective local databases and image data to the hard disk, which are then ready for clinical review.

2. *Trace the data flow through each component as described in item 1.* Trainees can observe the image flow from the logging messages on the screen of each component as well as from the PACS monitoring system.

3. *Query and retrieve images from WSs or Web clients.* Trainees can query and retrieve images from the viewing WSs and Web clients and observe the image flow messages on the screen of the WSs, Web clients, Web server, PACS server, and the PACS monitoring system.

4. *Review images at WSs.* Trainees can use image processing tools to enhance image interpretation.

5. *Induce failure in a component to observe its impact on the PACS operation.* Because the PACS simulator is stand-alone, trainees can manually induce failures to any component and observe their impact on the PACS operation. For example, trainees can disconnect the DICOM gateway from the network while the AMS is sending images to it. The images will not be archived at the PACS server and will not be able to be viewed; however, the PACS monitoring system will record such a failure event.

6. *Identify image data flow bottleneck.* Trainees can launch query/retrieve simultaneously at multiple workstations and Web clients and watch the image flow from the WSs. This training step can be executed because the PACS server and the Web server can process multiple tasks simultaneously. Usually the speed of image transmission will slow down even when only one WS launches the query/retrieve.

7. *Troubleshoot common problems encountered in the daily clinical PACS operation.* There might be some minor problems daily in running a clinical PACS, for example, a power cutoff from a DICOM gateway machine, disconnection of the network from a WS, or minor software bugs in some PACS components. These problems can be tested in the PACS simulator by trainees to learn how to troubleshoot them.

28.3 EXAMPLES OF PACS AND IMAGING INFORMATICS TRAINING PROGRAM

In this section we provide two examples on using the PACS simulator for training.

28.3.1 PACS Training in the Image Processing and Informatics Laboratory, University of Southern California

PACS and imaging informatics training was provided at the Image Processing and Informatics Laboratory (IPILab), Department of Radiology, University of Southern California (USC). The PACS simulator architecture used for the training is illustrated in Figure 28.3, and the hardware and software components and functions are given in Table 28.1. The USC PACS simulator is connected to the clinical PACS, which provides a supply of images to the acquisition modality simulator (AMS).

28.3.1.1 PACS Training for the Professional IPILab is both a training and research laboratory. The PACS simulator was developed as a stand-alone training and research tool for radiologists, clinicians, relevant healthcare providers, PACS administrators, IT personnel, and biomedical engineering students and fellows. With the in-house PACS simulator (with noninvasive connection to the clinical PACS)

Fault-Tolerant PACS Simulator

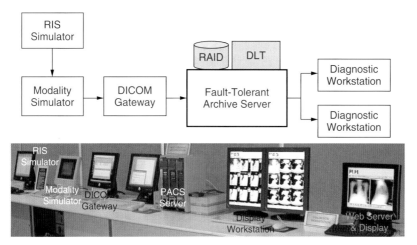

Figure 28.3   Architecture of PACS simulator at IPILab, University of Southern California with connection to the Clinical PACS for live images. Left to right: RIS simulator, modality simulator, DICOM GW, FT (Fault-Tolerance) PACS server, PACS WS, and Web server and WS. The bottom figure was taken at the InfoRAD Exhibit, RSNA 2002, Chicago.

and PACS expertise at various levels, clinical and engineering, the IPILab organized PACS training courses at both advanced and basic levels for the various categories of personnel using the PACS simulator. Table 28.2*A* gives an example of a comprehensive training curriculum for PACS administrators. Two types of PACS professionals were entered in this training:

1. *IT personnel training.* These trainees already had some IT knowledge above the basic level. The teaching approached used in the curriculum were lectures and tutorials, hands-on sessions, and clinical site visits. The training was more technically oriented with clinical components used as examples.
2. *PACS administrators' course.* The sessions included PACS implementation, fault tolerance, backup and upgrade of archive, data recovery solutions, and research applications of the PACS.

In the hands-on training, the PACS simulator was used to demonstrate the simulator functions described earlier. The PACS training classes were held as stand-alone one- or two-week workshops. A copy of the schedule for a recent two-week advanced level training for PACS administrators and radiographers/technicians is provided in Table 28.2*B*.

28.3.1.2   *PACS Simulator as a Laboratory Component in BME Graduate Courses*   In 2004, the IPILab developed an Imaging Processing and Imaging Informatics Master of Sciences Program within the Department of Biomedical

TABLE 28.1 PACS Simulator hardware and software components at IPILab, USC

PACS Components	Hardware	Software
1. RIS[a] Simulator	Dell Optiplex Gx 150: P III 1.8 GHz, 128 MB memory, 20 GB hard disk, 10/100 MB Ethernet card	System: Windows 2000/XP, ORACLE 8i Windows client[b], IE browser Application: RIS simulator software package
2. Acquisition modality simulator	Dell Optiplex Gx 150: PIII 1.8 GHz, 128 MB memory, 20 GB hard disk, 10/100 MB Ethernet card	System: Windows 2000/XP, ORACLE 8i Windows client[b], Microsoft Office 2000 Application: modality simulator software package
3. DICOM gateway	Dell Optiplex Gx 150: PIII 1.8 GHz, 256 MB memory, 40 GB hard disk, 10/100 MB Ethernet card	System: Windows 2000/XP, Microsoft Office 2000 Application: DICOM gateway software package
4. PACS server	SUN Ultra2: UltraSparc 300 MHz, 512 MB memory, 30 GB hard disk, 10/100 MB Ethernet card	System: Solaris 2.6/2.7/2.8, ORACLE Enterprise 8i for Solaris Application: PACS controller software package
6, 7. Viewing or Web client workstations	Dell Precision 330: PIII 2.0 GHz, 512 MB memory, 40 GB hard disk, 10/100 MB Ethernet card	System: Windows NT4.0/2000, Application: Cedara VR Read 4.0 or Web client software
5, 8. PACS workstations	Dell Optiplex Gx 150: PIII 1.8 GHz, 128 MB memory, 20 GB hard disk, 10/100 MB Ethernet card	System: Windows 2000/XP, ORACLE 8i Windows client,[b] IE browser, Microsoft Office 2000 Application: PACS monitor software package Application: Apache Web server

[a]Numerals represent the PACS simulator components shown in Figure 28.2.
[b]The system needs ORACLE Enterprise 8i server in Solaris.

Engineering (BME), School of Engineering, USC. After obtaining an MS degree, qualified students can enter the PhD program in medical imaging informatics. The details of this program are described in Section 28.4. Every student enrolled in this degree program has to take in the BME department two three-credit new courses: (1) BME 527—Integration of Medical Imaging Systems Technology—and (2) BME 528—Medical Imaging Informatics. The PACS simulator is being used as the laboratory component of these two courses. The first semester is to learn the basic PACS concept, and the second semester is for research topics development. Tables 28.3*A* and *B* describes the course contents of these two courses.

TABLE 28.2*A*   **Training curriculum for PACS administrators at IPILab, USC**

Mode of Training	Topics	Content
Lectures and tutorials	Introduction to computer systems and networks	UNIX/PC/Mac systems Networking basics Server processes Storage devices Database UNIX server and network administration basics System and network troubleshooting
	Basics of PACS	Basic concepts and standards PACS components: HIS/RIS, PACS broker, modality, DICOM gateway, PACS controller, diagnostic workstations, and Web server
	Clinical PACS workflow	Review of workflow Examples of workflow pitfalls Clinical perspective of display workstations and PACS workflow
	PACS implementation	Implementation methodology Identification of resources Implementation pitfalls
	Advanced technologies and teleradiology	Internet 2 Telemedicine and teleradiology
	Future PACS applications	Fault-tolerant PACS server Disaster recovery solution PACS archive upgrade PACS security ASP backup archive Design of PACS application server: Web, PC, UNIX PACS-based CAD server
Hands-on	PACS components	Demonstration and hands-on
	Adding components	Configuration and set up of components using PACS simulator
	Troubleshooting	Troubleshooting each component and the entire PACS simulator and workflow
	Fault-tolerant system	System faults and fail-over demonstration
	Archive	Backup and upgrade
Clinical site visits		Clinical PACS overview Follow through live clinical examinations Walk through daily PACS operations Troubleshooting clinical PACS: issues and examples

TABLE 28.2B. Advanced PACS and informatics training schedule at IPILab

Mon 9/1/08 Overview	Tue 9/2/08 Integration	Wed 9/3/08 Workflow and PACS Simulator	Thu 9/4/08 CAD	Fri 9/5/08 Data Migration, Security, and Fault Tolerance
9:30AM to 10:30AM Introduction & Icebreaker Activities HK Huang/Brent Liu	**8:30AM to 10:30AM** Lecture: HL7 & Its Usage Brent Liu Lecture: HIS/RIS/PACS Integration and the ePR Concept Brent Liu	**8:30AM to 10:30AM** Lecture: How to Divorce a PACS Manufacturer Case Study: USCRA Siemens to Fuji Kevin Wang, Brent Liu	**8:30AM to 10:30AM** Lecture: Introduction to PACS-Based CAD Brent Liu	**8:30AM to 10:30AM** Data Migration with Case Studies Brent Liu
10:30AM to 12:30PM Overview of USC Radiology, IPILab, BME, PACS Training Course Schedule & Goals Brent Liu	**10:30AM to 12:30PM** Lecture: Enterprise PACS & Single vs. Multiple Vendor Challenges Case Studies HK Huang	**10:30AM to 12:30PM** Clinical IT Ride-Along: HCC2 Kevin Wang, PACS IT Support Team	**10:30AM to 12:30PM** Lecture: Medical Imaging Informatics PACS-based CAD Case Study: Automatic Bone Age Assessment Dr. Lucy Zhang	**10:30AM to 12:30PM** Clinical IT Ride-Along: UH/Norris Kevin Wang, PACS IT Support Team
12:30PM to 2:00PM LUNCH	**12:30PM to 2:00PM** LUNCH	**12:30PM to 2:00PM** LUNCH	**12:30PM to 2:00PM** LUNCH	**12:30PM to 2:00PM** LUNCH

TABLE 28.2B. (*Continued*)

2:00PM to 4:00PM Lecture: The Role of IT in Radiology HK Huang	**2:00PM to 4:00PM** Lecture: Post-processing Workflow and Integration with PACS: Challenges and Pitfalls Bing Guo Lecture: PACS Simulator Brent Liu	**2:00PM to 4:00PM** Lecture: Data Mining Methods in PACS Dr. Lucy Zhang	**2:00PM to 5:00PM** BME 527 Graduate Course Lecture Week 2: HK Huang Opening Lecture
4:00PM to 6:00PM Program Adjustments HK Huang, Brent Liu	**4:00PM to 6:00PM:** Two-Day Review: Q&A Session Brent Liu	**4:00PM to 6:00PM** Hands-On Training: PACS Simulator Lab Jorge Documet, Anh Le, Kevin Ma	**4:00PM to 6:00PM** Lecture: How to Setup CAD in a Clinical Environment Case Study: BAA in the WCH Dr. Lucy Zhang Site Visit: WCH Dr. Lucy Zhang, Kevin Ma, Dr. Paymann Moin
			5:00PM Onward Site Visit: USC Main Campus

TABLE 28.2B. (*Continued*)

Mon 9/8/08 Data Grid	Tue 9/9/08 PACS Implementation and Tools	Wed 9/10/08 CAD/PACS Integration	Thu 9/11/08 UCLA Site Visit & Q&A Session	Fri 9/12/08 ePR for RT & Surgery
8:30AM to 10:30AM Lecture: Data Integrity and Security Jasper Lee Lecture: The Concept of the Data Grid Jasper Lee	**8:30AM to 10:30AM** Lecture: PACS Study Management Tools (Wireless, QC, Dashboard) Jorge Documet Lecture: Fault-Tolerance & Data Backup Solutions Brent Liu	**8:30AM to 10:30AM** Lecture: IHE Workflow Profiles Brent Liu Lecture: CAD-PACS Toolkit Anh Le	**8:30AM to 10:30AM** Site Visit: UCLA Medical Center Kinchi Kong	**8:30AM to 10:30AM** Lecture: Integration and Usage of DICOM-RT Objects Anh Le Hands-On Live Demo: DICOM-RT ePR System Anh Le
10:30AM to 12:30PM Clinical IT Ride-Along: UH/Norris Kevin Wang, PACS IT Support Team	**10:30AM to 12:30PM** Clinical IT Ride-Along: HCC2 Kevin Wang, PACS IT Support Team	**10:30AM to 12:30PM** Lecture: DICOM-SR Report and Applications Anh Le Hands-On Demo: PACS-CAD Toolkit Examples Anh Le, Kevin Ma	**10:30AM to 12:30PM** Site Visit: UCLA Medical Center Kinchi Kong	**10:30AM to 12:30PM** Lecture: Integration of Surgical Data in OR: Minimally Invasive Spinal Surgery HK Huang Hands-On Live Demo Jorge Documet
12:30PM to 2:00PM LUNCH	**12:30PM to 2:00PM** LUNCH	**12:30PM to 2:00PM** LUNCH	**12:30PM to 2:00PM** LUNCH in Westwood	**12:30PM to 2:00PM** LUNCH & Certificate Presentation HK Huang & Brent Liu

TABLE 28.2B. (*Continued*)

2:00PM to 4:00PM Lecture: Data Grid Applications—1) Tier 2 Storage 2) Imaging-Base Clinical Trials Jasper Lee	**2:00PM to 4:00PM** Lecture: Radiology Integrated Molecular Imaging Center—Grant Dagliyan et al	**2:00PM to 4:00PM** Visit California Spine Inst., Thousand Oaks, CA Dr. John Chiu: Minimally Invasive Spinal Surgery HK Huang, Brent Liu, Jorge Documet et al	**2:00PM to 4:00PM** Q&A Panel Topics: 1) Keys to a Successful PACS IT Administrator; 2) System Monitoring Tools for PACS IT Support; 3) Managing a Clinical IT Support Team Kevin Wang & Brent Liu	**2:00PM to 4:00PM** BME 527 Graduate Course Lecture Week 3: Medical Imaging Concepts Brent Liu
4:00PM to 6:00PM Hands-On Live Demo: The Data Grid Jasper Lee & Kevin Ma Six-Day Review: Q&A Session Brent Liu	**4:00PM to 6:00PM** Workshop: Case Studies on PACS Design, Acceptance Testing and Contingency Planning Brent Liu	**4:00PM to 6:00PM** Dinner at Bernie's house	**4:00PM to 6:00PM** Final Review: Q&A Session Brent Liu, HK Huang, All IPILab Members	**Farewell Dinner** HK Huang

TABLE 28.3A   BME 527 Fall: Integration of Medical Imaging Systems Technology

Course Outline (40 hours)

1. Special Opening Lecture—PCAS and Imaging Informatics
2. Introduction: (Medical Images, Clinical System Fundamentals, Introduction to Radiology Workflow) Medical Imaging Fundamentals (Image Quality, Spatial and Frequency Domains, Image Transformation)
3. Imaging Informatics of: Projection Radiography, CR, DR, Digital Mammography, Sectional Imaging: CT, MR, US, NM/PET/SPECT, Light Imaging
4. Medical Image Compression (Lossless, Lossy, Cosine Transform Wavelet Transform)
5. Health Care Information Industrial Standards & Workflow Protocols (DICOM, HL7, IHE)
6. Picture Archiving and Communication System (Concept, Components, Data Flow)
7. Image Acquisition Gateway, Healthcare Data Gateway, Display Workstation (Components, Types, Functions, GUI)
8. Midterm Exam Closed Book
9. PACS Server and Archive (Components, Software Design, Data Flow, Fault Tolerance)
10. Communication Networks (LAN and WAN, Wireless, Internet and Intranet, TCP/IP Protocols, Internet 2, PACS Networks, Teleradiology Networks) Integration of HIS, RIS, PACS, and ePR
11. Implementation of PACS in a Clinical Environment and PACS Acceptance Testing Design & Implementation
12. Telemedicine and Teleradiology (Components, Trade-off Parameters, Operation, Radiology & Clinical Impact)
13. Special Guest Lecture—Department of Radiology: A Clinical Perspective
14. Final Exam Open Book

Textbook: Huang, *PACS and Imaging Informatics*, Wiley & Sons, March 2004. DEN (Distance Education Network) enrollment available.
Homework: 30%, Midterm Exam: 30%, Final Exam: 40%

28.3.1.3   *PACS Simulator Used for Demonstration of Advanced PACS Concepts*

In addition to serving the training functions described, the PACS simulator has been used to test some advanced PACS concepts. An example is to add the fault-tolerance module to the PACS server (see Chapter 16). During the test the clinical environment under consideration was simulated by continuously feeding images from the modality simulator to the fault-tolerant PACS server 24 hours a day, 7 days a week for 3 months to test its continuous availability (CA). This test demonstrated that the PACS simulator can be a good stand-alone test bed for any new radiology imaging components, including software and hardware. Because the PACS simulator supports most DICOM-compliant devices or software, users can test whether the new components can be connected directly to an existing PACS system without the need to connect with a clinical PACS system during the laboratory stage of validation.

TABLE 28.3B   BME 528 Spring: Medical Imaging Informatics

Course Outline (40 hours)

1. Introduction to Medical Imaging Informatics Introduction of Special Class Project
2. Review Integration of HIS, RIS, PACS, and ePR
    i. Concept of PACS-Based Imaging Informatics
    ii. Computer-Aided Detection and Diagnosis
    iii. Special Class Project: Development of Teams and Tasks
3. Computer-Aided Diagnosis of Specific Neurological Pathologies
    i. Integration of CAD Results with PACS and Clinical Workflow
    ii. The CAD/PACS Integration Toolkit
4. Computer-Aided Diagnosis for Bone Age Assessment of Children and Clinical Applications
5. Computer-Aided Detection in CT Imaging and Clinical Applications
6. A DICOM RT Based ePR System with Knowledge Base for Decision Support in Radiation and Ion Therapy
7. Integrating Imaging Technologies for the Development of an ePR for Minimally Invasive and Image-Guided Spinal Surgery
8. Midterm Exam Closed Book
9. Imaging Informatics Research in a Clinical Environment: Tour of USC Radiology HCC2 Imaging Department (HIS/RIS/PACS/VR)
10. Fault-Tolerant Medical Imaging System Design & Applications
    i. Hands-on Experience of a FT System & PACS Simulator
    ii. Introduction to IPI Lab
    iii. Special Class Project: Second Update
11. Data Storage Grid for Clinical Image Data Applications
12. Image/Data Security and HIPAA Architecture for Securing Clinical Image Data
13. Imaging and Informatics System Integration
    i. Mobile Clinical Applications for Medical Imaging Systems
    ii. Physician's Dashboard for Radiology Workflow
14. Special Class Project Presentations
15. Final Exam Open Book

Textbook: Huang, *PACS and Imaging Informatics*, Wiley & Sons, March 2004, and current literature DEN (Distance Education Network) enrollment available
Special Project/Homework: 30%, Midterm: 30%, Take Home Final Exam: 40%

28.3.2   PACS Training Programs in the Hong Kong Polytechnic University

28.3.2.1   Background   The second example is the PACS and Imaging Informatics training program at Hong Kong Polytechnic University (PolyU). PolyU has a radiography division in the Department of Health Technology and Informatics. The Division offers a BSc (Hon) degree in radiography with a specialty in either medical imaging or radiation therapy for radiographers and radiation therapists, respectively.

It also offers MSc and PhD programs as continuing education courses. In addition to the academic programs, it operates a radiography clinic in joint venture with University Health Service, which provides general radiography, US, and mammography service for university staff and students. Clients from the public and private sectors may also have examinations performed under special arrangements.

28.3.2.2   PACS Simulator Infrastructure and the Health PACS   The installation of the PACS simulator at PolyU started in 2000. It was built on a generic PACS simulator with clinical imaging modalities such as CR, film scanner, mammography, and US scanners connected to it. The PACS simulator gradually grew to a functional small-scale clinical PACS. Figures 28.4*A* and *B* shows the system's workflow and major components of the health PACS in PolyU, respectively. Because the university does not have a CT or MR scanner, it relies on the modality simulator to generate those images for simulation. To streamline the workflow, there are three DICOM gateway machines for images from different modalities and for different applications. There are altogether 21 viewing workstations (10 in an Image Management Laboratory, 1 in the clinic and 1 in the PACS laboratory) with the Cedara I-Report software and other manufacturers' workstations installed for viewing images. The PACS server is connected to a Web server (Cedara, Toronto, Canada) for Web client's use. The PolyU PACS is also connected to a workstation with the I-View software in the University Health Service, using the university's network Ethernet at 100 Mbps, and to a teleradiology site for an external consultant radiologist using a broadband at 1.5 Mbps.

28.3.2.3   PACS Training at PolyU

Undergraduate Program   The PolyU PACS simulator and the health PACS are both training tools for the undergraduate and postgraduate programs, besides its application in clinical services. For the undergraduate program, the basic principles of the PACS are incorporated into a course called Medical Informatics. Students are briefed on the concept of PACS, and its components. In addition they practice image transmission, query, and retrieval using the workstations.

Postgraduate Program and Continuing Education Program   For the postgraduate and continuing education programs, the target audiences are the operators of PACS. Thus the direction of the training is geared toward the whole system with a clinical and practical emphasis. In the continuing education program, there are two training goals. The first is to provide the trainees with an understanding of the PACS and its workflow as a system. The second is to enable trainees to do some basic PACS troubleshooting. The training is planned at two levels, basic and advanced. The basic course is a refresher course to update radiography practitioners who have not been exposed to digital images or the PACS. The advanced level is for practitioners who will perform the daily operation of the PACS. Both courses have hands-on components. Tables 28.4 and 28.5 give an outline of the training content of both courses.

The trainees enjoy the various tasks they are able to perform during the hands-on sessions using the PACS simulator. They also make full use of those occasions to relate their learning to their work situation and discuss hypothetical problems

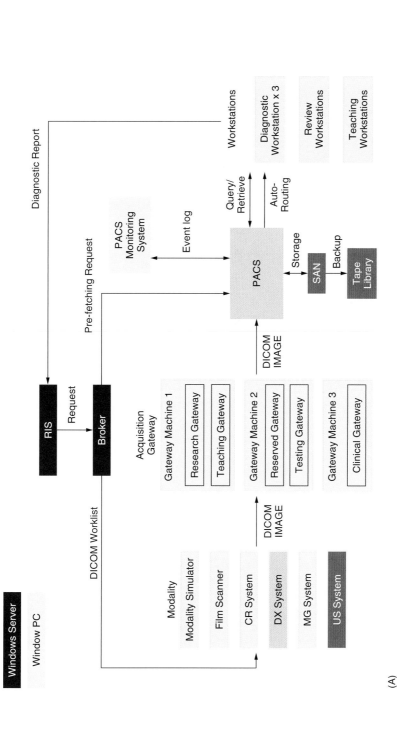

Figure 28.4 (A) Data flow of the PolyU PACS in the Department of Health Technology and Informatics, Hong Kong Polytechnic University. (B) Setting of the PACS Lab and Image Management Lab, and other imaging modalities at PolyU.

(A)

911

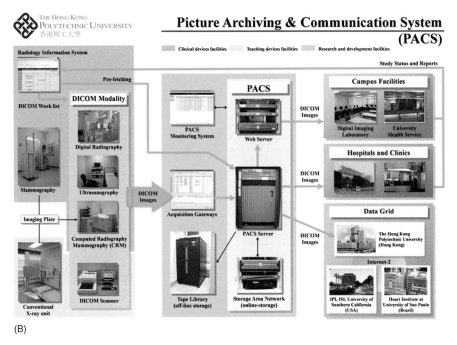

(B)

Figure 28.4 *(Continued)*

TABLE 28.4 Basic PACS training at PolyU: Course contents

Lectures	Hands-on Workshop
1. From film to filmless 2. Concept of digital images 3. PACS components and functions 4. IT concept in PACS: image size, network issues, and communication speed 5. Standards used: DICOM standards and TCP/IP, IHE concept 6. PACS workflow	1. (a) Acquiring and transmitting images from modalities: 　• CR 　• US 　• Scanner 　• Modality simulator 　(b) Monitoring completion of transmission at the PACS monitor 2. Nonstandard input of patient data (error simulation exercise) 3. Use of display software to query and retrieve images transmitted in 1 4. Comparing viewing monitors

with tutors. Trainees with different responsibilities and from different departments have different needs of their own. As expected, the courses so far have been found suitable for the PACS operator level. During class discussion trainees from the managerial level expressed more concern about the design and workflow planning,

TABLE 28.5   Advanced PACS training at PolyU: Course contents

Lectures	Hands-on Workshop
1. PACS data flow design and monitoring 2. DICOM SOP class and scheduled workflow in IHE 3. Basics in connecting imaging and computer components to the PACS using DICOM networking concepts and DICOM communications 4. Adding new modalities to PACS 5. PACS archive server 6. Teleradiology 7. PACS value-added application	Adding components to PACS Setup and configure PACS components • Adding different viewing stations • Adding digital scanner • Adding US scanner Hardware debugging • Simulation of hardware failure: network failure • Software debugging: wrong DICOM configuration, software Components Workflow design exercise or estimation of archive needed

potential problems in PACS implementation, and budgeting. They liked to exchange their experiences with different vendors. In view of this, cost analysis and implementation of PACS for managers could be another course offered in the education programs.

Through the years, PACS and imaging informatics training at PolyU have grown from continuing education to the healthcare professional to two different MSc degree programs: MSc in Health Technology (MIRS [Radiation Science]), and MSc in Health Informatics. The basic and advanced PACS training course contents as shown in Tables 28.4 and 28.5 had been consolidated to become a graduate course called Digital Imaging and PACS shown in Table 28.6.

28.3.3 Future Perspective in PACS Training

So far the discussion about PACS training has focused on its operation in radiology. However, PACS training can go beyond the WS operation level because PACS is an evolving tool with immense prospects for other applications. The current PACS with its standard DICOM format is still the early model of how medical images in radiology can be transmitted, displayed, and archived. The concept can be extended to other medical specialties where images are used for other purposes. Such extension can be found in the development of a radiation therapy (RT) ePR system (Chapter 23) and minimally invasive spinal surgery (MISS) ePR system (Chapter 24).

To cater for such future PACS applications, a comprehensive PACS education program for the professional should include imaging informatics that cover workflow design, outcome analysis, research methods, and applications using PACS. Figure 28.5 shows the hierarchy of a comprehensive PACS education. The PACS fundamentals and the advanced PACS are prerequisites to the three courses at the bottom of the hierarchy. The last three courses, PACS for Administrators, PACS for Managers, and Image Informatics and PACS Applications can be electives depending on the participant's career direction. The next section describes an even more ambitious program for career development in PACS and imaging informatics.

TABLE 28.6   PolyU Digital Imaging and PACS: Course Contents

Syllabus

Part I: Image Formation, Processing and Visualization

1. Concepts of digital image formation in various imaging modalities
    1.1 Formation of digital images
    1.2 Signal and image processing
2. Digital image analysis and visualization
    2.1 Statistical image analysis methods
    2.2 Advanced image segmentation methods
    2.3 Models for image visualization
    2.4 Limitations of image visualization

Part II: Picture Archiving and Communication System

3. PACS for imaging manager and administrators
    3.1 Streamlined workflow integration
    3.2 Requirements of system architecture
    3.3 Connectivity issues
    3.4 Image compression: wavelet conversion, JPEG, JPEG2000 considerations for local and teleradiology communications
    3.5 Security and ethical issues (e.g., encryption & decryption), HIPPA
    3.6 Considerations for PACS purchase
        - Trend of electronic storage: SAN, SATA disk, LTO tape
        - Choice of display workstations
    3.7 Image security: encryption & decryption, HIPPA
    3.8 Legal issues: law of personal information protection considerations for operating PACS, networking, workstations
    3.9 Management of medical image information system & network
4. PACS-based imaging applications and research

28.4 TRAINING MEDICAL IMAGING INFORMATICS FOR INTERDISCIPLINARY CANDIDATES

The IPILab, USC received a renewable five-year T32 training grant from the U.S. National Institute of Biomedical Imaging and Bioengineering (NIBIB), U.S. National Institutes of Health (NIH), DHHS, totaling about U.S.$1.6 million. The principal investigator (PI) and co-PI are Dr. H. K. Huang of Radiology and Dr. Michael Khoo of Biomedical Engineering (BME), respectively. The program emphasizes multidisciplinary training by bridging the gap between physicians and engineers, and considers candidates from the following four categories of applicants: USC radiology residents and fellows, USC biomedical engineering PhD students, USC MD/PhD program

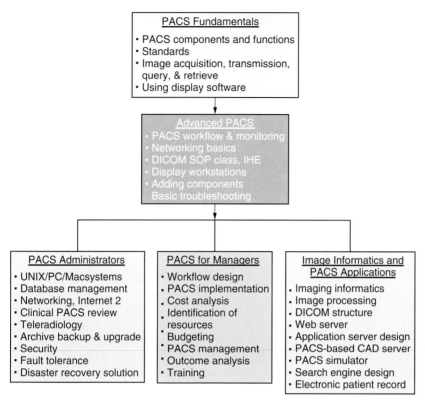

Figure 28.5 Hierarchy of a comprehensive PACS education program with five modules: fundamentals, advanced, administrators, managers, and applications. The fundamental and the advanced modules are mandatory with the administrators, managers, and applications as electives depending on the trainee's career goal.

students, and postdoctoral fellows and qualified candidates of the aforementioned fields from other institutions. Each year the available positions are (postdoctoral, Predoctoral) (2, 2), (3, 3), (3, 3), (3, 3), (3, 3), and selected candidates can be reappointed annually. Annual stipend and partial tuition/fees are provided for the successful candidates.

NIH has supported many training and research programs throughout the years as a way to guide potential candidates to leadership in selected fields. Examples are the two programs funded by the National Cancer Institute (NCI), NIH in the mid-1980s and the early 1990s when the concept of PACS had just started (entitled "Biomedical Physics Training Program" and "PACS in Radiology") to the author of this book. At that time he was with UCLA (University of California, Los Angeles) and later relocated to UCSF (University of California, San Francisco); and Professor Michael McNitt-Gray and Professor Hooshang Kangarloo of UCLA took over the principal investigatorship of the two programs, respectively. These two grants are still active, and have provided opportunities for a good number of individuals who are now the leaders in medical imaging and PACS. The "Biomedical Physics Training Program" has helped developing the Medical Imaging Division at UCLA; many trainees got their PhD and/or PD training credentials there and have since moved on to work on imaging informatics research. "PACS in Radiology" has helped developing the infrastructure of PACS, whose many components were then adopted by manufacturers in their commercial PACS products. The biomedical imaging informatics training program may become another means of contributing to the continuing growth of medical imaging and PACS over the next few years.

This section describes in full the training program, starting from the its goals, contents, recruitments, and proceeding to the guidance it can offer to those who may want to consider developing such a large-scale training program at their institutions through the U.S. National Institute of Health, or other institutes with similar capacity and interest around the world.

28.4.1 Objectives and Training Emphases

Medical Imaging Informatics is the branch of imaging science that studies image/data information gathering, processing, manipulation, storage, transmission, management, distribution, and visualization as well as knowledge discovery from large-scale biomedical image/data sets. Recent advances in medical imaging science and technology have made knowledge of imaging informatics an essential tool in the synthesis and management of medical images for patient care. Although there exist training programs in medical imaging and medical informatics, focused training dedicated to imaging informatics is limited because of its novelty.

This training program, leveraging the strengths of three existing academic structures, and one unique laboratory at the University of Southern California (USC), tailors to suit the needs and requirements of each trainee. The three programs are Biomedical Engineering Department (BME), School of Engineering (see Section 28.4.2.1); Radiology Department (see Section 28.4.2.2), and the Joint USC and California Institute of Technolog (CAL Tech) MD/PhD program (see Section 28.4.2.3); the latter two programs are located at the School of Medicine. In addition the unique facility in the Image Processing and Informatics Laboratory (IPI) within the Radiology Department serves as the cornerstone for this training program

The trainees benefit from the unique blending of two differing traditional educational cultures and methods at the engineering and medical schools, and as a group from interdisciplinary training derives optimal career development path, adjusted for each individual, through the mixed and rich training environments.

28.4.1.1 Objectives   The objective of this training program is to provide postgraduate students, radiology residents and fellows, and MD/PhD students the skills necessary to become leaders in medical imaging informatics. Four primary career perspectives are used to guide a trainee's development:

1. Academe
2. Healthcare delivery providers
3. Medical imaging industry
4. U.S. federal/military healthcare system

28.4.1.2 Training Emphases

1. Image processing and manipulation
2. Novel biomedical imaging devices
3. Medical imaging system integration
4. Imaging informatics technology
5. Informatics applications
6. Clinical integration/physician acceptance and regulatory issues

28.4.2 Description of Three Existing Academic Programs and the IPILab at USC

This training program is under the auspices of three academic programs at USC: Department of Biomedical Engineering, Viterbi School of Engineering; Department of Radiology, Keck School of Medicine; and USC MD/PhD Program. A predoctoral trainee, upon satisfying the specific training requirements, will be awarded a PhD degree in Medical Imaging and Informatics by the BME. Postdoctoral fellows trainee will be awarded a Fellowship Certificate by the Radiology Department. A radiologist resident who participates in the training program as a postdoctoral fellow can also obtained a MS degree from BME after satisfying all necessary BME requirements. This section describes the three established academic programs at USC.

28.4.2.1 The Department of Biomedical Engineering (BME)   The Department of Biomedical Engineering (BME), located on the USC main campus, has longstanding tradition of advancing biomedicine through the development and application of novel engineering ideas. Its 60 primary and affiliated faculty members conduct cutting-edge research in a wide variety of areas, including neuroengineering, biosystems and biosignal analysis, medical devices (e.g., bioMEMS and bionanotechnology), biomechanics, and bioimaging and imaging informatics. It has 180 graduate students with about 90 pursuing the MS degree and the other 90 for the PhD. It awards in average 10 PhDs a year. The T32 training grant recruits predoctoral candidates from students in the BME graduate program.

28.4.2.2 The Department of Radiology   The Department of Radiology (DOR) in the Keck School of Medicine, located at the USC Health Sciences campus, serves three hospitals—LAC (LA County) + USC Medical Center, USC Kenneth Norris Cancer Hospital and Research Institute, and USC University Hospital—and three imaging centers—LAC + USC Imaging Science Center, USC PET Imaging Science Center, and one outpatient imaging center. DOR performs over 500,000 radiological procedures a year.

There are 46 full-time faculty members as well as many affiliated clinical faculty. The program oversees the training of 16 radiology fellows and over 42 residents. The T32 training grant recruits postdoctoral fellows from these groups of residents and fellows.

28.4.2.3 The USC and Cal Tech MD/PhD Program   The USC/Cal Tech MD/PhD Program established in 1988 is an eight-year program in which each student

spends four years in pursuit of an MD degree, and four years for the PhD degree in an academic PhD granting department at USC or Cal Tech selected by the candidate. The student first takes two-year basic medical sciences, passing the basic sciences Board Exam. He/she then enrolls in a department for the PhD study. After the PhD degree (four years), the student returns to complete the clinical rotations necessary for the MD degree. The T32 training grant recruits predoctoral candidates from students in the MD/PhD Program.

28.4.2.4 The Imaging Processing and Informatics Laboratory (IPILab)

Image Processing and Informatics (IPI) Lab, Imaging Informatics Division, Department of Radiology is located at the Health Sciences campus, USC. Its mission is to perform R&D in medical imaging informatics for education, research, and clinical utilization, and to bridging the gap between the Schools of Engineering and Medicine with collaborative research. IPI was established in 2000 at USC, before USC it was at UCLA, UCSF and Berkeley since 1982. The Lab has three full-time faculty members with joint appointments in the Department of Radiology and Biomedical Engineering, five visiting faculty, four postdoctoral fellows and many graduate students, and consultants worldwide. Figure 28.6 shows the T32 training environment.

28.4.3 NIH T32 Training Program Description

28.4.3.1 Program Faculty
The following table shows the number of faculty participates in this training program:

T32 Training program faculty (total number of faculty)

Total	BME (13+44)	Radiology (46)	BME and Radiology Joint Appointment	Biostatistics/ Informatics
22	5	8	7	2

28.4.3.2 The Training Program
The PhD candidates are drawn from BME, USC MD/PhD, and USC radiology residency programs. Postdoctoral candidates are recruited from USC and other institutions' radiology residency program, as well as candidates with a PhD, MD, or other equivalent doctoral degrees in science, engineering, medicine, or other qualified disciplines from outside institutions. For a radiology resident, arrangement can been made at BME for the candidate to take image processing and imaging informatics courses and to obtain an MS degree by fulfilling the BME requirements.

One uniqueness of the T32 is that the training program has obtained the approval from the American Board of Radiology, the ACGME (Accreditation Council for Graduate Medical Education), and the Graduate Medical Education Department at USC, which allows a USC radiology resident to spend one year in imaging informatics training as an option to fulfill the four-year Diagnostic Radiology Residency Program.

28.4.3.3 PhD Degree
In the PhD degree track, the training program supports a candidate for the first two years after entering the PhD program. The candidate will seek a mentor from the faculty roster in the training program, continuing the PhD

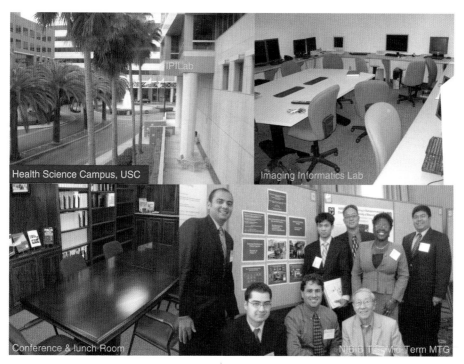

Figure 28.6 NIH T32 training environment at IPILab, USC. Top Left: Health Science campus, USC where IPILab is located. Top Right: Imaging Informatics Lab at the IPILab. Bottom Left: Conference and lunch room. Bottom Right: T32 trainees past and present attending the NIBIB Training Grantees Meeting, June 19–20, 2008 Silver Springs, Maryland. Starting from left, bottom row: James Fernandez, MD, Intern/1st year radiology resident; Paymann Moin, MD, 3rd year radiology resident; Mark Haney, MD, 1st year surgery resident; H. K. Huang, DSc, PI. Starting from right, top row: Kevin Ma, BME PhD candidate; Anika Joseph, BME PhD candidate; Brent Liu, PhD, T32 coordinator and investigator; Jasper Lee, BME PhD candidate.

research. The mentor will have the responsibility to support the trainee to complete the PhD requirements.

For a candidate who has been accepted by the USC MD/PhD program, if the candidate selects BME to pursue a PhD, he/she would have to first get accepted by the BME during the first two basic clinical science years. During the third year of the MD/PhD program, the candidate then becomes the first-year graduate student of BME, and completes the PhD in four to five years (past experience in the MD/PhD program has demonstrated that it may take more than four years for the PhD degree). The supporting conditions would be identical to that described in the aforementioned paragraphs. After the PhD degree, the candidate returns to the Medical School to complete the two-year clinical training and be awarded the MD degree by the Keck School of Medicine.

28.4.3.4 Postdoctoral Fellow The one- to two-year postdoctoral (PD) fellow training can correspond to one of the following plans depending on the background and interest of the trainee:

1. For standard postdoctoral training in biomedical imaging informatics, the trainee follows the guidance of a mentor to participate in the mentor's research field.

2. For a radiology resident, the trainee takes basic imaging informatics courses described in Section 28.4.4 and selects a mentor to learn about performing research. The goal is to have the trainee complete the draft of an individual training grant application targeted for submission to a particular Institute in NIH that accepts individual training grant application. If the resident completes all requirements of the master degree of BME, an MS can be granted by the BME Department to the trainee.

28.4.4 Courses Offered by the Medical Imaging and Imaging Informatics (MIII), BME, and Electives

The following courses are offered by the BME Department for the PhD and MS degrees:

BME-425: Basics of Biomedical Imaging (3 units)

BME-501: Systems Physiology (4 units)

BME-513: Signal and Systems Analysis (3 units)

BME-525: Advanced Biomedical Imaging (4 units)

BME-527: Medical Imaging System Integration (3 units)

BME-528: Medical Imaging Informatics (3 units)

BME-535: Ultrasound Imaging (3 units):

BME 533 Seminar in Bioengineering

BME 590 Direct Research in Imaging Informatics

BME 599 Special Topics in Imaging Informatics

BME 605 Experimental Projects in Biomedical Engineering including

BME 686 Introduction to Biomedical Research

BME 790 Research in Biomedical Engineering

BME 794a,b,c,d Doctoral Dissertation

28.4.5 Requirements for Advanced Degrees

28.4.5.1 PhD Degree Requirements in Biomedical Engineering   The doctor of philosophy (PhD) in biomedical engineering is designed to be completed in four to five years of full-time study beyond the bachelor of science degree (including summers). The first year is devoted primarily to formal coursework. Sixty units of credit beyond the BS, with a minimum grade point average of 3.0, are required for the PhD degree. PhD candidates must pass a screening exam at the end of their first year, a qualifying exam when they begin their dissertation research, and an oral defense of their dissertation at the end of the program.

28.4.5.2 MD/PhD Program   Candidates in the MD/PhD program follow the BME PhD requirements described in Section 28.4.5.1.

28.4.5.3 *Radiology Resident and Fellow Training Programs* To fit the candidate who is a radiology resident or fellow into the T32 training program, it will need the candidate to arrange time off from the residency program and/or the clinical service schedule during the informatics training. The arrangement is tailored to the trainee's interest and his/her clinical requirements and time slots.

A radiology resident or fellow can obtain an MS degree in imaging Informatics in BME by taking 30 units, including BME 425, 525, 527, 528, 590, 599, and other elective courses.

Figure 28.6 bottom right shows the past and current T32 fellows at IPILab who attended and gave their training experience presentations during the mid-term "All NIBIB T32 Training Programs Meeting" at Silver Spring, MD, June 19–20, 2008.

28.5 CHANGING PACS LEARNING WITH NEW INTERACTIVE AND MEDIA-RICH LEARNING ENVIRONMENTS

In this section we introduce an innovative technology of learning, called simPHYSIO (simulation physiology) using an interactive and media-rich learning environment. SimPHYSIO, originally designed for learning more difficult concepts in physiology, together with the concept of distance learning (see Table 28.3*A* and *B*, footnote) and the PACS simulator discussed in Section 28.2.3, may provide a means to facilitate PACS and media-rich imaging informatics learning in a fast-paced and always busy clinical environment.

28.5.1 SimPHYSIO and Distance Learning

28.5.1.1 *SimPHYSIO* PACS requires diversity in personnel to interface with the intricate and complex system. To successfully implement PACS, a comprehensive education program would enable personnel to interleave all its components seamlessly. SimPHYSIO's pedagogical design and methodologies can be applied to build an educational environment for all levels of personnel involved in the integrated PAC system. It is a suite of interactive on-line teaching media designed to integrate and dynamically teach complex systems with media-rich animations, real-time simulations, and virtual environments in physiology that has been proved to be successful in interactive learning of the subject at Stanford University and several universities in Sweden. The strength of simPHYSIO also includes Internet distribution, scalability, and content customization. It provides the convenience of anytime Web access and a modular structure that allows for personalization and customization of the learning material. Figure 28.7 shows the infrastructure of the simPHYSIO and how to connect the PACS learning modules to it. Figure 28.8 provides an example of a window in the Cranial Nerve Exam Simulator Neuro Module of the simPHYSIO. For details of the methods, readers are referred to C. Huang (2003).

28.5.1.2 *Distance Learning* Distance learning can be loosely defined as a student gaining knowledge on a workstation through a Web-based connection that is either physically or temporally distant from a live instructor. The ubiquity of computers and network technology targeting a wide audience can provide up-to-date information and, most important, promote student learning outside the classroom.

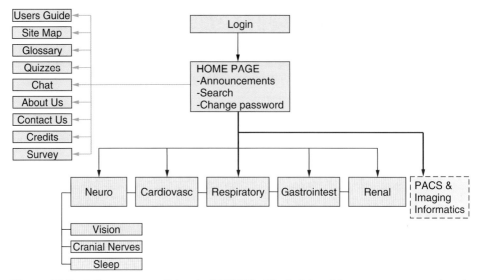

Figure 28.7 Infrastructure of the simPHYSIO. The left-hand boxes are supported tools and resources, and the bottom row contains existing modules. For example, the neuro module has three submodules: vision, cranial nerves, and sleep. PACS and imaging informatics learning can be a new module (rightmost: blue) with five submodules: fundamentals, advanced, managers, administrators, and applications (shown in Figure 28.5), all these modules can be supported by the tools and resources shown at the left. (Courtesy of Dr. C. Huang)

A prevailing method of distance learning is the use of on-line tutorials, with pedagogic complexity ranging from a digital textbook to high-end interactive simulations, as discussed in this chapter. Although the Web is sufficient for timely Intranet transmission of digital, textbook-style material within an institution, complex didactic media (i.e., time-based animations, interactive virtual laboratories, or mathematical-based simulations) will require higher bandwidth communications technology.

Once the PACS learning modules based on the contents described in this chapter, along with the multimedia techniques described in simPHYSIO, have been developed, it can be incorporated with simPHYSIO by using its infrastructure tools and resources. It can go live and be connected through broadband networks (e.g., Internet 2) to learners at remote distances, at home or other institutions. The two BME courses BME 527 and BME 528 are an experiment in distance learning through the DEN (Distance Education Network) facility at USC that has been ongoing for the past four years.

28.5.2 Perspective of Using simPHYSIO Technology for PACS Learning

Current training of the whole PACS involves taking courses like those discussed in this chapter or having an on-site trainer—both types of training require a devotion of time by the trainer in coordination with many related departments. The methodologies behind simPHYSIO can be applied to the development of an on-line training course for the integrated PACS based on the contents described in this chapter.

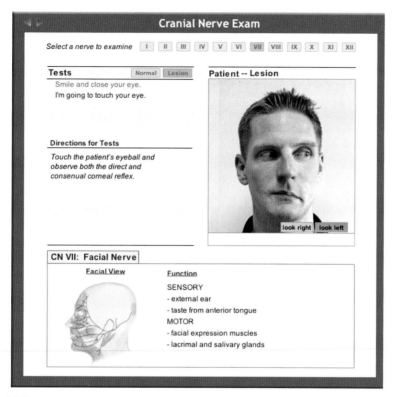

Figure 28.8   Example of a window in the Cranial Nerve Exam Simulator Neuro Module of the simPHYSIO (see Fig. 28.7, bottom). After the tutorial on learning the cranial nerves in the brain, the user can go to the patient simulator to apply the knowledge to a clinical setting. In this example, the student learns how to perform the diagnostic tests to a normal patient or a lesioned patient. (Courtesy of Drs. C. Huang and J. DeVoss)

We mentioned previously that the successful implementation of PACS requires a multidisciplinary team:

1. PACS manager: Needs to understand the whole PACS system including hardware, software, and data flow.
2. IT personnel: Need to know the components of the system, and system integration in order to address the problem of system failure and provide immediately solutions.
3. Hospital administrators: Need to understand the overall concept of PACS data flow through the hospital to maintain efficiency of the workflow.
4. Technologists: Need to know the workflow inside the PACS and how patient data moves from one point to another.
5. Radiologists: Need to learn how to use the workstation to acquire and read images.
6. Nurses and physicians: Need to know how to access the images at remote sites and find solutions to problems from IT or the administrators.

A centralized, interactive on-line training system for the integrated PACS based on the simPHYSIO technology would offer convenience, ease of distribution and access, customization/modularity, and efficient pedagogical training that would benefit its implementation and operation. A training system like simPHYSIO offers the convenience of learning the necessary training material whenever a time slot is available to a the PACS team member. Housing a tutorial on-line would provide anytime, anywhere access to the training material through a computer with an Internet Web browser. Because these tutorials are modular, they can be scaled and customized for each level of the team in terms of appropriateness and level of depth. An interactive training tutorial is also beneficial in terms of delivering high-quality content in a dynamic way using simulations. This strategy can engage the user in problem solving and understanding the whole PACS. The resulting benefit is the coordination of the knowledge base for the different hierarchies of background and thus improved workflow.

28.5.3 Beyond simPHYSIO and Distance Learning — The Virtual Labs Concept of Interactive Media

The use of interactive media in learning has been shown to engage students, increase performance, and help educators convey difficult concepts. In science curricula, PACS, and imaging informatics, interactive media can transform classroom instruction, making dynamic processes come alive and be interactive, while illustrating the connections among different disciplines. The creation of interactive media for science education has been prolific, but, the adoption of this media has been limited and disorganized. The concept of interactive media learning based on the simPHYSIO Virtual Labs is to consolidate all possible interactive media from PACS onto a single teaching resource website for distance distribution. Figure 28.9A shows the evolution from single display for teaching (top) to the beginning of the multiple displays (bottom). Figure 28.9B depicts the concept of consolidation of all teaching materials on a single subject, like PACS, into one Virtual Lab Web site.

28.6 SUMMARY OF PACS AND MEDICAL IMAGING INFORMATICS TRAINING

In PACS and imaging informatics there is a need of training for the users beyond how to use workstations to review images. As more and more PAC systems are being installed, many users are exploring to use PACS data for other image-intensive medical applications. Extending PACS education to other clinical specialties would promote better utilization of the PACS data and maximize the benefits of the PACS to all clinical departments. A more comprehensive education program treating PACS as a complete medical information system is required.

This chapter presents several topics, including new directions in PACS and imaging informatics education and training, using the PACS simulator as a training tool, combining interdisciplinary specialties training, and PACS training with interactive media methodology.

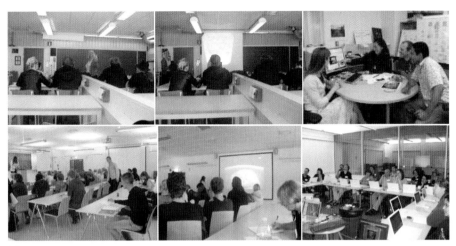

(A)

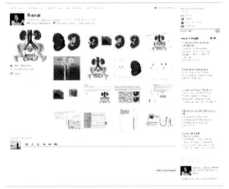 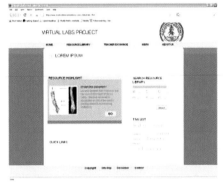

(B)

Figure 28.9   (*A*) Top: Traditional classroom teaching with chalkboard (left), overhead projector (middle), and trainer's laptop (right: Dr. C. Huang in dark dress, who developed the Virtual Lab simPHYSIO concept). Bottom: The twenty-first century classroom with both chalkboard and overhead projector (left); special designed classroom with rotating chairs for multiple displays (middle); and each learner uses a laptop computer (right). (*B*) Interactive media. Consolidation of different PACS modules in the future Virtual Lab Web site with search, tags, thematic arrangement of contents, downloadable or embeddable content. Left: Menu for searching; right: a single subject displayed. (Courtesy of Dr. C. Huang)

References

Beird LC. How to satisfy both clinical and information technology goals in designing a successful picture archiving and communication system. *J Digit Imag* 13(2 suppl 1): 10–2; 2000.

Beird LC. The importance of a picture archiving and communications system (PACS) manager for large-scale PACS installations. *J Digit Imag* 12(2 suppl 1): 37; 1999.

Carrino JA, Unkel PJ, Miller ID, Bowser CL, Freckleton MW, Johnson TG. Large-scale PACS implementation. *J Digit Imag* 11(3 suppl 1): 3–7; 1998.

Crivianu-Gaita D, Babyn P, Gilday D, O'Brien B, Charkot E. User acceptability—a critical success factor for picture archiving and communication system implementation. J *Digital Imag* 13(2 suppl 1): 13–6; 2000.

Edward B. How many people does it take to operate a picture archiving and communication system? *J Digit Imag* 14(2 suppl 1): 40–3; 2001.

Hirchom D, Eber C, Samuels P, Gujrathi S, Baker SR. Filmless in New Jersey, the New Jersey Medical School PACS project. *J Digit Imag* 15(suppl 1): 7–12; 2002.

http://virtuallabs.stanford.edu.

http://virtuallabs.stanford.edu/k12/got/.

Huang C. Changing learning with new interactive and media-rich instruction environments: virtual labs case study report. *Comput Med Imag Graph* V27(2–3): 157–64; 2003.

Huang C, Huang HK. Interactive Instruction of cellular physiology for remote learning. *Cell and Molecular Biology* 49(8): 1377–1384; 2003.

IHE demonstration participants 2001–2002. http://www.rsna.org/IHE/participation/index.shtml.

Integrating the Healthcare Enterprise. http://www.rsna.org/IHE/index.shtml.

Law MYY, Hunag HK. Concept of a PACS and imaging informatics-based server for radiation therapy. *Comp Med Imag Graph* 27: 1–9; 2003.

Law MYY, Tang FH, Cao F. A PACS and image informatics training. 87th Scientific Assembly and Annual Meeting, *Radiol Soc N Am*, 25–30 Nov, p. 120; 2001.

Mendelson DS, Bak PRG, Menschik E, Siegel E. Informatics in radiology. *RadioGraphics* 28: 1817–33; 2008.

Pilling J. Problems facing the radiologist tendering for a hospital wide PACS system. *Eur J Radiol* 32(2): 101–5; 1999.

Protopapas Z, Siegel EL, Reiner BI, Pomerantz SM, Pickar ER, Wilson M, Hooper FJ. Picture archiving and communication system training for physicians: lessons learned at the Baltimore VA Medical Center. *J Digit Imag.* 9(3): 131–6; 1996.

Tang FH, LAW MYY, Zhang J, Liu HL, Matsuda K, Cao F. Implementation of a PACS for radiography training and clinical service in a university setting through a multinational effort. In: Siegel EL, Huang HK, eds. *Medical Imaging 2001: PACS and Integrated Medical Information Systems: Design and Evaluation, Proc SPIE* 4323: 67–72; 2001.

Watkins J. A hospital-wide picture archiving and communication system (PACS): the views of users and providers of the radiology service at Hammersmith Hospital. *Eur J Radiol* 32(2): 106–12; 1999.

Backup archive The PACS archive server saves a patient's images for seven years. Since the archive has only one copy, a backup archive with one extra copy, preferably off site, is necessary to ensure data integrity. Should a natural disaster occur, the server can retrieve images immediately from the backup archive to maintain the clinical operation.

CAD–PACS integration The ultimate goal of developing a CAD (computer-aided diagnosis) system is to integrate CAD results into PACS to facilitate radiologists and healthcare providers for daily clinical practice. However, the value and effectiveness of CAD are still hindered by the inconvenience of the stand-alone CAD WS or server. Wider use of DICOM and IHE technologies as an integral part of PACS daily clinical operation could help overcome these obstacles. The CAD–PACS tools allow for such integration.

Communication networks PACS is a form of system integration; all components in PACS are connected using communication networks. The communication protocol the networks use is TCP/IP (transport control protocol/Internet protocol). If the networks are within the hospital (Intranet), they are called a local area network (LAN). If the networks are outside of the hospital (Internet), they are called a wide area network (WAN).

Data Grid Grid computing is the integrated use of geographically distributed computers, networks, and storage systems to create a virtual computing system for solving large-scale, data-intensive problems in science, engineering, and commerce. Data Grid is a subset of grid computing and ensures data integrity in grid computing. Three major applications of Data Grid in medical imaging informatics are large-scale enterprise PACS operation, integration of multiple PAC systems, and PACS disaster recovery.

DICOM Digital Imaging and Communication in Medicine (DICOM) is the de facto standard used in PACS for image and data communication. It has two components, communication protocol and image data format. The former is based on the TCP/IP protocol. All major imaging and related data manufacturer equipment are DICOM compliant. Every hospital should request this standard in its image-related equipment purchases.

DICOM RT ePR The DICOM standard has been extended for radiology to radiation therapy (RT) by ratifying seven DICOM RT objects, which helps set standard for data integration and interoperability between RT equipment from different vendors. DICOM RT ePR is a patient-centric integrated image-based RT planning and treatment system based on medical imaging informatics infrastructure for cancer treatment.

Enterprise PACS PACS was first developed for radiology subspecialities, then extended to the complete radiology department, and finally to the entire hospital. The current trend of hospitals merging and federating has resulted in many healthcare enterprises. Enterprise PACS is a very large-scale PACS in supporting of these federated or enterprise hospitals. The key functions in enterprise PACS are a fault-tolerant, backup archive and streamlining of data flow.

ePR The hospital information system (HIS) is organized by the functions of departments, wards, and specialties. HIS was designed for facilitating the hospital's business operations. This design is not patient oriented. Because, for a patient undergoing examinations and procedures, healthcare providers usually cannot trace the patient's medical history from a single information system, the electronic patient record (ePR) or electronic medical record (eMR) system is an effort to re-design or extract information from HIS with the focus on the patient. Most ePRs currently contain only textual information; the trend is to include images in the ePR.

ePR with image distribution The full potential of ePR in streamlining patient data distribution cannot be realized without images. ePR with image distribution is a natural extension of text-based ePR system in which radiological and other medical related images of the patient are also acquired, archived, and distributed through the Web-based ePR system.

Four-dimensional image With the time coordinate added to 3-D space, 4-D medical images can be generated from time sequences of 3-D images. The time duration can be very short, less than seconds, in order to capture the physiological changes like the blood flow or organ movements like the heart beat. On the other hand, the time duration can be very long, in weeks, like in molecular images and ultrasound fetus images.

Fault-tolerant PACS PACS has several single points of failure (SPOFs). When any SPOF fails, it can cripple the PACS operation or even render whole system failure. The fault-tolerant (FT) PACS is designed to minimize the SPOF and recover function gracefully to avoid a total system failure. The most critical features in FT PACS are the backup image data and the FT PACS server.

HIPAA HIPAA (Health Insurance Portability and Accountability Act) mandates the guidelines that healthcare providers follow to receive insurance payment. It became effective in April 2003. Its implications for PACS, among other things, are data privacy, security, and integrity. For these reasons the PACS design has to be fault tolerant or be continuously available in order to be HIPAA compliant.

HIS The hospital information system (HIS) is a healthcare information system designed to streamline hospital business operations. His is comprised of many health-related databases that have grown gradually through years. For large hospitals, HIS uses mainframe computers and depends on many staff members to operate.

HIS, RIS, PACS integration In order for PACS to operate effectively and efficiently, HIS, RIS, and PACS have to be integrated. They are usually integrated with a DICOM broker in which pertinent patient data and radiology reports are translated from one system to the other. HIS, RIS, PACS integration is necessary for the success of PACS operation, and for the design of ePR with image distribution.

HL7 Health Level 7 is a data format standard used for healthcare textual information. Data encoded in HL7 must be transparent to other healthcare system following the standard. The data transmission between two healthcare systems following HL7 normally uses TCP/IP as the communication protocol.

IHE IHE (Integrating Healthcare Enterprise) consists of hospital workflow profiles, including radiology and other medical specialties workflows. The number of profiles have been increasing annually. In radiology alone, IHE has 19 profiles. The goal of IHE is for manufacturers to use the DICOM standard and follow the workflow profiles so that their equipments can be easier to integrate with others in clinical environment.

Image acquisition gateway There are many imaging modalities in radiology operation. In general, they are not connected to the PACS server and archive server directly but to an image acquisition gateway(s) as a staging buffer. The gateway checks the DICOM compliance of the image and makes necessary correction if needed before it forwards the image to the PACS server. Several imaging modalities can share a gateway.

Image-guided (-assisted) surgical ePR Multimedia electronic patient record (ePR) system for image-assisted surgery consists of a mix of text, surgical forms, images, waveforms, and graphics. Multimedia includes not only data integration but also the data acquisition and integration performed in real time during surgery. This type of multimedia ePR is classified as the "dynamic multimedia." The real-time component has to be handled and managed differently from the static multimedia.

Image archive After an image is acquired from the modality, it goes to the image acquisition gateway, and then the PACS server and archive. In the archive, the database acknowledges the receipt of the image, updates the patient directory, and stores the image in the storage systems like SAN (storage area network) and RAID (redundant array of inexpensive disks) for the short term and tape or hard disk for the long term. Images in the short-term archive follow the first-in–first-out algorithm after a set time.

Image compression A 300 to 500 bed hospital can generate 5 to 10 terabytes of image data a year. For this reason image compression is necessary to save storage space and speed up the image transmission time. Compression can be lossless or lossy. Currently lossless is mostly used with a compression ratio of 2:1, which reduces 50% of the image size. In ePR with image distribution, the compression ratio in the ePR system may be 10:1 or even higher.

Image quality Image quality is an inherent property of the imaging modality device when it generates the image. Image quality is measured by three parameters: spatial resolution, density resolution, and the signal-to-noise ratio. When an image flows through various components of the PACS, the image quality is preserved except in lossy compression.

Image size The medical image size and the amount of data generated in an examination vary. The size of a medical image can be from 0.5 Mbytes (CT) to 40 Mbytes (digital mammogram). A typical chest examination with two images generates 20 Mbytes, a thin section CT examination can generate a thousand images of

500 Mbytes. In PACS implementation, care has to be taken to investigate the image load for the archive and communication requirements.

Image/data security Image/data security considers three parameters: *authenticity*—Who sends the image; *privacy*—who can access the image; and *integrity*—has the image be altered since it was generated? HIPAA compliance requires the healthcare providers to guarantee the image/data security.

Image-guided/assisted surgery and therapy In surgery and in radiation therapy, images are used to assist the operation procedure. In surgery, pre-surgical images can be used to simulate the surgical outcome, and 3-D rendering of CT/MR images to guide for surgery. In radiation therapy, CT simulation images are used to plan the therapeutic beams and predict radiation dose distribution. These images are normally obtained from the PACS archive server.

Image fusion Image fusion is to combine multimodality images into one single display. In order to optimize the display result, proper manipulation and matching the contrast of the lookup table of each modality image are critical. In addition, using pseudocolor on one modality image and gray scale on the second is important. For example, after two 3-D image sets, one anatomical and the second physiological, have been properly registered, they are laid one over the other and the results are displayed on a LCD monitor. The displayed results then show physiological data on top of anatomical data.

Imaging informatics Imaging informatics is a branch of science that studies how best to manage, extract, and process pertinent information from large image databases. Methods used in imaging informatics include image processing, statistics, data mining, graphical user interface, visualization, and display technologies. The source for large image databases is mostly PACS.

Imaging informatics training Medical imaging informatics is a branch of imaging science that studies image/data information gathering, processing, manipulation, storage, transmission, management, distribution, and visualization as well as knowledge discovery from large-scale biomedical image/data sets. Training programs separating medical imaging and medical informatics exist but they seldom combine imaging and informatics during the training. Recently the U.S. National Institutes of Health (NIH), launched a number of training programs in medical Imaging Informatics in interdisciplinary approach.

Internet/Intranet Internet is a technology used for network communication. TCP/IP is the most commonly used protocol. All PACS components are connected by TCP/IP. When the all PACS components connection is within the hospital networks, it is called Intranet. The data transmission speed can reach Gbits/s, and the cost is low. When the components connection requires public networks, it is called Internet; in this case the data transmission speed is slower and more expensive.

Location tracking and verification system A location tracking and verification system (LTVS) integrates biometric technologies with HIS/RIS/PACS data to automatically monitor and identify staff and patients in a healthcare image-based environment during clinical hours. LTVS therefore partially conforms to the HIPAA patient security requirement. The biometric technologies used include facial features recognition and fingerprint recognition. The time stamps of patient registration, procedure workflow, examination, and patient discharge in HIS/RIS/PACS data are used. Visualization and graphic tools are heavily utilized at the monitor system to locate and track the patient movement in the clinical environment.

Multimedia ePR Multimedia ePR system includes not only textual data but also images, video, waveform and other data from acquisition devices within and outside of radiology domain. The multimedia ePR data acquisition gateways collect and convert input data to proper standards so that the ePR workflow from input to archive, display and visualization is seamless.

PACS The Picture Archiving and Communication System (PACS) is a means of integrating imaging modalities from radiology and various information systems from hospitals for effective and efficient clinical operations. The major components of PACS are the radiology information system gateway, the image acquisition gateway, the PACS server and archive server, display workstations, application servers, communication networks, PACS monitoring, and PACS software.

PACS server and archive server PACS server and archive server has three major functions in PACS operation. It monitors the data flow of the complete system operation, archives all image and related data, and distributes them in a timely way to designated workstations and application servers for review and other clinical functions. In general, patient directory is kept in mirrored databases, and images are stored in short-term SAN and RAID, and long-term disk or digital tape storage devices. Image data normally requires a backup second copy. In the United States, the storage requirement of a patient's images is seven years.

PACS monitoring system Since PACS has many integrated components, the PACS server needs to keep track of the performance of every component and every transaction in the system. PACS monitor system is a software package that resides either inside the server or separately in a monitoring server. Tools are implemented in the monitoring system to analyze data flow and to streamline the PACS operation. The monitoring system can be used to detect system bottlenecks, speed up network performance, and trace and recover system or human errors.

PACS training PACS is neither a single modality nor a single information system; it is system integration of many imaging components in radiology and information systems from the hospital. In general, it takes a team effort to operate PACS, since no one person can comprehend all components. PACS training is therefore required to train the different users of the system, from the PACS manager, to radiologist, technologist, clinician, and other healthcare providers.

PACS-based CAD Computer-assisted (or -aided) detection or diagnosis (CAD) uses the computer to assist and facilitate the radiologist and clinician in their diagnoses. PACS-based CAD directly uses images and related patient information from PACS to perform CAD. Current successful clinical CAD systems are digital mammography and chest lung tumor detection on CT.

Projection X-ray image Digital projection X-ray images are generated from computed radiography (CR) and digital radiography (DR). A conventional X-ray film can be converted to a digital image by way of a laser film scanner. The size of these images is generally $2500 \times 2000 \times 12$ bits, or about 10 Mbytes per image. Projection X-ray images account for about 60% to 70% of radiology examinations.

RIS The radiology information system (RIS) is an information system tailor made for radiology operation. It connects to both HIS and PACS for effective and efficient clinical operation. Some radiology information systems are stand-alone with connection to HIS to obtain necessary patient information. Others are embedded in the HIS.

Sectional image Sectional images in radiology include computed tomography (CT), magnetic resonance image (MRI), ultrasound image (US), positron emission tomography (PET), and single photon emission tomography (SPECT). Each of these images is of the size from $256 \times 256 \times 12$ to $512 \times 512 \times 12$ bits. Sectional images account for about 30% to 40% of radiology examinations.

Teleradiology Teleradiology is the practice of radiology using both images from radiology and telecommunication technology. From the system design point of view, teleradiology is very similar to PACS except that the components connection is mostly WAN, and the equipment requirement in teleradiology, is general, less demanding compared to PACS.

Three-dimensional image Most three-dimensional (3-D) medical images are generated by using image reconstruction (tomography) techniques with data from projections that are collected from detectors coupled with various energy sources. If the projections are 1-D, then the image formed is a 2-D sectional image. A collection of combined multiple sectional images becomes a 3-D image volume. If the projections are 2-D, and z is the body axis, then the reconstruction result will be a fully 3-D image volume.

Web-based image distribution PACS images can be distributed throughout the hospital or healthcare enterprise using Web-based technology. Since most hospitals are equipped with many low-cost desktop computers throughout the campus, these computers with some upgrade, can be used as Web clients for receiving PACS images. The image quality using Web-based image distribution is not superior, but the cost of distribution is low.

Workstation The workstation (WS) is the component in PACS that the everyday user interacts with. Various types of image WS have been introduced to healthcare providers through different imaging modalities with negative results. For this reason users are very critical of the functionality of PACS WSs. The difficulty in WS design for PACS is that the PACS WS has to display different types of images as well as pertinent patient information used in clinical practice. Most diagnostic images required two 2000 line LCD monitors with 2 to 3 seconds per image display time. PACS WS is different from other health-related information displays in that it can display many images within large file sizes.